To Mary —
Thank you for being such an important member of our VCA team this year, and for always doing your best for your patients and clients.
Best wishes always —

Todd Tams

Handbook of

Small Animal Gastroenterology

Handbook of

Small Animal
Gastroenterology

Todd R. Tams, DVM

Diplomate ACVIM
Chief Medical Officer
VCA Antech, Inc.
Los Angeles, California

Staff Internist
VCA West Los Angeles Animal Hospital
West Los Angeles, California

Second Edition

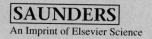

SAUNDERS
An Imprint of Elsevier Science

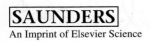

An Imprint of Elsevier Science

11830 Westline Industrial Drive
St. Louis, Missouri 63146

NOTICE

Veterinary Medicine is an ever-changing field. Standard safety precautions must be followed, but as new
research and clinical experience broaden our knowledge, changes in treatment and drug therapy may become
necessary or appropriate. Readers are advised to check the most current product information provided by the
manufacturer of each drug to be administered to verify the recommended dose, the method and duration of
administration, and contraindications. It is the responsibility of the licensed prescriber, relying on experience
and knowledge of the patient, to determine dosages and the best treatment for each individual patient.
Neither the publisher nor the author assumes any liability for any injury and/or damage to persons or
property arising from this publication.

Acquisitions Editor: Raymond Kersey
Developmental Editor: Denise LeMelledo
Publishing Services Manager: John Rogers
Project Manager: Mary Turner
Designer: Kathi Gosche
Cover Art: Kathi Gosche

Printed in United States of America

Last digit is the print number: 9   8   7   6   5   4   3   2   1

CONTRIBUTORS

Joseph W. Bartges, DVM, PhD

Diplomate ACVIM, ACVN
Professor of Medicine and Nutrition
The Acree Endowed Chair of Small Animal Research
Department of Small Animal Clinical Sciences
College of Veterinary Medicine
The University of Tennessee
Knoxville, Tennessee
Enteral and Parenteral Nutrition

Robert C. DeNovo, DVM, MS

Diplomate ACVIM
Professor and Head
Department of Small Animal Clinical Sciences
College of Veterinary Medicine
The University of Tennessee
Knoxville, Tennessee
Diseases of the Stomach

Pamela A. Green, DVM

Diplomate ACVR
Staff Radiologist
VCA West Los Angeles Animal Hospital
West Los Angeles, California
Radiology and Ultrasonography of the Digestive System

Linda J. Konde, DVM

Diplomate ACVR
Veterinary Radiologist
Diagnostic Imaging, PC
Aurora, Colorado
Radiology and Ultrasonography of the Digestive System

Michael R. Lappin, DVM, PhD

Diplomate ACVIM
Professor of Small Animal Medicine
Department of Clinical Sciences
Colorado State University
Fort Collins, Colorado
Acute Medical Diseases of the Small Intestine

Victoria S. Larson, DVM, MS

Diplomate ACVIM (Oncology)
Assistant Clinical Specialist
Small Animal Clinical Sciences
College of Veterinary Medicine
University of Minnesota
St. Paul, Minnesota
Oncologic Diseases of the Digestive System

Nicole F. Leibman, DVM, MS

Diplomate ACVIM (Oncology)
Staff Oncologist
Animal Medical Center
New York, New York
Oncologic Diseases of the Digestive System

Gregory K. Ogilvie, DVM

Diplomate ACVIM (Internal Medicine, Oncology)
Professor and Head of Medical Oncology
Animal Cancer Center
Colorado State University
Fort. Collins, Colorado
Oncologic Diseases of the Digestive System

Charles R. Pugh, MS, DVM

Diplomate ACVR
Veterinary Radiologist
Diagnostic Imaging, PC
Aurora, Colorado
Radiology and Ultrasonography of the Digestive System

Keith P. Richter, DVM

Diplomate ACVIM
Staff Internist
Veterinary Specialty Hospital of San Diego
Rancho Santa Fe, California
Diseases of the Liver and Hepatobiliary System

Howard B. Seim III, DVM

Diplomate ACVS
Professor of Small Animal Surgery
Department of Clinical Sciences
Colorado State University
Fort Collins, Colorado
Enteral and Parenteral Nutrition

Robert G. Sherding, DVM

Diplomate ACVIM
Professor and Department Chair
Department of Veterinary Clinical Sciences
College of Veterinary Medicine
The Ohio State University
Columbus, Ohio
Diseases of the Large Intestine

Kenneth W. Simpson, BVMS, PhD, MRCVS

Diplomate ACVIM, Diplomate ECVIM-CA
Associate Professor of Medicine
Department of Clinical Sciences
College of Veterinary Medicine
Cornell University
Ithaca, New York
Diseases of the Pancreas

Todd R. Tams, DVM

Diplomate ACVIM
Chief Medical Officer
VCA Antech, Inc.
Los Angeles, California;
Staff Internist
VCA West Los Angeles Animal Hospital
West Los Angeles, California
Gastrointestinal Symptoms
Endoscopy and Laparoscopy in Veterinary Gastroenterology
Diseases of the Esophagus
Chronic Diseases of the Small Intestine

Andrew Triolo, DVM

Diplomate ACVIM
Regional Medical Director
VCA Antech, Inc.
Los Angeles, California
Acute Medical Diseases of the Small Intestine

This book is dedicated to:

My late father, Roland.
My dad was a gentle spirit,
a man easy to love and respect.
He gave me a living example
of an honorable work ethic,
a gift beyond measure.

To my mother, Peg,
who made our house a home.

Thank you, Mom and Dad, for always being
there for me, and for teaching me
through your example.

My wife, Sazzy, and our 12-year-old son, "Snapper."
Thank you for all the love, joy, and humor you have brought to my life
and for the encouragement and support that you have always given me.
You make each day an adventure.

To my many colleagues in the veterinary profession—
doctors, veterinary technicians, and support staff—
with whom I have worked closely over the years.
We have accomplished much together
for the benefit of our
patients and their owners.
Thank you for caring so deeply.
Each of you in your own way
has contributed to me professionally and personally.

PREFACE

The practice of gastroenterology has changed dramatically in the last decade. The not-uncommon frustration that veterinarians and their clients experienced in the past when dealing with pets afflicted with chronic gastrointestinal disorders has given way to very satisfying results in many cases. This is in large part attributable to major advances that have been made both in our diagnostic capabilities and in the availability of more effective therapeutic agents. Most notably, with the advent of endoscopic instrumentation, it has become possible to directly examine a large portion of the gastrointestinal tract and to procure biopsy samples in a minimally invasive manner. Endoscopy has truly played a major role in enabling clinicians to diagnose many disorders that otherwise might have gone unrecognized until much later in their course. Laparoscopy is also being used much more commonly for minimally invasive procurement of liver and pancreatic tissue for histopathologic evaluation, for prophylactic gastropexy, and for other innovative techniques.

Additionally, advances in imaging techniques (ultrasonography, nuclear scintigraphy) have occurred, and more specific tests of liver function (e.g., bile acids assay), exocrine pancreatic insufficiency (trypsin-like immunoreactivity), and pancreatic inflammation (pancreatic lipase immunoreactivity assay) are now in routine use. These improvements, as well as others too numerous to list here, have enhanced our ability to approach digestive system problems more accurately and less invasively. In short, we can now do a much better job for our patients and their owners.

The second edition of the *Handbook of Small Animal Gastroenterology* meets the original goal of the first edition—it provides a practical update on small animal clinical gastroenterology that should serve as a useful reference in any practice setting. It is clearly recognized in veterinary practices throughout the world that digestive system disorders are among the most common reasons that pet owners seek veterinary consultation. The text is therefore directed particularly toward veterinary students, interns, residents in medicine and surgery, and primary care practitioners. Emphasis is placed on a practical diagnostic approach and development of well directed treatment plans for a majority of the gastrointestinal diseases that are encountered in practice. The second edition has been extensively revised and includes important updates throughout, and there is a new chapter, which provides a detailed review of neoplasia of the digestive system (Chapter 11).

The importance of directing very careful consideration to the patient's history when presented with animals exhibiting symptoms of a digestive system disorder cannot be overemphasized. Therefore an entire chapter (Chapter 1) has once again been devoted to a discussion of important symptoms and differential diagnosis. Chapters 2 and 3 complete the overview of diagnosis of digestive system diseases with information highlighting the clinical utility of four very important diagnostic modalities in gastroenterology: radiology and ultrasonography (Chapter 2) and endoscopy and laparoscopy (Chapter 3). The remaining chapters sequentially address the various anatomic regions of the digestive system individually. Newer tests and drugs are described throughout. Chapter 12 discusses enteral nutritional support, and this chapter has been expanded for the new edition.

I am indebted to the authors who contributed to this book. They are highly experienced clinicians with demonstrated expertise in either busy private or academic practices. They all share the common thread of being excellent teachers. I have the greatest respect for their contributions to our profession. I also acknowledge the excellent assistance of the staff at Elsevier, and in particular my editors, Raymond Kersey, Denise LeMelledo, and Mary Turner, for their encouragement, advice, and professionalism.

Todd R. Tams, DVM

CONTENTS

Seven 4-color plates precede chapter 1.

Handbook of

Small Animal
Gastroenterology

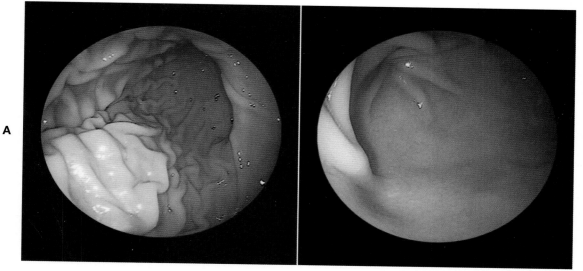

A | **B**

FIGURE 5-4 Normal stomach. **A,** Endoscopic appearance of a normal stomach. The smooth, pale-pink rugal folds of the greater curvature of the gastric body gradually become more linear distally at the junction with the pyloric antrum. The incisura angularis appears as a curved fold located at the 12 to 3 o'clock position. **B,** Appearance of a normal pyloric antrum *(foreground)* and pylorus *(upper left)*. The antral mucosa is smooth, pale pink, and without rugal folds. The closed pyloric orifice is located at the center of the converging mucosal folds.

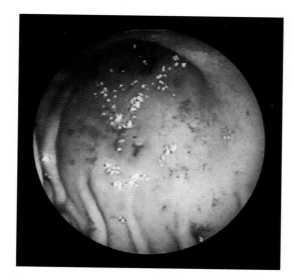

FIGURE 5-5 NSAID-induced ulcerative gastritis. Diffuse ulcerative gastritis in a 9-year-old German shepherd–mix with degenerative joint disease. The dog was being treated with aspirin (325 mg 2 times a day). Treatment began 2 months before presentation, but clinical signs of weakness, vomiting, melena caused by acute gastrointestinal blood loss, and anemia did not occur until the day of presentation.

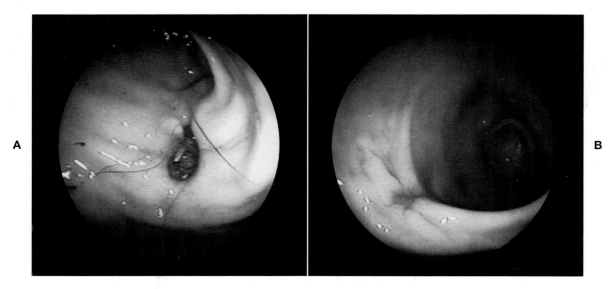

FIGURE 5-6 NSAID-induced gastric ulcer. **A,** Gastric ulcer in pyloric antrum of a 5-year-old Welsh corgi that had been treated for back pain with ibuprofen (325 mg every day for 5 days). The dog had an acute onset of vomiting and an episode of melena on the day of presentation. **B,** Healing gastric ulcer in the same patient after 7 days of treatment with omeprazole (0.3 mg/lb every day).

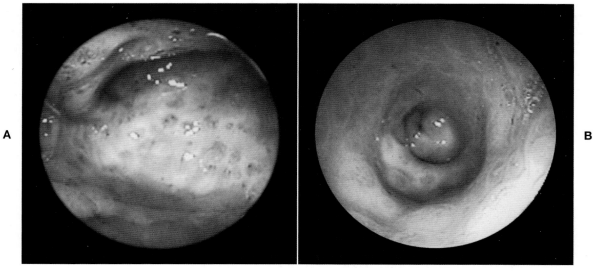

FIGURE 5-7 *Helicobacter* gastritis. **A,** Endoscopic view of the gastric body and incisura angularis in a 3-year-old English bulldog with chronic intermittent vomiting. Raised nodules, some with a central reddened craterlike appearance, were present throughout the body and antrum. **B,** Endoscopic view of the pyloric antrum from the same dog showing a diffusely nodular mucosa. The pylorus is seen distally in the center of the image. Biopsy revealed the nodules to be accumulations of lymphocytes. Urease-positive *Helicobacter* organisms were present on the surface musosa and extending into the gastric pits. Clinical signs resolved after treatment with omeprazole (0.3 mg/lb every day) in combination with amoxicillin (10 mg/lb 2 times a day) for 14 days.

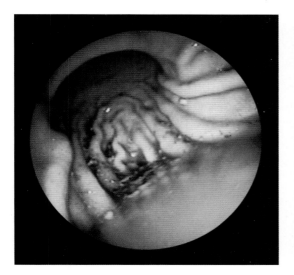

FIGURE 5-8 Gastric retention of food particles and bile-colored fluid in a 12-year-old miniature poodle with clinical signs of intermittent vomiting, regurgitation, inappetence, and bloating. The dog had no food or water for 14 hours before endoscopy. Results of gastric mucosal biopsies were normal, and the dog was diagnosed with primary (idiopathic) gastric motility disorder. Clinical signs improved, but did not resolve, when the dog was treated with cisapride and dietary management (small meals, fat-restricted food).

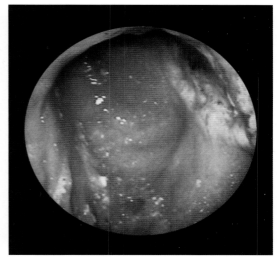

FIGURE 5-9 Malignant gastric ulcer located on the incisura angularis (1 to 3 o'clock position in the field of view) in a 13-year-old Weimaraner with a 2-month history of chronic vomiting and weight loss. The dog had hypochromic microcytic anemia. The raised edges and central crater of the ulcer were very firm and required that multiple biopsy specimens be obtained from each of several sites to ensure adequate depth of tissue was obtained. Histopathologic findings confirmed gastric adenocarcinoma.

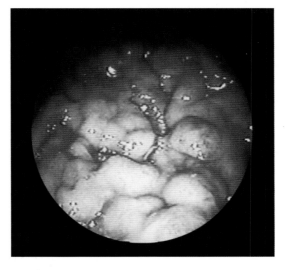

FIGURE 5-10 Diffuse nodular gastric lymphosarcoma in a 9-year-old beagle with intermittent vomiting of 2 weeks' duration and weight loss. Clinical signs resolved with chemotherapy (Adriamycin and L-asparaginase). After 6 months of remission, clinical signs reoccurred and the dog was euthanized.

GASTROINTESTINAL SYMPTOMS

Todd R. Tams

I consider this opening chapter to be a very important part of this text. My goal is to provide veterinary students and practicing veterinarians alike with a framework that can be used to approach diagnosis of digestive system disorders in an organized manner based on a thorough understanding of the patient's history. It is clearly recognized in veterinary practices throughout the world that gastrointestinal (GI) problems are among the most common reasons that pet owners seek veterinary consultation. In fact, probably only dermatologic disorders are evaluated more commonly on a daily basis. The challenge to the clinician who is presented with a patient exhibiting clinical signs of GI distress or dysfunction is to determine whether or not the problem represents an emergency or is potentially serious and subsequently to make appropriate decisions regarding **diagnostic evaluation** (may be limited to history and physical examination or may require limited or more extensive testing) and **treatment** (outpatient versus inpatient). It is well known that the digestive tract is a very resilient system, capable of withstanding a variety of challenges and insults with minimal untoward effect, and that in many pets with clinical signs such as acute vomiting or diarrhea the problem resolves uneventfully, with or without the benefit of routine supportive care. However, some patients that exhibit acute GI

symptomatology have potentially life-threatening disorders (e.g., gastric dilatation-volvulus, intestinal obstruction, pancreatitis, severe parvoviral enteritis, addisonian crisis), and failure by the clinician to recognize important historical and physical findings may lead to crucial errors in patient management.

It is also very important that the clinician make a timely determination regarding when patients with seemingly mild intermittent or chronic persistent signs due to an as yet undiagnosed disorder should undergo thorough diagnostic evaluation to define the problem more accurately. It concerns and saddens me that many patients with chronic GI disorders, which can often be associated with periods of discomfort caused by nausea, vomiting, abdominal cramping and/or pain, could often have had their problem resolved or controlled much earlier if only an accurate diagnosis had been established.

It is often stated that one of the most important steps in approaching a clinical problem is to obtain an accurate history and perform a thorough physical examination. Nothing could be more true about the digestive system, in which disorders can be associated with a wide variety of signs and symptoms. In light of the fact that disorders of other body systems can cause clinical signs of GI dysfunction (e.g., hyperthyroidism, renal

1

failure, feline heartworm disease, hypoadrenocorticism), the need for careful initial screening becomes even more important. It is essential that the patient's history be well understood so that diagnostic evaluation addresses the problem as directly as possible.

This chapter provides an overview of the diagnostic approach to GI disorders based on the presenting signs and symptoms. Emphasis is placed on the meaning of various historical and physical examination findings. Once an accurate review of the history has been established, a concise list of most likely **differential diagnoses** can be established. A list of clinical signs that are associated with digestive system problems appears in Box 1-1. Definitions of symptoms of GI disorders are listed in Table 1-1. Symptoms discussed in this chapter include dysphagia; regurgitation; vomiting; grass ingestion/coprophagy/pica; diarrhea; borborygmus and flatulence; bloating, fullness, and abdominal discomfort; fecal incontinence; and constipation. Additional symptoms are discussed

in other chapters throughout the text. Vomiting and diarrhea, the clinical signs that occur most commonly with GI disease, are given the most emphasis in this chapter.

BOX 1-1	Symptoms of Gastrointestinal Disease
Salivation	Change in appetite
Halitosis	Anorexia
Regurgitation	Polyphagia
Dysphagia	Pica
Nausea	Coprophagy
Vomiting	Borborygmus
Hematemesis	Flatus
Diarrhea	Weight loss
Melena	Polyuria/polydypsia (PU/PD)
Hematochezia	Anemia
Dyschezia	Shock
Tenesmus	Abdominal pain
Constipation	Abnormal mentation

TABLE 1-1	Definitions of Symptoms of Gastrointestinal Disorders
Anorexia	Lack or loss of appetite for food
Borborygmus	A rumbling noise caused by the propulsion of gas through the stomach and intestines
Constipation	Infrequent or difficult evacuation of the feces
Coprophagy	The ingestion of feces
Diarrhea	The passage of feces that contain an excess amount of water, resulting in an abnormal increase in stool liquidity and weight
Dyschezia	Difficult or painful evacuation of feces from the rectum
Dysphagia	Difficulty in swallowing
Flatulence	The presence of excessive amounts of air or gases in the stomach or intestine, leading to distention of the organs
Flatus	Gas or air expelled through the anus
Hematemesis	The vomiting of blood
Hematochezia	The passage of bright-red blood with the stools
Jaundice	A syndrome characterized by hyperbilirubinemia and deposition of bile pigment in the skin, mucous membranes, and sclera with resulting yellow appearance of the patient (also called icterus)
Melena	The passage of black, tarry stools resulting from digested blood
Obstipation	Intractable constipation resulting from prolonged constipation, with progressive enlargement, drying, and hardening of the fecal mass
Odynophagia	Pain on swallowing
Pica	A craving for unnatural articles of food; a depraved appetite
Polyphagia	Excessive or voracious eating
Pseudocoprostasis	A mechanical obstruction of the anus by hair matted with drying fecal material
Pseudoptyalism	Failure to swallow saliva produced in normal amounts
Ptyalism	Excessive secretion of saliva (also called hypersalivation, sialorrhea)
Regurgitation	The effortless expulsion of ingesta from the esophagus
Tenesmus	Straining, especially ineffectual and painful straining, to pass stool (or urine)
Vomiting	The forcible expulsion of the contents of the stomach through the mouth
Xerostomia	Dryness of the mouth from lack of secretions

DYSPHAGIA

Dysphagia is defined as difficult or painful swallowing. It may be due to obstruction, motility disturbance, or pain. Although dysphagia most commonly indicates a disorder involving the oral cavity or pharynx, esophageal disorders can cause this clinical sign as well. Oropharyngeal dysphagia can generally be differentiated from esophageal dysphagia on the basis of history. Characteristic signs of oropharyngeal disorders include acute gagging, exaggerated swallowing movements, and increased frequency of swallowing. Food is frequently dropped from the mouth within seconds of prehension. In contrast, patients with esophageal dysphagia do not exhibit exaggerated swallowing motions and food is not dropped from the mouth. If clinical signs are acute and persistent or progressive, a morphologic lesion (e.g., foreign body, mass, inflammation) should be suspected. Intermittent occurrence of clinical signs is usually consistent with a motility disturbance.

The causes of oropharyngeal dysphagia are listed in Box 1-2. A careful review of the history and observation of the patient as it eats will confirm the presence of dysphagia, identify its primary anatomic location (oropharyngeal in most cases), and help determine a diagnostic plan. Typically patients with oropharyngeal dysphagia eat readily but have trouble swallowing the food normally. If the tongue is not functioning normally, there may be problems with prehension and mastication as well. Affected patients may extend, ventroflex, or throw their heads back during exaggerated efforts to swallow. Additional signs that may be observed include salivation (related to inability to swallow and/or secondary to pain), nasal discharge secondary to passage of liquid and food into the nasopharynx and nasal cavity, and coughing resulting from aspiration of food retained in the pharynx. Weight loss or failure to grow may also occur in some cases.

The initial step in diagnosis is to differentiate among oral, pharyngeal, and cricopharyngeal dysphagias. Signalment, clinical course (i.e., acute and persistent versus gradual onset), and physical findings are reviewed first. Clinical signs associated with cricopharyngeal achalasia are generally initially observed at the time of weaning onto solid food and, if not this early, almost always by 1 year of age. Dogs with congenitally short or cleft palate will also exhibit signs at a very young age. Young to middle-age patients are most prone to

---

BOX 1-2 Causes of Oropharyngeal Dysphagia

ORAL PAIN

Stomatitis/glossitis/pharyngitis
  Feline viral rhinotracheitis, calcivirus
  FeLV infection
  FIV infection
  Immune-mediated disease (e.g., pemphigus, SLE)
  Foreign body
  Uremic glossitis
  Sepsis
  Ingestion of caustic agents (acids, alkalis, thallium)
Tooth-related problems
  Periodontitis
  Tooth root abscess
  Fractured teeth
Fractured bones
Osteomyelitis
Electric cord burns
Retrobulbar abscess

ORAL MASS

Neoplasia (benign or malignant)
  Squamous cell carcinoma
  Fibrosarcoma
  Melanoma
Eosinophilic granuloma
  Foreign body obstruction (oral, pharyngeal, nasopharyngeal, proximal esophageal)
  Sialocele

NEUROMUSCULAR DISEASE

Myasthenia gravis (focal or generalized)
Acute polyradiculoneuritis
Tick paralysis
Botulism
Oral, pharyngeal, cricopharyngeal dysfunction
Polymyositis
Temporomandibular joint disease

NEUROLOGIC DISORDERS

Rabies
Trigeminal paralysis
Neuropathies of cranial nerves VII, IX, X, XII
CNS lesions (brainstem lesions)

FeLV, Feline leukemia virus; *FIV*, feline immunodeficiency virus; *SLE*, systemic lupus erythematosus; *CNS*, central nervous system.

---

lodgment of foreign bodies in the mouth and pharynx and accidental ingestion of caustic materials (such as petroleum products or alkalis), and signs of dysphagia are acute and persistent until definitive treatment is administered. Older dogs with an insidious onset of clinical signs are more likely to be afflicted with neoplasia (e.g., glossal neoplasia, pharyngeal tumors such as squamous cell carcinoma, fibrosarcoma, melanoma, tonsillar carcinoma, retropharyngeal mass causing compression). Weight loss and reluctance to eat are generally present in chronic cases. Presence of systemic signs, such as weakness that worsens with exercise, with or without cough and dyspnea, suggests myasthenia gravis. Signs of myasthenia gravis may be limited to pharyngeal dysfunction. Weakness may also be caused by polymyositis or central nervous system disease. Dysphagia occurring in conjunction with dementia suggests cerebral disease as the underlying problem. Rabies vaccination history and potential for exposure (environment) must always be determined early in the evaluation of any patient with dysphagia.

Thorough physical examination will successfully identify the cause of dysphagia in some cases. Physical signs may also alert the clinician to the presence of any significant complications (e.g., pneumonia) and help determine specific tests that should be done to establish a definitive diagnosis. Physical examination should include a thorough evaluation of the head (temporal muscle atrophy, pain associated with muscles of mastication, ocular areas for inflammation or proptosis of one of the eyes to suggest retrobulbar mass or cellulitis), oral cavity, external pharyngeal and cervical soft tissue areas for any mass effect, lymphadenopathy, or draining tract; recognition of any pain related to opening of the mouth (e.g., masticatory muscle myositis, retrobulbar inflammation, temporomandibular joint disease); and a neurologic examination. Specific neurologic tests include evaluation of cranial nerves IX (glossopharyngeal) and X (vagus) by checking the swallow and gag reflexes, respectively, evaluation of cranial nerve XII (hypoglossal) via observation and palpation of the tongue, and evaluation of gait and strength. Focal lesions of the medulla oblongata and diffuse neuromuscular disease may cause ataxia, conscious proprioception deficits, and limb weakness. Patients that exhibit any evidence of systemic signs (e.g., weakness, polyuria/polydypsia [PU/PD], muscle pain) in conjunction with dysphagia should initially be evaluated by complete blood count (CBC) (infection, inflammation, anemia of chronic disease), biochemical profile (including creatine phosphokinase [CPK] for polymyositis), and urinalysis. For example, a biochemical profile and urinalysis may confirm that lingual ulceration or necrosis is due to uremia.

Sedation or general anesthesia is often required for *thorough* examination of the oral cavity, pharynx, and larynx. The dental arcade, tongue (including frenulum area), palate, tonsils, and tonsillar crypts should be carefully evaluated for the presence of inflammation, mass, or foreign body. Biopsies of masses should be deep to determine diagnosis and prognosis accurately. A superficial biopsy may fail to harvest neoplastic cells from a cancerous mass because the changes at the surface may be limited to inflammation and necrosis. Electrocautery can be used to control postbiopsy hemorrhage. It is important to evaluate the nasopharynx (for significant inflammation, foreign body, mass) and the proximal esophagus as well. On occasion I have found foreign bodies such as long blades of grass, peanut shells, or small needles lodged in the nasopharynx and not extending caudal to the free border of the soft palate (i.e., not readily visible on initial oral examination). *Use of a flexible endoscope that is small enough to allow retroflexion over the soft palate greatly facilitates examination of the nasopharynx* (Figure 1-1). **Survey pharyngeal radiographs** may be indicated as part of the preliminary work-up if history or physical examination suggests that a mass, foreign body, or injury (e.g., hyoid bone fracture) may be present. **Contrast radiographic studies with fluoroscopy** while observing swallowing of both liquids and food are required for differentiation of pharyngeal and cricopharyngeal dysphagia.

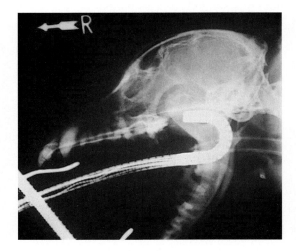

FIGURE 1-1 Lateral skull radiograph of a dog, demonstrating correct placement of a flexible endoscope for posterior rhinoscopy. Examination of the nasopharynx and choanae is facilitated by the use of a scope with a tip deflection capability of 180 degrees or more.

An **acetylcholine receptor antibody titer test** (see Chapter 4) should be run if there is any possibility of myasthenia gravis (signs of *focal* myasthenia gravis may be limited to pharyngeal dysfunction and regurgitation). A **Tensilon (edrophonium chloride) test** could also be done, but the clinician should observe carefully for and be prepared to treat cholinergic overstimulation if it occurs. If central nervous system disease is suspected, testing may include **cerebrospinal fluid analysis, nuclear scintigraphy**, and/or **computed axial tomography** or **magnetic resonance imaging (MRI)**.

▌REGURGITATION

Regurgitation refers to a *passive*, retrograde movement of ingested material to a level proximal to the upper esophageal sphincter. Usually this occurs before ingested material reaches the stomach. Regurgitation is not associated with the same spectrum of premonitory signs that often precede vomiting and retching. Although regurgitation may occur during or shortly after eating, it is essential that the clinician recognize that regurgitation may not occur until at least several hours after eating in some patients, especially those with megaesophagus. Regurgitation is a clinical sign of many disorders and should not be considered a primary disease. Regurgitation is a problem that occurs uncommonly in cats. Significant complications of regurgitation include aspiration pneumonia and chronic wasting disease. The term **reflux** refers to movement of gastric or duodenal contents into the esophagus without associated eructation or vomiting. This process may or may not produce symptoms. The term **expectoration** refers to expulsion of material from the respiratory tract, an event that is usually associated with coughing. Box 1-3 provides a differential list for the problem of regurgitation.

Regurgitation is usually a clinical sign of an esophageal disorder. In most cases it results from abnormal esophageal peristalsis or esophageal obstruction. The most common cause of regurgitation seen in clinical practice is megaesophagus. **Megaesophagus** refers to a specific syndrome characterized by a dilated, hypoperistalic esophagus. By definition and for use in this text, megaesophagus is differentiated from other causes of esophageal dilation (e.g., esophageal foreign body, vascular ring anomaly, neoplasia) that may or may not be characterized by abnormal peristalsis. Megaesophagus is discussed in detail in Chapter 4.

Many patients with disorders causing regurgitation have owners who incorrectly but understandably interpret the problem as vomiting. *Regardless of the owner's terminology, the clinician must carefully differentiate the clinical signs of regurgitation and vomiting.* Characteristics of regurgitation and vomiting are summarized in Table 1-2. Too often, dogs with megaesophagus are incorrectly diagnosed and treated for chronic vomiting because the clinician failed to thoroughly review the history. Regurgitation involves *passive* ejection of material that usually includes undigested food that is often in tubular shape and devoid of bile. If there is no food in the esophagus, regurgitated material may

---

BOX 1-3 ▌ Causes of Regurgitation

Megaesophagus—idiopathic
Megaesophagus—secondary
  Myasthenia gravis (focal or generalized)
  Hypoadrenocorticism
  Polyneuropathy (giant axonal neuropathy—canine;
    Key-Gaskell syndrome—feline)
  Canine distemper
  Systemic lupus erythematosus
  Polymyositis
  Hypothyroidism
  Lead toxicosis
  Organophosphate toxicity
  Thallium toxicosis
Motility disorder—segmental

Foreign body
Stricture
  Intraluminal lesion
  Extraluminal compression (vascular ring anomaly,
    anterior mediastinal mass, other intrathoracic
    tumors, hilar lymphadenopathy, abscess)
Esophagitis
Hiatal disorder
Neoplasia of esophagus
  Primary
  Metastatic
Granuloma
  e.g., *Spirocerca lupi*
Esophageal diverticulum

From Tams TR: Vomiting, regurgitation, and dysphagia. In Ettinger SJ, ed: *Textbook of veterinary internal medicine*, ed 4, vol 1, Philadelphia, 1995, WB Saunders.

TABLE 1-2	Vomiting or Regurgitation? A Checklist for Differentiation
Regurgitation	**Vomiting**
Passive process; sometimes almost effortless expulsion of esophageal contents	Active process, usually with vigorous abdominal contractions (retching)
Few additional premonitory signs except ptyalism in esophageal inflammatory or obstructive disease	Premonitory signs pronounced; including ptyalism, pacing, swallowing, and tachycardia (nausea)
Semiformed food material usually obvious and may smell "fermented"; often contains mucus (saliva), but blood is rare; never bile stained	No characteristic consistency; varies from freshly ingested food to liquid bile, blood, and mucus; may contain grass
pH of esophageal contents variable—unreliable indicator	pH of gastric contents variable—unreliable indicator

From Burrows CF: Vomiting and regurgitation in the dog: a clinical perspective. In *Viewpoints in veterinary medicine*, ed 2, Lehigh Valley, Pa, 1993, Alpo Pet Foods.

consist entirely of thick white foam. The frequency of regurgitation can vary dramatically, from as few as 1 to 2 episodes per week in some patients with megaesophagus to as often as 10 to 15 times per day.

Vomiting involves *active* expulsion of food and/or fluid. Vomiting is accompanied by retching and active abdominal contractions. Frequently signs of nausea (salivation, restlessness, increased swallowing motions) occur prior to retching. Occurrence of any of these associated signs should be discussed with the owner as the history is reviewed. Vomited material may include bile, and food may be present in various states of digestion. Vomiting may occur seconds to minutes to many hours after eating. With regard to incidence, patients with vomiting disorders far outnumber those with disorders associated with regurgitation. It is important to note that some patients with a history more *suggestive* of regurgitation may actually be vomiting. If it is unclear based on the history or clinical impression whether or not the patient is actually regurgitating rather than vomiting, a survey thoracic radiograph should be made at the outset to look for evidence of esophageal dilation. A barium swallow may be necessary to rule out esophageal dilation.

In evaluation of a patient with regurgitation, important historical factors to be considered by the clinician include signalment; nature of onset of clinical signs (i.e., acute and persistent versus intermittent [recent or chronic]); environment (e.g., likelihood of foreign body or toxin ingestion); pertinent history (e.g., recent anesthetic event suggesting possible development of a reflux-related esophageal stricture); presence of any systemic signs, such as weakness (e.g., myasthenia gravis, hypoadrenocorticism, polymyositis) or vomiting (e.g., hypoadrenocorticism, toxin ingestion such as lead); and whether there are any signs of complications from regurgitation (e.g., coughing or dyspnea, suggesting that an aspiration event with subsequent development of pneumonia has occurred). Because the patient's history is the major factor in determining the extent of the diagnostic work-up, it should be thoroughly investigated. *The importance of careful consideration of the history is highlighted by the fact that some causes of regurgitation, including certain disorders that result in megaesophagus, are reversible if recognized and treated appropriately early enough in their course. Missed diagnosis may result in significant worsening of the patient's long-term prognosis.*

Signalment

The signalment, particularly age and breed, provides important diagnostic clues. If regurgitation begins at the time of weaning onto solid food, a vascular ring anomaly (e.g., persistent right aortic arch) or congenital megaesophagus should be suspected. Regurgitation is persistent, and affected patients are often malnourished and weak. Dog breeds most commonly affected with vascular ring anomalies include the German shepherd, Irish setter, English bulldog, and Boston terrier. Vascular ring anomalies are extremely uncommon in cats.

Idiopathic megaesophagus is the most common cause of regurgitation in dogs, including puppies. Idiopathic megaesophagus is now recognized somewhat more frequently in adults than in young patients. Idiopathic megaesophagus is known to be hereditary in wirehaired fox terriers and miniature schnauzers. A breed predisposition for idiopathic megaesophagus exists for the German shepherd, Great Dane, Irish setter, and golden retriever. Although idiopathic megaesophagus can occur at any age, a later age of onset (8 to 12 years) seems to predominate. A recent study has shown that dogs with acquired megaesophagus and focal myasthenia gravis have a bimodal age of onset of clinical signs, with a younger group of dogs showing clinical signs at 2 to 4 years of age and an older group at 9 to 13 years of age. Although megaesophagus related to focal myasthenia gravis has been reported in a number of breeds, it may be more common in golden retrievers and German shepherds.

Megaesophagus may rarely occur secondary to hypoadrenocorticism. Retrospective studies have shown that hypoadrenocorticism is more common in young to middle-age female dogs (with a majority younger than 7 years of age at the time of diagnosis). Dogs with megaesophagus and hypoadrenocorticism often present with vomiting and diarrhea, as well as regurgitation.

Nature of Clinical Signs

Regurgitation that begins *acutely* at a time other than weaning is most often due to an esophageal foreign body. Most esophageal foreign bodies that cause nearly complete or complete obstruction are bones (e.g., steak, chicken, pork chop). If the esophageal lumen is only partially obstructed, regurgitation may occur only after ingestion of solids. Although an acute onset of regurgitation may also occur as a developing esophageal stricture results in significant narrowing of the esophageal lumen, generally there is a more gradual onset over a period of 2 to 3 days, with regurgitation of solids then becoming more persistent.

If regurgitation begins acutely, the owner should be questioned carefully about the possibility of foreign body ingestion. Frequently owners will relate that a bone was purposely fed or that they observed their pet on a foray into the garbage or saw evidence after the fact that the garbage had been invaded. If the patient has been free outdoors, there may be no known history of foreign body ingestion.

Because a majority of esophageal strictures develop within 1 to 3 weeks of a general anesthetic event, the history should be reviewed carefully regarding any recent anesthetic procedures. In addition, strictures occasionally develop in cats within 1 to 2 weeks after significant difficulty is experienced in vomiting a large hairball and in dogs or cats as a sequela to frequent vomiting. An esophageal stricture may also develop as a sequela to caustic acid or alkali ingestion, foreign body trauma, lodgment of tablet or capsule medication in the esophagus (e.g., doxycycline tablets in cats), and thermal burns. Whereas esophageal strictures may develop at any age, a majority of foreign body obstruction cases occur in patients 2 to 3 years of age or younger. Patients with strictures generally demonstrate signs such as vomiting, dysphagia, persistent gulping, and salivation *before* the onset of regurgitation. Because many esophageal foreign bodies are radiodense, the screening procedure that is most likely to readily differentiate acute regurgitation caused by a foreign body from that of an esophageal stricture is a survey thoracic radiograph. Contrast studies and/or esophagoscopy may be required to confirm the diagnosis in some cases.

Most disorders other than vascular ring anomaly, congenital megaesophagus, esophageal foreign body obstruction, and esophageal stricture cause a gradual onset of clinical signs. The clinician should inquire about details that might suggest a systemic disorder. Although idiopathic megaesophagus is the most common cause of regurgitation, every effort is still made to identify a potentially treatable cause. Inquiries should be made about potential exposure to toxins such as lead or thallium or exposure to carrion that could cause botulism. Any clinical signs such as weakness, collapse, vomiting, and diarrhea should be discussed, looking for evidence to support a likely diagnosis of such disorders as myasthenia gravis, hypoadrenocorticism, polymyositis, or systemic lupus erythematosus.

Physical Examination

Physical examination findings may vary considerably. If dysphagia, as well as regurgitation, is present, the same steps in physical examination previously outlined for evaluation of dysphagia should be followed (oral examination, external palpation). Excessive salivation may suggest odynophagia associated with an esophageal foreign body or esophagitis. Many megaesophagus patients are thin and in poor condition. A Heimlich type of maneuver on the thorax or anterior abdomen may produce an externally visible bulge on the left side of the neck resulting from a gas-filled flaccid cervical esophagus. Occlusion of the nostrils with compression of the thorax may also allow visualization of a dilated cervical esophagus. Gurgling sounds and halitosis might result from fermentation of food in a hypomotile esophagus. Thoracic auscultation may reveal pulmonary crackles secondary to aspiration pneumonia. Fever, mucopurulent nasal discharge, coughing, and dyspnea also suggest the presence of pneumonia.

Patients with intraluminal esophageal strictures are often normal on physical examination. Other examination findings, such as weakness and/or decreased palpebral reflex (myasthenia gravis), weakness and bradycardia (hypoadrenocorticism), muscle pain (polymyositis), and signs that may include joint pain and shifting limb lameness (systemic lupus erythematosus), erosive glossitis, and others, often occur with systemic disorders. Cats that regurgitate secondary to an anterior mediastinal mass often have a noncompressible anterior chest cavity. Physical findings in cats with Key-Gaskell syndrome, a neurologic disorder characterized in part by regurgitation due to megaesophagus, include persistent pupillary dilation, decreased nasal and lacrimal secretions, bradycardia, and constipation.

Diagnostic Studies

Survey radiography of the esophagus is the first and most important step in the diagnosis of a regurgitation disorder. Radiographs are evaluated for evidence of esophageal dilation, presence of a foreign body, or thoracic mass. If survey radiographs fail to provide a definitive diagnosis, a **barium esophagram** should be performed to evaluate the cervical and thoracic esophagus. Barium paste offers the best mucosal coating and should be used to evaluate suspected mucosal or mass lesions. Esophageal dilation is best detected with liquid barium suspension. Liquid barium mixed with food is best for evaluating disorders of motility and examining for esophageal stricture (strictures often allow fluid but not food to pass).

Although young patients with congenital megaesophagus are not usually evaluated with detailed diagnostic tests, patients with acquired megaesophagus should be evaluated as thoroughly as possible. Baseline tests should include a **CBC, biochemical profile, serum thyroid hormone analysis, urinalysis,** and **fecal examination** for *Spirocerca lupi* ova (in endemic areas). Specific tests to evaluate for systemic disorders such as hypoadrenocorticism (**adrenocorticotropic hormone [ACTH] stimulation),** systemic lupus erythe-matosus (**antinuclear antibody),** and myasthenia gravis (**acetylcholine receptor antibody titer, Tensilon test)** are done if the history, physical examination, or baseline tests indicate that these primary disorders may exist. It is recommended that the acetylcholine receptor antibody titer test be run in any patient with acquired megaesophagus because many with focal myasthenia gravis do not show classic signs associated with generalized myasthenia gravis (weakness, collapse). **Serum lead levels** are indicated if lead toxicity is considered a possibility.

Endoscopic examination of the esophagus (esophagoscopy) is a valuable diagnostic and therapeutic tool. Endoscopy is most effective in diagnosis of disorders that affect the mucosa (esophagitis, mass lesions, strictures), for retrieval of foreign bodies, in management of esophageal strictures with guided bougienage or balloon dilation, and as an adjunctive step in diagnosis of hiatal hernia. Hiatal hernia is best diagnosed using a combination of contrast radiography (with fluoroscopy if available) and endoscopy (looking for anatomic and secondary inflammatory changes [esophagitis]). In most patients with megaesophagus, endoscopic examination is not necessary for diagnosis and is rarely of benefit in determining a cause. Esophageal motility disorders in which clear radiographic evidence of marked esophageal dilation is lacking are best recognized by **esophageal fluoroscopy** and **manometry studies**. If this equipment is not available, esophagoscopy may be beneficial; in some cases pooling of fluid or mild esophageal dilation can be identified.

▌VOMITING

Most small animal practitioners agree that vomiting is one of the most common reasons that dogs and cats are presented for diagnosis and treatment. Vomiting refers to a forceful ejection of gastric and often proximal small intestinal contents through the mouth. The vomiting act involves three stages: nausea, retching, and vomiting. It is emphasized that vomiting is simply a *clinical sign* of any of a number of disorders that can involve any organ system in the body. Vomiting does not constitute a diagnosis in itself.

Clinical Features

Because a wide variety of disorders and stimuli can cause vomiting (Box 1-4), it may present the clinician with a major diagnostic challenge. Although

BOX 1-4   Causes of Vomiting

DIETARY PROBLEMS
1. Sudden diet change
2. Ingestion of foreign material (e.g., garbage, grass, plant leaves)
3. Eating too rapidly
4. Intolerance to specific foods
5. Food allergy

DRUGS
1. Intolerance (e.g., antineoplastic drugs, cardiac glycosides, antimicrobial drugs [e.g., erythromycin, tetracycline], arsenical compounds)
2. Blockage of prostaglandin biosynthesis (non-steroidal antiinflammatory drugs)
3. Injudicious use of anticholinergics
4. Accidental overdosage

TOXINS
1. Lead
2. Ethylene glycol
3. Zinc
4. Others

METABOLIC DISORDERS
1. Diabetes mellitus
2. Hypoadrenocorticism
3. Renal disease
4. Hepatic disease
5. Sepsis
6. Acidosis
7. Hyperkalemia
8. Hypokalemia
9. Hypercalcemia
10. Hypocalcemia
11. Hypomagnesemia
12. Heatstroke

DISORDERS OF THE STOMACH
1. Obstruction (e.g., foreign body, pyloric mucosal hypertrophy, external compression)
2. Chronic gastritis (superficial, atrophic, hypertrophic)
3. Parasites (*Physaloptera* spp.—dog and cat; *Ollulanus tricuspis*—cat)
4. Gastric hypomotility
5. Bilious vomiting syndrome
6. Gastric ulcers
7. Gastric polyps
8. Gastric neoplasia
9. Gastric dilatation
10. Gastric dilatation-volvulus

DISORDERS OF THE GASTROESOPHAGEAL JUNCTION
Hiatal hernia (axial, paraesophageal, diaphragmatic herniation, gastroesophageal intussusception)

DISORDERS OF THE SMALL INTESTINE
1. Parasitism
2. Enteritis
3. Intraluminal obstruction (foreign body, intussusception, neoplasia)
4. Inflammatory bowel disease—idiopathic
5. Diffuse intramural neoplasia (lymphosarcoma)
6. Fungal disease
7. Intestinal volvulus
8. Paralytic ileus

DISORDERS OF THE LARGE INTESTINE
1. Colitis
2. Obstipation
3. Irritable bowel syndrome

ABDOMINAL DISORDERS
1. Pancreatitis
2. Zollinger-Ellison syndrome (gastrinoma of pancreas)
3. Peritonitis (any cause, including feline infectious peritonitis)
4. Inflammatory liver disease
5. Bile duct obstruction
6. Steatitis
7. Prostatitis
8. Pyelonephritis
9. Pyometra
10. Urinary obstruction
11. Diaphragmatic hernia
12. Neoplasia

NEUROLOGIC DISORDERS
1. Psychogenic (pain, fear, excitement)
2. Motion sickness (rotation or unequal input from the labyrinths)
3. Inflammatory lesions (e.g., vestibular)
4. Edema (head trauma)
5. Autonomic or visceral epilepsy
6. Neoplasia

MISCELLANEOUS CAUSES OF VOMITING
1. Heartworm disease (feline)
2. Hyperthyroidism (feline)

Modified from Tams TR: Vomiting, regurgitation, and dysphagia. In Ettinger SJ, ed: *Textbook of veterinary internal medicine*, ed 4, vol 1, Philadelphia, 1995, WB Saunders.

vomiting does not always signify the presence of a serious disorder, it may be the first indication of intestinal obstruction, renal failure, pancreatitis, parvovirus enteritis, addisonian crisis, drug toxicity, neoplasia, and others. A complete historical review with emphasis on all body systems is essential for determining a realistic and effective initial work-up plan and treatment protocol. All too often, early concentration on only the GI tract leads to a misdiagnosis and inappropriate treatment for the cause of the vomiting.

As previously discussed, it is essential that the clinician make a clear differentiation between *regurgitation* and *vomiting* at the outset. If there is uncertainty about whether or not regurgitation is occurring after the history is reviewed, survey thoracic radiographs should be made to evaluate for possible esophageal dilation. Contrast studies may occasionally be necessary to identify the presence of esophageal dilation.

Consideration of the following historical features is often useful in assessing and diagnosing disorders that cause vomiting (Box 1-5):

- Duration of signs and systems review
- Content of the vomitus
- Time relation to eating
- Nature (e.g., type, frequency) of vomiting
- Dietary and environmental history

The line of questioning should begin with determining if the vomiting is an acute problem or is chronic (longer than 2 weeks in duration) and whether there has been any blood in the vomitus. The signalment, immediate signs, past pertinent history, and beneficial or deleterious effects of any drugs that may have been administered (either for the immediate symptoms or as treatment for another disorder) should be reviewed. In particular it should be determined whether any nonsteroidal antiinflammatory drugs (e.g., aspirin, carprofen, etodolac, flunixin meglumine [Banamine], phenylbutazone, ibuprofen [Motrin, Nuprin], piroxicam [Feldene]) have been used. Gastric and intestinal erosions and potentially serious ulceration may develop in conjunction with their use. Nephrotoxicity may also

---

BOX 1-5   Important Historical Considerations in the Investigation of Vomiting

I. Duration and frequency of vomiting
  A. Acute
    1. Dietary indiscretion or incorrect feeding practice of any type? (e.g., foreign body, garbage ingestion, fatty meal, overfeeding)
    2. Drug administration? (any drug can potentially cause vomiting, but the most commonly involved offending drugs include NSAIDs, antibiotics [especially tetracycline, erythromycin], chemotherapeutic agents, cardiac glycosides)
    3. Any exposure to infectious organisms? (parvovirus most common)
    4. Any specific associated symptoms? (e.g., diarrhea, lethargy, fever, signs of abdominal pain, anorexia, vestibular symptoms)
  B. Chronic (more than 2 weeks)
    1. Intermittent, with no significant associated symptoms such as inappetence, weight loss, lethargy?
    2. Increasing frequency? (this is often an indicator that a work-up should be pursued in patients that have a history of chronic intermittent vomiting)
    3. Persistent vomiting?
    4. Any pertinent environmental considerations? (e.g., cat from an endemic heartworm area, review likelihood of foreign body ingestion)
    5. Associated symptoms present? (general systems review—e.g., PU/PD, dyschezia or dysuria)
II. Content of vomitus
  A. Food
    1. State of digestion?
    2. Time relation to eating?
  B. Mucus
    1. Salivary or gastric
  C. Bile
    1. Bilious vomiting syndrome, persistent or forceful vomiting, intestinal obstruction
    2. Large volumes of green fluid with acute onset and frequent vomiting most consistent with a proximal to mid small bowel obstruction

BOX 1-5 Important Historical Considerations in the Investigation of Vomiting—cont'd

D. Grass
   1. Nausea, gastric problems
E. Blood
   1. Fresh blood? Coffee grounds?
   2. Acute or chronic gastritis, ulcer, neoplasia (especially older dogs), shock, renal disease, hepatic disease
F. Parasites
   1. Presence indicates probable cause of vomiting (roundworms, *Physaloptera* most commonly involved)
G. Fecal odor or material (uncommon)
   1. Intestinal obstruction, peritonitis with ileus, ischemic injury to the intestine, or stasis with bacterial overgrowth

III. Timing of vomiting
A. Immediately or within 30 minutes after eating—most commonly associated with acute or chronic gastritis, gastric parasitism (especially *Physaloptera*)
B. Vomiting more than 7 to 10 hours after eating—consistent with gastric outlet obstruction from any cause or gastric hypomotility
C. Early morning only—most commonly associated with bilious vomiting syndrome in small breeds of dogs; also seen in some dogs with gastric hypomotility or inflammatory bowel disease

IV. Nature of vomiting
A. Projectile
   1. Pyloric outflow obstruction

B. Unproductive
   1. Impaction of stomach (e.g., large gastric trichobezoar in a cat)
   2. Gastric dilatation-volvulus
   3. Persistent vomiting

V. Dietary considerations
A. Specific foods fed?
B. Amount and frequency?
C. Any opportunities for indiscretion by either the owner or the patient itself?
D. Is the timing of feeding associated in any way with periods of excitement (e.g., exercise) or stress (e.g., conflictual situations with other animals that might lead to too rapid ingestion of food, or nervousness that could precipitate vomiting)?
E. Does the patient bolt certain favorite foods that it only occasionally receives? (e.g., cats that receive mostly dry food may eat canned or semimoist foods too rapidly on the occasions when they receive them—this may lead to vomiting of the food soon after it is ingested)

VI. Environmental considerations
A. Scavenging opportunities?
B. Contact with toxins? (e.g., ethylene glycol, lead)
C. Regional infectious disorders (e.g., heartworms in cats; *Physaloptera*, gastric parasite of dogs and occasionally cats—Midwest, East, South most common areas of the United States; liver fluke *(Platynosomum concinnum)* infection in cats—Florida, Gulf states, Hawaii)

NSAIDs, Nonsteroidal antiinflammatory drugs; *PU/PD*, polyuria/polydypsia.

occur. Inhibition of renal prostaglandins can be associated with renal ischemia and acute renal failure. Fortunately this syndrome is uncommon. However, patients with hypovolemia, congestive heart failure, or preexisting renal insufficiency may be at increased risk. Acute pancreatitis may be a component of a drug reaction; agents that have been implicated include azathioprine (Imuran), thiazide diuretics, furosemide, sulfonamides, tetracycline, L-asparaginase, and others.

Occasionally a chronic asymptomatic disorder is first manifested by an acute onset of vomiting, which may then persist as either a frequent or a sporadic problem until definitive treatment is instituted. Inflammatory bowel disease is an example of a common disorder that may present in this way. Specific information regarding diet (type of food, number and timing of feedings each day, amount fed per meal, any recent changes); vaccinations (consider systemic disorders such as distemper, parvovirus, feline infectious peritonitis); travel history; and environment (e.g., exposure to toxins, ingestion of spoiled food or foreign bodies, likelihood of GI parasites or infectious problem such as parvovirus enteritis, feline patient from an endemic heartworm area) is obtained in all cases. A **thorough systems review** with questions investigating any significant occurrence of potentially important signs such as PU/PD, coughing and sneezing, dysuria, or dyschezia should also be addressed. This routine systematic approach will help to alleviate diagnostic "tunnel vision" on the part of the clinician. For example, a history of PU/PD and acute vomiting in an older intact female dog immediately suggests the possibility of pyometra (also rule out primary renal disease), and the presence of dyschezia in conjunction with vomiting may be consistent with vomiting secondary to colitis (approximately 30% to 35% of dogs with colitis also have vomiting, which may occur before or in conjunction with the onset of large bowel signs).

A description of the vomiting episodes, including any association with eating or drinking, yields important information in some cases. Normally all food should be evacuated from the stomach by 7 to 10 hours after ingestion. The presence of food and its state of digestion will depend on dietary composition (with high-fat diets the stomach empties more slowly), gastric secretions and motility, presence of any gastric outflow obstruction, and time elapsed since ingestion. Vomiting shortly after eating most commonly suggests dietary indiscretion or food intolerance, overeating, stress or excitement, gastritis, or a hiatal disorder. Vomiting of undigested or partially digested food more than 7 to 10 hours after eating is an important clinical sign that usually indicates a gastric motility disorder or gastric outflow obstruction. Dogs with hypomotility may vomit undigested food several hours to 10 to 18 hours or more after eating and often exhibit a cyclic pattern of clinical signs. This disorder has been recognized much more frequently in recent years. Misconceptions commonly lead to misdiagnosis and mismanagement of affected patients. It is often incorrectly assumed that gastric retention means gastric outflow obstruction, and unnecessary surgery such as pyloromyotomy may be performed. It is now well recognized that pyloromyotomy procedures are *not* commonly indicated in dogs or cats with chronic vomiting.

Causes of gastric outflow obstruction include foreign bodies, antral and/or pyloric mucosal hypertrophy, gastric and duodenal ulcers, antral or pyloric neoplasia or polyps, and external compression on the antrum and pylorus (e.g., abscess, mass). Foreign bodies are identified much more commonly than the other disorders listed in Box 1-4. All are characterized by vomiting, which may occur shortly or a number of hours after eating, and occasionally projectile vomiting occurs.

Significant information can often be obtained from a complete description of the color and consistency of the vomitus, especially when interpretation is made in conjunction with a review of clinical signs. As previously discussed, if food is present, the degree of digestion and time since the most recent meal should be determined. Presence of bile in the vomitus is not unusual because vomiting begins with jejunal retroperistalsis and intestinal contents are swept into the stomach before the actual act of vomiting. Bile may appear as a yellow or green coloration. Bile is often present when vomiting is due to inflammatory bowel disease, idiopathic or secondary gastric hypomotility (bile alone or bile with food), intestinal foreign bodies, and pancreatitis. Chronic intermittent bilious vomiting in small breeds of dogs, especially when it occurs mostly in the early morning hours, is most suggestive of reflux gastritis. The presence of bile helps to rule out a complete pyloric obstruction.

Expulsion of large amounts of predominantly greenish-colored fluid from a patient with acute vomiting is most consistent with a proximal to mid small bowel obstruction. Lethargy, dehydration, and abdominal pain are generally present in affected patients. *In general, the more proximal a bowel obstruction is located, the more fulminant the clinical signs will be.* Small amounts of blood may be present in any case of gastric or duodenal mucosal compromise with erosions or ulceration (e.g., hypovolemia with resultant loss of integrity of the gastric mucosal barrier, drug-induced damage, acute or chronic gastritis or inflammatory bowel disease, gastric or duodenal ulceration, or neoplasia). Hematemesis may also be caused by a coagulopathy or ingestion of blood from another site (e.g., mouth, nasal sinuses, lungs). Large clots of blood or "coffee grounds" (blood altered by and mixed with gastric juice) usually indicate a more significant degree of erosions or ulceration. Fresh blood is usually altered in the stomach to the dark brown or black color known as "coffee grounds" in a matter of minutes. Presence of bright-red blood in the vomitus thus indicates very recent or active hemorrhage.

Clinicians should be aware that not all patients with gastric ulcers have hematemesis or even vomit. This fact highlights the importance of obtaining a thorough history to determine if any "ulcerogenic factors" could be present. Recent onset of hematemesis in a patient with *chronic* vomiting is often a sign that a potentially serious and worsening disorder is present. Such conditions as neoplasia with ulceration, uremic gastritis, or chronic severe gastritis with erosive changes should be considered, and diagnostic evaluation to determine the cause should be expedited. Potential causes of hematemesis are listed in Box 1-6.

A fecal odor suggests intestinal obstruction, peritonitis with ileus, ischemic injury to the intestine, or stasis with bacterial overgrowth. **Projectile** vomiting is an imprecise term that is used to describe forceful ejection of vomitus from the mouth, which is expelled a considerable distance. Its occurrence suggests a significant degree of gastric or proximal small bowel obstruction (foreign body, large antral or pyloric polyps, neoplasia, pyloric hypertrophy). In my experience this clinical sign occurs infrequently.

Chronic intermittent vomiting is a common presenting complaint in veterinary medicine. Often there is no specific time relation to eating, the content of the vomitus varies, and the occurrence of vomiting may be very cyclic in nature. Depending on the disorder, other signs, such as diarrhea, lethargy, inappetence, weight loss, and

salivation (nausea), may occur as well. When presented with this pattern of clinical signs in patients in which metabolic disorders, GI parasitism, and adverse food reactions have been ruled out, the clinician should strongly consider chronic gastritis, inflammatory bowel disease, irritable bowel syndrome, and gastric motility disorders as leading differential diagnoses. A detailed work-up, including gastric and intestinal biopsies, is often required for definitive diagnosis in these cases. It is important to note that chronic intermittent vomiting is a *common* clinical sign of inflammatory bowel disease in both dogs and cats. Diarrhea may or may not be a concurrent problem in patients with inflammatory bowel disease. Vomiting from systemic or metabolic causes may be an acute or chronic sign, and generally there is no direct correlation with eating and no predictable vomitus content.

The concomitant presence of diarrhea with vomiting often provides important diagnostic clues. Vomiting preceding diarrhea suggests toxic ingestion, a progressively severe disease of the small intestine such as viral enteritis (e.g., due to parvovirus or rotavirus), pancreatitis, or acute colitis. Also, infections with parasites, including *Giardia* and roundworms, can cause vomiting that precedes the

---

BOX 1-6 Causes of Hematemesis

COAGULOPATHY (UNCOMMON CAUSE)
Thrombocytopenia
Clotting factor deficiency
Disseminated intravascular coagulation

ALIMENTARY TRACT LESION
Gastrointestinal ulceration
  Infiltrative disease
    Neoplasia (especially older dogs)
    Pythiosis (younger dogs in southeastern United States)
  "Stress" ulceration
    Hypovolemic shock (common cause)
    Septic shock
  Hyperacidity
    Mast cell tumor
    Gastrinoma (rare)
  Drug induced
    Nonsteroidal antiinflammatory drugs (common cause)
    Corticosteroids (especially dexamethasone or if combined with nonsteroidal antiinflammatory drugs)

Other causes
  Hepatic disease (common cause)
  Renal disease (not a common cause)
  Inflammatory bowel disease
  Foreign objects (rarely a primary cause, but will worsen preexisting ulceration/erosion)
  Idiopathic
Gastritis
  Acute gastritis (very common cause)
  Hemorrhagic gastroenteritis
Esophageal disease (uncommon cause)
  Tumor
  Inflammatory disease
Bleeding oral lesion
Gallbladder disease (rare)

EXTRAALIMENTARY TRACT LESION (RARE CAUSE)
Respiratory tract
  Lung lobe torsion
  Pulmonary tumor
  Posterior nares lesion

From Willard M: Clinical manifestations of gastrointestinal disorders. In Nelson RW, Couto CG, eds: *Essentials of small animal internal medicine*, St. Louis, 1992, Mosby–Year Book.

onset of diarrhea. Occasionally *Giardia* may cause chronic intermittent vomiting without diarrhea or with only sporadic bouts of abnormal stools. Diarrhea preceding vomiting usually suggests primary but progressive intestinal damage, and vomiting is generally a secondary event in these patients. This includes patients that have gastric hypomotility secondary to inflammatory bowel disease.

Physical Examination

It is important to stress the enormous significance of a complete history and physical examination in evaluation of a vomiting patient. An all too frequent error in clinical practice is to make a diagnosis based on an incomplete history and cursory examination. This may lead to use of unnecessary diagnostic tests and inappropriate treatment. Essential early diagnosis of a serious disorder may be missed. A systematic approach can be both thorough and time efficient. Areas to receive emphasis in a vomiting patient are listed here.

The first step in physical examination is to assess the patient's overall attitude, posture, and energy level (i.e., active versus lethargic). This will often assist the clinician in determining to some degree the seriousness of the patient's condition and its degree of discomfort, if any exists. Observe the patient! Will any pain relief or antiemetic medication to control nausea be needed? It is often very reassuring to the owner when the clinician begins the examination by showing interest in how the patient has been acting and feeling. Patients that are experiencing a significant degree of nausea often have a forlorn expression, swallow frequently, and salivate (Figure 1-2). Patients with intestinal foreign body obstruction, pancreatitis, gastric neoplasia, and other serious conditions are often quite subdued at the time of presentation. These types of observations can often be made as the history is being discussed and recorded. Careful observation should be continued throughout any subsequent period of hospitalization.

The mucous membranes are evaluated for evidence of blood loss, dehydration, sepsis, shock, and jaundice. Salivation suggests the presence of nausea (common causes of salivation are listed in Box 1-7). An oral examination may reveal a part of an oral or pharyngeal foreign body that may extend to the stomach or intestine. The best example of this is a linear foreign body in a cat in which a portion of the foreign material loops around the tongue at the frenulum, with the free

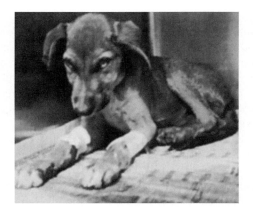

FIGURE 1-2 Typical appearance of a puppy quite ill from parvovirus enteritis. This puppy was depressed, reluctant to move, and nauseated. Watery diarrhea was present in the cage.

ends subsequently advancing along the intestinal lumen as a result of progressive peristalsis. Intestinal plication with potential for perforation results. *It is extremely important that an oral examination with careful evaluation of the frenulum area be done in all vomiting cats.* In some cases, mild tranquilization (e.g., ketamine 5 to 8 mg intravenously) is required so that a definitive examination can be done (Figure 1-3). Dogs occasionally have similar foreign body positioning, so a careful oral examination is important in this species as well. The cervical soft tissues of vomiting cats should be palpated for an enlarged thyroid nodule or nodules (hyperthyroidism commonly causes vomiting). Hyperthyroidism should be considered in any cat 5 years of age and older. Cardiac auscultation may reveal rate and rhythm abnormalities that can

---

BOX 1-7	**Causes of Salivation**

Nausea
Stomatitis (including chronic feline gingivitis/ stomatitis/pharyngitis)
Direct oral stimulation (e.g., ingestion of caustic materials, foreign body, electric cord injury, oral neoplasia)
Chemical poisoning (organophosphates, carbamates, metaldehyde)
Esophagitis
Esophageal foreign body
Portosystemic shunt (especially in cats)
Medications (especially in cats; e.g., trimethoprim/ sulfadiazine)
Rabies
Conditioned reflex (Pavlovian response)

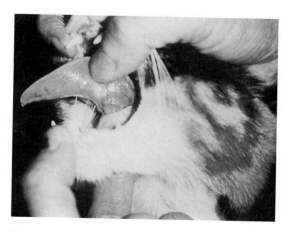

FIGURE 1-3 Linear foreign body (dental floss) under the tongue of a cat that was tranquilized in order to facilitate a thorough oral examination. The cat was presented because of acute vomiting, anorexia, and lethargy.

occur with metabolic disturbances such as hypoadrenocorticism (bradycardia, weak femoral pulses), infectious enteritis with septic shock (tachycardia, weak pulses), or gastric dilatation-volvulus (tachycardia, weak pulses, pulse deficits).

A careful assessment is made for either generalized or localized abdominal pain (e.g., pancreatitis, foreign body, pyelonephritis, hepatic disease, regional inflammation in inflammatory bowel disease). Other abdominal factors to evaluate include abnormal organ size (e.g., hepatomegaly, small or large kidneys), presence of a mass (foreign body, intussusception, lymphadenopathy, neoplasia), degree of gastric distention (increased with gastric dilatation, gastric dilatation-volvulus, gastric retention due to hypomotility or outflow obstruction), and altered bowel sounds.

Auscultation of the abdomen may occasionally be useful. Bowel sounds are often absent in peritonitis and increased in acute inflammatory disorders. An increased pitch suggests distention of intestinal loops. **Serial palpation** may be required to detect problems in some patients, including those with tensing of the abdominal wall due to pain or nervousness and when a foreign body, mass, or intussusception (especially sliding or ileocolic intussusceptions) is located in the craniodorsal abdomen, where the ribs prevent careful manipulation. It is often helpful to have someone hold the patient with the front end elevated so that the anterior abdominal organs shift caudally a little, into a more palpable position. It is also recommended that a two-hand palpation technique be

used, starting with gentle extension of one hand under each side of the rib cage. Finally, if history or radiographs strongly suggest the possibility of a foreign body or intussusception that has eluded initial palpation efforts, it may be useful to sedate the patient so that further *gentle* palpation can be done. Difficult-to-find foreign bodies can often be readily palpated with the assistance of sedation or general anesthesia. *Clinicians need to exercise great care when palpating patients that may have sharp intestinal linear foreign bodies or a large turgid uterus due to pyometra—forceful palpation could cause perforation of the intestine or uterus in these situations!*

A rectal examination is *always* done in dogs to evaluate stool characteristics for fresh blood or mucus, melena, or presence of foreign material; to obtain a fresh stool sample for parasite and possibly cytologic examination; and to evaluate the mucosa for sensitivity and abnormal texture. Serial rectal examinations are most important when GI bleeding is either suspected or has been identified. Because patient size precludes rectal examination in many small cats, careful assessment of stool characteristics is done instead in such patients.

Diagnostic Plan

Vomiting patients in some cases require an extensive work-up, but an organized approach will help to minimize the tests necessary for an early diagnosis. The most important initial considerations in determining what tests to perform are (1) signalment, (2) duration (acute [less than 7 to 14 days] versus chronic), (3) frequency of vomiting, (4) degree of symptoms (mild versus moderate to severe illness, i.e., life-threatening), (5) other clinical signs (e.g., shock, melena, abdominal pain), and (6) physical examination findings. Diagnostic studies and their possible results are summarized in Table 1-3.

If reasonable concern is established, a minimum database, including **CBC, biochemical profile** (or specific tests for evaluation of liver, kidneys, pancreas, electrolytes), complete **urinalysis** (determination of pretreatment urine specific gravity is extremely important for accurate differentiation of prerenal azotemia and primary renal disease), and **fecal examination,** is essential. Intestinal parasites, including *Giardia*, can cause vomiting and diarrhea. **Survey abdominal radiographs** are indicated if historical information suggests that they should be done or if thorough abdominal palpation is not possible or suggests an abnormality

TABLE 1-3 Diagnostic Studies in the Vomiting Patient

Test	Interpretation
Hemogram	
PCV, Hb, RBC	Increased: dehydration
	Decreased: gastrointestinal blood loss, decreased nutrient absorption (intestinal disease), anemia of chronic disease (e.g., severe inflammatory bowel disease), hypoadrenocorticism
WBC	Increased: inflammation, infection
	Decreased: sequestration or loss into gut (e.g., salmonellosis or viral infection)
Blood chemistries	
Na, Cl	Normal or decreased: outlet obstruction
	Decreased in most hypoadrenocorticism patients
K	Normal in most patients
	Decreased: outlet obstruction, severe vomiting, anorexia
	Increased: azotemia or hypoadrenocorticism
Total CO_2	Increased: gastric outlet obstruction
	Decreased: acidosis
BUN	Increased: gastrointestinal bleeding or azotemia
	Decreased: hepatic insufficiency, anorexia
Creatinine	Increased: azotemia
ALT, ALP	Increased: hepatic disease, pancreatitis, or intestinal disease
Serum proteins	Increased: dehydration, inflammation
	Decreased: protein-losing enteropathy, glomerular disease, blood loss, chronic liver disease, and possibly ascites
Triglycerides	Increased: pancreatitis
Cholesterol	Increased: pancreatitis, diabetes mellitus
	Decreased: protein-losing enteropathy, congenital portosystemic shunt
Amylase/lipase	Increased: pancreatitis, azotemia, gastrointestinal disease (with increased intestinal permeability), duodenal obstruction, neoplasia
Ca	Increased: dehydration (hyperalbuminemia), neoplasia
	Decreased: protein-losing enteropathy (hypoalbuminemia), ethylene glycol toxicity, necrotizing pancreatitis, hypoadrenocorticism
Glucose	Increased: diabetes mellitus
	Decreased: sepsis, neoplasia
TLI	Increased: acute pancreatitis, infiltrative bowel disease, renal failure
PLI	Increased: pancreatitis
T_4	Increased: hyperthyroidism
	Decreased: hypothyroidism (gastric hypomotility)
Urinalysis	Low specific gravity with dehydration suggests azotemia; biliuria suggests liver disease (especially in cats); glucosuria and ketonuria support diagnosis of diabetes mellitus
Fecal examination	Gastrointestinal parasites
Radiographic studies	
Survey abdominal films	Gastric distention, foreign body, mass, visceral displacement, effusion, ileus
Upper gastrointestinal contrast study	Delayed gastric emptying, filling defect, foreign body, mucosal irregularity, obstruction
BIPS	Delayed gastric emptying, obstruction
Ultrasonography	Liver and gallbladder disorders, gastrointestinal foreign bodies, intestinal and gastric wall thickening, intestinal masses, intussusception, kidney disorders, pancreatitis
Endoscopy and mucosal biopsy	Direct examination, biopsy of lesion, foreign body removal
Exploratory surgery	Examination, biopsy, therapeutic intervention

Modified from Burrows CF: Vomiting and regurgitation in the dog: a clinical perspective. In *Viewpoints in veterinary medicine,* ed 2, Lehigh Valley, Pa, 1993, Alpo Pet Foods.
PCV, Packed cell volume; *Hb,* hemoglobin; *RBC,* red blood cell count; *WBC,* white blood cell count; *Na,* sodium; *Cl,* chloride; *K,* potassium; *CO_2,* carbon dioxide; *BUN,* blood urea nitrogen; *ALT,* alanine aminotransferase; *ALP,* alkaline phosphatase; *Ca,* calcium; *TLI,* trypsin-like immunoreactivity; *PLI,* canine pancreatic lipase immunoreactivity; *T_4,* thyroxine; *BIPS,* barium-impregnated polyethylene spheres.

(e.g., foreign body, pancreatitis, pyometra). Unfortunately these tests are often not done early enough. Even if baseline results are unremarkable, such studies are more than justified because they help to rule out serious problems at the outset (e.g., vomiting due to renal failure, diabetes mellitus, liver disease). Alternatively, any abnormalities provide direction for initial treatment and further diagnostics.

A recently developed test, **canine and feline pancreatic lipase immunoreactivity (cPLI, fPLI),** is now available for diagnosis of pancreatitis in dogs and cats. This assay specifically measures the concentration of lipase originating from the exocrine pancreas. Because there are many lipases from different cellular origins, running total serum lipase levels is not specific enough for diagnosing pancreatitis. The assay for pancreatic lipase immunoreactivity uses specific antibodies directed against pancreatic lipase and therefore directly measures pancreatic lipase. Preliminary studies have shown that serum PLI concentration is both very specific and sensitive for diagnosis of pancreatic inflammation. The test is available at The GI Laboratory at Texas A&M University in College Station, Texas.

The decision to perform more in-depth diagnostic tests is based on ongoing clinical signs, response to therapy, and initial test results. These tests may include an **ACTH stimulation** test to confirm hypoadrenocorticism in a patient with an abnormal sodium-potassium ratio (Na:K) or suggestive CBC changes (anemia, lymphocytosis, and eosinophilia in a stressed patient) or to investigate for this disorder if electrolytes are normal (approximately 10% of dogs with hypoadrenocorticism do not present with abnormal electrolyte levels). Hypoadrenocorticism is more common in young to middle-age female dogs. A **complete barium series** is useful for identification of a gastric or intestinal foreign body, gastric hypomotility, gastric outflow obstruction, and partial or complete intestinal obstruction. Liquid barium contrast studies may be normal in patients with gastric hypomotility disorders. Measuring the emptying of barium mixed with food is a better test for evaluating gastric motility. Solids empty by a different mechanism from that for liquids, and it is not uncommon for patients with a known gastric emptying disorder to empty a liquid meal in a timely manner.

Alternatively, small, **nondigestible radiopaque markers (e.g., BIPS*) can be mixed with food for a radiographic series to study motility.**

BIPS are inert, white, radiopaque, barium-impregnated polyethylene spheres (BIPS). They have a density similar to food but are sufficiently radio-dense to show clearly on abdominal radiographs (Figure 1-4). All animals receive exactly the same dose of BIPS. They can be administered with or without food, depending on the clinical situation. BIPS are dispensed in capsule form. There are two sphere sizes contained in each dose application. There are 10 larger spheres (5 mm in diameter) and 30 smaller spheres (1.5 mm in diameter). The primary function of the large BIPS is the detection of GI tract obstructions. The small BIPS mimic the passage of food, and their transit through the GI tract provides an accurate estimate of the gastric emptying rate and intestinal transit time of food. Instructions on the use of BIPS are available from the distributor. Also, references are listed at the end of this chapter.

An **air contrast gastrogram** is often very useful for identifying gastric foreign bodies in cases in which survey films alone are not diagnostic (Figure 1-5). Confirmation of presence of a gastric foreign body may not be made in some

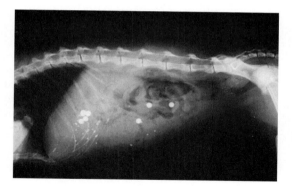

FIGURE 1-4 Lateral abdominal radiograph of a 15-year-old cat taken 24 hours after the start of a BIPS study to evaluate GI motility. This cat had presenting symptoms of intermittent vomiting and diarrhea. Many BIPS spheres remain in the stomach many hours after they would have exited the stomach of a cat with normal motility. The stomach should be completely empty after a meal by 7 to 10 hours. Small bowel transit time was also prolonged. This scattered pattern of BIPS is consistent with ileus. Endoscopy was subsequently performed, and moderate to severe inflammatory bowel disease was diagnosed. It was thought that the delayed motility resulted from the infiltrative bowel disease. Initial treatment included corticosteroids, cisapride (for GI promotility effect), and a diet featuring a protein source that was novel to this cat.

Medical ID Systems, Inc, Grand Rapids, MI 49512–3942.

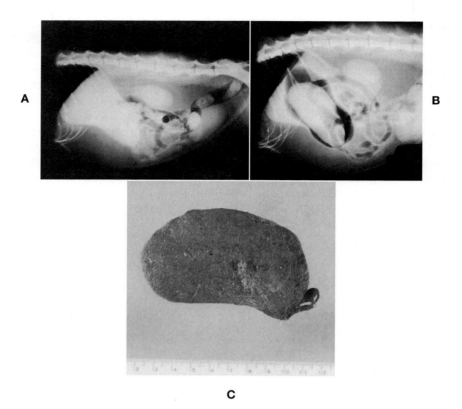

FIGURE 1-5 A, Lateral abdominal radiograph from a 10-year-old feline immunodeficiency virus (FIV)–positive cat with intestinal lymphoma. The cat had a gradually decreasing appetite, recent onset of intermittent vomiting, and occasional episodes of nonproductive retching. Abdominal palpation revealed a doughy mass in the region of the stomach. This radiograph shows that the stomach is distended and has a soft tissue/fluid opacity. The small intestine and colon are normal. **B,** Air gastrogram (40 ml of air was injected through a small feeding tube into the stomach while the cat was lightly tranquilized). A large mass density within the lumen of the stomach is consistent with a gastric trichobezoar. This simple procedure allowed rapid confirmation that a foreign body was present in the stomach. **C,** Trichobezoar that was surgically removed from the cat. The trichobezoar was 9 cm in length, and its configuration was similar to the inside of the stomach.

cases in which a barium series is done until most of the barium has left the stomach because a large barium pool often obscures foreign objects. **Barium swallow with fluoroscopy** is often necessary for diagnosis of hiatal hernia disorders and gastroesophageal reflux disease. **Endoscopy** is also useful for identifying these disorders.

Serum bile acids assay is used to assess for significant hepatic disease, including portosystemic shunts and chronic severe liver disease, when the liver enzymes are normal or only mildly elevated. Because vomiting is a frequent presenting sign in cats with heartworm disease, a **feline heartworm antibody test** should be done to investigate this possibility. In endemic areas testing cats for heartworm disease should be considered part of the minimum database. Because most cats with heartworm disease are amicrofilaremic, tests for microfilaria are usually negative. Antigen tests are also frequently negative. **Thoracic radiographs** may provide important clues in a cat with heartworm disease. Suggestive findings include right ventricular enlargement, pulmonary lobar artery enlargement, and pulmonary parenchymal disease. The caudal lobar arteries usually show the earliest radiographic changes, with the left and the right being equally affected. These changes are best recognized on the ventrodorsal or dorsoventral views. Some cats also have hyperglobulinemia. The presence of both peripheral eosinophilia and basophilia is also suggestive of heartworm disease in cats.

Thyroid testing should also be done on vomiting cats 5 years of age and older to evaluate for hyperthyroidism. It is important to remember that cats with hyperthyroidism may have thyroid hormone levels that fluctuate into the normal range for several days at a time early in the course of the disease. If hyperthyroidism is still suspected after an initial serum thyroxine (T_4) level is shown to be normal, either the test should be repeated in 1 to 3 weeks or, alternatively, other tests can be run. Alternative tests include the triiodothyronine (T_3) **suppression test, free T_4 by equilibrium dialysis (fT_4ED), TRH stimulation test,** or performance of a **technetium scan**. In cats with a total T_4 (TT_4) in the upper 50% of the basal resting range, an elevated fT_4ED in the face of clinical signs is highly predictive of hyperthyroidism. Due to the simplicity of running an fT_4ED versus performing a T_3 suppression test or TRH response test, fT_4ED should be the first test run for diagnosis of cats with hormonally occult (normal TT_4) hyperthyroidism.

Chronic vomiting in cats is occasionally due to infection with the gastric parasite *Ollulanus tricuspis*. Young, free-roaming cats are most often affected. Diagnosis is made by evaluation of gastric contents via the **Baermann technique** or by **examination of filtered vomitus** using a ×40 or dissecting microscope for detection of the nematode (Figure 1-6). Xylazine (Rompun) can be administered at 1 mg/lb intramuscularly to stimulate vomiting in order to collect the gastric secretions.

Serum gastrin levels are run if a gastrinoma (Zollinger-Ellison syndrome) is suspected. Gastrinoma, a gastrin-secreting tumor usually found in the pancreas, is infrequently seen in clinical practice. Clinical signs include chronic vomiting and/or diarrhea, weight loss, and anorexia. Middle-age to older dogs are most commonly affected (gastrinomas are quite rare in cats). The clinician should consider running a serum gastrin level in patients with chronic vomiting and wasting disease that are not readily explained by more routine diagnostic testing (i.e., baseline blood tests, urinalysis, radiography, and endoscopy).

One of the most reliable and cost-efficient diagnostic tools currently available for evaluation of vomiting is **flexible endoscopy**. Endoscopy allows for direct gastric and duodenal examination, mucosal biopsy from these areas, and in many cases gastric foreign body retrieval. Endoscopy is considerably more reliable than barium series for diagnosis of gastric erosions, ulceration, chronic gastritis, gastric neoplasia, and inflammatory bowel disease. Vomiting due to presence in the upper GI tract of the parasite *Physaloptera* is best diagnosed via direct visualization at endoscopy. The nema-

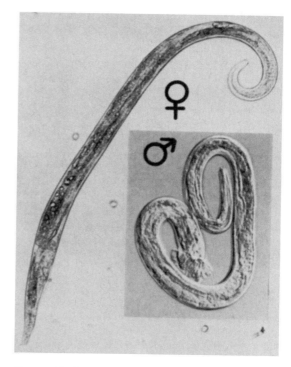

FIGURE 1-6 *Ollulanus tricuspis* from a leopard (×140). Diagnosis is usually based on finding adult specimens of this viviparous species in vomitus. (From Georgi JR: Helminths. In Georgi JR, Georgi ME, eds: *Parasitology for veterinarians*, ed 5, Philadelphia, 1990, WB Saunders.)

tode parasites can be readily seen on the surface of the gastric mucosa and retrieved through the endoscope working channel for definitive identification (Figure 1-7). It is stressed that biopsy samples should always be obtained from the stomach and, whenever possible, the small intestine during endoscopic procedures regardless of gross mucosal appearance. Normal gastric biopsy results may support gastric motility abnormalities, psychogenic vomiting, or irritable bowel syndrome or may be noncontributory (i.e., look elsewhere for diagnosis). *Many dogs and cats with vomiting due to inflammatory bowel disease have no abnormalities on gastric examination or biopsy. If only gastric biopsies are performed, the diagnosis may be missed.* As previously mentioned, some patients with colitis both vomit and have diarrhea. If large bowel symptoms are present in conjunction with vomiting, the colon should be examined and biopsies performed as well. Flexible endoscopy equipment should be used whenever possible so that the entire colon, including ascending colon, cecum, and terminal ileum, can be examined. Diagnosis of the rare ileocolic or cecocolic intussusception case that may

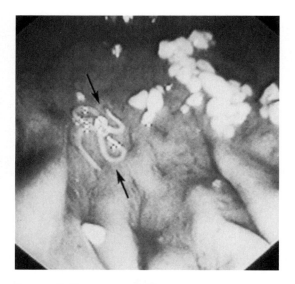

FIGURE 1-7 Multiple *Physaloptera* nematodes *(arrows)* lying on the gastric mucosa in a dog. These nematodes may cause the chronic vomiting and histologic lesions of lymphocytic-plasmacytic gastritis. (From Jergens AE, Moore FM: Endoscopic biopsy specimen collection and histopathologic considerations. In Tams TR, ed: *Small animal endoscopy*, ed 2, St. Louis, 1999, Mosby.)

have eluded diagnosis up to this point can be readily made on direct visualization of these areas. Examination or biopsy may also reveal typhlitis.

Ultrasonography can be useful in the diagnostic work-up of a number of disorders that can cause vomiting (see Chapter 2). Among the problems that may be detected with ultrasonography are certain disorders of the liver (e.g., inflammatory diseases, abscessation, cirrhosis, neoplasia, vascular problems) and gallbladder and bile ducts (cholecystitis, choleliths, bile duct obstruction), GI foreign bodies, intestinal and gastric wall thickening, intestinal masses, intussusception, kidney disorders, pancreatitis, and others. Needle aspirations and/or biopsies can be done at many sites under ultrasound guidance.

Abdominal exploratory is indicated for a variety of problems, including foreign body removal, intussusception, gastric mucosal hypertrophy syndromes, procurement of biopsy samples, and resection of neoplasia. If the diagnosis is unclear on examination, gastric and small intestinal (two to three samples total) biopsies must be performed. In a majority of dogs and cats with gastritis and inflammatory bowel disease, no gross abnormalities are detected at exploratory. Samples should also be obtained from liver and any

enlarged lymph nodes. Also, any visible abnormalities in the pancreas warrant biopsy of this organ. Pancreas biopsy is a safe procedure when done properly.

Timing of Work-up

The frequency and duration of vomiting can vary from weeks to years. In animals with chronic, slowly progressive disorders, vomiting may be only a sporadic event with or without occasional periods of increased frequency or severity possibly associated with flare-ups of the disease process. *Clinicians often ask when a patient with a disorder characterized by intermittent vomiting should undergo a detailed diagnostic work-up.* Indeed, it is not unusual for some cats, several of my own included, to vomit once or twice every 1 to 2 weeks or so for many months or years without any apparent untoward effect. A variety of factors are usually involved in the decision-making process regarding when diagnostic evaluation should be undertaken. The foremost factors include development of any concurrent worrisome signs, such as inappetence, weight loss, signs of abdominal discomfort such as cramping, presence of leukocytosis and/or hypoproteinemia, any signs of hyperthyroidism in cats to suggest advancing inflammatory bowel disease, and, very importantly, the degree of the owner's concern and level of interest in finding answers regarding his or her pet's problem.

In general, I recommend that a work-up be started if the frequency of vomiting or degree of any signs associated with the vomiting (e.g., lethargy, discomfort, inappetence) begins to increase. Always keep in mind that as disease processes worsen they are frequently more difficult to bring under control. With the availability of endoscopy and our ability to utilize it for examination and biopsy of the stomach and small intestine, in a significantly noninvasive manner when compared with surgery, it is definitely reasonable to recommend its use even in patients with mild clinical signs. A countless number of my patients from over the years come to mind during this discussion, but two in particular should help make a lasting point here. Both demonstrated only mild clinical signs, which included intermittent vomiting and mild *occasional* lethargy. Each, however, had a serious life-threatening problem that was fortunately diagnosed early enough for the patient to undergo meaningful treatment. A brief account of their histories follows.

In early 1988 I examined a 10-year-old neutered male domestic short hair (DSH) cat with a history of intermittent vomiting of 7 weeks' duration. There was a gradual increase in frequency over the last 2 weeks, no weight loss, and a normal appetite. Although the owner did not have a great deal of money to spend, he expressed concern about his cat's well-being and requested that we try to find out what was wrong while keeping his cost-containment concerns in mind. The cat weighed 12 lb, and physical examination was unremarkable other than signs of vague anterior abdominal discomfort. A CBC, biochemical profile, serum T_4, feline leukemia virus (FeLV), feline immunodeficiency virus (FIV) test, and a urinalysis

were run. Radiography was bypassed in favor of endoscopy (greater sensitivity and likelihood of definitive diagnosis). Endoscopy revealed a large mass in the fundus of the stomach, which was found to be lymphoma (Figure 1-8). Intestinal biopsy specimens revealed moderate lymphocytic-plasmacytic enteritis. After 5 months of chemotherapy (no surgery was done), the mass was no longer detectable at endoscopy (Figure 1-9). After 1 year of chemotherapy there was no histologic evidence of lymphoma and chemotherapy was discontinued. Subsequent yearly endoscopic examination and biopsy of the stomach and duodenum revealed no evidence of recurrence of the lymphoma. Interestingly, the cat still had a

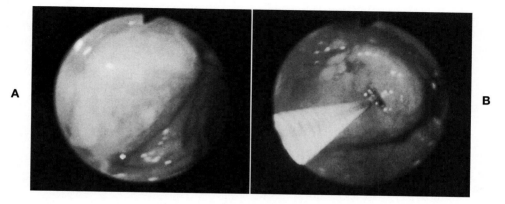

FIGURE 1-8 A, Close-up endoscopic view of a large mass in the gastric fundus of a 10-year-old cat with a 7-week history of intermittent vomiting. **B,** Biopsy forceps are advanced into the mass under endoscopic guidance. The histologic diagnosis was lymphoma. (From Tams TR: Gastroscopy. In Tams TR, ed: *Small animal endoscopy*, ed 2, St. Louis, 1999, Mosby.)

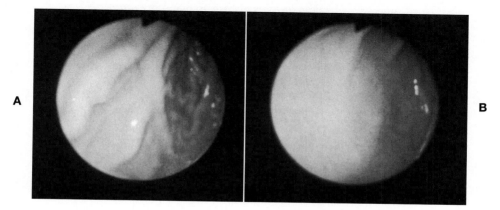

FIGURE 1-9 Five-month follow-up endoscopic examination of the cat described in Figure 1-8. Treatment involved chemotherapy (prednisone, cyclophosphamide, vincristine) alone. No surgery was done. **A,** Forward view of proximal stomach at mild distention. The mass is no longer visible, and the rugal folds are smooth. **B,** Same site as **A** with moderate distention. The mucosa at the original site of the mass appears whiter than the surrounding mucosa. (From Tams TR: Gastroscopy. In Tams TR, ed: *Small animal endoscopy*, ed 2, St. Louis, 1999, Mosby.)

moderate degree of inflammatory bowel disease, and antiinflammatory therapy (prednisone) was maintained. If the dose was decreased too much, vomiting began to recur. The cat lived to the age of 17 years, 7 years beyond the diagnosis of gastric lymphoma.

In 1992 I evaluated a 9-year-old neutered male Bouvier with a history of intermittent vomiting of 5 months' duration (only one to two episodes per week and with no worrisome associated signs). The owners became concerned because they felt the dog was sleeping a little more than normal, and they requested that their regular veterinarian begin investigating the problem. A CBC, biochemical profile, serum T_4, urinalysis, fecal examination for parasites, and survey radiographs of the thorax and abdomen were unremarkable. The dog was then referred for endoscopy, which revealed a large proliferative mass involving the entire pyloric canal and the proximal duodenum just aboral to

the pylorus (Figure 1-10). The pyloric canal was occluded an estimated 300 degrees. The remainder of the stomach and duodenum were grossly and histologically normal. Histologic examination of the mass revealed it to be an adenocarcinoma. The distal antrum, pylorus, and proximal duodenum were resected, and the dog recovered uneventfully. This patient experienced an excellent quality of life. Upper GI endoscopy was performed at 6-month intervals to examine the stomach and proximal small intestine, and there were no gross or histologic abnormalities detected (Figure 1-11). There was also an exploratory laparotomy done at one point for removal of a cloth linear foreign body. This allowed a thorough examination of the abdominal cavity, and there was no evidence of recurrence of neoplasia. The dog lived 30 months beyond the diagnosis of gastric neoplasia, and there was never any recurrence of adenocarcinoma in the stomach region. Unfortunately, euthanasia was

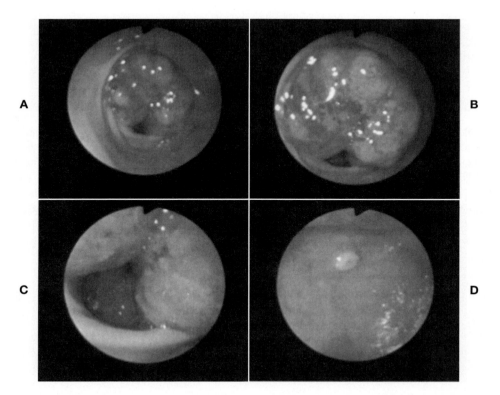

FIGURE 1-10 Endoscopic views of the stomach and proximal duodenum of a 9-year-old male Bouvier with a history of intermittent vomiting of 5 months' duration. **A,** The antral walls are normal. A proliferative mass is visualized in the pyloric orifice. **B,** Close-up view of the pyloric mass. The mass is occluding a majority of the pyloric orifice. The remaining orifice space is visualized at the six o'clock position. **C,** Pyloric canal near the pyloroduodenal junction. The mass extended into the proximal duodenum. The histologic diagnosis was adenocarcinoma. **D,** The major duodenal papilla is visualized in the upper center in the field of view.

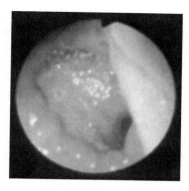

FIGURE 1-11 Six-month follow-up endoscopic view from the dog described in Figure 1-10. The anastomosis site between the proximal gastric antrum and the duodenum is in the field of view (note ridged area extending from five o'clock to twelve o'clock position). There was no gross or histologic evidence of tumor recurrence.

performed at 30 months because of prostatic adenocarcinoma.

These two case histories clearly demonstrate the value of timely diagnosis of potentially life-threatening problems. Frequently dogs and cats with intermittent vomiting have much more minor problems; however, it is difficult to anticipate which are the patients that will have the more severe problems. One of the clinician's most important roles is to advise and educate owners in a responsible manner. Shouldn't we as clinicians at the very least make owners aware of the diagnostic capabilities that we have at our disposal today? There is no question that a *majority* of our canine and feline patients with GI symptoms have treatable disorders. *The important point is that we diagnose the chronic and potentially serious disorders early enough to make a difference.*

Summary

The cause of chronic vomiting can be determined in most dogs and cats, and early diagnosis is facilitated when a systematic diagnostic approach is followed. In my experience, once adverse food reactions, GI parasites, drug reactions, and metabolic causes have been ruled out, the *most common* causes of chronic vomiting encountered in practice are inflammatory disorders (gastritis, inflammatory bowel disease), gastric hypomotility, obstructive disorders (foreign bodies, hypertrophy syndromes), and neoplasia. The most clinically useful (i.e., high yield of important information

while being cost-effective) diagnostic procedures include hemogram and biochemical profile evaluation, thyroid and feline heartworm testing in cats, urinalysis, fecal examination, survey abdominal radiography, ultrasonography, and endoscopy.

GRASS INGESTION/ COPROPHAGY/PICA

It is not uncommon for dogs and cats to ingest grass and for dogs to demonstrate a tendency toward coprophagy or pica. Occasionally, certain cats may excessively lick materials such as soil, litter, wool, and other items. Although the tendency to do this may be related to a group of syndromes termed ingestive behavior problems, these conditions may also occur as a result of some type of digestive system disorder. Questions are frequently asked about the significance of these activities, especially grass ingestion and coprophagy. A brief discussion of each problem follows.

Grass Ingestion

Many dogs and some cats enjoy eating grass for no proven reason and with no apparent untoward effects. For some it may represent a normal physiologic event. Perhaps these animals simply enjoy "grazing," or they may be seeking a source of roughage to supply minerals or fiber. If grass ingestion is *not* associated with any immediate symptoms of a GI disturbance, such as nausea, bloating, or vomiting, its significance is probably minor and there is no need for concern on the part of the owner. Cats that do not get vegetable matter in their diets may have a tendency to eat parts of house plants. This problem can often be successfully eliminated by providing a small flower pot with grass for the cat to eat. For cats that develop an undesirable habit of eating certain house plants, measures such as removal of the plant or aversion taste-smell conditioning with pepper sauce or vinegar often work. Plant ingestion may cause vomiting from irritant or toxic effects, and it should certainly be discouraged if these symptoms develop.

I commonly encounter canine patients that are reported to ingest grass only at times when they seem to be experiencing some type of distress related to the digestive system. The most common of these is nausea, exhibited by such signs as licking of the lips, exaggerated swallowing motions, salivation, and often disinterest in eating food.

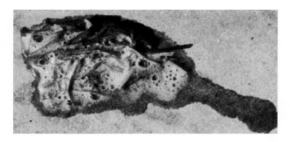

FIGURE 1-12 Grass and bile fluid vomited by a dog that was demonstrating symptoms of nausea before ingesting the grass.

Frequently the dog, when allowed outside, moves quickly to a grassy area and begins ingesting grass. Shortly thereafter, the grass, usually along with fluid that is often bilious (Figure 1-12), is vomited, and the dog often subjectively appears to feel much better after the stomach has emptied (based on improved appetite and energy). In my experience this is not an uncommon occurrence in dogs with the bilious vomiting syndrome, which is frequently associated with some degree of gastric hypomotility. Dogs with this syndrome that eat grass often do so more in the early morning hours (although it can occur at any time). They most likely awaken from a period of sleep while experiencing nausea, and they tend to pace around until they can gain outdoor access, where they often head directly to a grassy area.

Some large-breed dogs will impulsively eat large quantities of grass in the early stages of a gastric dilatation event. Perhaps grass has some type of soothing property for dogs and cats with esophageal or gastric irritation that can result from any of a number of causes. These may include gastroesophageal reflux, erosive gastritis, superficial irritation from bile reflux, vomiting related to chronic gastritis or inflammatory bowel disease, and others. For many years it has been theorized by laypeople that dogs with GI upset may eat grass because they have a sense that doing so will help them vomit. Dogs that eat grass as a result of a digestive system disorder generally do so only on an intermittent basis that often coincides with their periods of discomfort. I definitely consider this to be a meaningful clinical sign, and I make a point of asking owners whose pets are presented for evaluation of disorders characterized by inappetence, nausea, or vomiting if they ever see their dog eating grass during periods of apparent GI discomfort. Not uncommonly the answer is yes. In

fact, the act of grass ingestion can actually become a valuable monitoring tool for owners, providing an indication that their pet is uncomfortable and in need of some type of treatment.

My own Doberman pinscher, which was afflicted with a gastric hypomotility disorder for much of her life, demonstrated very clear signs of nausea with subsequent grass ingestion, followed by vomiting, on days on which I failed to medicate her properly (she was on lifelong twice-daily metoclopramide therapy to improve gastric motility) or to feed her on time. On occasion even when I did administer the medication in a timely manner, she would still exhibit signs of nausea and have a propensity to eat grass. My response, which often seemed to provide relief, was to increase the frequency of metoclopramide to three times a day and to add an H_2-receptor antagonist (famotidine) to lower gastric acid levels, both for several days. She rarely showed any interest in eating grass when her GI symptoms were well controlled.

Other veterinarians have recounted stories to me about their own dogs that have had grass-eating tendencies. Some have not shown any concurrent GI symptoms such as nausea or vomiting but dramatically decreased or stopped altogether the grass ingestion when they were treated with H_2-receptor antagonist therapy on an empirical basis. In some, as soon as this medication was stopped, the grass ingestion behavior was resumed. Ideally these dogs should undergo upper GI endoscopy to examine for evidence of reflux esophagitis, gastritis, bile retention in the stomach, upper small bowel inflammation, and other conditions. One can only speculate that for these particular dogs the ingestion of grass may truly have some type of therapeutic effect. The difficulty for us in working with our patients, of course, is in clearly determining whether or not there is any significant reason for a particular patient to ingest grass, especially when there are no obvious associated symptoms. Certainly care must be taken not to overinterpret the significance of grass ingestion. Further investigation is needed before any conclusions can be drawn.

Coprophagy

Coprophagy is the ingestion of feces. This is common behavior in some species, most notably rabbits, and in the young of most species. Cats rarely become coprophagic, but to the dismay of many dog owners it is a frequently occurring canine misbehavior. The idea of coprophagy is revolting to most humans, and there is potential for its occurrence to seriously alter an owner's attitude toward his or her dog. Most will try any suggestions offered by their veterinarian, trainer, or any other opinionated person. Some owners, however, come to accept their dog's habit. Many dogs also display a great preference for ingesting cat feces. Potential causes of coprophagy are listed in Box 1-8.

Many theories, none scientifically accepted, about why coprophagy occurs in dogs have been proposed by veterinarians and laypeople. It is adaptive behavior during the first 3 weeks of nursing for the mother to keep the nest free of urine and feces. It is possible that, for some dogs, consuming the feces of the young may predispose them to coprophagy in nonmaternal situations. It is also possible that the habit of coprophagy may be an example of neonety, that is, the retention of juvenile behavior in the adult dog.

Common reasons for coprophagy probably include boredom, lack of attention from an owner, unresolved conflictual situations in the environment, insufficient exercise, consumption of nutritionally incomplete rations, poor hygiene in the environment, and digestive system disorders that result in malabsorption or maldigestion. Bored or fastidious dogs might first begin ingesting their

feces during confinement situations (e.g., cage confinement in a kennel). Coprophagy may then become a habit. Dogs with exocrine pancreatic insufficiency (EPI) may become coprophagic, probably secondary to polyphagia and as a consequence of specific nutritional deficiencies. In fact, any disorder that causes polyphagia can also potentially cause coprophagy. In addition to malassimilation disorders, other problems that have been reported to be associated with coprophagy include hyperadrenocorticism, intestinal parasitism, and hyperthyroidism; glucocorticoid therapy also appears to be associated with coprophagy.

A few significant deleterious consequences are usually associated with coprophagy. The severe halitosis that results is particularly offensive to most owners. Depending on the timing of their activity, dogs may find themselves relegated to areas where they are unable to gain access to the owner. The potential for acquiring parasitic infections from ingesting stools always exists. Bacterial and viral infections can also be transmitted in this way. Occasionally dogs with access to horse manure are presented in acute distress that results from partial or complete intestinal obstruction. Surgery is sometimes necessary to relieve these impactions.

The diagnostic evaluation for the problem of coprophagy starts with obtaining a thorough history. A differential diagnosis should be made regarding the likelihood of the presence of a significant medical problem versus environmental problems or primary behavior tendencies. The quality of the diet should be assessed. If a poor quality diet is being fed, it may simply be enough to change to a higher quality ration, preferably one with a high digestibility ratio. Dogs that are fed only one meal per day may have a lesser tendency toward coprophagy if food is provided two to three times a day.

Questioning regarding the environment includes information about hygiene practices, level of daily exercise that patient gets, amount of interaction with humans or other animals, and whether there are any known stresses or conflicts that the patient undergoes in its environment. Delayed cleanup and disposal of stools can contribute to the initiation and maintenance of a habit of coprophagy. Efforts must be made by the owner to remove stools from the environment as quickly as possible. Boredom can be a contributing factor to coprophagy. Dogs that spend much of their time alone all day, especially outdoors, may eventually

---

BOX 1-8	Possible Causes of Coprophagy

BEHAVIORAL
Learned habits from puppyhood
Carryover of maternal behavior to nonmaternal situations

ENVIRONMENTAL/BEHAVIORAL
Poor sanitation
Unresolved conflictual situations
Boredom (lack of sufficient exercise and interaction with humans and other animals)
Confinement in close quarters (e.g., boarding [kennel] situations)

MEDICAL DISORDERS
Parasitism
Nutritional deficiency
Exocrine pancreatic insufficiency
Intestinal malabsorption
Hyperadrenocorticism
Hyperthyroidism
Any cause of polyphagia

get into the habit of eating their stools. Extra exercise and human interaction every morning and evening, which includes walks and periods of play with the owner, as well as providing another animal with which to interact, may be of some help in these situations. Proffering the dog fresh rawhides on a daily basis may help lessen the tendency for coprophagy.

If coprophagy involves ingestion of cat feces from litter boxes, the only realistic methods of control include placing the litter boxes in areas where dogs are unable to gain access, using covered litter containers, and cleaning the litter as frequently as possible.

If the history suggests that there may be a medical disorder present, appropriate diagnostic evaluation should be undertaken to identify or rule out any potential problems. Treatment is then directed toward whatever problem is identified. Examinations for intestinal parasites should be done routinely. If there is any possibility of EPI, a trypsin-like immunoreactivity (TLI) assay should be run. It should be noted that some dogs with EPI only infrequently have diarrhea. The canine TLI test is readily available at many commercial labs and is highly diagnostic for EPI. Treatment includes pancreatic enzyme replacement therapy and dietary management (mild to moderate fat restriction and low fiber content). Coprophagic tendencies often stop in dogs with EPI once appropriate therapy is instituted.

Myriad compounds that can be added to the food in an attempt to decrease or alleviate coprophagic behavior have been recommended and tried over the years. These compounds include various types of digestive enzymes and vitamins used to improve digestion and subsequent absorption of nutrients, or chemicals that are added to the food to make stools that are subsequently passed less desirable to eat for coprophagic dogs by creating an offensive taste. In my experience this approach unfortunately rarely works. However, these ideas should be discussed with owners who are willing to try anything to curb their dog's habit of coprophagy. A list of various enzymes or chemicals that have been recommended by veterinarians, breeders, and behavior specialists appears in Box 1-9.

Once the habit of coprophagy is started, it can be very difficult to break. Treatment may require retraining the patient. Use of a muzzle to prevent prehension of stool may be a useful starting point in the retraining process. Moreover, several recently

BOX 1-9	**Partial List of Food Additives Suggested for Prevention of Coprophagy***

Various pancreatic or digestive enzymes (e.g., Pancrezyme, Viokase, Prozyme, meat tenderizers, crushed pineapple)
B-complex vitamins
Sulfur
Glutamic acid
Monosodium glutamate (MSG)
Oil of anise
Sauerkraut
Canned pumpkin
Forbid

*There is no doubt many compounds that have been tried by someone, somewhere, do not appear on this list.

proposed behavior modification techniques, used alone or in combination, have shown promise in fairly consistently stopping coprophagic tendencies in dogs whose problem has been found to be behavioral rather than medical. First, an owner may condition a dog to expect a treat immediately after stooling. In this fashion its expectation of a delicious food treat may inhibit the tendency to feed on stools. Second, a way may be found to punish the activity or make the activity aversive. One method is to inject the commercial product Bitter Apple *into* the stool. Simply spraying this product on the surface of the stool will not be likely to have any lasting effect because the dog will shy away before it touches the stool. The element of surprise is lost if this is done. Biting into stool that is impregnated with Bitter Apple will often cause a very significant aversive sensation. Dose depends on the size of the stool, but a general range of 1 to 3 ml is suggested. This method may also help prevent a dog from ingesting cat feces. An alternative would be to inject the feces with the emetic drug apomorphine. Ingestion of feces followed shortly by a strong sensation of nausea and then vomiting may suffice to cause a strong aversion to the stool.

As a last resort, owners who strongly desire to stop coprophagic behavior can try remote punishment with a shock collar. Remote punishment is applied the moment the dog begins to explore or prehend stool. Behavior modification with shock collars has been reported to be very effective. It must be noted that this method of treatment should be carefully discussed with any owner who expresses interest in trying it. The owner's ethical concerns and other issues surrounding the application of this procedure need to be taken into consideration. For some this form of treatment may be unacceptable. The reader should consult the references at the end of the chapter for an overview of using this kind of treatment to solve behavioral problems.

Pica

Pica is defined as a craving for and ingestion of unnatural articles of food. Dogs may eat dirt (geophagy), cloth, carpet, rocks, sticks, cat litter, or other materials or may show a distinct interest in licking carpet or concrete. Cats may eat soil, grass, or even cat litter. Anemic cats sometimes lick soil, litter, walls, or rusty objects. Wool sucking is an abnormal behavior disorder known to occur in Siamese, part-Siamese, and Burmese cats. Cats with this tendency may actually destroy woolen articles by sucking or chewing on them.

Nutritional deficiencies should be corrected if they exist. The diagnostic approach is similar to that followed for coprophagy. Dietary and environmental factors should be investigated. Occasionally, geophagic animals are found to be iron deficient. Dogs that lick or chew on foreign objects may have acute or chronic vomiting that may be related to the presence of a gastric or intestinal foreign body. I have seen dogs with large clumps of carpet fibers that probably took weeks to months to build up before endoscopic retrieval or gastrotomy became necessary to remove the material.

Most of the time, animals with pica have a behavioral tendency rather than a true medical disorder. Treatment usually involves preventing access, if at all possible, to favored objects or limiting access to one to two items. Taste aversion methods can also be tried. Thyroid hormone supplementation works well in some wool-sucking cats.

▌ DIARRHEA

In addition to vomiting, diarrhea is one of the most common presenting complaints that veterinarians deal with on a daily basis. Surveys have confirmed that a majority of practicing veterinarians rank definitive diagnosis and management of chronic intermittent and chronic persistent diarrhea as one of the most challenging and frustrating aspects of their medical practices.

Decisions frequently revolve around such questions as, What are the most meaningful initial clinical tests? When and for how long should empirical treatment be tried? What are the most appropriate medications to use for empirical treatment trials? When should a detailed diagnostic work-up, which often includes GI function testing and intestinal biopsies, be recommended? This section and the chapters on small intestinal (Chapters 6 and 7) and large intestinal (Chapter 8) disorders describe an organized approach to the problem of diarrhea that is applicable to any practice setting.

Diarrhea is defined simply as passage of feces that contain an excess amount of water. This results in an abnormal increase in stool liquidity and weight. In some patients there may simply be an increase in frequency of defecation. Diarrhea has also been described in broad, simple terms as "the too rapid evacuation of too loose stools." Definitions notwithstanding, however, it is most important that the clinician carefully determine exactly what the owner means when the term *diarrhea* is used. The owner's interpretation is often not as encompassing as the clinician's. To some people diarrhea indicates only profuse, watery stools. In fact, any variance from what is considered normal for a patient in terms of frequency and consistency should be considered potentially abnormal and worthy of discussion.

Although a variety of symptoms can be caused by intestinal disorders, diarrhea is the hallmark sign of intestinal dysfunction. It can result from primary intestinal disease (e.g., parasitism, various inflammatory disorders, infectious problems, neoplasia), disorders of the liver or pancreas that affect normal intestinal digestive and absorptive processes, and a number of other factors or conditions that adversely affect intestinal function in some way (e.g., dietary indiscretion, adverse food reactions, drugs [e.g., antibiotics, cardiac glycosides], systemic disorders including renal failure, hypoadrenocorticism).

Diarrhea is often classified according to **location** (small or large intestinal in origin), **mechanism(s)** of diarrhea (**osmotic**—decreased solute absorption, **secretory**—hypersecretion of ions, **exudative**—increased permeability, and **abnormal motility**), and **etiology.** Most small animals with diarrhea can be successfully treated. Clinicians are cautioned, however, that patients with diarrhea that do not respond satisfactorily to routine care within a reasonable period of time, as determined by the patient's overall condition, frequency of clinical signs (increasing?), and presence of any significant laboratory abnormalities, should be thoroughly investigated to determine the cause of the problem before it becomes significantly chronic and potentially nonresponsive to any treatment that is administered. *Intestinal biopsy is often required for diagnosis in patients with chronic, poorly responsive diarrhea.*

Historical Findings—Overview

It is clear that a great number of problems can cause diarrhea. The clinician is faced with the tasks of formulating a well-directed diagnostic plan from a variety of available clinical tests and accurately selecting an effective therapeutic regimen from a wide array of diets and pharmaceuticals. This all too often has to be accomplished with cost-containment factors foremost in the owner's mind. As a result it is extremely important that a thorough history be obtained so that a limited list of most likely diagnostic possibilities can be accurately determined. This is best done by asking a broad-based series of questions in an orderly manner. Box 1-10 provides a list of questions to ask when interrogating an owner whose pet has diarrhea.

The first step involves establishing the **duration** of clinical signs as clearly as possible. It is important to ascertain how frequently a patient's stools are actually observed. Patients that live primarily outdoors or that are only casually watched when they are outside may have been experiencing abnormal defecations longer or more persistently than the owner may actually realize. Emphasis is also placed on a review of the **clinical course** (e.g., acute and short duration, acute onset and then persistent for several weeks or more, intermittent initially but now more persistent, chronic [more than 1 month] and unrelenting).

Next, a clear description of the nature and character of the stool is obtained. This will help differentiate small bowel from large bowel disorders (Table 1-4). Tests and treatment often vary for small and large intestinal disorders, making this initial characterization very important. Because large bowel type of problems occur so commonly, I often begin by asking questions relative to this area of the GI tract. Specifically, the presence or absence of mucus (Figure 1-13),

fresh blood, straining, and any change in frequency of defecation are discussed. A rough estimate of fecal water content is made (e.g., Are the stools profuse and watery in nature? Generally soft formed?). Small bowel diarrhea is characterized by passage of increased volumes of fecal material.

The vaccination history, dietary history, and environmental history (potential for dietary indiscretion, exposure to any infectious or parasitic agents) are always discussed, and valuable diagnostic clues are often elucidated, especially in patients with acute diarrhea. Any recent history of drug administration should also be reviewed, because some pharmaceuticals could be implicated as causative agents (more so in patients with acute diarrhea). Sometimes the patient's lifestyle plays an important role in the development of diarrhea. For example, working dogs such as sled or police dogs may experience diarrheal episodes during stressful times. Sled dogs sometimes exhibit explosive diarrhea, with or without blood, at the start of or during a race. In police dogs (frequently German shepherds), diarrhea, which may be consistent with either small or large bowel type of signs, and other GI symptoms can be related to intense work situations. Home environment and a patient's individual personality type (e.g., excitable, aggressive) may play a role in causing diarrhea in dogs with irritable bowel syndrome.

The initial phase of the interview is completed with an assessment of the patient's overall condition, with emphasis on attitude (alert/responsive/active versus variable degrees of lethargy) and whether there has been any weight loss. The clinician has now had an opportunity to gain perspective regarding how the case should be approached diagnostically and therapeutically and, very importantly, whether or not there should be some sense of urgency in expediting the initial plan (e.g., parvoviral enteritis, intussusception, symptoms including abdominal pain, chronic wasting disease associated with a severe protein-losing enteropathy condition). More detailed information regarding the meaning of historical findings is provided in the following discussion.

Stool Characteristics

Table 1-4 outlines historical and gross fecal characteristics useful in differentiation of small and

BOX 1-10   Questions to Ask in the Investigation of Diarrhea

1. **Was the onset recent and acute?** If so:
   a. Is this a young patient that was just obtained from a locality where there was close contact with other animals (e.g., pet store, kennel, humane shelter)? If so, assume parasitism (including *Giardia*) and/or viral infection as most likely causes.
   b. Are any contact animals in the immediate home environment affected?
   c. Has the patient recently been to any area frequented by other animals (e.g., parks, pet shows)?
   d. Is the vaccination history current?
   e. Has the patient had access to drinking pond or stream water? Strongly consider *Giardia* in endemic areas.
   f. Could the patient have ingested garbage, spoiled food, or any toxins? Concomitant systemic signs are often present (e.g., vomiting, lethargy).
   g. Can administration of any drugs, especially antibiotics, be temporally related to the onset of diarrhea?
   h. Has there been a sudden diet change, especially to a high-fat, meat-based canned food?
   i. Can any stress factors be associated with the onset of diarrhea (e.g., boarding, conflictual problems in the home environment, any situation that causes apprehension)?
   j. Is the diarrhea associated with other symptoms (fever, vomiting, lethargy, weakness)? Diagnostic tests and supportive care are often indicated.

2. **Is the diarrhea of chronic duration (longer than 2 to 3 weeks)?** If so:
   a. For how long a period of time?
   b. Intermittent? Persistent?
   c. Has there been a change in appetite (ravenous, decreased, intermittent changes, pica)?
   d. Has there been any weight loss? Chronic wasting disease with a decreased appetite suggests possibility of benign moderate to severe infiltrative disease or neoplasia.
   e. Is there any history of flatulence or borborygmus?
   f. What is the patient's normal environment like (indoors versus outdoors, contact with parasite-infected environment, working dog or pet, identifiable stressful events in patient's environment)? Has the patient lived in or traveled to any areas where histoplasmosis is known to be a problem? Parasitism can be a factor in any patient with diarrhea, acute or chronic.
   g. Has the patient been eating a poor-quality diet?
   h. What is the patient's breed and character? German shepherds have a high incidence of inflammatory small intestinal disease, intestinal bacterial overgrowth, and pancreatic disease. Shar-peis have a high incidence of inflammatory small intestinal disease and intestinal bacterial overgrowth. Hyperexcitable or nervous dogs may be prone to irritable bowel syndrome.
   i. Is the patient a cat 5 or more years of age? Hyperthyroidism must be considered.

3. **What are the characteristics of the stools?**
   a. Size and volume?
   b. Consistency? Watery? Soft formed? Are any of the stools or portions of stools that are passed during a given day normal?
   c. Is there any undigested food present?
   d. Frequency?
   e. Is any blood or mucus present?
   f. Is there any incidence of tenesmus? Tenesmus suggests distal colonic, rectal, or anal disease.
   g. Timing? Is there a need to defecate frequently during the night? Urgency?
   h. If the patient is a cat, does it discharge abnormal stools next to or at a distance from the litter box? This often suggests a large intestinal problem such as colitis.

large bowel disorders. When asking owners questions about stool characteristics, it is often necessary for clinicians to describe what they mean *in simple terms*. For example, owners sometimes misinterpret questions about presence of mucus in the stool. If there is uncertainty, it is useful for the clinician to use such descriptive terms as "clear gel," "appearance of a clear coating around the stool," or even "appearance of 'gloppiness' to the stool." Owners who initially denied presence of mucus may change their answer to a more accurate one once they have a better understanding of what mucus in fecal material may look like. Indeed, sometimes mucus is difficult to identify, especially in liquid stools in which there is thorough admixture of mucus with water or when loose stool is mixed in with cat litter. Occasionally patients with frequent urgency to defecate will expel only clear mucus. This might be described by the owner as a "thick, ropy, clear liquid." I have on occasion observed owners entering the examination room with a thick strand of clear mucus on their arm, having been deposited there by their cat or small dog as they

TABLE 1-4	Differentiation of Small Intestinal From Large Intestinal Diarrhea	
Parameter	**Small Intestine**	**Large Intestine**
Feces		
Mucus	Rarely present	Frequently present
Hematochezia	Absent, except in hemorrhagic gastroenteritis syndrome	May be present. Often appears as streaks of bright-red blood on surface of stool or admixed with loose stool.
Volume	Increased	Normal to decreased
Quality of stool	Varies from nearly formed to quite watery. Often appears soft formed ("cowpile"). Undigested food or fat droplets or globules may be present. Malodorous.	Loose to nearly formed. Mucus may be absent or be present in small amounts, or constitute nearly the entire volume of material expelled. No undigested food.
Shape	Variable—depends on amount of water present in feces	May be normal or reduced in diameter (narrowed)
Steatorrhea	Present with maldigestive or malabsorptive disorders	Absent
Melena	May be present—appears as black, tarry stool	Absent
Color	Considerable variation—tan to dark brown, black (not always indicative of melena), grayish brown. May be altered by certain medications.	Variable—usually brown, may be nearly clear (increased mucus) or laced with bright-red blood
Defecation		
Frequency	Usually increased to 2-4 times a day but may remain normal in some patients	Almost always increased. May be as frequent as 3-10 times per day (average 3-5). The combination of increased frequency of defecation and passage of decreased amounts of stool strongly suggests large intestinal involvement.
Dyschezia	Absent	Frequent in dogs, less common in cats
Tenesmus	Absent	Frequent in dogs, less common in cats
Urgency	May be present in cases of acute severe enteritis, with rapid transit of large volumes of fluid through the gastrointestinal tract	Frequent. Common reason for owner being awakened during the night to allow a dog outdoors to defecate. Often causes restless or anxious behavior in well-trained house dogs as they await an opportunity to get outdoors.
Associated Signs		
Weight loss	Usually occurs as disease becomes more chronic. Occurs with both malabsorptive and maldigestive disease processes.	Unusual. May occur in conjunction with severe colitis, diffuse neoplasia, or histoplasmosis. If both small and large bowel signs are present, any weight loss that has occurred is more likely due to the small intestinal disease component
Vomiting	*Common* in patients with inflammatory bowel disorders and acute infectious disorders	May occur in 30%-35% of patients with acute colitis. Sometimes occurs *before* onset of abnormal stools.
Appetite	Usually normal or decreased. May be cyclic, often decreasing in conjunction with flare-ups of symptoms. May be ravenous in some	Usually remains normal. May be decreased if disease is severe (neoplasia, histoplasmosis).

TABLE 1-4	Differentiation of Small Intestinal From Large Intestinal Diarrhea—*cont'd*	
Parameter	**Small Intestine**	**Large Intestine**
Appetite—*cont'd*	dogs with inflammatory bowel disease (especially shar-peis). Appetite may be increased in cats with inflammatory bowel disease or lymphoma (transiently in the latter).	
Halitosis	May be associated with maldigestive or malabsorptive diseases	Absent
Borborygmus	May be present	Absent
Flatulence	May be present	Absent
Fecal incontinence	Rare—would only be associated with severe enteritis and rapid transit of large volumes of watery diarrhea	May be present
"Scooting" or chewing at perianal area	Absent	Occasionally present—may be quite pronounced in some patients with proctitis

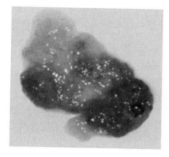

FIGURE 1-13 Stool passed by a dog exhibiting a sense of urgency. Diarrhea had begun several days earlier. A majority of the stool is mucus, a characteristic that is consistent with a large bowel disorder.

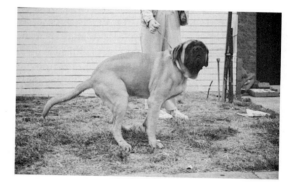

FIGURE 1-14 Two-year-old mastiff with signs consistent with chronic large bowel diarrhea. One of the major clinical signs was dyschezia (straining to defecate), which had been occurring over the last year. Typically the dog would crouch for several minutes, as is shown here, while passing only a small amount of stool. The dog would then walk around for a few minutes and then crouch to try to pass stool again. Only small amounts of stool were passed at a time. These signs were consistent with a chronic large intestinal disorder. Colon biopsies were obtained at colonoscopy and revealed chronic moderate to severe lymphocytic-plasmacytic colitis. A stool sample was also positive for *Clostridium perfringens* enterotoxin. Treatment included both sulfasalazine for chronic colitis and tylosin for *C. perfringens* enterotoxicosis. Dietary therapy included fiber supplementation.

held it in their arms in the waiting room. The initial line of questioning is readily apparent when this occurs!

Two of the most useful questions to ask relative to presence of a large bowel disorder are whether there is any fresh blood (bright-red blood) in the stool or any evidence of straining to defecate (Figure 1-14). Once again, communicating a clear description of our interpretation of these findings, without leading the owner into an answer, is very important. *The owner must be made comfortable enough to acknowledge when he or she is not certain of the answer.* If the history is unclear, the patient can be hospitalized for further evaluation or the owner can, newly armed with specific ideas about what to look

for, observe more closely in the home environment.

When asked if there has been blood in the stool, the owner may picture large pools of blood, when in fact blood in the stools of patients with a large bowel disorder often appears as small droplets or streaks that could easily be missed by a nondiscerning observer. This is compounded by the fact that blood may be present only intermittently. A differentiation must also be made regarding stool color when blood is present (hematochezia versus melena). The origin of bright-red blood (**hematochezia**) is generally anal, rectal, or descending colon. The cause of hematochezia can usually be more clearly determined by asking if the stools are consistently formed, with blood present on the surface of the stool, or loose, with blood on the surface or admixed in the stool. Dogs that pass formed stools with blood on the surface usually have rectal polyps (passage of stool over a polyp often causes it to bleed) (Figure 1-15), whereas those that pass soft stools with blood most often have some type of inflammatory or irritative disorder. Passage of formed stools with fresh blood in cats is most often related to the presence of abrasive material (e.g., hair, particulate matter from ingestion of prey) passing along the colonic mucosa (Figure 1-16). Rectal polyps are extremely uncommon in cats. Occasionally cats with colitis will pass consistently formed stool with blood on the surface (this is unusual in dogs).

The various causes of hematochezia are summarized in Box 1-11. **Melena** describes dark, tarry stools resulting from digested blood. The origin may be from the pharynx, lungs (i.e., coughed up and swallowed), esophagus, stomach, or upper

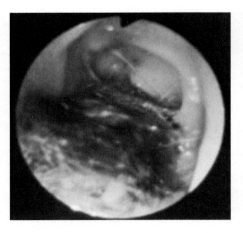

FIGURE 1-16 Abrasive clumps of hair in the colon of a cat with intermittent hematochezia and mild lymphocytic-plasmacytic colitis. Commonly the cat's stools were formed but had blood on the surface and contained hair. The hematochezia was thought to be primarily a result of the abrasive effect of hair on the colonic mucosa. The hair clumps observed in this photograph remained after two warm-water enemas were administered in preparation for colonoscopy. (From Leib MS: Colonoscopy. In Tams TR, ed: *Small animal endoscopy,* St. Louis, 1990, Mosby.)

small intestine. Tarry stools result from bacterial breakdown of hemoglobin. *There must be a sufficiently large amount of blood present before stools will appear tarry.* In one retrospective study that evaluated 43 dogs with gastric and/or duodenal ulceration, it was found that only 40% of the dogs had melena. It must also be noted that not all patients with dark stool have melena.

Dyschezia is defined as difficult and/or painful defecation. **Tenesmus** refers to persistent or prolonged straining that is usually ineffectual. It generally indicates a sense of urgency. Both dyschezia and tenesmus can be associated with alimentary, as well as genitourinary, disorders. The most common alimentary tract causes are colitis, proctitis (inflammation of rectal mucosa), and constipation. *Because owners frequently interpret straining to indicate constipation, it is essential that the clinician differentiate constipation from the straining that is often associated with large bowel inflammation and diarrhea at the outset.* Experienced clinicians recognize that many telephone calls involving a request for advice on how to treat a constipated pet at home actually involve an inaccurate assumption by the owner. Frequently tenesmus is caused by colitis and/or proctitis in these patients. The differentia-

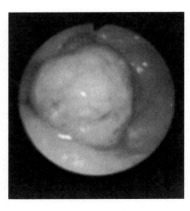

FIGURE 1-15 Close-up endoscopic view of a large rectal polyp with a friable surface in a 10-year-old neutered male Great Dane. The primary clinical sign was passage of consistently formed stools that occasionally had streaks of fresh blood on the surface. The polyp was exteriorized through the anus and excised.

BOX 1-11	Causes of Hematochezia

ANAL CANAL
Fissures
Anal sacculitis
Trauma
Neoplasia

RECTUM AND COLON
Proctitis
Colitis
  Idiopathic
  Infectious
    Campylobacter
    Clostridium perfringens
    Parvovirus
  Parasitism
    Whipworms
    Coccidia
    Hookworms
Mucosal trauma
  Passage of foreign material (common cause of
    hematochezia associated with formed stools
    in cats—especially hair)
  Automobile trauma
  Iatrogenic (e.g., thermometer or enema tube
    damage)
Prolapsed rectum
Neoplasia
  Rectal polyp (common cause of hematochezia
    associated with formed stools in dogs)
  Rectal adenocarcinoma
  Lymphoma

ILEOCECOCOLIC AREA
Ileocolic intussusception
Cecocolic intussusception

described is whether the stools and act of defecation (if observed) are normal or abnormal. Frequently information to support existence of a large bowel diarrhea disorder will be elucidated. If the stools are consistently normal, a behavior disorder should be suspected (e.g., cognitive dysfunction syndrome in older dogs and cats). Diagnostic work-up and/or initial empirical treatment can then be accurately directed.

Small bowel diarrhea is often characterized by an increased frequency of defecation with evacuation of larger than normal amounts of soft-to-watery stool. Color variations range from light tan to darker brown to orange to black (melena). Dyschezia and tenesmus are not characteristics of a small bowel disorder and are apparent only if a large bowel disorder is present as well (this is an important historical point, indicating probable diffuse intestinal involvement). Urgency may be present in *acute* small bowel disorders or in those associated with cramping. Generally, rapid evacuation of a large volume of watery diarrhea ensues (as opposed to large bowel problems in which only a small volume is passed). Steatorrhea may cause the feces to have an oily appearance and/or a grayish coloration. Presence of undigested food indicates maldigestion, which is generally due to either EPI or rapid bowel transit time. Weight loss that occurs in conjunction with chronic diarrhea is most often due to a significant disorder of malabsorption or maldigestion and may be associated with a guarded prognosis. Diagnostic testing sufficient to determine a definitive diagnosis should be expedited.

Associated Clinical Signs

Clinical signs that occur in conjunction with diarrhea often provide important clues regarding area of involvement and the potential seriousness of the condition. Important ancillary clinical signs that the clinician should ask about when reviewing the history include vomiting, weight loss, appetite change, flatulence, and borborygmus. Flatulence and borborygmus most often indicate small intestinal dysfunction. These symptoms are discussed in detail later in this chapter. Whereas vomiting commonly occurs in patients with small intestinal disease, especially inflammatory and parasitic disorders, it is also sometimes observed in patients with large intestinal problems. It is estimated that up to 35% of dogs with acute colitis vomit in addition to exhibiting typical signs of large bowel diarrhea. A majority of these patients that undergo

tion is readily made through a review of the history and physical examination.

Other important clues that indicate the onset of a large bowel diarrhea disorder include increased frequency of defecation with evacuation of only small amounts of stool (and in some patients eventually only mucus), defecating in abnormal places (cats), well-trained house dogs acting out of character by defecating in the house (usually due to a sense of urgency to defecate) while the owner is away or unavailable to allow them outside, and dogs waking their owner frequently during the night to go outside (sense of urgency) when normally they sleep through the night. Sometimes cats with colitis will defecate next to but not in the litterbox. The first question to ask if any of these abnormal patterns is gastroscopy and colonoscopy have normal findings on stomach biopsy. In fact, in some of these patients, vomiting actually precedes the onset of diarrhea by several hours to 1 to 2 days. Vomiting and inappetence often precede the onset of diarrhea in dogs with parvovirus enteritis. These facts highlight the importance of looking for physical evidence of intestinal disorders in patients presented for acute vomiting. This is accomplished through a physical examination, which must include a rectal examination to evaluate for increased mucosal sensitivity (suggestive of proctitis/colitis) and stool characteristics. Dogs with severe enteritis that have not yet passed any stool may release a large amount of watery, bloody diarrhea as soon as a rectal examination is performed.

The presence of weight loss and inappetence in conjunction with chronic diarrhea suggests a significant small intestinal disorder (e.g., inflammatory bowel disease, lymphangiectasia, histoplasmosis, neoplasia), and their presence should hasten the clinician's efforts toward making a definitive diagnosis. The combination of chronic diarrhea, weight loss, and *increased* appetite in cats suggests hyperthyroidism, inflammatory bowel disease, EPI, (rare in cats), and occasionally lymphosarcoma (some cats with GI lymphoma actually have an increased rather than decreased appetite). This combination of signs in dogs is most consistent with EPI. Characteristics of diarrhea in patients with EPI include voluminous "cowpile"-consistency stools that are often rancid in nature. Coprophagy is an ancillary sign that frequently occurs in dogs with EPI. Weight loss and inappetence rarely occur in dogs and cats with intestinal disorders limited to the large bowel.

Young to middle-age dogs that have chronic unrelenting diarrhea with minimal to no weight loss and a consistently normal appetite most often have a more significant problem in the large intestine than in the small bowel. I have found that the large bowel signs in these patients are often mild to subtle (e.g., mild dyschezia with transient flare-ups, soft stools that only occasionally contain blood, intermittent passage of mucus). The prevailing sign is that the stools are never consistently normal. If small bowel disease is present as well it is generally mild, so inappetence and weight loss would not be expected. The most common combination of findings is mild to moderate colitis, mild inflammatory bowel disease of the small intestine, and intestinal bacterial overgrowth. Each of these problems needs to be treated appropriately before adequate

resolution of signs can be expected. Significant weight loss and/or inappetence occur in association with primary large bowel disorders only when they are severe (e.g., severe colitis, including histiocytic ulcerative colitis of boxer dogs, diffuse neoplasia, or histoplasmosis).

Physical Examination

Physical examination of patients with diarrhea is similar to the thorough evaluation that is done on vomiting patients (see earlier discussion). Along with the history, physical findings help direct the clinician regarding what specific tests, if any, should be done and how quickly work-up should be expedited. Particular attention is paid to the patient's attitude, hydration, and posture. Depression and dehydration occurring in conjunction with acute diarrhea suggest an infectious or toxicity-related cause. Careful evaluation for any signs of sepsis (fever or hypothermia, tachycardia, tachypnea, and signs of shock, which may include changes in mucous membrane color to brick red or, alternatively, pale, cool extremities and injected membranes) is conducted initially and at any indication that a patient's condition may be destabilizing again. Abnormal posture (e.g., arched back) may indicate abdominal pain that can be associated with acute or chronic disorders. The neck should be carefully palpated in cats with diarrhea for evidence of an enlarged thyroid nodule (indicating hyperthyroidism). Body weight and overall physical stature should be noted. The act of defecation, especially if there is a history of dyschezia or tenesmus, should be observed by the clinician whenever possible.

Careful abdominal palpation is done to examine for thickened bowel (inflammatory or neoplastic infiltration), intussusception, presence of a mass that could be causing partial intestinal obstruction with resultant diarrhea, and lymphadenopathy (benign or neoplastic). Hepatomegaly suggests the possibility of hepatic disease in a causative role, and patients with acute or chronic severe small bowel diarrhea may have markedly increased fluid in the small bowel. Sensitivity localized to the caudal dorsal abdomen can often be detected in patients with colitis. This area is often not palpated carefully enough by veterinary clinicians.

A rectal examination is always done in dogs to examine for increased mucosal sensitivity, presence of narrowing (e.g., infiltrative disease, stricture), foreign body, or mass effect, and to obtain a fresh stool sample for gross examination. The finger should be rotated 360 degrees in the rectal canal so that as much mucosal contact as possible is made. Rectal polyps, which are often soft, can easily be missed on cursory examination. The perineal area is also examined for evidence of perianal fistulas, perineal hernia, and anal gland disease, all of which can cause symptoms of large bowel disease.

Diagnostic Plan

Specific diagnostic studies performed in patients with diarrhea are generally determined by the following considerations: (1) duration (acute versus chronic [2 to 3 weeks or more]); (2) presence of associated clinical signs such as inappetence, weight loss, frequent vomiting, severe bloody diarrhea, listless behavior (expedite diagnostic efforts if any of these signs are present); (3) environmental history; (4) signalment; (5) localization of the diarrhea to either small or large bowel or both; (6) frequency of diarrhea (intermittent versus chronic and persistent); and (7) physical examination findings. This will help the clinician determine whether a conservative step-by-step approach is feasible (e.g., diagnostic dietary trials, empirical treatment for parasites if screening fecal examinations are negative for parasites, treatment for mild acute colitis) or a more aggressive diagnostic effort is indicated. When evaluating patients with chronic diarrhea, the list of diagnostic tests need not be extensive, just well directed (Figure 1-17).

Acute Diarrhea

Diet-induced problems, viral infections, and parasites are the major causes of acute diarrhea in dogs and cats. Because intestinal parasites may be a factor in any diarrheic state, **fecal examinations (direct and flotation)** should be routinely done in all patients. Multiple examinations may be required to identify *Giardia* and *Trichuris* infections. Examination of **fresh saline smears** may identify ova, larvae, or motile protozoan parasites. High magnification with moderate light intensity should be used. Adding a drop of iodine may enhance the visibility of *Giardia* trophozoites and will stop any motion of the organism. Unfortunately, saline smears are not very reliable for diagnosis of *Giardia* infections (only 40% of dogs infected with *Giardia* were diagnosed in one study when saline smears were done using fresh stool on 3 separate days). The most accurate practical test for *Giardia* is **zinc sulfate centrifugal flotation** for identification of

Giardia cysts. Examination of duodenal lavage fluid, obtained via endoscopy or at laparotomy, for trophozoites may also be done but is impractical as an early diagnostic test. A **fecal enzyme-linked immunosorbent assay (ELISA)** for *Giardia*-specific antigen has also become available (Figure 1-18). This is a sensitive test and can be easily performed in-house or at commercial laboratories. My preference when examining for parasites in patients with acute diarrhea is to run both a zinc sulfate assay and a test for *Giardia* antigen. This gives me a high level of confidence in my efforts to more accurately determine whether or not intestinal parasites are present. Empirical treatment for parasites using such drugs as fenbendazole (Panacur) or febantel (contained in Drontal Plus, Bayer, along with pyrantel pamoate and praziquantel) for whipworms and giardiasis may also suggest a diagnosis if their use is successful in resolving the diarrhea.

Although diet-induced enteropathies are common, they are sometimes difficult to diagnose definitively. Acute diarrhea may result from overeating, a sudden change in diet (especially to a canned meat-based food), ingestion of spoiled food, food intolerance, or food sensitivity. The diagnosis is most likely to be made based on **history, ruling out other causes,** and **response to treatment.** Strict dietary trials with hypoallergenic diets are indicated more for patients with more chronic signs (e.g., 2 weeks or longer in duration). **Dietary therapy** for patients with acute diarrhea includes dietary restriction for 24 to 48 hours (to place the intestinal tract in a state of physiologic rest) followed by gradual reintroduction of food using a bland, readily digestible but low-fat diet (e.g., chicken and rice or boiled hamburger and rice in a 1:4 ratio, or a commercial diet of similar formulation) provided in small, frequently fed amounts for several days. Finally, either the regular diet is resumed or a change is made to a new maintenance diet if the previous food is considered unsatisfactory or is thought to have played a causative role in development of the diarrhea.

Patients with such signs as depression, dehydration, and fever in conjunction with acute diarrhea, with or without blood, should be evaluated for systemic abnormalities. The minimum database always includes a **CBC,** looking for leukocytosis or leukopenia, presence or absence of left shift, and supportive evidence for dehydration (elevated packed cell volume [PCV] and total solids). A blood smear can be evaluated quickly and easily

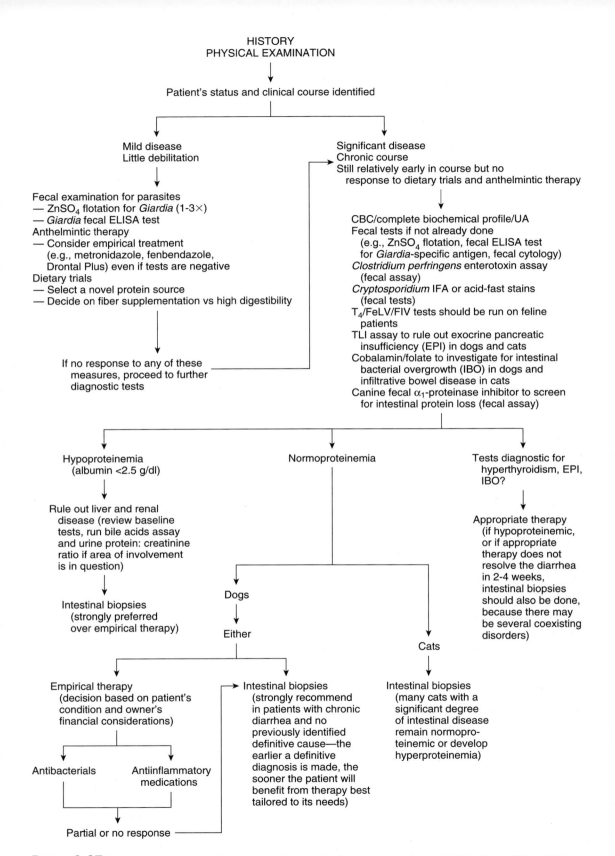

FIGURE 1-17 Sequential diagnosis of chronic small bowel diarrhea in dogs and cats. *ZnSO₄,* Zinc sulfate; *CBC,* complete blood count; *UA,* urinalysis; *ELISA,* enzyme-linked immunosorbent assay; *T₄,* thyroxine; *FeLV,* feline leukemia virus; *FIV,* feline immunodeficiency virus; *TLI,* trypsin–like immunoreactivity.

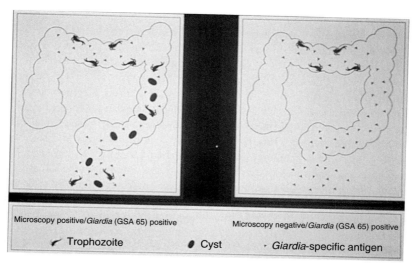

FIGURE 1-18 This schematic illustrates how the *Giardia* antigen test works (ProspecT *Giardia* Rapid Assay, Remel). On the left side there is a depiction of an intestine that contains *Giardia* trophozoites, *Giardia* cysts (the oval objects), and *Giardia* antigen (the small triangles). All three are being passed in the stool, and a direct saline smear for trophozoites, a zinc sulfate test for *Giardia* cysts, and a *Giardia* antigen test could all be positive. The right schematic shows a patient that has *Giardia* trophozoites in the intestine, but there are no trophozoites or cysts being passed in the feces. The only test that will be positive in this situation is an antigen test. Humans and animals that are infected with *Giardia* can shed cysts intermittently. Therefore, if an antigen test is not done, the diagnosis will be missed if there are no cysts present in the stool sample. I prefer to run this test in addition to running a zinc sulfate test to help make an accurate diagnosis for *Giardia*. This test can also be used after a course of treatment to check to see if a *Giardia* infection has been successfully eradicated (the test is run 14 days after the conclusion of therapy).

for an estimated white blood cell count. In patients with hemorrhagic gastroenteritis, there may be a dramatic increase in PCV to levels as high as 70% to 75%. This degree of increase in PCV contrasts with that in parvovirus infection and is the key to diagnosis of hemorrhagic gastroenteritis. If CBC results will not be readily available, a blood smear should be examined for estimation of the white blood cell count. **Serial blood counts** may be necessary because leukocytosis or leukopenia may be transient. A CBC may also suggest a possible diagnosis of hypoadrenocorticism (lymphocytosis, eosinophilia, mild anemia). **Electrolytes** (including sodium and potassium), **serial blood glucose** assessments for evidence of sepsis, and urinalysis both for baseline evaluation of renal function and for serial urine specific gravity levels as an aid in monitoring hydration in patients with normal renal function should also be run.

Hemagglutination, hemagglutination inhibition, or ELISA tests are used to test for **fecal shedding of viral antigen.** In-office ELISA tests have proven useful in detecting fecal shedding of parvovirus in acute cases and are probably more sensitive and specific than is hemagglutination.

Fecal shedding of viral particles often decreases rapidly, however, so a negative result does not rule out infection. **Fecal cultures** to examine for *Salmonella* spp., *Campylobacter jejuni, Yersinia enterocolitica,* and *Shigella* are indicated in some situations (e.g., kennel outbreaks, patients recently obtained from pet stores or shelters, households where more than one animal has diarrhea). It is extremely important that proper technique be used when obtaining feces for stool culture (see Chapter 6).

Chronic Diarrhea

Diarrhea that has not responded to conventional therapy within 2 or 3 weeks can be considered chronic. It is then appropriate to recommend that the problem be more thoroughly evaluated by using specific diagnostic tests. Considerable expense may be involved in some cases, so it is always best to start by reviewing the history once again (including differentiation between small and large intestinal involvement or determining that both areas are likely involved) to be as accurate as possible in selecting tests that are likely to provide useful information. Suggested diagnostic strategies for small intestinal and large intestinal diarrhea are presented separately here. An algorithm for sequential diagnosis of chronic small bowel diarrhea is presented in Figure 1-17.

Small Intestinal Diarrhea

Chronic small intestinal diarrhea can be broadly categorized into three groups: **maldigestive disease, malabsorptive disease,** and **functional disorders.** A majority of canine and feline patients with chronic small intestinal diarrhea seen in clinical practice have malabsorptive type of problems. There are many causes of intestinal malabsorption. Maldigestive disease is principally caused by EPI.

Maldigestive Disease

EPI is uncommon in dogs and cats. In the past EPI was greatly overdiagnosed and many patients were needlessly and ineffectually placed on pancreatic enzyme replacement therapy. Much of the confusion was caused by the lack of a reliable and definitive test for EPI. Tests commonly used in the past, including the x-ray film digestion test for fecal trypsin activity and the fat (lipomul) absorption test, proved to be insensitive and extremely unreliable. Tests for steatorrhea (staining feces for fat with Sudan stain), amylorrhea (staining for starch with Lugol's solution), and creatorrhea (staining for protein with standard stains) are reasonable and inexpensive in-house screening tests that can be run, but a significant drawback is that there can be false-negative and false-positive results. The **bentiromide (BT-PABA) test** is sensitive and reliable but cumbersome to perform.

Without question the most sensitive and specific test for EPI is the **serum trypsin-like immunoreactivity (TLI) assay.** This test simply involves obtaining a serum sample after fasting the patient for 12 to 18 hours (see Chapter 10). Serum TLI has been validated for use in both dogs and cats. Previously the fecal proteolytic activity (FPA) assay was the test of choice in cats. Although EPI is an uncommon disease, it is recommended that a TLI test be run in patients with chronic diarrhea so that EPI can be definitively ruled out early in the course of diagnostic evaluation. Failure to run this simple and inexpensive test may result in needless intestinal biopsies for diagnosis of a suspected malabsorption disorder.

Malabsorptive Disease

Malabsorptive intestinal disease can be divided into **protein-losing** and **non–protein-losing** enteropathies. Use of this classification scheme helps the clinician determine to some extent the current degree of seriousness of the condition and thus aids in the decision regarding whether a detailed work-up, including intestinal biopsies, should be expedited versus the feasibility of pursuing conservative therapeutic trials first (e.g., time-consuming strict dietary trials). In general, dogs with GI signs and a total protein of less than 5.5 g/dl should undergo intestinal biopsy. Dogs with mild hypoproteinemia (5.5 to 5.9 g/dl) should be watched carefully. Cats develop hypoproteinemia much less commonly than dogs. Hypoproteinemia usually indicates a significant degree of disease in cats, and intestinal biopsies should definitely be done if the intestine is considered to be the likely source of the problem.

Baseline tests, including **CBC** to identify leukocytosis (which suggests inflammatory disease), eosinophilia (eosinophilic enteritis, chronic previously undiagnosed endoparasitism), absolute lymphopenia (often observed in lymphangiectasia), and anemia (blood loss, anemia of chronic disease, nutrient malabsorption); **biochemical profile** (e.g., hypoalbuminemia, hypoproteinemia, abnormal liver enzymes, exclusion of metabolic disorders); and **urinalysis** to evaluate renal function and check for proteinuria, should be run in all patients with chronic diarrhea. Even if a CBC and biochemical profile were run previously, during the early days of onset of the diarrhea, it is often useful to repeat these tests at a later time because tests that were previously normal may then be found to be abnormal (see example in Table 1-5).

Hypoproteinemia most often results from disorders of the small intestine (protein loss involves albumin or both albumin and globulin), liver (primarily hypoalbuminemia due to decreased production), and protein-losing glomerulonephropathy (primarily hypoalbuminemia). Although the combination of chronic diarrhea and hypoproteinemia is usually consistent with small intestinal disease, there may still be concurrent disease in the liver or kidneys. It may therefore be necessary in some cases to evaluate these organs thoroughly (e.g., **bile acids assay** for liver function, **urine protein: creatinine ratio** to more accurately identify degree of proteinuria).

Fecal cytology may be useful in evaluating patients with chronic diarrhea. A thin smear of stool is stained (e.g., with new methylene blue, Diff-Quik, Wright's) and examined under high power or oil immersion for the presence of inflammatory cells. Increased numbers of neutrophils appear with inflammatory small or large

TABLE 1-5	Laboratory Data From a 4-Year-Old Spayed Female Shar-pei With a History of Chronic Small Bowel Diarrhea (8 Weeks), Ravenous Appetite, and Mild Weight Loss	
Test	**Initial (2 Weeks After Onset of Diarrhea)**	**6 Weeks**
PCV	41%	40%
WBC	17,600	22,400
Neutrophils/mm³	14,784	19,936
Lymphocytes/mm³	1,936	2,016
Eosinophils/mm³	528	
Monocytes/mm³	352	448
Total protein (n = 6–7.6 g/dl)	6.1	4.3
Albumin (n = 2.8–3.8 g/dl)	3.0	2.2
Globulin (n = 2.5–5.2 g/dl)	3.1	2.1
ALT (IU/L)	75	28
SAP (IU/L)	85	20
Glucose (mg/dl)	90	88
TLI (n = 5–35 µg/L)		13.5
Cobalamin (n = 225–660 ng/L)		126.2
Folate (n = 6.7–17.4 µg/L)		9

PCV, Packed cell volume; *WBC*, white blood cell count; *n*, normal values; *ALT*, alanine aminotransferase; *SAP*, serum alkaline phosphatase; *TLI*, trypsin-like immunoreactivity.

*Note the marked decrease in protein levels over the 6-week time period between sampling, indicating the presence of a significant degree of disease. Intestinal biopsies obtained via endoscopy revealed moderate lymphocytic-plasmacytic duodenitis and ileitis. A TLI test was normal. The low cobalamin level suggests the possibility of intestinal bacterial overgrowth.

intestinal disease or secondary to invasive bacterial enteritis.

The clinician or owner may reasonably elect to try **therapeutic trials** as the next step in noncompromised normoproteinemic patients. Therapeutic trials could include treating for adverse food reactions (dietary intolerance, food sensitivity); occult parasitic infections (especially giardiasis and whipworm infestation) if this has not already been done (also, successful treatment of giardiasis may require longer than one course of treatment); small intestinal bacterial overgrowth; and *Clostridium perfringens* enterotoxicosis (usually causes large bowel diarrhea). **Dietary trials** using hypoallergenic diets or high-quality commercial foods with a novel protein source are the primary diagnostic tool for identifying adverse food reactions. **Radioallergosorbent tests,** which determine serum levels of antigen-specific immunoglobulin E, have shown poor correlation with oral challenge, skin, and intragastric tests for food allergy. A response to treatment for any of the conditions listed above supports a diagnosis and precludes further work-up. Dietary trials are generally prescribed for 3 to 4 weeks in patients with GI disorders. Some patients will respond favorably within 3 to 14 days.

The next step in diagnosis of suspected malabsorptive disease, after baseline evaluation has been completed, is to look for evidence of intestinal bacterial overgrowth. The most accurate means of diagnosis is to obtain samples of duodenal fluid for both qualitative and quantitative analysis. This must be done using meticulous sterile technique either at laparotomy or with endoscopic instrumentation. Quantitative duodenal culture is expensive and cumbersome and is generally available only in academic institutions. The most practical method of testing for intestinal bacterial overgrowth is by measuring serum concentrations of **vitamin B$_{12}$** (cobalamin) and **folate** (see Chapter 7). These assays can be done in both dogs and cats. Because bacterial overgrowth is not uncommon in patients with pancreatic insufficiency, the cobalamin and folate assays should be run if this disorder is suspected. In fact, I generally submit enough serum to run all three special assays (TLI, cobalamin, and folate) rather than running just one or two of the tests. If intestinal bacterial overgrowth is diagnosed, it may be the primary problem or it may be present secondary to some other abnormality that has allowed it to persist. Treatment for bacterial overgrowth involves antibiotics, which may have to be administered for as little time as 1 to 2 weeks or as long as many weeks to months. If a decision is made to treat for bacterial overgrowth rather than do further tests, 2 to 3 weeks is an adequate trial period. If the problem is not resolved at this point, it is generally best to move ahead and look for other concurrent problems.

In addition to intestinal bacterial overgrowth and EPI, low serum cobalamin concentrations have been observed in dogs and cats with severe intestinal disease, in giant schnauzers with inappetence and failure to thrive and the laboratory findings of anemia, leukopenia, and methylmalonyl aciduria, and in many shar-peis with intestinal disease. It is important to evaluate serum cobalamin levels in cats with chronic GI disorders because supplemention with cobalamin by injection can be quite beneficial therapeutically (see Chapter 7).

At this stage the next best step is usually to perform intestinal biopsies. Other procedures that might be indicated in some patients include **contrast radiography** and **abdominal ultrasonography.** Contrast studies of the small intestine may help identify segmental lesions, tumors, or foreign bodies. Accurate interpretation of mucosal lesions on contrast studies is very difficult. The decision regarding whether or not a contrast study is done is usually based on physical examination findings (suggestion of a mass or well-localized pain) and survey radiographs. Ultrasonography is frequently recommended over contrast radiography in patients with suspected intestinal disease because intestinal wall thickness can be much more accurately assessed and lesions such as masses and enlarged lymph nodes can be readily detected and also aspirated under ultrasonographic guidance.

Ultrasound scanning of the intestinal tract provides an evaluation of peristalsis, wall thickness and diameter, lesion location, and appearance of luminal contents. Ultrasound is particularly useful in identification of obstruction and its various causes (e.g., masses, foreign objects, inflammatory disease, intussusception). Thickening of the bowel wall can occur in either inflammatory or neoplastic disease processes. Probably the greatest value in performing contrast radiography and/or abdominal ultrasonography in a patient with chronic diarrhea lies in helping make a decision on whether endoscopy will be adequate for obtaining diagnostic intestinal biopsy samples or whether exploratory surgery is indicated (e.g., if there are focal intestinal

lesions that may not be reached with endoscopic instrumentation, a mass is present, or there is lymphadenopathy or an intussusception).

The definitive diagnostic step in many patients with chronic, nonresponsive diarrhea is to perform **intestinal biopsies** either via endoscopy or surgery. *In a majority of cats and dogs with chronic diarrhea that exists with or without associated clinical signs (e.g., vomiting, appetite change, weight loss), a definitive diagnosis can be established based on endoscopic examination and biopsies.* The advantages and limitations of endoscopy are discussed in detail in Chapter 3. In most patients with chronic diarrhea, it is preferred that *both* upper and lower endoscopy be done so that sections from *both* the small and the large intestine can be evaluated histologically to determine the extent of a disease process as accurately as possible. In addition, in a majority of dogs weighing more than 8 to 10 lb, a pediatric endoscope can be advanced into the ileum via the colon by an experienced operator. Thus, complete colonoscopy followed by ileoscopy allows for more detailed evaluation of the small intestine (i.e., both upper and lower small intestine are examined and sampled for biopsy). This is especially important in cases in which a disease process may not yet diffusely involve the small intestine (e.g., occasionally, benign inflammatory disease or lymphoma will be found in the ileum but not in the duodenum). Ileum biopsy samples can often be obtained from cats by advancing the biopsy forceps through the ileocolic junction area with the endoscope tip situated in the ascending colon. Multiple forceps biopsy samples (6 to 10) are obtained from each area of intestine examined.

If an exploratory laparotomy is done to obtain intestinal biopsies, the entire bowel should be carefully evaluated. Biopsies of focally abnormal areas should be performed (full-thickness samples) along with one to two normal areas. *Many patients with chronic small bowel diarrhea have grossly normal intestine as observed at surgery. Biopsy samples must still be procured!* Two or three full-thickness samples are obtained (duodenum and ileum, or duodenum, jejunum, and ileum). A biopsy of any other tissue that appears abnormal (e.g., liver, pancreas, stomach, lymph nodes) should also be performed during exploratory laparotomy.

Biopsies are not often performed as early as they should be in patients with chronic GI disorders. Although the availability of endoscopy and its minimal risk in obtaining tissue samples is well recognized, some clinicians still wait too long to advise owners that a biopsy procedure is *definitely* needed. Progressive symptoms such as persistent or worsening diarrhea, weight loss, and decrease in appetite, as well as abnormal laboratory parameters such as hypoproteinemia, are reliable indicators that biopsies should be performed. It is important to remember, however, that some chronic intestinal disorders may manifest with only mild symptoms until the disease becomes serious. The patient's condition may then rapidly decline. Routine tests such as a hemogram and biochemical profile are generally very useful in screening for significant intestinal problems. For example, hypoproteinemia should be thoroughly investigated whether or not a patient is demonstrating significant symptoms. If screening tests indicate that the intestinal tract is most likely involved, a strong effort should be made to obtain biopsy samples. A representative case example is illustrated in Table 1-6. This patient should have undergone a small intestinal biopsy procedure much closer to the time the total protein and albumin levels were determined to be 4.1 g/dl and 1.6 g/dl, respectively, rather than 10 weeks later, when the protein level dropped to 2.8 g/dl and the patient was in a somewhat more compromised

TABLE 1-6	Laboratory Data From a 7–Year-Old Neutered Male Airedale With a 10-Week History of Small Bowel Diarrhea of Variable Consistency (Watery to Soft Formed) and Increased Volume and Frequency*	
Test	**Initial (3 Days After First Symptoms of Diarrhea)**	**10 Weeks**
PCV	53%	45%
WBC	9,600	11,500
Neutrophils	8,160	10,235
Lymphocytes	768	1,265
Monocytes	288	
Eosinophils	384	
Total protein (n = 6–7.6 g/dl)	4.1	2.8
Albumin (n = 2.8–3.8 g/dl)	1.6	1.4
Globulin (n = 2.5–5.2 g/dl)	2.5	1.4
ALT (IU/L)	22	159
SAP (IU/L)	19	50
Glucose (mg/dl)	84	96
Cholesterol (mg/dl)	60	48
Creatinine (mg/dl)	1.1	1.2
BUN (mg/dl)	15	18
Urinalysis	No proteinuria	
Bile acids (μmol/L)		
Resting (n = <5)	4	
Postprandial (n = <10)	9	
TLI (n = 5–35 μg/L)		9
Cobalamin (n = 225–660 μg/L)		175.3
Folate (n = 6.7–17.4 μg/L)		>24

PCV, Packed cell volume; *WBC*, white blood cell count; *n*, normal values; *ALT*, alanine aminotransferase; *SAP*, serum alkaline phosphatase; *BUN*, blood urea nitrogen; *TLI*, trypsin-like immunoreactivity.
*The appetite was fair to good and there was mild weight loss. Initial blood tests 3 days after the *onset* of diarrhea revealed marked hypoproteinemia (total protein 4.1 g/dl). *Based on the degree of hypoproteinemia and hypocholesterolemia, strong consideration should have been given to obtaining small intestinal biopsies at that time rather than waiting to see what type of response could be achieved using empirical treatment.* Not all patients with protein-losing enteropathy have chronic diarrhea and/or vomiting. The total protein level dropped to 2.8 g/dl by 10 weeks after the initial tests. Endoscopic biopsies were then obtained from the duodenum and ileum. The diagnosis was lymphangiectasia and mild lymphocytic-plasmacytic enteritis. Note that the absolute lymphocyte levels were subnormal on the initial test and low normal on the follow-up. Many lymphangiectasia patients have an absolute lymphopenia or persistently low normal lymphocyte numbers. The cobalamin and folate levels were consistent with intestinal bacterial overgrowth.

condition. Screening tests for liver and kidney disease done during the initial screening period were normal.

Treatment is then based on a review of the laboratory tests and biopsy results. It is emphasized that some patients with chronic diarrhea may have several disorders at the same time (e.g., inflammatory small bowel disease, intestinal bacterial overgrowth, colitis). A thorough work-up will lead to diagnosis of each disorder, with subsequent development of a comprehensive treatment plan. The likelihood of more rapid resolution of symptoms is much greater when each existing problem is properly treated.

Large Intestinal Diarrhea

As previously stated, large bowel disorders are common in dogs and cats. In mild cases, a diagnosis is often established based on **fecal parasite examination** (e.g., hookworms, whipworms, coccidia, and *Giardia*); **positive response to empirical treatment for difficult-to-diagnose parasite problems** (*Giardia* and whipworms); **response to dietary trials** (high-fiber diet, elimination diets); or **response to empirical treatment for acute colitis.**

Diagnostic tests for chronic large bowel diarrhea principally involve the following:

1. **Fecal cytology** to look for increased numbers of C. perfringens spores and inflammatory cells (specifically neutrophils), which suggest bacterial or primary inflammatory disease. Fecal or rectal scrape cytology is also useful in identifying Histoplasma organisms.
2. **Fecal culture** if history or fecal cytology suggests the possibility that bacterial infectious disease exists *(Campylobacter, Salmonella).*
3. **Enterotoxin assay** on stool to evaluate for *C. perfringens* enterotoxicosis.
4. **Colon biopsy** via colonoscopy (preferred technique) or surgery.

Complete colonoscopy with examination of the rectum, descending, transverse, and ascending colon, cecum, and ileocolic orifice area is preferred. Although examination and biopsy of the descending colon with a rigid colonoscope is commonly diagnostic in patients with large bowel diarrhea, such problems as occult trichuriasis, in which whipworms may be grossly evident in the cecum but not in the descending colon, ileocolic or cecocolic intussusception, typhlitis, or neoplasia that is localized in the transverse or ascending colon may be missed unless a complete examination of the colon is done with a flexible endoscope. Another advantage of using a flexible endoscope is that ileoscopy may be accomplished in many dogs after complete colonoscopy. Biopsy samples should *always* be obtained during colonoscopy, regardless of gross appearance. Indeed, it is not uncommon for patients with histologic evidence of colitis to have grossly normal colonic mucosa. If biopsy samples are not obtained, the diagnosis may well be missed.

Although it is a sound idea to evaluate patients with chronic large bowel diarrhea thoroughly by including a CBC, biochemical profile, urinalysis, and survey abdominal radiographs in the work-up, it is not always financially feasible for the owner to approve this detailed approach. If cost containment is essential, emphasis should be placed on a thorough history, physical examination with careful abdominal palpation and rectal examination, serial fecal examinations for parasites (preferably using zinc sulfate concentration with centrifugation because this test is more reliable for detecting *Giardia*), fecal or rectal scrape cytology, and colonoscopy with biopsy. A great majority of patients with disease *localized* to the large intestine will be diagnosed correctly if this approach is followed. However, if there is any evidence of systemic signs, such as PU/PD, inappetence, weight loss, or vomiting, in addition to large bowel diarrhea, baseline data, including CBC, biochemical profile, urinalysis, and survey abdominal radiographs, should be obtained. The scope of any further work-up is then expanded based on these results (e.g., panhypoproteinemia suggests that a small intestinal disorder is concurrently present, azotemia and low urine specific gravity indicate renal disease). It is once again emphasized that if there is any possibility that both small and large intestinal disease are present, biopsies of both regions should be performed. All too often, incomplete diagnosis and only partially effective treatment regimens are established if a less than thorough approach is made once the step of intestinal biopsies is reached.

BORBORYGMUS AND FLATULENCE

Borborygmus is a term used to describe a rumbling type of gut sound. Borborygmi are due to a moving gas-fluid interface in the gut. These sounds usually originate in the stomach. Borborygmi most commonly affect the dog. They are rarely heard emanating from cats. Borborygmus and flatulence commonly result from dietary indiscretion; however, these signs may be exaggerated in malassimilation or in any condition that promotes bacterial fermentation of malabsorbed carbohydrates and proteins. They may also occur as a matter of course in some normal patients or in association with functional bowel disorders (e.g., irritable bowel syndrome). Owners of patients that display these symptoms, especially flatulence, invariably highlight information about their occurrence as they discuss their pet's history. Indeed, sometimes offensive flatulence is the primary reason for seeking veterinary consultation.

Gas is normally present in the GI tract. The two most common sources of intestinal gas in humans and animals are swallowed air and bacterial fermentation. In adult humans the volume of intraluminal intestinal gas present at any one time varies from 140 to 260 ml. No such figures are available for animals. Most (99%) of the gas present in the GI tract is composed of five gases: nitrogen, oxygen, carbon dioxide, hydrogen, and methane. All of these gases are odorless. The unpleasant odor that may be detected in flatus is probably imparted by other gases that are present in trace amounts and by hydrogen sulfide and mercaptans metabolized from sulfur-containing substances present in certain foods.

The upper GI tract contains oxygen, nitrogen, and carbon dioxide, whereas the colon contains hydrogen, methane, and carbon dioxide. The source of oxygen and nitrogen is inspired air. Carbon dioxide is produced by the interaction of acid and alkaline substances in the stomach. Much of the carbon dioxide generated is absorbed through the bloodstream. Gas generated in the lower intestinal tract is the result of bacterial fermentation. Fermentation by the colon flora results in the production of variable amounts of hydrogen, methane, carbon dioxide, and oxygen.

The GI transit time for gas is considerably shorter than for liquids or solids. Gas introduced to the stomach of humans can be passed in as little time as 15 minutes. Overdistention of the GI tract with gas can potentially lead to significant discomfort. Patients will frequently continue to shift positions or assume an arched stance when experiencing gas-related discomfort.

Historical Features

The complaints described by owners of dogs with "gaseousness" problems include the pet's (1) ten-

dency to bloat, with or without belching, (2) assumption of an arched back stance, which might indicate cramping, and (3) excessive expulsion of flatus. Generally these symptoms occur only individually in a patient. It is rare for any single patient to exhibit all three of these main symptoms.

These symptoms should not be treated cavalierly or be dismissed too rapidly as insignificant by the clinician. Although in some patients the problem may simply be related to aerophagia, as may be caused by excitement, eating too rapidly, or eating foods that are high "gas producers," in other patients a more serious disorder may be present. For example, some dogs with gastric hypomotility disease or gastric outflow obstruction tend to experience bloating or a feeling of abdominal distention. Many of these dogs exhibit intermittent to frequent signs of nausea, and vomiting frequently occurs. Pronounced borborygmi may be present. There may be intermittent inappetence as well. Early in the course of the disorder there may be minimal symptoms, but as the disorder progresses, there may be significant patient discomfort. This is also true of the patient with inflammatory bowel disease or irritable bowel syndrome that tends to stand at times with an arched back because of abdominal discomfort related to gas pain. Diagnostic efforts should be undertaken to determine the cause of the symptoms in these patients. Treatment often provides significant relief. Although patients with excessive flatus do not often exhibit signs of discomfort, they may be affected by a malassimilation disorder that warrants diagnostic efforts.

Diagnosis

Diagnosis involves a review of historical factors, physical examination, and selected tests based on the primary symptoms and the degree of significance that the clinician affords them. The evaluation of a patient with flatulence includes determination of the daily diet and whether there exist opportunities for dietary indiscretion. Legumes, such as soybean meal, and vegetables such as beans, cabbage, lentils, and brussel sprouts are known as "gas producers." Legumes contain large quantities of oligosaccharides that are indigestible because the normal gut lacks the enzymes necessary to metabolize them. Ten percent to 20% of ingested carbohydrates may be malabsorbed, and protein substrates, when fermented, may contribute to gaseous constituents.

Spoiled foods are likely to yield increased quantities of odiferous gases. Milk products may cause gaseousness in patients with lactase deficiency. The owner should also be questioned about the patient's eating habits. Excessive aerophagia may occur when liquid or solid food is bolted or eaten rapidly. For some patients this may simply be habit, whereas in others it may result from a sense of competition with other animals in the immediate vicinity for rights to the food. Patients that are quite active (e.g., working dogs) may have a tendency to be aerophagic and produce excessive flatus as a result.

When the flatulence is fairly recent in occurrence and is accompanied by other signs, such as inappetence, weight loss, evidence of abdominal discomfort, and diarrhea, a detailed work-up is in order. Depending on the patient's environment and the dominant symptoms, this may include **fecal analysis** for evidence of *Giardi* (both zinc sulfate centrifugal flotation and a *Giardia* antigen test), **TLI assay** to investigate for EPI, **cobalamin and folate assays** for intestinal bacterial overgrowth, **survey** and possibly **contrast radiographs** of the GI tract (with particular attention paid to transit time, as well as to any morphologic abnormalities), and **endoscopy** to obtain gastric and intestinal biopsy samples (rule out infiltrative disorders).

Treatment often involves dietary manipulation (with change to foods that are highly digestible and low in fiber, with a moderate protein content and a novel protein source), feeding smaller meals more frequently if too rapid ingestion of food is considered a problem, and treatment of any primary disorder that might be identified by the tests listed above. Occasionally, gas-reducing drugs are used. Pharmacologic management attempts may include adsorbents, antifoaming agents, or various enzyme preparations. Response to these products is often variable. Charcoal is an adsorbent that has been commonly used in humans. Simethicone is an antifoaming agent that reduces surface tension and promotes coalescence of bubbles so that they can be more easily passed. Simethicone is not absorbed from the GI tract and can be used safely in dogs and cats, although its effectiveness is unknown.

An antiflatulence treat preparation was studied and shown to be beneficial for reduction of the offensive odor of flatulence in dogs. The treats included activated charcoal, *Yucca schidigera*, and zinc acetate. Treated dogs experienced a signifi-cant reduction in the percentage of highly odoriferous episodes. In vivo hydrogen sulfide levels were significantly reduced. Treatment for excessive flatus is discussed in more detail in Chapter 7.

BLOATING, FULLNESS, AND ABDOMINAL DISCOMFORT

Bloating, fullness, and abdominal discomfort are nonspecific symptoms that may be encountered in both organic and "functional" (e.g., irritable bowel syndrome, disorders characterized by deranged motility) digestive tract disorders. These syndromes do not seem to occur as commonly in animals as they do in humans. Although in human medicine they have been presumed over the years to be associated with a central problem of increased gaseousness, it is now known that most of these patients' symptoms do not originate in *excessive* intestinal gas. Rather, the responsible mechanisms appear to involve disordered intestinal motility and a heightened pain response to intestinal distention. It is now thought that gas, even in small volumes, may trigger symptoms even though the total quantity of gas in the intestinal tract is not greater than in asymptomatic subjects. Patients with these problems may be symptomatic more often if they tend to be aerophagic as well.

The symptom complex of bloating, fullness, and abdominal discomfort certainly is recognized to occur in dogs but can be difficult to detect unless the owner is an astute observer. Clinicians are cautioned to not overlook the possibility that patients with these vague symptoms have a significant disorder, not in terms of being life-threatening, because this is rarely the case, but rather in terms of causing significant discomfort.

Disorders that tend to cause these symptoms in dogs include gastric and/or intestinal motility derangement and inflammatory bowel disease. **Diagnostic tests** that should be considered include **survey abdominal radiographs** to examine for presence of excessive bowel gas (rarely positive), **radiographic studies** to evaluate intestinal motility (e.g., BIPS, nuclear scintigraphy), and both **upper and lower GI endoscopy** to obtain small and large bowel biopsy samples. Normal intestinal biopsy results support a diagnosis of dysmotility (irritable bowel syndrome), whereas abnormal biopsy results are generally consistent with some degree of inflammatory bowel disease.

Treatment is often based on biopsy results and clinical interpretation of the symptom complex exhibited by the patient. Dietary manipulation, including use of high-fiber diets for irritable bowel syndrome, and various types of pharmacologic management are usually employed. Inflammatory bowel disease is discussed in Chapter 7. Irritable bowel syndrome is discussed in Chapter 8.

FECAL INCONTINENCE

Fecal incontinence denotes uncontrolled release of rectal contents. Although it is not a common disorder in dogs and only rarely occurs in cats, the ramifications of this problem for a household pet and its owner are highly significant. Pets with a fecal incontinence problem that cannot be reasonably controlled are often euthanized because of the impracticality of maintaining the animal on a long-term basis in terms of the problems associated with fecal soiling.

There are many potential causes of fecal incontinence (Box 1-12). Most incontinence disorders can be classified as neurogenic or nonneurogenic. Causes include anatomic disruption of the anal sphincters or pudendal nerve trauma resulting from surgery (e.g., perineal hernia repair, perianal fistula repair, anal sac removal, tumor removal), obstetric trauma or other injuries (e.g., lacerations, bite wound trauma with subsequent ascending bacterial neuritis as may occur from a cat fight injury), and various non–surgery-related neuro-

logic problems. Neurologic problems may include peripheral neuropathies, cauda equina syndrome, and congenital defects of the caudal vertebral column and spinal cord (e.g., sacrocaudal agenesis of Manx cats). Incontinence may be related to aging in some patients. Also, any disease that causes rapid transit of large volumes of diarrhea (e.g., severe enteritis) may produce transient fecal incontinence in patients with healthy continence mechanisms.

The mechanisms of anal continence are complex, and a detailed description is beyond the scope of this discussion. In the dog and cat the internal and external anal sphincter muscles and the puborectalis muscle (the caudal portion of the levator ani muscle) play major roles in maintaining continence. The most important muscle in maintaining the sphincter component of the continence mechanism may be the puborectalis muscle. The external anal sphincter is innervated by the caudal rectal branch of the pudendal nerve, originating from the sacral spinal cord segments (S1 to S3). Bilateral transection of the pudendal nerve or sacral cord lesions will result in fecal incontinence. However, unilateral transection usually does not lead to major dysfunction because the remainder of the innervated external anal sphincter muscle can compensate for the denervation. Surgical procedures involving full-thickness circumferential resection at the anorectal area always carry the risk of ensuing fecal incontinence. The internal anal sphincter is innervated by branches of the pelvic

---

BOX 1-12	**Causes of Fecal Incontinence**

NEUROGENIC	**NONNEUROGENIC**
Iatrogenic (inadvertent damage to caudal rectal nerves related to surgical manipulation)	Urgency
Anal sacculectomy	Acute severe enteritis
Perianal fistulectomy	Bacterial proctocolitis
Perineal hernia repair	Inflammatory disorders (proctitis, colitis, anusitis)
Other invasive perirectal procedures	Irritable bowel syndrome
Peripheral neuropathies	Neoplasia
Cauda equina syndrome	Traumatic
Congenital defects of the caudal vertebral column and spinal cord (e.g., sacrocaudal agenesis of Manx cats)	Anal fistulation (either presurgical or associated with iatrogenic mass lesions resulting from surgical procedures)
Trauma (orthopedic)	Neoplastic infiltration of the sphincter apparatus, rectum, or anus
Fight wounds (especially cats with deep tailhead bites and subsequent ascending bacterial myelitis)	Fight wounds
"Idiopathic" (primary neurogenic)	Iatrogenic (surgical damage)
Aging	Miscellaneous
Chronic constipation	Behavior abnormality
	Perineal hernia (mechanism is most likely external anal sphincter incompetence)

nerve (afferent and efferent) and pudendal and hypogastric nerves (efferent).

The colon also plays an important role in helping to maintain fecal continence through its reservoir function. Reflex activity in the colon appears to allow the external anal sphincter to retain fecal material while the internal anal sphincter relaxes, thereby allowing the colon to dilate and accommodate increases in fecal mass. Simultaneously there is a brief (several minutes) decrease in propulsive contractions in the colon, which also helps facilitate the accommodation process. The colon continues to readapt with subsequent peristaltic delivery of fecal material until a time when defecation is appropriate. If the colon is presented with large volumes of watery fecal material in a short period of time, as may occur in patients with severe viral or bacterial enteritis, this reservoir function can become overwhelmed and transient incontinence (urge incontinence) may result. Urge incontinence can also be associated with moderate to severe proctitis or colitis, in which the patient experiences significant discomfort (perhaps a "burning" sensation) with a resultant sense of urgency to defecate and overriding of the continence mechanism.

The internal and external anal sphincter muscles and the puborectalis muscle are primarily responsible for maintaining a high-pressure zone in the terminal rectum that maintains continence at rest. Studies have shown that the internal anal sphincter contributes 50% to 80% of the resting tone in the high-pressure zone. The primary function of the external anal sphincter is to actively contract over short periods of time to resist the action of peristaltic waves.

Diagnosis

Important factors in diagnosis include obtaining a detailed history so that any potential causative factors (e.g., trauma, difficult whelping, history of significant constipation problems) can be elucidated, physical examination (including neurologic assessment), and completion of any indicated diagnostic tests.

The signalment is very important in evaluating a patient with fecal incontinence. Manx and other tailless cats and Old English sheepdogs, bulldogs, and Boston terriers may be affected with an agenesis of the sacrocaudal vertebrae and spinal cord. The neurologic deficit is present from birth but is often first noted at weaning. Clinical signs

include both urinary and fecal soiling and irritation around the perineal and abdominal skin. Occasionally there is complete paralysis of the pelvic limbs as well. Aging patients with gradual onset of incontinence are most likely to have some type of neurologic problem.

Once the existence of incontinence has been established, the clinical evaluation begins with an assessment of the frequency, severity, and circumstances surrounding the incontinent episodes. How acute are the symptoms? Are the episodes associated with urgency, or is there no prior warning? The owner should be asked whether or not the dog still assumes an appropriate posture for defecation, and, if so, does this take place at an appropriate time and place? Some dogs with mild incontinence still do this on a fairly routine basis but on occasion will inappropriately release stool when asleep, during periods of relaxation, or while on a walk. These episodes may occur in response to increased rectal pressure related to the presence of stool that overrides a now compromised continence mechanism.

Excitement may also cause spontaneous evacuation of stool. In some patients incontinence episodes become much more frequent (i.e., major incontinence versus partial), and this suggests a severe anorectal sensory disorder. Unconscious anal dribbling of small amounts of fluid and residue may become common, especially during periods of increased abdominal or rectal pressure (e.g., associated with coughing, excitement, or exercise).

The owner should also be asked if the patient can urinate normally. Because micturition relies on nerve pathways similar to those involved in fecal continence, abnormalities involving both functions suggest that the fecal incontinence is of neurologic origin.

If the fecal incontinence has been a very recent development, questions regarding trauma are asked. Lumbosacral and sacrocaudal fracture, subluxation, and luxation can cause fecal incontinence (distended bladder and atonic tail often result as well). In cats these injuries are commonly associated with getting their tails caught by something. Cats with bite wounds around the tailhead may develop abscessation and ascending bacterial neuritis and meningomyelitis of the caudal spinal cord. Any history of anorectal surgery is reviewed. Generally symptoms develop and are reported shortly after any surgery in which nerve damage occurs. Any incidence of significant straining episodes should also be discussed. Severe proctitis, for example, may cause so much irritation that urge incontinence occurs.

In my experience one of the most common presentations for the complaint of fecal incontinence is an aging dog with no obvious predisposing history of major trauma, anorectal disease, or neurologic disease. Careful studies using electromyography and other neurophysiologic techniques in human patients with "idiopathic" incontinence have identified striated muscle denervation damage in the majority. Detailed studies have not been done in animals, but it is suspected that a similar mechanism exists.

Physical Examination

The most important aspects of the physical examination in a patient with fecal incontinence include close perianal inspection and digital examination of the anorectum. The skin in the perianal and perineal regions may show evidence of irritation from fecal or urinary soiling. Perianal fistulas, which may be accompanied by mild leakage of residue from the rectum, are readily identified on visual inspection. Rectal examination may reveal evidence of proctitis (e.g., increased sensitivity on palpation, irregular rectal mucosa) or a perineal hernia. Fecal incontinence has been documented as a potential complication of perineal herniation, most likely occurring secondary to external anal sphincter incompetence. Anal tone is assessed during digital palpation, but it should be noted that this provides only a crude assessment (unless there is loss of tone altogether) of true anal sphincter function. The presence of fecal impaction and tumors can also be determined. Abdominal palpation is done to assess bladder tone (a large, distended, easily expressed bladder found in conjunction with fecal incontinence and a dilated anus supports diagnosis of a neurogenic disorder), colon content, and any sensitivity of the colon that might suggest colitis. Signs of hindlimb paresthesia and hyperesthesia suggest the possibility of cauda equina syndrome.

Neurologic examination includes evaluation of gait, pelvic limb postural reactions and proprioception, and spinal reflexes of the pelvic limbs, anus, tail, and bladder. The anal reflex is elicited by pinching or touching the anus and observing contracture of the anal sphincter. If the S1 to S3 spinal segments or nerve roots are damaged, the anus is dilated and unresponsive.

Diagnostic Testing

Baseline analysis of patients with fecal incontinence without a readily explainable cause includes **survey radiography** of the lumbar spine and lumbosacral and tailhead areas and **proctoscopy** with examination and biopsy of the rectum and colon. **Myelography** or **epidurography** can be done to help diagnose spinal cord and cauda equina disorders. **Electrodiagnostic evaluation** by **electromyography (EMG)** of the muscles of continence is very useful and may reveal denervation or myopathy. In patients with incontinence associated with an acute diarrheal illness, diagnostic evaluation usually requires no specific anorectal evaluation other than evaluation of the diarrhea itself.

Treatment

The treatment of fecal incontinence is directed toward the underlying cause if one can be identified. The prognosis for resolution or adequate control of incontinence also varies with the type and extent of involvement, but, in general, it is somewhat worse when neurogenic disorders (especially those resulting from surgical damage) are present.

General treatment principles include dietary manipulation, pharmacologic therapy to increase anal tone and decrease colonic transit rate (opiate derivatives), and proper supportive care for any injuries that may have been incurred.

The goal of dietary therapy is to minimize fecal volume. This is best accomplished through feeding a low-residue, highly digestible diet. Homemade diets consisting of cottage cheese and rice or tofu and rice often work well. Commercial diets such as Eukanuba Low-Residue (Iams), IVD Select Care Sensitive and Canine Vegetarian Formula diets, or Prescription Diet Canine i/d (Hill's) may also be effective. Two to three small meals rather than one large meal should be fed each day.

When fecal incontinence is associated with chronic diarrhea, urgency, or decreased anal tone as may be seen in aging patients, symptomatic improvement can often be effected with opiate derivatives (diphenoxylate [Lomotil], loperamide [Imodium]). Solid stools are much easier to retain than liquid stools, and thus antidiarrheal therapy alone may eliminate all symptoms in patients with loose stools. Several human studies have suggested that loperamide is superior to diphenoxylate in reducing soiling and improving continence of rectally infused saline. Pharmacologic actions include increased anal tone, increased fluid absorption in the colon, decreased secretions, and increased rhythmic segmentation in the bowel, thereby decreasing colonic transit rate. These drugs can be safely administered on a long-term basis if necessary. I have had good success in managing geriatric patients with age-related incontinence with low-residue diets used in conjunction with loperamide. Dosage recommendations for these drugs are presented in Chapter 8. It may also be useful to manage geriatric patients with incontinence problems with periodic enemas in an effort to decrease fecal volume in the rectum and colon, as well as to help decrease episodes of fecal soiling.

Inflammatory disorders (colitis, proctitis, anusitis) are treated with antiinflammatory medications used either singly or in combination. The most commonly used drugs include sulfasalazine (Azulfidine), metronidazole (Flagyl), and prednisone. Use of these drugs for large bowel disorders is discussed in detail in Chapter 8. Loperamide or diphenoxylate may be used in conjunction with any of these drugs as well. Dietary therapy in the form of a highly digestible low-residue diet, as discussed previously, is also used.

Surgical intervention is indicated for patients with incontinence related to perineal herniation or anal or rectal neoplasia and for some with diseases of the lumbosacral spine. The prognosis is guarded when profound urinary and anal sphincter disturbances exist. Attempts have been made to correct complete neurogenic fecal incontinence surgically with such techniques as fascia slings or silicone elastomer slings. However, results have not been encouraging, and these procedures are not commonly recommended.

CONSTIPATION

Constipation is defined as absent, infrequent, or difficult defecation. Obstipation is intractable constipation and results in severe fecal impaction throughout the rectum and colon (Figure 1-19). Both conditions should be differentiated from megacolon, which is a clinical disorder characterized by chronic dilation and hypomotility of the colon and rectum. Not all patients with constipation have megacolon. Constipation is a common problem in dogs and cats. This problem is discussed in detail in Chapter 8. The causes and treatment of constipation are listed in Tables 8-3 and 8-4, respectively.

The main consideration discussed here is the importance of a careful review of the history and

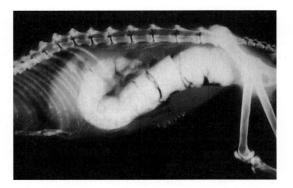

FIGURE 1-19 Severe obstipation in a 16-year-old cat with idiopathic megacolon.

physical examination by the clinician when an owner believes that his or her pet is constipated. Whenever possible, owners who telephone the clinician to describe their pet's symptoms of straining should be encouraged to bring their pets for an examination unless past pertinent history is well known by the clinician and the likelihood of what the problem is can be accurately assessed without an examination. It is extremely important that urethral obstruction in cats and dogs (a potentially life-threatening problem) be differentiated from straining related to constipation, proctitis, colitis, or other less worrisome causes. The caudal abdomen is palpated for evidence of an enlarged and difficult-to-express urinary bladder, distended colon with hardened stool, colonic sensitivity (often increased in patients with colitis), and any masses that might be present. A small, painful bladder suggests cystitis or cystic calculi. If the alimentary tract seems to be the cause of the problem, a rectal examination is mandatory to evaluate mucosal sensitivity and texture, to evaluate presence and consistency of fecal material in the rectal canal, and to look for evidence of obstruction (stricture, mass, prostatomegaly, foreign body, perineal hernia).

Once the initial physical assessment is completed, a more detailed line of questioning can begin based on the problem that has been identified (i.e., constipation versus some other cause of straining). Important areas to investigate for the problem of constipation include diet, environment (e.g., likelihood of ingestion of foreign body material, ready access to clean litter for cats), normal defecation habits, exercise patterns, drug therapy, and any history of sacrocaudal or pelvic trauma. Because some patients with constipation do not strain to defecate, it is important that owners become familiar with their pet's normal defecation patterns (frequency, amount, time of day). This is especially important regarding cats with megacolon. It is useful to teach owners of cats with a history of a constipation problem how to palpate the colon so that they can recognize a state of constipation early enough to seek treatment, well before development of obstipation.

Diagnostic testing during the initial detailed assessment of the patient should include a **CBC, biochemical profile, urinalysis,** and **thyroid studies.** These tests are done to investigate for systemic problems that can cause colonic inertia (peripheral neuropathies, hypercalcemia, hypokalemia, hypothyroidism). **Survey radiographs** of the abdomen, lumbosacral spine, and pelvis are made to confirm the presence and assess the degree of constipation and to look for evidence of such causes as prostatomegaly, enlarged sublumbar lymph node, presence of a mass, narrowed pelvic canal, and stricture (Figure 1-20). Colonoscopy is *not* commonly required in patients with constipation. The primary indication would be to evaluate an intraluminal mass or stricture site. **Ultrasonography** may be useful for localizing a site of obstruction.

Treatment

The treatment of constipation and obstipation is reviewed in detail in Chapter 8. Treatment often involves dietary manipulation (high-fiber diets) used alone or in combination with stool softeners. The promotility drug cisapride, used in conjunction with a stool softener such as lactulose, is often effective in managing colonic inertia problems. Manual deobstipation under general anesthesia is generally required in dogs and cats with severe constipation or obstipation. Balloon catheters for dilation of colonic strictures are available and are used under endoscopic guidance. Surgery is required for removal of masses, severe benign strictures and any malignant stricture, and some foreign body impaction cases. Colectomy may be indicated for the occasional cat with megacolon that does not respond to combination therapy using cisapride, stool softeners, and dietary management.

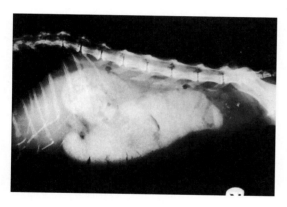

FIGURE 1-20 Severe obstipation in a 13-year-old spayed female DSH cat. Note that the fecal column ends abruptly ventral to L6. There are small radiopaque densities posterior to the fecal column that are presumably in the colon. Enemas and transabdominal manual manipulation performed under sedation failed to move the fecal mass any closer to the anus. Exploratory laparotomy revealed an annular constricting lesion in the colon approximately 4 cm proximal to the rectum. The histologic diagnosis was adenocarcinoma. Mesenteric lymphadenopathy and extensive nodular involvement in the mesentery were also found. The annular adenocarcinoma in the colon caused nearly complete obstruction of the descending colon. In cats with idiopathic constipation and obstipation, the fecal mass generally extends into the rectum (see Figure 1-19).

REFERENCES

Beaver BV: Feline ingestive behavior. In Beaver BV, ed: *Feline behavior: a guide for veterinarians*, Philadelphia, 1992, WB Saunders.

Berk JE: Gaseousness. In Berk JE, Haubrich WS, eds: *Gastrointestinal symptoms*, Philadelphia, 1991, BC Decker.

Burbridge HM, Guilford WG: Barium-impregnated polyethylene spheres (BIPS): clinical observations, *Vet Radiol Ultrasound* 37:79, 1996.

Burrows CF: Diarrhea in the dog: a clinical perspective. In *Viewpoints in veterinary medicine*, ed 2, Lehigh Valley, Pa, 1993, Alpo Petfoods.

Burrows CF: Vomiting and regurgitation in the dog: a clinical perspective. In: *Viewpoints in veterinary medicine*, ed 2, Lehigh Valley, Pa, 1993, Alpo Petfoods.

Dean PW, Bojrab MJ: Defecation and fecal continence. In Bojrab MJ, ed: *Disease mechanisms in small animal surgery*, Philadelphia, 1993, Lea & Febiger.

Friedman G: Diet and irritable bowel syndrome. In Friedman G, ed: The irritable bowel syndrome: realities and trends, *Gastroenterol Clin North Am* 20:313, 1991.

Giffard CJ et al.: Administration of charcoal, *Yucca schidigera*, and zinc acetate to reduce malodorous flatulence in dogs, *J Am Vet Med Assoc* 218(6):892, 2001.

Guilford WG: Approach to clinical problems in gastroenterology. In Guilford et al., eds: *Strombeck's small animal gastroenterology*, ed 3, Philadelphia, 1996, WB Saunders.

Giulford WG, Lawoko C: Validation of radiopaque markers for assessment of gastric emptying rates of food in dogs, *J Vet Intern Med* 10:170, 1996.

Hedlund CS: Surgery of the perineum, rectum, and anus. In Fossum TW, ed: *Small animal surgery*, St. Louis, 1997, Mosby.

Lorenz MD: Coprophagy and pica. In Lorenz MD, Cornelius LM, eds: *Small animal medical diagnosis*. Philadelphia, 1987, JB Lippincott.

Luescher UA, McKeown DB, Halip J: Stereotypic or obsessive-compulsive disorders in dogs and cats. In Voith V, Marder A, eds: Advances in companion animal behavior, *Vet Clin North Am Small Anim Pract* 21:401, 1991.

Niebauer GW: Rectoanal disease. In Bojrab MJ, ed: *Disease mechanisms in small animal surgery*, Philadelphia, 1993, Lea & Febiger.

Polsky R: Electric shock collars: are they worth the risks? *J Am Anim Hosp Assoc* 30:463, 1994.

Richter KP: Diseases of the rectum and anus. In Kirk RW, Bonagura JB, eds: *Current veterinary therapy XI*, Philadelphia, 1992, WB Saunders.

Tams TR: Endoscopic examination of the small intestine. In Tams TR, ed: *Small animal endoscopy*, ed 2, St. Louis, 1999, Mosby.

Tams TR: Gastroscopy. In Tams TR, ed: *Small animal endoscopy*, ed 2, St. Louis, 1999, Mosby.

Tams TR: Vomiting, regurgitation, and dysphagia. In Ettinger SJ, ed: *Textbook of veterinary internal medicine*, ed 4, Philadelphia, 1995, WB Saunders.

Willard M: Clinical manifestations of gastrointestinal disorders. In Nelson RW, Couto CG, eds: *Small animal internal medicine*, ed 2, St. Louis, 1998, Mosby.

2

RADIOLOGY AND ULTRASONOGRAPHY OF THE DIGESTIVE SYSTEM

Linda J. Konde
Pamela A. Green
Charles R. Pugh

RADIOLOGY OF THE DIGESTIVE SYSTEM

Pharynx
Radiographic Anatomy

The air-filled pharynx provides contrast for visualization of the soft palate, epiglottis, hyoid apparatus, and retropharyngeal area. Therefore any changes in shape, size, or opacity of these structures can be readily discerned. The pharynx is divided into four anatomic regions (Figure 2-1): nasopharynx—the area between the soft palate and the base of the skull; oropharynx—the area between the soft palate and the base of the tongue; pharyngeal isthmus—caudal to the soft palate and cranial to the larynx; and laryngopharynx—dorsal to the larynx and ventral to the second cervical

vertebra (position varies slightly in different species and breeds).

The craniocaudal limits of the retropharynx extend from the caudal border of the pharyngeal isthmus to the level of the third cervical vertebra. The dorsoventral limits are ventral to the cranial cervical vertebra and dorsal to the larynx. A general guideline for the normal dorsoventral dimension of the retropharynx is that it should be no greater than the length of the third cervical vertebra (see Figure 2-1).

Swallowing is a dynamic process that is best assessed fluoroscopically while administering radiopaque contrast medium. There are three phases in normal swallowing: oral—action of the tongue forms the bolus; pharyngeal—propulsion of the bolus from the base of the tongue to the

51

FIGURE 2-1 Normal pharynx: nasopharynx *(N)*, soft palate *(SP)*, oropharynx *(O)*, pharyngeal isthmus *(I)*, and laryngopharynx *(L)*. The width of the retropharyngeal area should be no greater than the length of the third cervical vertebra *(arrows)*.

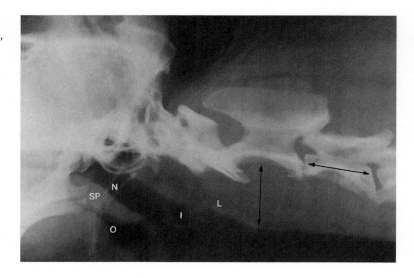

laryngopharynx; and cricopharyngeal—the cricopharyngeal sphincter opens as the isthmus contracts, to allow passage of the bolus into the esophagus. The sphincter rapidly closes after the bolus moves into the esophagus.

Pharyngeal Contrast Study

Indications include dysphagia, excess salivation, cough, pain, visible tissue swelling, and suspected foreign object.

The following materials are needed for a pharyngeal contrast study: thick barium paste,* 100% micropulverized barium sulfate or barium-food mixture†; water-soluble iodinated contrast (used if perforation is suspected)‡; and a dose syringe.

Administer the contrast medium orally in the buccal pouch. Obtain lateral and ventrodorsal (VD) views. Make the exposures while the patient is swallowing.

A normal-appearing contrast study of the pharynx shows smooth coating of the pharyngeal mucosa, absence of pooled contrast medium in the pharynx, and no reflux of contrast medium into the nasopharynx or trachea.

Radiographic Signs of Pharyngeal Disease

Mass Lesions. Common causes of mass lesions in the pharynx include abscess, neoplasia, cyst, foreign object, granuloma, and inflammation.

Abnormal location of soft tissue or mixed opacities (mineral, fat, fluid, and/or gas) may be visualized. These opacities may cause compression

of or may impinge on the normally gas-filled pharynx (Figure 2-2). Closely evaluate the VD view for asymmetric opacities in the pharyngeal and laryngeal areas (many lesions are unilateral). Contrast studies may show compression or extravasation.

Swallowing Disorders. *Oral* dysphagia is related to functional impairment of tongue movement. Radiographically, poor bolus formation is seen

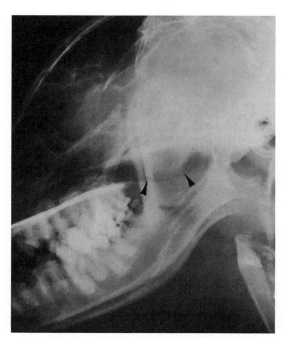

FIGURE 2-2 A soft tissue mass is seen impinging on the nasopharynx *(arrowheads)*. This mass was a tonsillar carcinoma.

*E Z EM, Inc. Westbury, NY 11590-5021.
†Novopaque. Picker International, Denver, CO 80239.
‡Oral Hypaque Sodium. Picker International, Denver, CO 80239.

from the base of the tongue caudally. Aspiration pneumonia is rare in oral dysphagia.

Pharyngeal dysphagia results in decreased pharyngeal peristalsis. Weakened contractility impairs movement of a bolus through the pharynx. On the survey film the pharynx may appear distended with gas. Contrast medium is retained in the oropharynx, pharyngeal isthmus, laryngopharynx, and piriform recesses. Contrast medium can be seen in the trachea. Aspiration pneumonia is often seen in pharyngeal dysphagia.

Cricopharyngeal dysphagia is due to insufficient relaxation of the cricopharyngeal sphincter. This is the most common form of oropharyngeal dysphagia (Figure 2-3). On the survey film, gas may be seen in the cervical esophagus. There is contrast reflux into the nasopharynx and trachea, and there is contrast retention in all other pharyngeal regions. Aspiration pneumonia may be seen in cricopharyngeal dysphagia.

Esophagus
Radiographic Anatomy

Because the esophagus has the same opacity as that of surrounding soft tissue structures in the neck and mediastinum, it is not usually seen on survey radiographs. However, normal transient dilation of an air-filled esophagus may be visualized. Common nonpathologic causes of air in the esophagus include aerophagia, anxiety, dyspnea, and anesthesia.

On the lateral view the cranial thoracic esophagus is dorsal to the trachea, and caudally it is located about halfway between the aorta and the vena cava. On the VD view the esophagus is to the left of the trachea, approximately on midline.

Esophagram

Indications include regurgitation of undigested food, persistent vomiting or gagging, suspected foreign object or mass, and assessment of position or compression of the esophagus.

The following materials are needed for an esophagram:

1. A dose syringe.
2. Barium paste, micropulverized barium suspension, or a food-barium mixture. Barium paste offers the best mucosal coating and should be used to evaluate suspected mucosal or mass lesions. Liquid barium suspension is used to evaluate an enlarged esophagus because a large volume may be required to fill the esophagus. A food-barium mixture is used to evaluate motility because peristalsis may be adequate for liquids and insufficient for solid food. Some strictures may allow fluid to pass normally but will restrict passage of solid food.
3. Aqueous organic iodide (used if perforation is suspected).

Administer the contrast medium orally in the buccal pouch. The dose is approximately 10 to 20 ml, to be administered before each exposure. Obtain lateral and VD oblique views (esophagus and spine are superimposed on the straight VD view).

In the dog a normal esophagram shows barium outlining longitudinal, parallel folds and a small diverticulum at the thoracic inlet (Figure 2-4); the diverticulum is more pronounced in brachycephalic breeds.

In the cat a normal esophagram shows a cranial esophageal mucosal pattern that is similar to that of the dog; caudally the mucosa has transverse mucosal folds, referred to as a herringbone pattern (Figure 2-5). Esophageal distention by a bolus of contrast medium in transit may be seen in all patients.

Radiographic Signs of Esophageal Disease

Megaesophagus (Figure 2-6). Megaesophagus appears as an enlarged esophagus containing fluid, ingesta, or air. There is ventral deviation of the trachea. A "tracheoesophageal stripe"—a thickened soft tissue opacity composed of dorsal tracheal wall and ventral esophageal wall—is more often seen on the left lateral view. The "stripe" is visible when there is air in the esophagus, as well as in the trachea. On the VD view the terminal esophagus

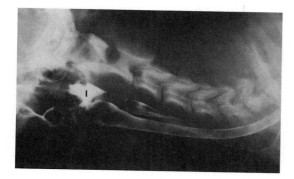

FIGURE 2-3 A dog with cricopharyngeal achalasia. There is accumulation of contrast medium in the pharyngeal isthmus *(I)*. Some contrast medium is present in the esophagus, but there is considerable accumulation in the trachea.

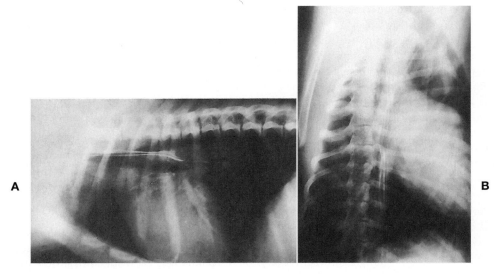

FIGURE 2-4 A, Lateral view of a normal canine esophagram. Note the normal longitudinal folds outlined by contrast medium. **B,** Ventrodorsal oblique view of a normal canine esophagram. The patient is at an oblique angle to avoid summation of the spine and esophagus.

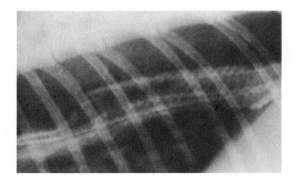

FIGURE 2-5 Close-up view of a normal barium study of the caudal feline esophagus. Note the normal transverse mucosal folds outlined by barium.

tapers into the diaphragm. Evidence of aspiration pneumonia may be present.

Vascular Ring Anomalies (Figure 2-7). Dilation of the esophagus cranial to the heart base is seen. The caudal esophagus is usually of normal size but may be enlarged. There is ventral depression of the trachea. The aorta may descend on the right side. The contrast study shows stricture at the heart base, and the aorta compresses the esophagus on the right side. Evidence of aspiration pneumonia may be present.

Esophageal Foreign Objects (Figure 2-8). A radiopaque foreign object is often visible. Esophageal dilation may be seen proximal to the obstruction. There may be mediastinitis, pleuritis,

and pneumomediastinum if the esophagus has been perforated. On the esophagram, barium surrounds the intraluminal filling defect. Esophageal stricture is a potential sequela.

Esophagitis. On the contrast study there is prolonged retention or pooling of barium in the affected area of the esophagus. The normal linear mucosal pattern is indistinct, blurred, or completely absent. Abnormal motility is present on fluoroscopy.

Esophageal Neoplasia (Figures 2-9 and 2-10). A soft tissue mass may be seen on survey radiographs in the area of the esophagus. The opacity may be homogeneous or may contain air or calcification. Dilation proximal to the mass may be present. Diverse changes seen on the contrast study, depending on the nature of the mass, include irregular or smooth mucosal pattern, wall rigidity, wall thickening, luminal lucent filling defect (protruding mass), and extravasation of contrast medium into the mass.

Stomach
Radiographic Anatomy
Complete evaluation of the lateral abdominal view includes appraisal of the stomach axis. The stomach axis is a line drawn from the fundus to the body of the stomach. The normal axis is roughly parallel to the ribs. Changes in the stomach axis correspond to changes in liver size. The pylorus and body are displaced caudally if the liver is enlarged, and they are displaced cranially if the

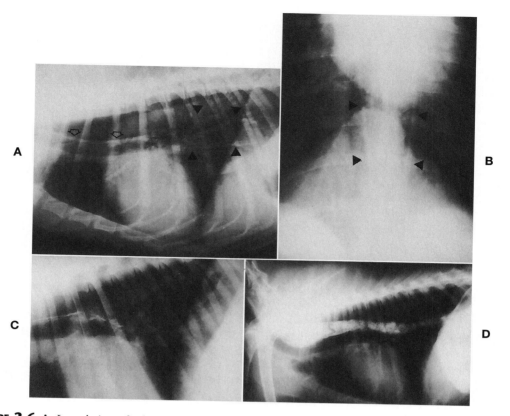

FIGURE 2-6 A, Lateral view of a dog with megaesophagus. The trachea is ventrally depressed by an enlarged, air-filled esophagus. Note the "tracheoesophageal stripe" *(open arrows),* which is seen when air is in the esophagus as well as in the trachea. Dorsal and ventral esophageal walls are seen caudally *(arrowheads).* **B,** Ventrodorsal view of the dog in **A.** This view is centered on the caudal esophagus. The air-filled esophagus appears as two linear opacities on either side of midline that taper into the diaphragm *(arrowheads).* **C,** Lateral view of a dog with mild megaesophagus. No abnormalities are seen with barium liquid. **D,** Same dog as in **C.** When food-barium mixture is used, esophageal dilation is seen, suggesting abnormal esophageal motility. Use of food mixed with barium should be considered when evaluating esophageal swallowing dysfunction.

liver is small or has herniated through the diaphragm into the thorax.

On the VD view the stomach position in the dog is slightly different from that in the cat: In the dog the fundus is cranial-left, the body is midline, and the pylorus is cranial-right. In the cat the fundus and body are cranial-left and the pylorus is midline or slightly to the right of the spine.

Stomach location varies with stomach distention, but the stomach is usually between the tenth and thirteenth ribs. Competent assessment of liver size and diagnosis of liver masses depend on knowledge of normal stomach position.

The variably sized stomach may contain nonpersistent air, fluid, or mineral opacities. The wall of the fundus has pronounced rugal folds that appear uniform and parallel in a distended stomach and undulant and tortuous in a nondistended stomach. The rugal pattern is negligible in the body and pyloric areas of a normal stomach.

Gastrogram

Indications include chronic vomiting, hematemesis, suspected foreign object or mass, pyloric disease, and identification of stomach position.

The following materials are needed for a gastrogram: micropulverized barium suspension diluted to 50% with warm water; gas source (room air, carbonated beverage, gas-producing tablets or granules); water-soluble iodinated contrast medium (used only if a gastric perforation or rupture is suspected); and a stomach tube, mouth gag, and large-dose syringe.

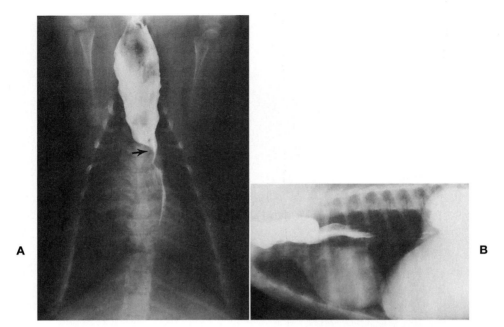

FIGURE 2-7 A, Ventrodorsal view of a cat with persistent right aortic arch. Note the abrupt change in diameter of the esophagus at the heart base. The right aortic arch compresses the esophagus, causing deviation of contrast medium to the left *(arrow)*. **B,** Lateral view of a dog with persistent right aortic arch. Contrast medium outlines the dilated cranial thoracic esophagus. There is a change in esophageal diameter at the heart base. The esophagus is partially dilated caudal to the vascular ring anomaly.

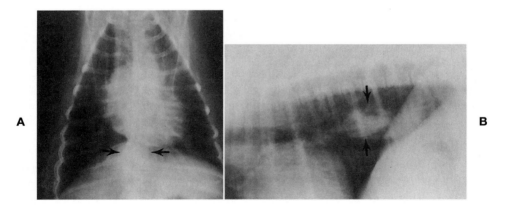

FIGURE 2-8 Survey ventrodorsal **(A)** and lateral **(B)** views of a dog with an esophageal foreign object. An opacity is located in the area of the caudal esophagus on both views *(arrows)*. Two views are necessary to determine the exact location of soft tissue opacity.

In a *positive or negative gastrogram* the following technique is best used to identify stomach position or gastric foreign objects:

1. The stomach should be empty.
2. Use the following doses: for barium, 1.5 to 2 ml of previously diluted (50%) micropulverized barium per lb; for room air, 1.5 to 2 ml of air per lb; for oral iodinated contrast, 0.7 ml of iodinated contrast mixed with 0.7 ml warm water per lb.
3. Administer the contrast medium via a stomach tube rather than orally to achieve maximum stomach distention. *Make sure that the tube is not in the trachea* (by palpation or radiograph).
4. Obtain right and left lateral views, VD and dorsoventral views, and additional oblique views as needed.

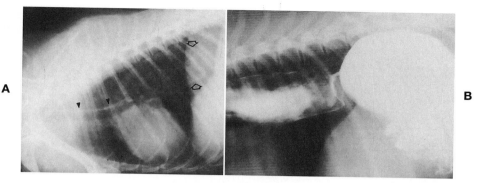

FIGURE 2-9 A, Lateral view of a dog with megaesophagus. The trachea is ventrally depressed by an air–filled esophagus. A "tracheoesophageal stripe" is seen *(closed arrowheads),* and the caudal esophagus is dilated *(open arrows).* No obvious cause for the dilated esophagus is seen. **B,** Lateral esophagram of dog in **A.** A smooth, curvilinear filling defect is in the caudal esophagus, which is caused by an intramural esophageal mass located proximal to the gastroesophageal junction. Contrast studies should be performed to determine the cause of megaesophagus. Diagnosis was leiomyosarcoma.

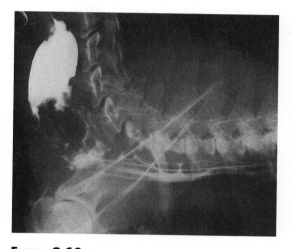

FIGURE 2-10 Lateral view of a cat with esophageal neoplasia. Irregular and asymmetric filling defects are in the midcervical esophagus. Contrast medium extends around the mass, suggesting a broad-based intramural mass. Diagnosis was an esophageal carcinoma.

In a *double-contrast gastrogram,* which is the best method for evaluating mucosal lesions, mural masses, and ulcerations, the following technique is used:

1. The stomach must be empty.
2. Via a stomach tube, give 0.25 ml diluted (50%) barium per lb followed by 1 to 1.4 ml gas per lb.
3. Obtain right and left lateral views, VD and dorsoventral views, and additional oblique views as needed.

A normal-appearing gastrogram (Figure 2-11) shows even gastric distention; smooth parallel rugal folds in the fundus, not in the body or pylorus (guideline: a rugal fold should be no thicker than the space between the folds); smooth mucosal surface; transient peristalsis in the body and pyloric areas; and stomach beginning to empty within 30 minutes and empty by 1 to 4 hours (normal stomach emptying of food is 5 to 6 hours but may be as long as 8 to 10 hours in some patients and still be considered normal).

Radiographic Signs of Gastric Disease

Pylorospasm. A pylorospasm is indicated by delayed gastric emptying and gastric dilatation with visible peristalsis.

Pyloric Stenosis. This disease may be congenital or acquired. Common causes of acquired stenosis include pyloric neoplasia, chronic hypertrophic gastritis, and uremic gastritis (Figure 2-12). Radiographic signs are delayed gastric emptying; gastric dilatation with peristalsis usually present; narrowed pylorus with contrast medium projecting into the pyloric canal (beak sign); and often the development of a distinct bulge in the stomach immediately proximal to the pyloric canal, especially on the lesser curvature.

Gastric Foreign Objects (Figures 2-13 and 2-14). Radiopaque foreign objects are often visible on survey radiographs. On a barium study soft tissue or air-filled foreign objects appear as lucent filling defects. The foreign object is usually freely movable in the stomach and changes location on different radiographic views.

Gastritis. This diagnosis is suggested when one or more of the following radiographic changes are evident (Figure 2-15):

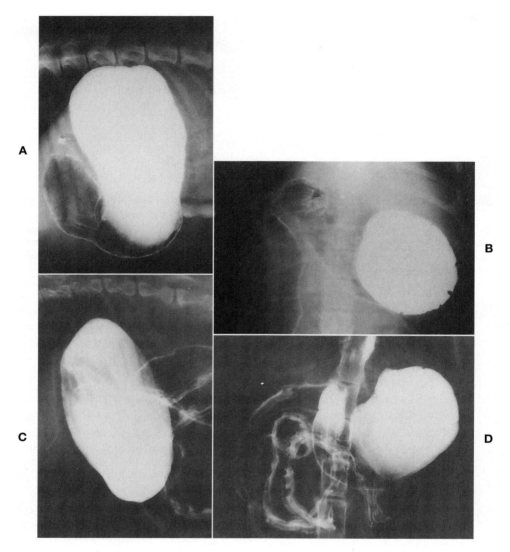

FIGURE 2-11 Lateral (**A**) and ventrodorsal (**B**) views of normal canine double-contrast gastrogram. Contrast medium is pooling in the fundus. Note the smooth mucosal surface and peristalsis in the body of the stomach. Filling defects seen in the wall of the fundus on the ventrodorsal view are normal rugal folds. Lateral (**C**) and ventrodorsal (**D**) views of normal feline double-contrast gastrogram. Rugal pattern, seen as lucent linear filling defects, is normally more evident in the fundus. Note that the cardiac area is slightly irregular. This is a normal finding in cats.

1. Thickened, irregular, or indistinct rugal folds
2. Prominent rugal folds in the pylorus and body
3. Rigid stomach wall that is nondistensible, is often thickened, and lacks peristalsis
4. Hyperperistalsis or hypoperistalsis
5. Barium precipitation caused by abnormal stomach contents, such as blood, excess mucus, or incorrect pH
6. Stomach emptying that is delayed or more rapid than normal
7. Calcification of gastric mucosa, secondary to chronic renal disease, appearing as faint linear

opacities that accentuate rugal folds on survey radiographs

Gastric Dilatation-Volvulus (Figures 2-16 and 2-17). The following radiographic signs indicate gastric dilatation-volvulus:

1. Gastric dilatation.
2. Compartmentalization of the stomach (double bubble sign) due to the stomach's folding on itself.
3. Pylorus located dorsally and to the left of midline, and fundus located ventrally and to the

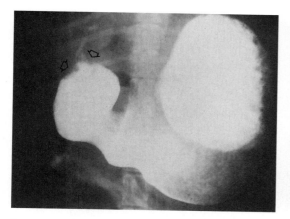

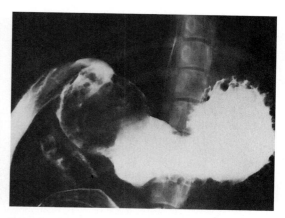

FIGURE 2-12 A dog with pyloric hypertrophy. A small, annular filling defect *(arrows)* extends into the pyloric antrum just proximal to the pylorus. A small amount of barium extends into the pyloric canal.

FIGURE 2-13 Gastrogram of a dog with a gastric foreign object (ball). The ball appeared as a soft tissue opacity on survey radiographs. When surrounded by barium, the ball appears radiolucent. The lucent filling defect is completely surrounded by barium, suggesting an intraluminal foreign object.

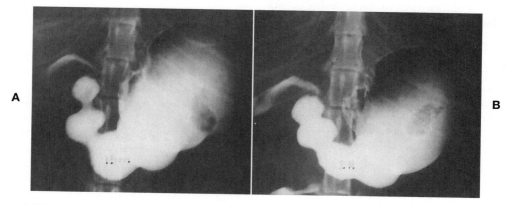

FIGURE 2-14 **A** and **B,** Ventrodorsal views of a cat that swallowed a toy fish. Note the normal irregular cardia. The toy fish is clearly seen as a lucent filling defect in the stomach. Between the two views the position of the toy has changed. This mobility indicates that the object is intraluminal.

right of midline. The fundus is the larger of the two "bubbles" and has a rugal pattern.

4. Splenomegaly caused by venous congestion or possible torsion.
5. Small liver and caudal vena cava caused by portal vein and caval compression by the enlarged stomach.
6. Small intestinal ileus.
7. Dilated esophagus.

Gastric Masses. Gastric masses usually require a barium study for identification and evaluation. Oblique views may be necessary. Because masses vary markedly in appearance, the signs listed below represent possible radiographic appearances (Figures 2-18 to 2-20):

1. Mural thickening.
2. Ulceration, which may be seen as an outpouching of barium beyond the lumen; focal pooling of barium beyond the lumen; or wall rigidity adjacent to the ulcer with a radiating rugal pattern from the site of the ulcer. The rugal pattern may be indistinct, and there may be evidence of perforation and peritonitis.
3. Rigid, nondistensible areas in the stomach.
4. Barium filling defect (lucency) if the mass protrudes into the lumen. The filling defect does not move with gravity on positional studies.
5. Smooth or irregular mucosal surface.

Ruptured Stomach. The radiographic signs of a ruptured stomach include the following:

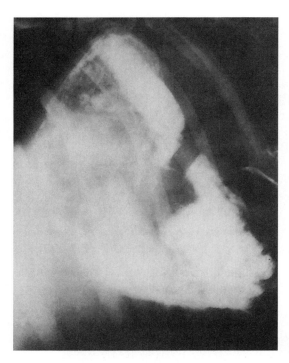

FIGURE 2-15 Lateral view of a dog with severe ulcerative gastritis. The mucosal margin is irregular, with spicules of barium extending into small ulcers in the stomach wall. This is primarily seen in the body and pyloric antrum. Barium appears smudged, suggesting poor mixing of contrast medium. This is probably due to abnormal stomach contents.

1. Free gas in the abdomen. Small amounts of free gas appear as bubbles outside the lumen and often in abnormal locations, such as near the kidneys or bladder. Larger amounts of free gas outline serosal surfaces of the stomach, intestine, liver lobes, and diaphragm.
2. Ingesta in the abdomen.
3. Indistinct stomach border is seen with large rupture.
4. Poor abdominal visceral detail caused by fluid and/or peritonitis.
5. Contrast extravasation into the abdomen. Use water-soluble iodinated contrast if intestinal rupture is suspected.

Small Intestine
Radiographic Anatomy
The duodenum is located about halfway between the spine and the ventral body wall on the lateral view. It descends along the right body wall and ascends in the midabdomen on the VD view. Jejunum is evenly distributed throughout the abdomen. The ileum is that portion of the distal small intestine that joins with the colon and is located in the right midabdomen.

Intestinal shape is uniform and tubular with transient narrowings due to peristalsis. Intestinal contents include *nonpersistent* air, fluid, or mineral opacity.

A general guideline used to evaluate intestinal size is that the diameter should be no larger than one to two rib widths or no larger than the height of a lumbar vertebral body (not the vertebral arch or dorsal spine, just the body).

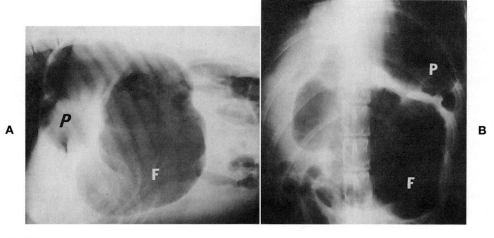

FIGURE 2-16 Lateral **(A)** and ventrodorsal **(B)** views of a dog with gastric dilatation-volvulus. There is compartmentalization of the stomach. The fundus *(F)* is the largest compartment. The pylorus *(P)* is displaced dorsally and to the left.

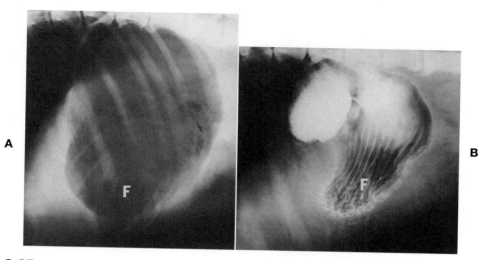

FIGURE 2-17 Lateral survey **(A)** and contrast study **(B)** of a dog with gastric dilatation–volvulus. Rugal folds are identified in the ventrally displaced fundus *(F)*. Pattern of rugal folds is helpful in identifying fundus of stomach.

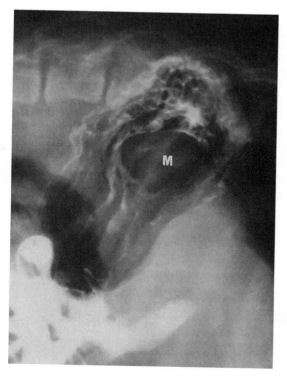

FIGURE 2-18 Lateral view of a dog with a fundic mass *(M)* protruding into stomach lumen. The mass causes a lucent filling defect in contrast medium. Rugal folds are distorted by the mass.

Small Intestinal Contrast Study

Indications include persistent vomiting and/or diarrhea, hematemesis, melena, and suspected foreign object or obstruction.

The materials needed for a small intestinal contrast study are micropulverized barium diluted to 50% concentration with warm tap water; water-soluble iodinated contrast if intestinal perforation is suspected; and a stomach tube, large syringe, and mouth gag.

The following technique is used:

1. Administer barium (0.7 to 1.4 ml/lb) orally in swallows or by stomach tube. Use the lower dose for larger dogs to avoid having too much barium in multiple bowel loops and thus to allow adequate evaluation of individual bowel loops.
2. Administer organic iodide (0.25 ml/lb) diluted with tap water (0.5 to 1 ml/lb) orally or by stomach tube. Undiluted organic iodides are extremely hypertonic and can lead to severe dehydration and shock in a compromised patient.
3. If sedation is necessary, studies have shown that acepromazine or triflupromazine can be used in dogs without significantly affecting gastrointestinal (GI) transit time. Recommended sedatives for cats are a ketamine/acepromazine combination or ketamine alone when motility is not a primary concern (both regimens cause more rapid transit of barium through the GI tract) or ketamine/diazepam if a motility problem is suspected, because there is no significant effect on GI transit time (each sedative should be administered in a separate syringe).

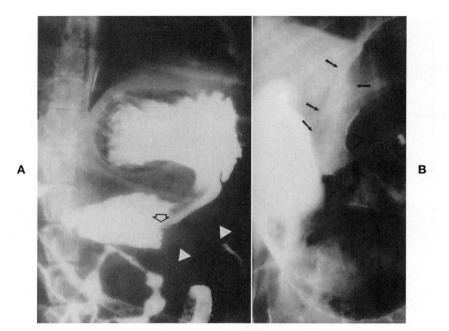

FIGURE 2-19 A, Ventrodorsal view of a dog with an intramural gastric mass. There is an abrupt change in diameter of stomach lumen *(open arrow)*. This is referred to as a "shelf sign." Stomach wall is markedly thickened *(closed arrowheads)*. **B,** An intramural mass is seen on the lesser curvature of the stomach body *(arrows)*. Barium is adherent to an irregular mucosal surface.

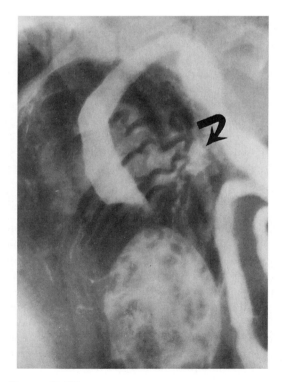

FIGURE 2-20 Barium pools in an ulcer in the gastric fundus *(arrow)*. Note how the rugae radiate from the area of the ulcer.

4. Make exposures in right lateral and VD positions at 0, 15, 30, and 60 minutes (45-minute films may be needed if transit time is rapid). Take films hourly thereafter until the contrast medium reaches the colon.

In a normal-appearing small intestinal contrast study:

1. The mucosal surface is either smooth or finely fimbriated (Figure 2-21).
2. Bowel is evenly distributed throughout the abdomen.
3. The normal feline duodenum may appear hyperperistaltic with multiple simultaneous contractions, giving the appearance of a "string of beads" (Figure 2-22).
4. The normal canine duodenum often has outpouchings in areas of lymphoid follicles (pseudoulcers) (Figure 2-23).
5. Normal canine small intestinal transit time is 3 to 5 hours for barium to reach the colon.
6. Normal feline small intestinal transit time is 15 to 60 minutes for barium to reach the colon.
7. Organic iodides are irritating and cause hyperperistalsis, so transit time is rapid. Iodinated contrast agents usually reach the colon within 1 hour.

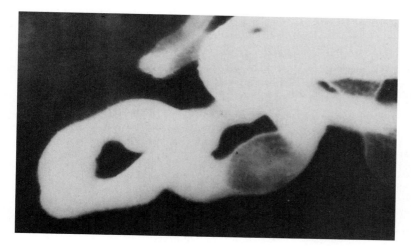

FIGURE 2-21 Barium contrast study of normal small intestine. The mucosal surface is slightly fimbriated. Lucent areas in the intestine are gas in the lumen. This is differentiated from foreign objects on serial films. Gas opacities are nonpersistent.

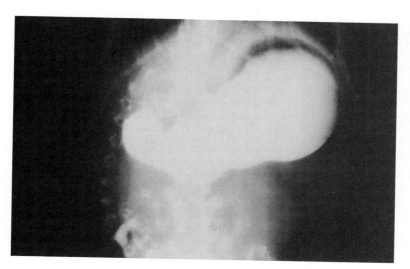

FIGURE 2-22 Normal feline duodenum with contrast medium. Duodenal hyperperistalsis is a normal finding in many cats. This is referred to as "string of beads" and must not be confused with a linear foreign object (see Figure 2-26).

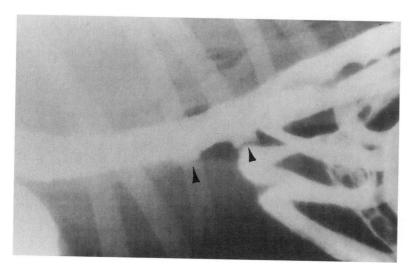

FIGURE 2-23 Pseudoulcers *(arrowheads)* are normal in the canine duodenum. These appear somewhat conical or square when filled with barium.

Radiographic Signs of Small Intestinal Disease

Excess Gas. Causes of excess gas in the small intestine *without* dilation include aerophagia, enteritis, anorexia, recent enema, and incomplete or high obstruction where vomition relieves gas/fluid distention; and, with dilation, paralytic ileus, obstructive ileus due to foreign objects, neoplasia, abscess, and granuloma.

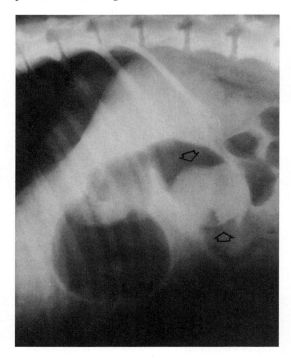

FIGURE 2-24 There is a smooth soft tissue opacity (foreign object) in the descending duodenum *(arrows)*. This opacity is visible because it is surrounded by air. The duodenum proximal to the foreign object is dilated.

FIGURE 2-25 Barium study of a cat that swallowed a backgammon chip. The duodenum is dilated proximal to the foreign object. Barium surrounds the object *(arrows)* and then passes into bowel of normal diameter.

Foreign Objects. Radiopaque foreign objects are visible on survey radiographs (Figure 2-24). Radiolucent foreign objects may be seen on survey radiographs. On a contrast study, foreign objects cause a lucent intraluminal filling defect in the contrast medium (Figure 2-25).

Bowel proximal to the foreign object may be dilated with fluid or gas. If bowel has been perforated, there may be free abdominal gas, loss of abdominal visceral detail, and fluid opacity in the abdomen.

Linear Foreign Objects. Survey radiographs may show numerous end-on loops of small intestine. This is not a definitive sign because hyperperistalsis may give this appearance.

A contrast study reveals plication or gathering of small intestinal loops (Figure 2-26). *Do not* confuse plication with the normal "string of beads" sign in cats. The "string of beads" appears as a symmetric widening and narrowing of the intestinal lumen. Plicated intestine has a serpentine appearance.

Perforation may occur, causing free gas and/or peritonitis.

Enteritis—Nonulcerative. Radiographic signs of nonulcerative enteritis include rapid intestinal transit time; severe accentuation of the fimbriated villous pattern; persistent narrowing or "stringing" of small intestinal lumen diameter, not to be confused with normal peristalsis; hypercontractility or hyperperistalsis; and precipitation of barium due to abnormal luminal contents, such as blood, excess mucus, or abnormal pH.

Enteritis—Ulcerative (Figure 2-27). Radiographic signs of ulcerative enteritis include severe

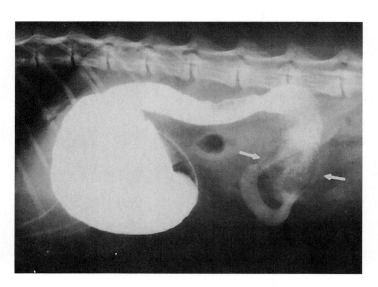

bowel spasticity or rigidity and irregular mucosal surface, with contrast medium extending beyond the lumen (in a spiculated pattern if ulcerations are small and diffuse, and with conical, rounded, or squared outlines if the ulcers are larger).

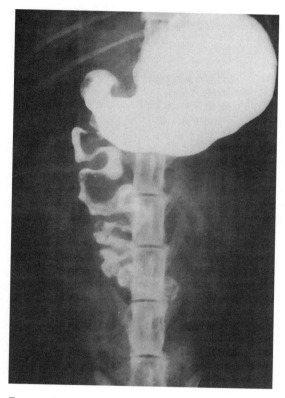

FIGURE 2-26 Ventrodorsal barium study of a cat with a linear foreign object. Contrast in intestine shows classic accordionated or plicated appearance associated with linear foreign object.

Intussusception. An intussusception is invagination of a segment of intestine into the lumen of an adjoining part of the intestine—usually the proximal segment enters the lumen of the distal segment. The intussusceptum is the invaginated segment. The intussuscipiens is the receiving segment.

On survey radiographs one may see intestinal distention and the intussusceptum may be identified if surrounded by gas.

On an upper GI contrast study, the intestinal transit time is markedly delayed, there is abrupt narrowing of intestinal lumen as barium enters the intussusceptum (Figure 2-28), and intestine proximal to the intussusception is usually dilated.

Intramural Lesions. These can be solitary, multiple, or diffuse. Common causes include neoplasia, granuloma, abscessation, stricture, and adhesions. Radiographic appearance is variable (Figures 2-29 and 2-30):

1. Wall thickness is difficult to assess on survey radiographs because fluid in the lumen adjacent to intestinal mucosa can mimic mural thickening. A contrast study or ultrasound examination is the best way to noninvasively determine actual wall thickness.
2. A mass is visible on survey radiographs.
3. A contrast study may show diffuse or focal increase in wall thickness.
4. A mass may impinge on the lumen concentrically or eccentrically, causing luminal narrowing.
5. Abnormal luminal dilation is seen.
6. A smooth, irregular, or ulcerative mucosal surface is seen. A "scalloped" surface is common

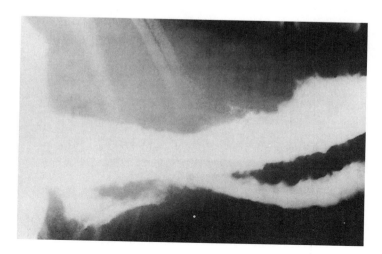

FIGURE 2-27 Dog with ulcerative enteritis. Mucosal surface has a spiculated appearance due to barium accumulating in small ulcers.

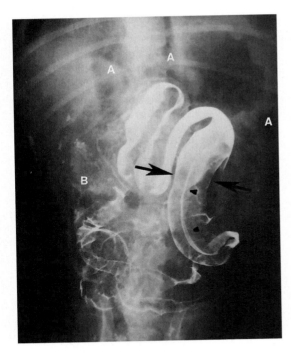

FIGURE 2-28 Ventrodorsal view of a dog that had surgery 3 days previously to correct an intussusception. Free air *(A)* is seen in the abdomen, presumably caused by the surgery. A second barium study was performed because of suspected recurrence of intussusception. *Arrows* indicate lumen of intussuscipiens; *arrowheads* show lumen of intussusceptum. Free barium seen in the abdomen *(B)* indicates intestinal rupture.

in multifocal intramural diseases such as lymphosarcoma, pyogranulomatous disease, and diffuse infiltrative diseases.

7. The lesion *must* be present on more than one film in a barium study to be significant because the radiographic appearance during peristalsis and spasms may mimic that in intramural disease.

Intestinal Perforation (Figures 2-31 and 2-32). Radiographic signs of intestinal perforation include loss of abdominal visceral detail and/or free fluid in the abdomen (suggesting peritonitis); ileus; and free abdominal gas. Small amounts of free gas appear as small extraluminal gas bubbles, usually seen in odd locations, such as near the kidneys or bladder. Larger amounts of free gas outline liver lobes, diaphragm, kidney borders, and serosal surfaces of intestine. A left lateral recumbent view obtained with a horizontal beam shows small amounts of free gas against the right abdominal wall.

Large Intestine
Radiographic Anatomy

The cecum and ascending colon are located in the right midabdomen. The transverse colon parallels the caudal border of the greater curvature of the stomach. The descending colon is in the left abdomen, and the rectum descends into the pelvic canal. The large intestine assumes the shape of a question mark (?) on the VD view. On the lateral view the regions of large intestine are usually superimposed in the midabdomen.

FIGURE 2-29 Jejunal intramural mass *(arrows)* is annular and has an irregular mucosal surface. There is minimal distention of intestine proximal to the mass.

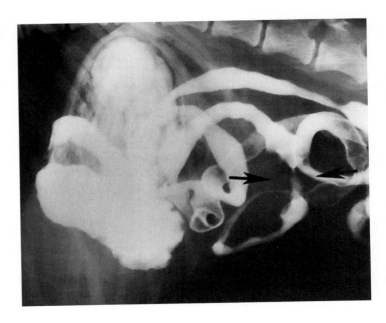

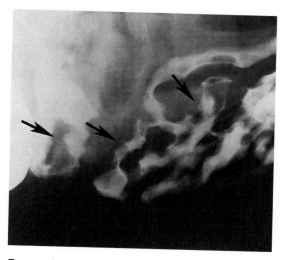

FIGURE 2-30 Dog with diffuse intestinal lymphosarcoma. The mucosal surface is irregular, with asymmetric filling defects and narrowed areas of small intestine *(arrows)*.

The canine cecum is very large, having a spiral or **C** shape, whereas the feline cecum is a small blind sac. In the cat there is no distinct border between the cecum and the ascending colon. The junction is defined only by viewing the site where the ileum joins the colon.

Normal size and opacity are extremely variable. Formed feces of heterogeneous opacity, including mineral or bone material, are commonly seen. A large amount of air in the colon can be normal.

Barium Enema

The large intestine should *not* be assessed on a small intestinal contrast study. Filling is incomplete, and barium inadequately coats large intestinal mucosa.

Indications for a barium enema include recurrent or persistent large bowel diarrhea; fresh blood in the feces; chronic constipation; suspected large bowel obstruction, pelvic masses, colonic or rectal masses, or intussusception; and chronic

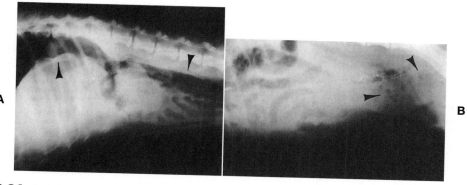

FIGURE 2-31 A, A large amount of free abdominal gas is present *(arrowheads)*. Gas outlines serosa of stomach, abdominal surface of diaphragm, and dorsal caudal abdomen. There is loss of abdominal visceral detail. **B,** Small amounts of free abdominal gas are more difficult to discern. Several small gas accumulations are seen superimposed over the bladder *(arrowheads)*. These gas opacities are not associated with bowel. There is loss of abdominal detail due to peritonitis and free abdominal fluid.

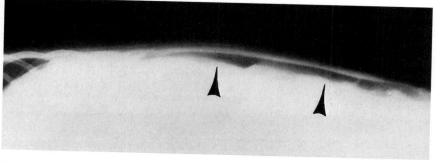

FIGURE 2-32 Positional studies are of value in determining the presence of small amounts of free abdominal gas. The patient is placed in left lateral recumbency, and an exposure is made using a horizontal beam. Free abdominal gas accumulates against the abdominal wall *(arrowheads)*.

inflammatory large bowel disease. Do not perform a barium enema within 2 hours of enema (spasms induced), 6 to 12 hours after colonoscopy (spasms induced), or within 3 to 4 days after colon biopsy (may rupture colon).

The following materials are needed for a barium enema:

1. Pediatric or adult-sized balloon catheters.*
2. Gravity-flow enema bag with tubing† or dose syringe with adapter and three-way valve.
3. Micropulverized barium diluted to 50% with warm tap water.
4. Aqueous organic iodides diluted to 50% with tap water, used only if perforation is suspected. Barium is the contrast medium of choice to achieve satisfactory mucosal definition.
5. Room air.

The following technique is employed for a barium enema:

1. A 24-hour fast is desirable, and multiple high-volume, warm-water enemas are essential to clean out the large intestine. Feces in the colon can obscure small lesions and mimic mass lesions.
2. General anesthesia is desirable to eliminate colonic spasms, facilitate manipulation and positioning, and alleviate patient anxiety and discomfort.
3. *Avoid* using narcotics that induce severe colonic spasms.
4. Use 2.3 ml/lb of diluted (50%) barium liquid as a general guideline because the dose is extremely variable. Infuse contrast medium slowly through an inflated balloon catheter.
5. Obtain a VD film after 2.3 ml/lb is administered or if there is resistance to flow. Administer more contrast medium as required.
6. Obtain lateral, VD, and two oblique views.
7. Perform a double-contrast study, best for evaluating mucosal detail, by removing most of the positive contrast medium and slowly infusing room air into the colon. Repeat exposures in lateral, VD, and oblique positions.
8. If a rectal lesion is suspected, the balloon catheter may obscure the lesion. A method to outline rectal lesions, if endoscopy is not available, is to inflate the balloon catheter cranial to the lesion, place a purse-string suture around the anus, and tighten the suture after positioning the tip of an additional catheter just inside the anus. A small amount of contrast medium given through the second catheter will outline the extent of a rectal lesion.

A normal-appearing barium enema study (Figure 2-33) shows uniform distention of the colon and cecum and a smooth mucosal surface. A redundant or long convoluted colon is a normal variant, and a spasm at the catheter tip is common.

Radiographic Signs of Large Intestinal Disease

Megacolon or Dilation of Large Intestine. This disease has numerous causes: neurologic disease such as trauma to the spine, spinal neoplasia, or congenital spinal abnormalities; mechanical obstruction such as neoplasia, foreign objects, extrinsic masses compressing or infiltrating the colon wall, or narrowed pelvic canal from malunion of pelvic fractures; abnormal diet; and psychogenic factors. There are no published guidelines for determining megacolon, so diagnosis of abnormal colonic dilation is subjective.

Colitis and Typhlitis (Figure 2-34). Radiographic signs of these diseases include mucosal irregularity ("cobblestone" appearance); increased wall thickness; spasticity and shortening of colon and/or cecum; and mucosal ulceration.

Emphysematous Colitis. Survey radiographs show gas in the bowel wall. Extensive amounts of gas in the wall parallel luminal gas, in a linear fashion, distinctly showing mucosal surfaces.

On a barium study contrast covers the mucosal surface and gas in the colon wall is still visible.

Ileocolic Intussusception. On survey films a tubular soft tissue mass outlined by colonic gas may be seen. The leading edge of the intussusceptum has an oval or rounded shape (Figure 2-35).

On a contrast study barium surrounds the intussusceptum, which appears as an intraluminal radiolucent filling defect. Barium may define linear bands, sometimes referred to as a "coil spring" appearance, in the wall of the intussuscipiens, as it contracts on the intussusceptum (Figure 2-36).

Colonic or Cecal Intramural Masses. These vary widely in appearance (Figure 2-37). On survey films fecal impaction may occur proximal to the mass. A solid soft tissue mass may be seen; the mass may be focal or diffuse. There is annular constriction or eccentric invasion of the colon by a mass.

---

*Picker Enema Tubes. Picker International, Denver, CO 80239.
†Rapidfil Enema System. Picker International, Denver, CO 80239.

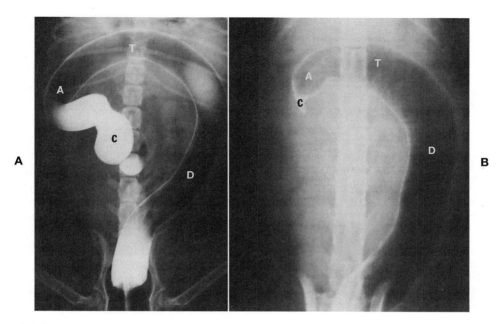

FIGURE 2-33 Normal dog **(A)** and cat **(B)** barium enema. There is smooth mucosal coating by contrast medium and even distention of the large intestine. Note the question mark configuration of the canine and feline colon. *A,* Ascending colon; *C,* cecum; *D,* descending colon; *T,* transverse colon.

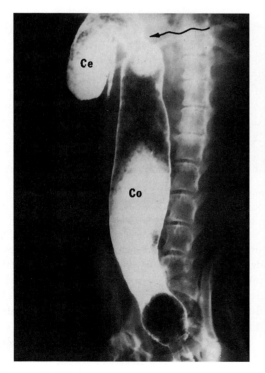

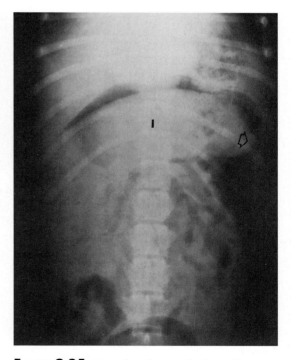

FIGURE 2-34 Ventrodorsal view of a dog with severe typhlitis and colitis. Small filling defects are seen protruding into the lumen of the cecum *(Ce)* and colon *(Co).* The colon is markedly shortened, and the cecum no longer has a normal shape. *Arrow* indicates ileocolic junction.

FIGURE 2-35 Ventrodorsal view of a dog with an ileocolic intussusception. The intussusceptum *(I)* appears as a large soft tissue opacity that is surrounded by air in the intussuscipiens. Note the round contour of the leading edge of the intussusceptum *(arrow).* Visualization of this abnormal shape is usually associated with intussusception or intestinal foreign object.

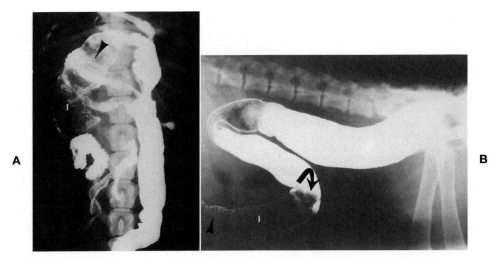

FIGURE 2-36 **A** and **B,** Two examples of ileocolic intussusception identified on a barium enema. The intussusceptum *(I)* appears as lucent filling defect within the colon. Abnormal rounded leading edge is visible *(curved arrow).* Faint linear bands in the intussuscipiens are outlined by barium *(arrowheads).*

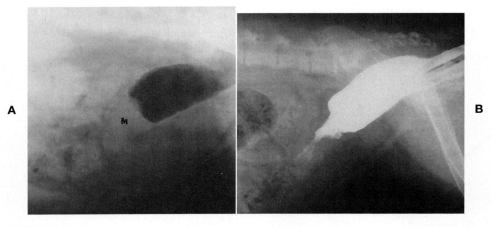

FIGURE 2-37 **A,** Survey radiograph of a dog with an intramural colonic mass. Gas is seen in the colon distal to the mass *(M),* and feces can be seen proximal to the mass. **B,** Same dog as in **A.** Barium enema shows an annular colonic mass. Note the abrupt change in colonic diameter caused by the nondistensible intramural mass.

On a barium study an irregular or smooth mucosal surface is seen. Ulceration may be diffuse and spiculated or large and cavitated. Polypoid masses cause luminal lucent filling defects on barium study.

Liver

Normal Anatomy

The liver has a soft tissue opacity; therefore internal structures are not defined. Much of the liver is silhouetted by the diaphragm, stomach, and right kidney, making it difficult to evaluate the liver borders. The ventrocaudal liver border is usually well visualized on the lateral view, with sharply defined edges and a triangular shape that projects just beyond the ribs. In the cat the ventrocaudal liver border is often displaced dorsally by falciform fat and may be located in the cranial midabdomen.

Normal liver size is best defined by the location of the stomach. On the lateral view the stomach axis from the fundus to the body should be parallel to the ribs, although this varies somewhat with breed, body conformation, and stomach distention. On the VD view an empty stomach is usually located between the tenth and thirteenth ribs. The pylorus and body are located more on midline in the cat.

Angiography of the Portal Venous System

This is an invasive procedure and is employed less frequently now that ultrasound and nuclear medicine scans are capable of diagnosing vascular anomalies.

Indications include suspected congenital or acquired portal vein anomalies, such as patent ductus venosus, portocaval shunts, or portosystemic shunts; and suspected arteriovenous fistulas.

The following techniques are used in angiography of the portal venous system:

1. Selective catheterization of the cranial mesenteric artery under fluoroscopic guidance. Because this method requires equipment that is prohibitively expensive for routine private practice, it is not described here.
2. Surgical catheterization of a mesenteric vein, which is invasive but will impart necessary information concerning liver vascular supply.
3. Percutaneous splenic puncture, using an 18-gauge styletted spinal needle,[*] on a patient that is heavily sedated or anesthetized, which will outline most portal shunts. Blood should be easily aspirated before contrast injection into splenic pulp, and then slow infusion of 10 to

---

[*]Tru-Fit spinal needles. Picker International, Denver, CO 80239.
[†]Hypaque 76. Picker International, Denver, CO 80239.

20 ml of sterile, water-soluble iodinated contrast medium is performed.[†] Three to four lateral radiographs, exposed 7 to 10 seconds after injection, should be obtained at 1- to 2-second intervals. This is possible with any radiographic equipment if a "tunnel" is constructed. The patient is placed on a Plexiglas board, which is elevated off the table high enough to allow easy passage of x-ray cassettes. Cassettes can be rapidly pushed through the "tunnel" using an object as simple as a broomstick. To ensure correct cassette placement under the abdomen, markers should be placed at appropriate locations on the broomstick before the initiation of the procedure.

On a normal-appearing angiogram, mesenteric or splenic veins normally drain into the portal vein, the portal vein branches with the liver (Figure 2-38), and hepatic venous blood flows into the caudal vena cava.

Radiographic Signs of Liver Disease

Hepatomegaly. Radiographic signs of hepatomegaly include the following:

1. Stomach displacement is usually more evident in the body and pyloric regions. The stomach is displaced caudally and dorsally, causing the stomach axis to be more horizontal.
2. With symmetric, diffuse liver enlargement, liver borders are often rounded and extend well beyond the ribs. Because the liver is larger on

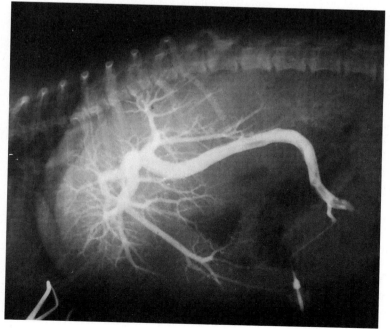

FIGURE 2-38 Normal hepatic portal venogram. Contrast medium was injected into a mesenteric vein, which drains into the portal vein. Note the extensive branching of the portal vein in the liver. (Courtesy Dr. Kathy Spaulding, North Carolina State University Veterinary Teaching Hospital, Raleigh, NC.)

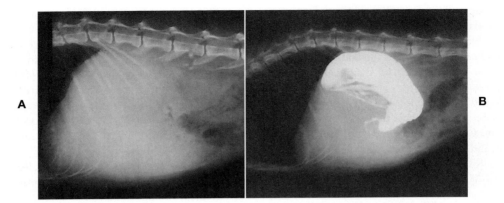

FIGURE 2-39 A, Lateral radiograph of a cat with an enlarged liver. On the survey film there is increased soft tissue opacity in the cranial abdomen. Liver cannot be delineated. **B,** Same cat as in **A.** Contrast medium in the stomach shows caudodorsal gastric displacement by an enlarged liver.

the right side, there is often axial displacement of the stomach on the VD view.

3. Asymmetric liver enlargement is usually due to liver masses. Concurrent displacement of the stomach, kidneys, spleen, and colon is directly influenced by the location of the mass. The liver borders are often spherical or nodular.

Positive or negative contrast in the stomach can aid in evaluating liver size (Figure 2-39).

Small Liver. This is commonly due to chronic liver disease and cirrhosis, portal vein anomalies, or physical displacement of the liver into the chest (diaphragmatic hernia). On the radiographic study, the stomach axis becomes more vertical or may be directed cranially, liver borders may be sharply defined or nodular, and free abdominal fluid often occurs secondary to chronic cirrhosis. With diaphragmatic hernia, soft tissue opacity is present in the thorax and the diaphragmatic outline is not well defined.

Portal Vein Anomalies—Angiography. On angiography a patent ductus venosus or other portosystemic shunt may be identified (Figures 2-40 and 2-41). Portal circulation in portocaval or portosystemic shunts is decreased or absent.

Gallbladder Diseases. These are difficult to diagnose on a survey radiograph. Changes in size and shape are not usually perceived. Only changes in opacity can be consistently detected radiographically.

Mineral opacity in the area of the gallbladder or biliary system is usually due to calculus formation, which is a rare occurrence in the dog and cat. Gas in the area of the gallbladder also is rare and is most likely associated with emphysematous cholecystitis.

Pancreas
Normal Anatomy

The normal pancreas is not visible radiographically. The pancreas is located medial to the descending duodenum and caudal to the pylorus

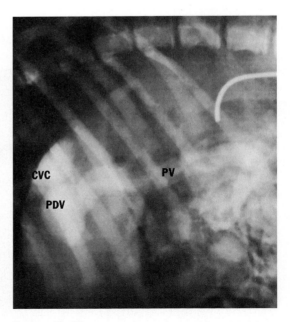

FIGURE 2-40 Venous phase of a cranial mesenteric arterial injection of contrast medium. The portal vein *(PV)* bypasses the liver through a patent ductus venosus *(PDV)* to empty into the caudal vena cava *(CVC)*. Normal portal circulation through the liver is not seen.

and greater curvature of the stomach. The transverse colon lies caudal to the area of the pancreas. Any significant pancreatic enlargement may be appreciated in these areas.

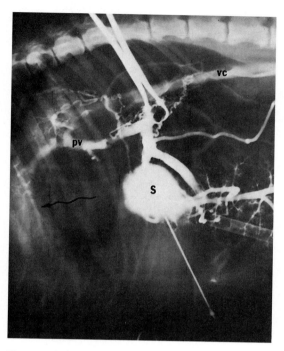

FIGURE 2-41 Percutaneous splenic portography shows numerous tortuous splenic veins draining into both the portal vein *(pv)* and the caudal vena cava *(vc)*. There is some portal blood flow through the liver *(arrow)*. *S,* Spleen.

Radiographic Diagnosis of Pancreatic Disease

Unfortunately, more than 50% of dogs with pancreatic disease have no detectable radiographic abnormalities. Any radiographic changes seen in pancreatic disease are nonspecific, with similar changes detected in acute or chronic pancreatitis and pancreatic neoplasia. The ill-defined increased opacity in the pancreatic region can be related to edema, necrosis, fibrosis, abscessation, or tumor spread. Changes include the following:

1. Loss of detail and increased soft tissue opacity in the area of the pancreas. This loss of detail may be subtle, and diagnosis relies heavily on judgment and experience in evaluating radiographs. Close comparison of other areas of the abdomen, such as the spleen and fundic border of the stomach, with the pancreatic area may facilitate the diagnosis (Figure 2-42).
2. On the VD view the pylorus may be displaced toward midline and the duodenum displaced to the right abdominal wall. This causes an increase in the size or width of the cranial duodenal flexure. A barium study may be necessary to confirm this finding.
3. The transverse colon may be displaced caudally away from the greater curvature of the stomach on both the lateral and the VD views.

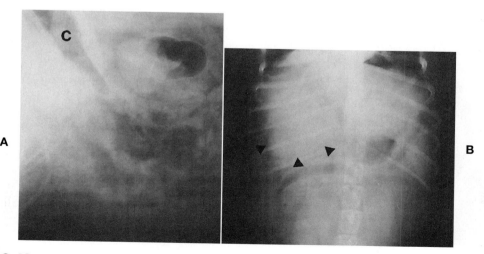

FIGURE 2-42 A, Lateral radiograph of a dog with clinical signs of pancreatitis. There is loss of abdominal visceral detail in the cranial ventral abdomen. A hazy, streaky fluid opacity is apparent in this region. *C,* Transverse colon. **B,** Ventrodorsal radiograph of a dog with clinical signs of pancreatitis. There is an increased soft tissue opacity in the area of the pancreas *(arrowheads)*.

4. The duodenum may be displaced dorsally or ventrally on the lateral view.
5. The duodenum may have persistent gas dilation or may appear "fixed" in position on serial radiographic studies.
6. A barium study may show the duodenum to have a thickened wall, corrugation or spasm, stricture formation, ulceration, and/or atonicity (Figure 2-43). These changes are nonspecific and cannot be considered as definitive evidence of pancreatic disease.

ULTRASONOGRAPHY OF THE DIGESTIVE SYSTEM

Terminology

Sonographic terms refer to television monitor images produced by returning echoes from tissue, fluid, or gas interfaces that appear as shades of white, gray, or black dots against a black background.

1. Hyperechoic—a tissue that produces echoes of high intensity, when compared with those of surrounding tissue, resulting in echoes that are very bright or white
2. Hypoechoic—a tissue that produces low-intensity echoes, when compared with those of surrounding tissue, resulting in echoes that are dark gray
3. Anechoic—an area in which there is no echo formation, resulting in a black image
4. Isoechoic—a tissue that produces echoes that are the same as those of surrounding tissues
5. Complex or heterogeneous echogenicity—a mixture of any of the above echo patterns

Scanning Technique

The following steps are followed in sonography of the digestive system:

1. Shave ventral and lateral abdominal hair.
2. Generously apply water-soluble acoustic coupling gel to the skin surface.★
3. Employ 3.5-, 5.0-, 7.5-, and 10-MHz transducers, depending on the depth of penetration necessary. Better resolution is obtained with higher-frequency transducers, but depth penetration is poor. Therefore use the highest-frequency transducer that gives adequate penetration to obtain the best resolution. For example, a 130-lb dog may require a 3.5-MHz transducer to image the dorsal area of the liver, but the pancreas or GI tract in the same dog may be imaged using a 7.5-MHz transducer. In most small dogs and cats optimal images of the entire abdomen can be obtained with a 7.5-MHz transducer.
4. Real-time sector or curved linear transducers are preferable to many of the linear array transducers because the smaller scanhead requires a smaller acoustic window. This is particularly useful in intercostal imaging.
5. Obtain sagittal and transverse images routinely. Scan additional planes as necessary, depending on body shape and organ position. To image the liver and stomach, place the transducer caudal to the sternum and last rib and angle cranially. The liver, stomach, pancreas, duodenum, and gallbladder can also be imaged through the intercostal spaces or from the right lateral aspect of the patient.
6. Place the patient in dorsal recumbency in a padded V-shaped trough with limbs restrained,

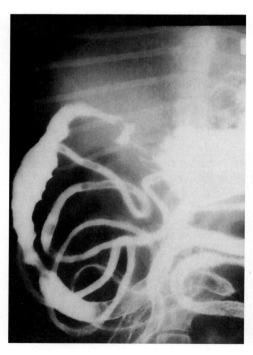

FIGURE 2-43 Barium contrast study on a dog with pancreatitis. The duodenum is slightly dilated and has an irregular, spastic-appearing mucosal surface. The pylorus is axially displaced.

★ Aquasonic 100 Transmission Gel. Parker Laboratories, Inc., Orange, NJ 07050.

or image in lateral recumbency with the top hindleg pulled away from the body. Breed conformation and GI gas affect transducer and patient positioning. Transducer and patient positioning vary, depending on the structure or disease processes imaged. For example, patent ductus venosus, small liver, pancreas, and gallbladder diseases are often best imaged from the right lateral abdomen.

7. To avoid the problem of gastric or intestinal gas shadowing, perform imaging early in the morning (before feeding or significant aerophagia), fill the stomach with water, or perform positional studies to circumvent the gas interference problem. Images are difficult to obtain and interpret if contrast medium is in the stomach or GI tract.

Normal Sonographic Anatomy of the Gastrointestinal Tract

The GI tract is composed of four major histologic layers. Each layer is sonographically displayed as alternating hyperechoic and hypoechoic bands. Five distinct layers may be seen with high-frequency transducers:

1. Lumen and mucosal surface—hyperechoic
2. Mucosa—hypoechoic
3. Submucosa—hyperechoic
4. Muscularis—hypoechoic
5. Serosa—hyperechoic

Often, only three layers are distinguished when the transducer frequency is 5.0 MHz or less: mucosal surface, muscular layer, and serosa.

Real-time scanning of the GI tract allows evaluation of individual wall layers, peristalsis, wall thickness and diameter, lesion location, and appearance of luminal contents. The presence of intraluminal bowel gas does not preclude evaluation of the bowel wall located between the lumen gas and the transducer.

Normal gastric wall thickness is 3 to 5 mm in dogs (Figure 2-44) and 1.1 to 3.6 mm in cats; small intestinal wall thickness in dogs is 3 to 4.5 mm (Figure 2-45) and 1.6 to 2.6 mm in cats; and colon wall thickness is 2.5 to 3 mm in dogs and 1.3 to 2.5 mm in cats.

The proximal duodenum can usually be identified by its continuity with the pylorus. The colon and cecum may be identified by relative location, size, and shape; these often contain considerable gas and/or feces.

The jejunum is randomly arranged. Therefore it is best to perform a survey scan of the jejunum and then isolate and trace individual loops.

Sonographic Diagnosis of Gastrointestinal Disease

Thickening of the gastric or bowel wall is the most common abnormality detected. This change is considered a nonspecific finding because it can occur in inflammatory and neoplastic bowel wall disease. Bowel wall thickening may be diffuse or focal, and focal thickening may be eccentric or concentric. As a rule the layered appearance of bowel wall tends to be conserved in inflammatory disease and disrupted by neoplasia. Asymmetric, focal change is common with neoplasia. Diffuse,

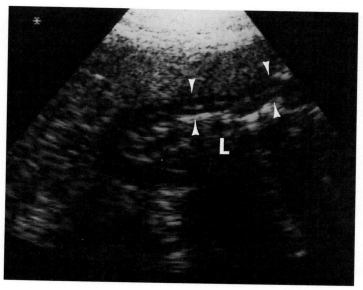

FIGURE 2-44 Normal scan of a canine stomach. Five distinct layers of stomach wall (between *arrowheads*) are seen. *L*, Stomach lumen.

FIGURE 2-45 Scan of a normal loop of small intestine *(arrows)*. Intestinal lumen and mucosal surface account for the central linear echogenicity. Five distinct layers of intestinal wall (between "+" marks) are seen.

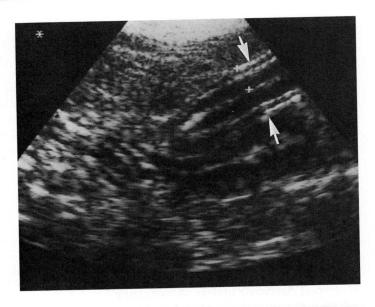

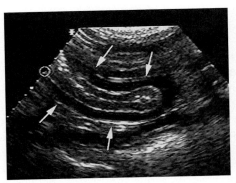

FIGURE 2-46 Sagittal scan of a small intestinal loop *(arrows)* in a 7-year-old domestic short hair cat with chronic vomiting. The wall layers are visible, but the hypoechoic muscle layer is moderately thickened. Inflammatory bowel disease was diagnosed.

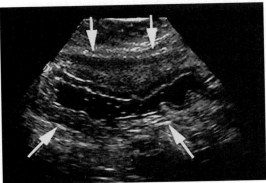

FIGURE 2-47 Transverse scan of the stomach *(arrows)* in a 13-year-old tabby cat with a history of anorexia and vomiting. The stomach wall is markedly thickened with maintained visualization of wall layers. Diagnosis was lymphosarcoma.

symmetric thickening is typical of inflammatory bowel disease (Figure 2-46) but can be seen with diffuse neoplasia, such as lymphosarcoma (Figure 2-47). Inflammatory bowel disease (IBD) in cats can appear as normal wall thickness or can show mild to moderate wall thickening, primarily involving the muscle layer. Enlarged mesenteric lymph nodes have been associated with IBD, so biopsy is very important to differentiate IBD from neoplasia. Cats with IBD may have concurrent cholangiohepatitis and pancreatitis. Disruptive, asymmetric changes can occur with hematoma or abscessation. Carcinomas are usually disruptive and concentric. Mucosal irregularity may be present in either neoplastic or inflammatory disease. Masses with a mixed echo pattern are more commonly associated with neoplasia, hematoma, abscess, and granuloma. Motility is usually decreased or absent through the affected area. A biopsy is needed for definitive diagnosis because benign and malignant lesions can appear similar on ultrasound. Some examples of GI tract neoplasia are seen in Figures 2-48, 2-49, 2-50, and 2-51.

Adynamic (nonobstructive, paralytic) ileus is indicated by distended loops of small intestine and variable peristalsis. Dynamic (obstructive) ileus is indicated by distended loops of small intestine larger than in adynamic ileus (Figure 2-52), minimal deformity from adjacent structures, and variable

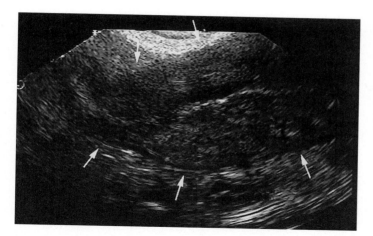

FIGURE 2-48 Sagittal scan of a small intestinal loop *(arrows)* in a 10-year-old mixed-breed dog with vomiting and diarrhea. The intestinal walls are severely thickened with loss of normal wall layers. The central linear hyperechogenicity is the lumen. Diagnosis was adenocarcinoma.

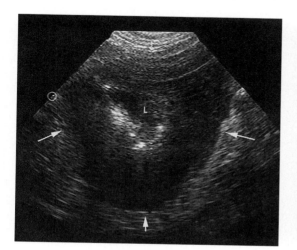

FIGURE 2-49 Transverse scan of the stomach *(arrows)* in a 12-year-old Siamese cat with weight loss, vomiting, diarrhea, and decreased appetite. White blood cell count (WBC) was 28,300 with a neutrophilia. The stomach wall is severely thickened and nonhomogeneous with loss of normal wall layers. The hyperechoic focus off center in the stomach is gas in the lumen. Diagnosis was lymphosarcoma.

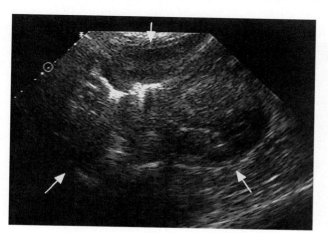

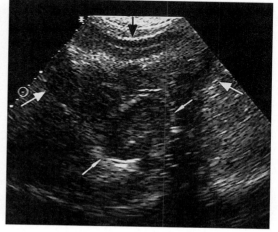

FIGURE 2-50 Transverse scan of the stomach *(arrows)* in a 9-year-old shih tzu with anorexia, intermittent vomiting, and weight loss. The stomach wall is markedly thickened and diffusely hypoechoic with loss of wall layers. Diagnosis was adenocarcinoma. *L,* Lumen.

FIGURE 2-51 Transverse scan of the cardia region of the stomach *(large arrows)* in a 16-year-old Lhasa apso with hematuria and vomiting once with possible blood in the vomitus. A circumscribed, oval, hypoechoic mass *(small arrows)* with a hyperechoic margin is seen at the cardia of the stomach. The mucosa appears intact over the mass. Diagnosis was leiomyoma.

FIGURE 2-52 Scan of a Doberman pinscher puppy presented for vomiting of 2 weeks' duration. Dilated, transverse segment of small intestine is seen *(arrows)*. Wall thickness is normal, with five layers seen *(arrowheads)*. Lumen *(L)* is filled with echoic material suspended in fluid. Echogenicity in the lumen was determined to be due to fluid, because movement of the echoic material was noted. Cause of ileus was an intraluminal foreign object.

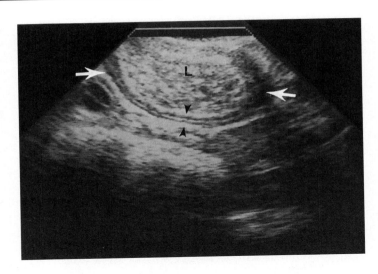

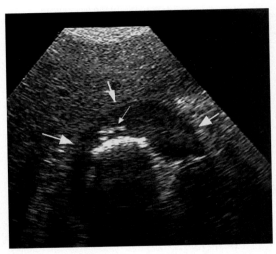

FIGURE 2-53 Transverse scan of the stomach *(large arrows)* in a 12-year-old cocker spaniel with a history of vomiting blood and melena. The stomach wall is markedly thickened with loss of wall layers. The small arrow points to hyperechoic foci within the stomach wall, determined to be gas in small ulcerations. The larger, linear hyperechogenicity is gas in the stomach lumen. Diagnosis was severe ulcerative gastritis.

peristalsis. Cause of obstruction—masses, foreign objects, inflammatory disease—can be imaged.

Ulcerative lesions that are small may be difficult to identify (Figure 2-53). Large ulcers have been observed as outpouchings of the GI tract filled with fluid or echogenic material (Figure 2-54). End-on ulcers may appear as a "target" lesion. Color Doppler imaging may show an actively bleeding ulcer. Adjacent free fluid, gas, and/or hyperechoic tissue (Figure 2-55, *A* and *B*) may be seen with perforating ulcers.

Intussusception is described as a double-concentric, hypoechoic ring with a hyperechoic center on cross section. The central echogenic area is the mucosa of the intussusceptum, which is surrounded by its hypoechoic muscle layer. The next hyperechoic ring is created by the intussusceptum serosa, mesenteric fat, and intussuscipiens mucosal surface. The outer rings are the hypoechoic mucosa and muscular layers and hyperechoic serosal layer of the intussuscipiens (Figure 2-56, *A* and *B*).

Ultrasound appearance of foreign objects is variable, depending on the composition of the object and degree of obstruction (Figures 2-56, *B,* 2-57, and 2-58). Small bowel dilation is common and should be traced to the area of obstruction. The specific type of foreign object cannot be determined because they all can have a similar appearance of a well-defined, usually hyperechoic focus, with distinct acoustic shadowing deep to the object. Linear foreign body will appear as plicated bowel, and usually a hyperechoic line can be traced through the affected bowel loops. The bowel can be mildly or markedly dilated.

Volvulus is seen as dynamic ileus with layering of U-shaped bowel loops. A cross-sectional image may show C-shaped anechoic masses, due to dilated bowel, with mesentery and mesenteric bowel wall, causing a central hyperechogenicity. At this time volvulus is better diagnosed with radiography.

Normal Sonographic Anatomy of the Liver

Individual liver lobes are difficult to identify, except for the caudate lobe, which is in contact with the right kidney. The quadrate and right

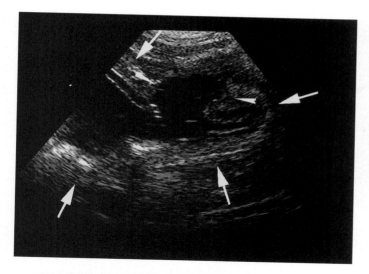

FIGURE 2-54 Transverse scan of the stomach *(large arrows)* in a 15-year-old domestic long hair cat with intermittent vomiting of 2 months' duration. Some episodes included blood. A large ulcer *(arrowheads)* is seen in the stomach wall. The ulcer is filled with anechoic fluid from the stomach lumen. The wall is mildly thickened with maintained wall layers. Histopathologic analysis was not performed, so the cause of the ulcer was undetermined.

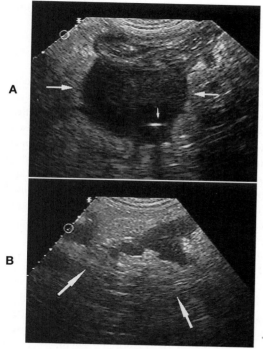

FIGURE 2-55 A, Oblique scan of the cecum *(large arrows)* in an 11-year-old mixed-breed dog presented for acute onset of vomiting and diarrhea, shaking, and tender abdomen. There is a well-defined hypoechoic mass arising from the cecum. Within the mass is a small hyperechoic focus *(small arrow)* that was suspected to be either gas or mineralization. **B,** Scan of mesentery adjacent to the cecal mass seen in **A.** There is hypoechoic tissue intermixed with hyperechoic tissue. This appearance is suggestive of hyperechoic reactive mesentery surrounding hypoechoic tissue that might be hemorrhage, necrosis, abscessation, or neoplastic implants. Diagnosis was mast cell tumor of the cecum with localized peritonitis from ulceration.

medial liver lobes lie on either side of the gallbladder. The cranial extent of the liver is delineated by the highly echogenic diaphragm. Caudal margins are partially bordered by the stomach and right kidney (Figure 2-59).

Normal liver parenchyma in the dog has a coarse echogenicity of medium intensity. It is usually more echogenic than renal cortices and less echogenic than spleen. In the cat, hyperechoic portal vessel walls are more prominent than in the dog (Figure 2-60). Normal feline liver echogenicity should be similar to falciform fat; however, increased body fat can cause the liver to be more echogenic than falciform in some cats, without clinical signs of disease.

Portal veins and hepatic veins appear as anechoic tubular, branching structures. Portal vein walls are hyperechoic, whereas hepatic vein walls are usually not visualized. Hepatic biliary ducts are normally not visible.

The main portal vein is ventral and axial to the vena cava. The porta hepatis, which is the site of bifurcation of the portal vein into right and left branches, images as a bright echogenic structure in the midliver. The increased echogenicity is due to fat deposition surrounding the structures in the porta hepatis.

The gallbladder is imaged to the right of midline between the quadrate and the right medial liver lobes. It is anechoic and usually shows distal enhancement. The gallbladder wall may or may not be seen as an echogenic linear structure. Echoic material is commonly found within the lumen of the gallbladder. The size of the gallbladder is variable. Gallbladder shape in dogs and most cats is ovoid, tapering to the neck of the gallblad-

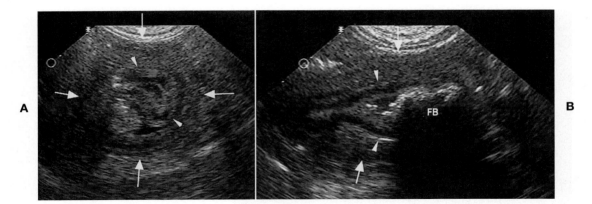

FIGURE 2-56 A, Transverse scan of small intestine *(large arrows)* in a 5-year-old Labrador retriever with nonspecific signs of abdominal pain and anorexia. One loop of small intestine *(arrowheads)* is surrounded by another loop *(arrows),* consistent with intussusception. **B,** Same dog as in **A.** Foreign material *(FB),* seen within the intussusceptum *(arrowheads),* surrounded by the intusscipiens *(arrows),* shows as a slightly irregular hyperechoic linear echogenicity with intense acoustic shadowing deep to the foreign material. Surgery confirmed the intussusception and the presence of cloth in the affected small bowel, which may have caused the intussusception.

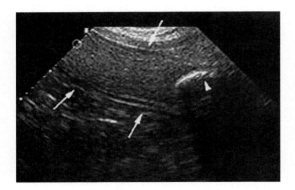

FIGURE 2-57 Sagittal scan of small intestine *(arrows)* in a 3-year-old domestic long hair cat with acute onset of lethargy and anorexia. The cat vomited bile 12 times overnight. The abdomen was tender to palpation. The small intestine is markedly dilated and filled with echoic fluid. A hyperechoic, curved focus that has acoustic shadowing is seen within the bowel lumen. Diagnosis was intestinal obstruction from hair, grass, and other foreign material.

der. Some cats may have bilobed gallbladders, but these are not considered clinically significant. The gallbladder neck is caudal to the body and connects with the cystic duct. Hepatic ducts empty into the cystic duct, at which point it becomes the common bile duct. Intrahepatic ducts are not normally imaged.

The common bile duct is ventral to the portal vein. It is not usually seen in normal dogs but may be imaged in some cats. The common bile duct may measure up to 4 mm in normal cats. Because

of its small size, it is difficult to visualize with low-frequency transducers.

Assessment of liver size is subjective. In most dogs the caudal ventral liver margin should be at or just caudal to the xiphoid. Body conformation will affect the normal position; for example, deep-chested breeds can have normal liver size, yet the liver can be imaged only from an intercostal location. Any intrathoracic process that results in the diaphragm and liver being caudally displaced can cause the liver to appear enlarged. Assessment of liver size is more accurate on radiographs than with ultrasound.

Sonographic Diagnosis of Liver Disease

Hepatic Parenchymal Disease

Ultrasound is an excellent way to evaluate liver parenchyma. It is particularly useful in differentiating focal from diffuse disease, differentiating cystic from solid masses, and identifying the presence and cause of biliary obstruction. Although ultrasound is sensitive in showing architectural parenchymal changes, it is not specific as to the cause of these changes. Therefore, an abnormality is seen, but the final diagnosis requires a liver biopsy. Multiple samples should be obtained because concurrent disease processes may be present in the liver; for example, lipidosis may be present along with cholangiohepatitis or neoplasia. Aspirates can be obtained but may not accurately reflect all changes occurring in the liver. Diffuse hepatic disease can exist without altering the normal sonographic appearance of the liver.

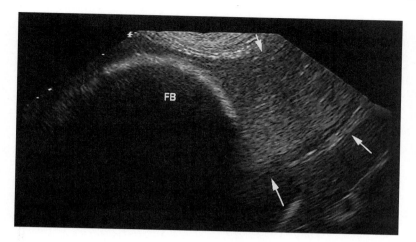

FIGURE 2-58 Scan of the stomach *(arrows)* in a 9-year-old Labrador retriever with a history of anorexia and lethargy. A large, curved, faintly echogenic structure with acoustic shadowing *(FB)* is seen within the stomach lumen. Surgery discovered a portion of a ball in the stomach.

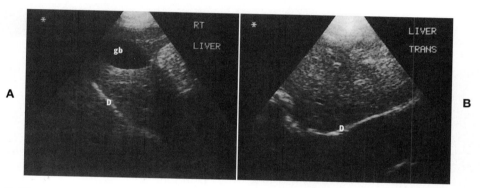

FIGURE 2-59 Sagittal **(A)** and transverse **(B)** scans of a normal canine liver. *D*, Diaphragm; *gb*, gallbladder.

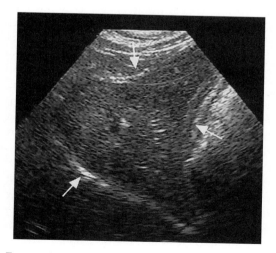

FIGURE 2-60 Sagittal scan of a normal feline liver *(arrows)*. The liver is homogeneous with prominent portal vessel wall and is slightly hypoechoic to falciform fat.

Indications for hepatic ultrasound include the following:

1. Elevated liver enzymes—Ultrasound images often show focal or diffuse hepatic disease not visible on radiographs.
2. Free abdominal fluid—Sonography can help differentiate among neoplastic masses, diffuse hepatic disease such as cirrhosis, and hepatic venous congestion.
3. To determine extent of hepatic neoplasia—Sonography can determine if the tumor is confined to one or multiple liver lobes or if there is extension to lymph nodes or other abdominal organs. This provides information that is used to determine if the patient has a lesion that can be surgically excised.
4. To differentiate obstructive from nonobstructive icterus—Dilation of the common bile duct, cystic duct, or hepatic ducts is readily visualized with ultrasound. Causes of the obstruction (e.g., calculi, masses, pancreatitis) can be imaged.

FIGURE 2-61 Sagittal scan of the liver *(arrows)* in an 8-year-old mixed-breed dog with a history of abdominal distension and anorexia for 2 days. Liver enzyme levels were markedly elevated, total bilirubin level was 1.8, and WBC was 19,000. The liver margins are irregular and nodular. Liver echogenicity is nonhomogeneous with patchy hyperechoic and hypoechoic regions and hypoechoic nodules. Anechoic free abdominal fluid surrounds the liver. Diagnosis was hepatic cirrhosis with nodular hyperplasia.

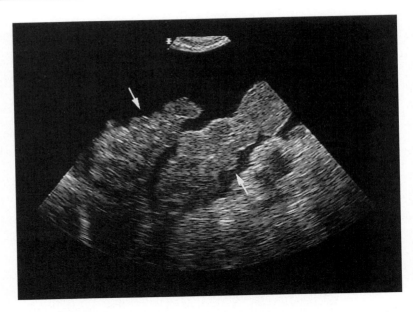

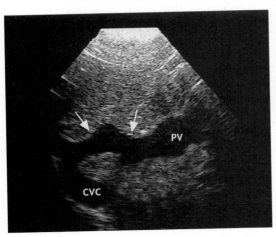

FIGURE 2-62 Sagittal scan of the liver in a 4-year-old springer spaniel mix with vomiting, diarrhea, weight loss, and decreased appetite. Liver enzyme levels were mildly elevated. The liver imaged very small, and an intrahepatic shunt *(arrows)* was discovered connecting the portal vein *(PV)* to the caudal vena cava *(CVC)*.

5. To differentiate cystic from solid masses— Benign cysts are anechoic, have thin, defined walls, and show increased echogenicity deep to the cyst.
6. To identify gallbladder calculi, cholecystitis, or ruptured gallbladder.
7. To image congenital or acquired portocaval or portosystemic shunts—This requires meticulous inspection of the abdomen using various scanning planes.
8. Biopsy—Ultrasound-guided hepatic biopsy allows precise direction of the biopsy needle to

the area of abnormal tissue and avoidance of large vessels, the gallbladder, and the GI tract.

Diffuse Liver Disease

The liver may appear sonographically normal despite the presence of liver disease. However, subjective assessment of liver size, shape, and echogenicity is helpful in determining the presence of a diffuse disorder.

Liver Size

Small livers are detected with chronic hepatitis, cirrhosis (Figure 2-61), liver shunts (Figure 2-62), liver atrophy, and diaphragmatic hernias. Enlarged livers can be seen with metabolic disease, neoplasia, granulomatous disease, hepatobiliary inflammation, feline lipidosis, venous congestion, cystic disease, abscesses, nodular hyperplasia, and biliary disease.

Liver Shape

Irregular liver shape or margin is frequently associated with cirrhosis, hyperplasia, neoplasia, abscesses, and granulomas. Sometimes it is necessary to use a 7.5-mHz or higher transducer, even on a large dog, to image the ventral liver margin to detect subtle margin irregularity.

Liver Echogenicity

In diffuse disease, changes in echogenicity include homogeneously hypoechoic, homogeneously hyperechoic, and patchy hypoechoic and hyperechoic zones or nodules. One lobe, multiple lobes, or segments of lobes may be affected.

Hypoechogenicity of the liver is a subjective assessment, but comparing liver with known surrounding normal tissues is helpful. Renal cortex and falciform fat are usually less echogenic than is

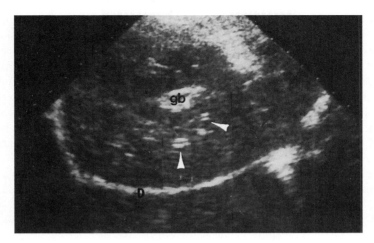

FIGURE 2-63 Liver scan of an Irish wolfhound presented for depression and icterus with elevated bilirubin and alkaline phosphatase. There is a very thick hyperechoic gallbladder wall. The gallbladder *(gb)* is not distended. The entire liver is hypoechoic. Multiple anechoic tubular structures with defined hyperechoic walls are seen throughout the liver *(arrowheads)*. These most likely represent portal veins that are better visualized owing to surrounding hypoechoic liver. Sonographic changes suggest cholecystitis and cholangiohepatitis. Surgery showed a diffusely enlarged liver filled with dark, inspissated bile. Diagnosis was cholangiohepatitis with severe canalicular bile stasis, consistent with a toxic insult. *D,* Diaphragm.

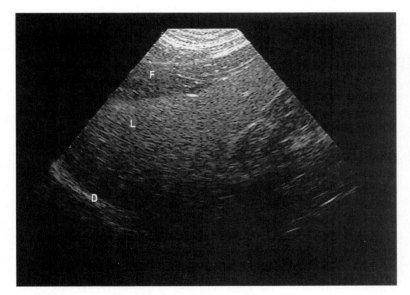

FIGURE 2-64 Sagittal scan of the liver in an 8-year-old domestic medium hair cat with some vomiting and diarrhea, anorexia for 1 week, and icterus. Liver enzyme levels were elevated, total bilirubin level was 12.3, and WBC was normal. The liver *(L)* is hyperechoic with loss of visualization of portal vessel walls and sound beam attenuation in the deeper portions of the liver. Falciform fat *(F)* appears hypoechoic to liver echogencity. Diagnosis was hepatic lipidosis. *D,* Diaphragm.

liver in dogs. Vessel walls appear more echogenic and more numerous, and gallbladder wall may be more prominent or thickened. Hypoechoic livers have been associated with diseases that accumulate fluid in hepatocytes, such as acute hepatitis, cholangiohepatitis (Figure 2-63), hepatic venous congestion (will also see dilated hepatic veins and caudal vena cava), and hepatic necrosis. Lymphosarcoma may also appear diffusely hypoechoic. These disorders are the more common causes for hypoechoic livers, but other processes are possible.

Inflammation or infection of other organs, such as pancreatitis, prostatitis, or gastroenteritis, may also cause the liver to appear diffusely hypoechoic, possibly secondary to septicemia.

Hyperechogenicity of the liver is subjectively determined by comparison with known surrounding normal tissues and decreased visualization of hepatic vasculature. Some infiltrative processes, particularly feline lipidosis, will cause attenuation of the sound beam in the deeper parts of the liver (Figure 2-64). Disease processes that are associated with hyperechoic liver include lipidosis, steroid hepatopathy (due to increased glycogen storage), cholangiohepatitis, chronic hepatitis, cirrhosis, diabetes mellitus, and lymphosarcoma. This list is not all-inclusive, and other processes are possible.

Patchy liver echo patterns with mixed hypoechoic, hyperechoic, and isoechoic regions are a nonspecific change that suggests a diffuse disorder. Some of the areas may show or mimic nodularity. The changes may reflect a mixture of normal liver, inflammation, fatty infiltration, hepatopathy, hepatic necrosis, hyperplasia, neoplasia, and other disease processes (Figure 2-65). Histologic diagnosis is necessary for definitive diagnosis. Hepatocutaneous syndrome has a fairly characteristic diffuse echopattern of hyperechoic, "lacey" strands that surround ovoid to spherical hypoechoic zones (Figure 2-66).

Focal Liver Disease

Ultrasound is useful to describe the appearance of focal lesions in the liver. The size, shape, number, margin definition, and echogenicity are easily characterized, except for very small masses, such as seen with carcinomatosis, which may not be detected. Focal lesions in the liver can appear hypoechoic, hyperechoic, anechoic, or isoechoic or have a combination of any of these echogenicities. Ultrasound can help determine the number and location of lesions and association with structures such as the portal vein, caudal vena cava, and gallbladder, which may affect the decision on whether to attempt surgical excision.

Anechoic focal lesions can be caused by true cysts, biliary pseudocysts, parasitic cysts, enlarged end-on bile ducts, abscesses, and arteriovenous fistulas (Figure 2-67). Hyperechoic, hypoechoic, and mixed echoic masses can be caused by metastatic or primary neoplasia, lymphosarcoma, abscesses, granulomas, nodular hyperplasia, biliary cystadenomas, and hematomas (Figures 2-68 to 2-75). Correlating history and clinical findings is helpful in forming a differential diagnosis, but biopsy is needed for definitive diagnosis.

Gallbladder Disease

1. Extrahepatic biliary obstruction (experimental) results in the following:
   a. Rapid gallbladder distention
   b. Bile duct enlargement by 48 hours
   c. Extrahepatic duct dilation by 3 days

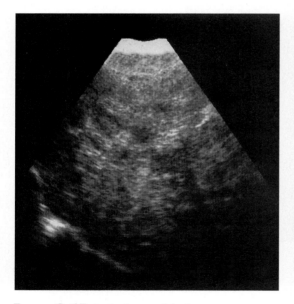

FIGURE 2-65 Sagittal scan of the liver in an 8-year-old German shepherd–mix that was on long-term phenobarbital for seizures. Liver enzyme levels were elevated. Ultrasound shows a nonhomogeneous liver echogenicity with patchy hyperechoic zones throughout the liver. Diagnosis was moderate hepatitis with nodular hyperplasia and vacuolar hepatopathy, possibly secondary to chronic phenobarbital administration.

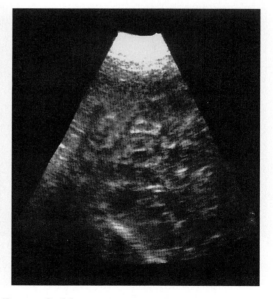

FIGURE 2-66 Sagittal scan of the liver in an 11-year-old Skye terrier with a 3- to 4-week history of severely inflamed, thickened, painful footpads on all four feet. Liver enzyme levels were elevated. The liver is diffusely nonhomogeneous with numerous hypoechoic nodules intermixed with hyperechoic strands. Overall liver texture appears coarse and has been described as a "Swiss cheese–like" or "honeycomb" appearance. Diagnosis was hepatocutaneous syndrome.

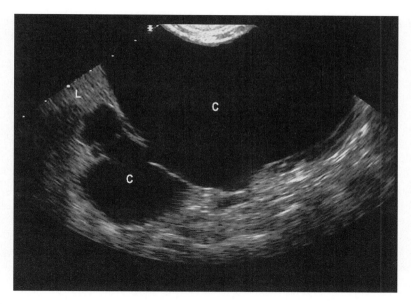

FIGURE 2-67 Transverse scan of the liver in a 10-year-old domestic short hair cat presented for routine vaccinations. A mass was palpated in the cranial abdomen. Ultrasound shows a large, thin-walled, anechoic structure *(C)* with a small connecting anechoic structure *(C)*. A small portion of liver *(L)* is seen. Diagnosis was probable congenital hepatic cyst.

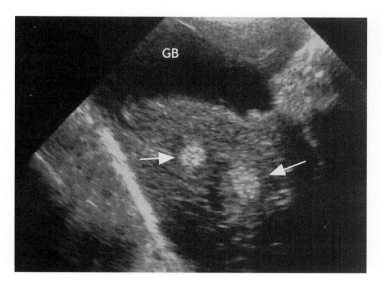

FIGURE 2-68 Sagittal scan of the liver in a 14-year-old German shepherd with multiple splenic and hepatic masses. Hyperechoic nodules *(arrows)* are seen in the liver, near the gallbladder *(GB)*. Diagnosis was metastatic hemangiosarcoma.

    d. Intrahepatic duct dilation by 7 days (Figure 2-76).

Pathologic biliary obstruction is usually mechanical secondary to liver, biliary, pancreatic, or duodenal inflammatory or neoplastic disease. These diseases can be sonographically visualized. Obstruction from biliary calculi is rare but is easily imaged. Mild intrahepatic duct dilation is seen on an ultrasound image as two parallel, anechoic channels in close proximity to each other. One channel is a portal vessel, and the other is a bile duct. The duct may have a tortuous appearance. Large intrahepatic duct dilations can be tubular or may look cystic, due to cross-sectioning of the duct.

2. Thickened gallbladder wall
    a. Diffusely hyperechoic wall, with or without shadowing, is often seen with cholecystitis, calcification or fibrosis, acute hepatitis, and cholangiohepatitis.

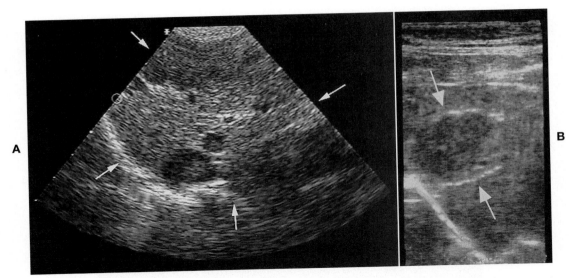

FIGURE 2-69 A, Transverse scan of the liver *(arrows)* in a 13-year-old springer spaniel with a history of weight loss and anorexia for 2 days. Focal, hypoechoic masses are seen within the liver. A large, mixed echoic mass was seen on another scan of a different area of liver. Diagnosis was metastatic hepatocellular carcinoma. **B,** Sagittal scan of the liver in an 11-year-old domestic short hair cat. A circumscribed, hypoechoic mass *(arrows)* is apparent. Diagnosis was metastasis from a cecal adenocarcinoma.

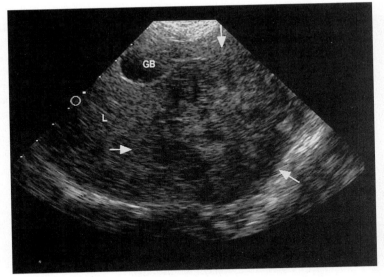

FIGURE 2-70 Transverse scan of the liver *(L)* in a 13-year-old golden retriever with vague signs of lethargy and anorexia. A mixed hypoechoic and patchy anechoic mass *(arrows)* is seen in the midliver and left liver. Margins on the mass are not sharply defined. Diagnosis was hepatocellular carcinoma.

b. Focal hyperechoic areas, with or without shadowing, are commonly associated with mineralization, fibrosis, or calculi.

c. "Halo" or double rim around gallbladder wall usually indicates wall edema or inflammation but can be seen with free abdominal fluid. Abdominal imaging should help differentiate wall edema from abdominal fluid (Figure 2-77).

d. Generalized wall thickening, with or without irregular mucosa, is consistent with inflammation (Figure 2-78). Nondistended

gallbladder walls may appear slightly thickened in normal patients.
3. Gallbladder and bile duct masses
   a. Calculi/concretions are hyperechoic and usually show shadowing deep to the calculus (Figure 2-79).
   b. Neoplasia is variable with circumscribed or ill-defined echogenicity in area of gallbladder or bile duct, with or without biliary obstruction (Figure 2-80).

   c. Polypoid, echoic masses in gallbladder may be due to glandular cystic hypertrophy.
   d. Biliary sludge may mimic mass lesions. If necessary, positional (gravitational) sonographic studies should be performed to further characterize gallbladder echoes.

Normal Sonographic Anatomy of the Pancreas

The pancreas can be imaged in normal dogs, cats, and most ferrets.

The right limb of the pancreas is found dorsomedial to the descending duodenum. The presence of the pancreaticoduodenal vein within the pancreas facilitates pancreatic identification (Figure 2-81). The left limb is more difficult to image in the dog because of its close relationship with the stomach and transverse colon and overlying gas; however, with perseverance it can often be located. The left limb is usually visualized in the cat between the transverse colon and the stomach (Figure 2-82).

Gross adjacent anatomic landmarks are described as follows: The right lobe is found dorsal or dorsomedial to the duodenum, cranioventral to the right kidney, ventrolateral to the portal vein, and between the ninth and tenth intercostal spaces to the level of the fourth lumbar vertebra. The left lobe is found dorsocaudal to the stomach, dorsocranial to the transverse colon, ventrolateral to the portal vein, ventral to the aorta and caudal vena cava, and dorsomedial to the spleen.

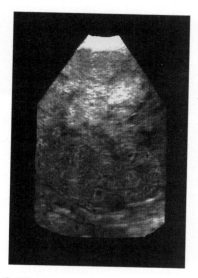

FIGURE 2-71 Scan of a large liver mass in a 12-year-old German Shepherd–mix with normal liver enzyme levels. The mass constitutes most of this image, with no normal liver parenchyma visible. It has a mixed hyperechoic and hypoechoic echo pattern and poorly defined margins. Diagnosis was hepatocellular carcinoma.

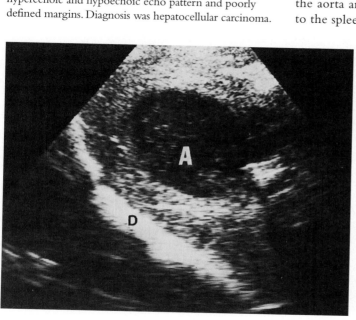

FIGURE 2-72 Sagittal liver scan of a Doberman pinscher with a history of gastric dilatation-volvulus and subsequent gastric rupture. A large, well-circumscribed hypoechoic mass (A) is seen in the midliver. A liver abscess was suspected and was confirmed at surgery. D, Diaphragm.

FIGURE 2-73 A, Sagittal scan
of the liver in a 10-year-old
Gordon setter with a history of
lethargy and an elevated
temperature of 105.6° F. The
WBC was normal, but liver
enzyme levels were mildly
elevated. There is a large mass in
the liver *(arrows)* that has mixed
echogenicity with a large central
anechoic region. Purulent
material was drained from the
mass. Culture indicated a hepatic
abscess due to hemolytic
Staphylococcus. Diagnosis based on
a biopsy specimen of the mass
was also chronic hepatic abscess.
B, One-month repeat ultrasound
of the area in **A** after antibiotic
therapy. The mass is still visible
but appears smaller and more
homogeneous with no evidence
of fluid within the mass.

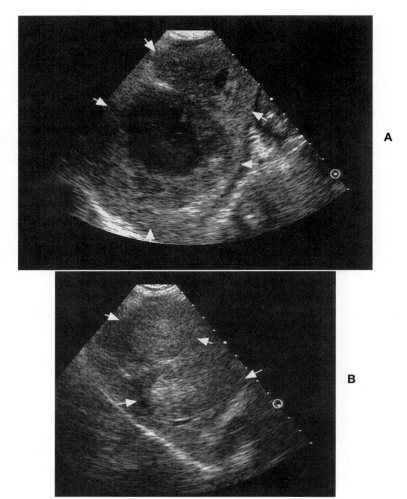

FIGURE 2-74 Transverse scan
of the liver in a 14-year-old
Persian cat with hematuria.
The hyperechoic liver mass
contains tiny cysts. It has a
defined but irregular margin.
Diagnosis was biliary
cystadenoma. Cystadenomas
have been reported to have
variable ultrasound patterns
that usually include
hyperechogenicity with
variable-sized cyst or cysts.
They can be multifocal or
singular. *GB,* Gallbladder.

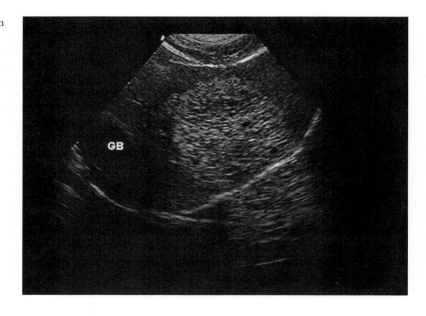

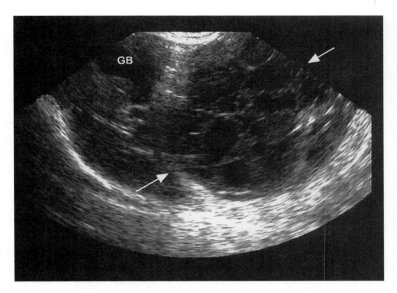

FIGURE 2-75 Oblique scan of the liver in a 14-year-old domestic short hair cat with vomiting and lethargy. Liver enzyme levels were mildly elevated; values for BUN, creatinine, and phosphorus were also elevated. The scan shows a very large, multicystic mass *(arrows)*. Biopsy of the mass was not performed, but sonographic differential diagnoses included primary neoplasia such as hepatocellular or biliary carcinoma, cystadenoma, hematoma, abscess, and nodular hyperplasia.

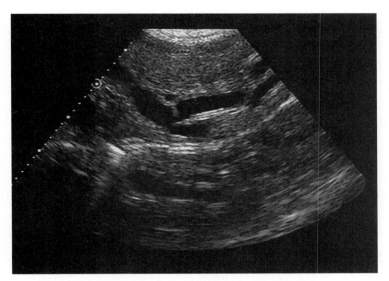

FIGURE 2-76 Transverse scan of the liver in a 4-year-old domestic short hair cat with intermittent vomiting and lethargy for 3 months and weight loss. There were marked elevations in liver enzyme levels, minor total bilirubin level elevation, and normal WBC. The anechoic tubular structures seen represent moderately dilated intrahepatic bile ducts. The dilation was due to a benign mass in the common bile duct (see Figure 2-80).

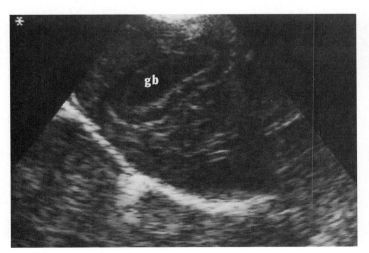

FIGURE 2-77 Sagittal scan of a Chihuahua. Gallbladder *(gb)* has a well-defined hypoechoic rim. This change is associated with gallbladder wall edema and/or inflammation.

FIGURE 2-78 Sagittal scan of the gallbladder in a 16-year-old domestic short hair cat that was vomiting and not eating for 3 days. Liver enzyme levels were moderately elevated, and total bilirubin level was mildly elevated. The gallbladder wall is mildly thickened with irregular mucosal surface. Gallbladder size appears normal. The tiny hyperechoic foci deep to the gallbladder are biliary stones. Changes were consistent with either cholecystitis and/or mucinous hyperplasia.

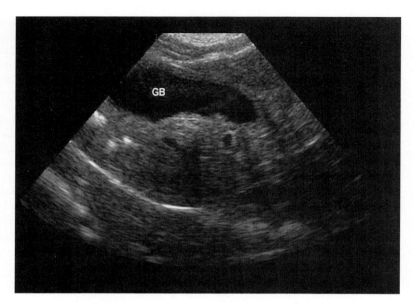

FIGURE 2-79 **A,** Sagittal scan of the common bile duct in the cat seen in Figure 2-78. The bile duct is markedly dilated with obstruction distally by a hyperechoic focus with acoustic shadowing, most likely a calculus. **B,** Oblique scan of the liver in the cat seen in **A** and in Figure 2-78. Numerous hyperechoic foci are seen throughout the liver, some following a linear course, most likely intrahepatic biliary calculi.

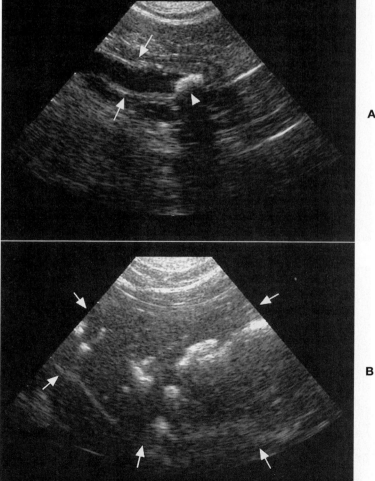

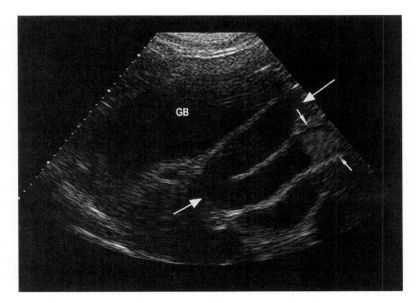

FIGURE 2-80 Oblique scan of the gallbladder *(GB)* and common bile duct *(large arrows)* in the cat seen in Figure 2-76. The bile duct is markedly dilated and is obstructed by an echogenic mass *(small arrows)* that appears to be intraluminal. The mass was determined to be benign fibroplasia of unknown cause.

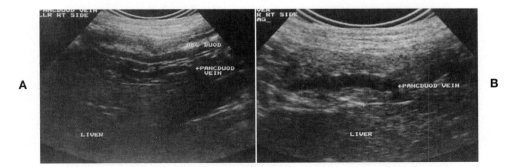

FIGURE 2-81 Sagittal scan of a normal dog pancreas showing the dorsal relationship to the duodenum **(A)** and the anechoic pancreaticoduodenal vein present within the pancreas **(B).**

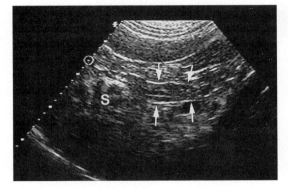

FIGURE 2-82 Sagittal scan of the left limb of the pancreas *(arrows)* in a normal cat. *S,* Stomach.

Pancreatic parenchyma is isoechoic to slightly hyperechoic compared with hepatic parenchyma, with a homogeneous echo pattern.

The right limb of the pancreas is best imaged with the patient in left lateral recumbency. A right intercostal approach is frequently necessary.

Sonographic Diagnosis of Pancreatic Disease

Acute Pancreatitis

Mild, acute pancreatitis may not be easily differentiated from normal pancreatic tissue, but in some cases the pancreas can be seen as mildly enlarged

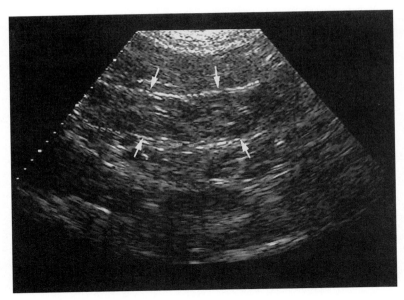

FIGURE 2-83 Sagittal scan of the pancreas *(arrows)* in an 8-year-old tortiseshell cat with a history of anorexia and hiding. The pancreas is mildly enlarged and nonhomogeneous with patchy hypoechoic zones and has slightly irregular margins. Sonographic diagnosis was pancreatic inflammation. The cat's signs resolved with medical therapy.

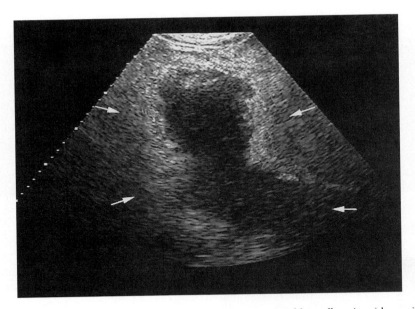

FIGURE 2-84 Oblique scan through the area of the pancreas in a 9-year-old poodle-mix with vomiting, diarrhea, shaking, anorexia, and fever. The WBC was 20,700, and the alkaline phosphatase level was mildly elevated. The pancreas is markedly enlarged, hypoechoic to anechoic, irregular in shape, and surrounded by hyperechoic tissue. Sonographic diagnosis was acute pancreatitis with localized peripancreatic inflammation. The dog recovered following 1 week of medical therapy.

and nonhomogeneous (Figure 2-83). The pancreas usually enlarges and is hypoechoic in moderate to severe pancreatitis. Anechoic cavitations may occur owing to necrosis, abscess, or hemorrhage (Figures 2-84 and 2-85). Peripancreatic hyperechoic mesentery and/or anechoic fluid may be visible. Decreased motility or thickening of proximal duodenum may be apparent. Intrahepatic and extra-

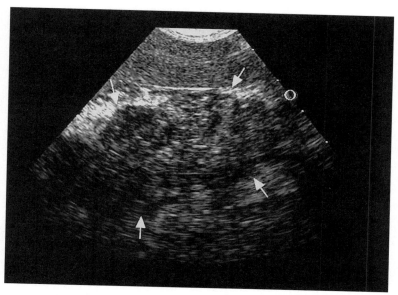

FIGURE 2-85 Oblique scan of the pancreas *(arrows)* in an 8-year-old Irish setter with shaking, groaning, and abdominal pain. Ingestion of garbage had occurred 2 days previously. There was mild elevation of alkaline phosphatase level. The pancreas appears markedly enlarged with mixed hypoechoic and anechoic zones surrounded by echogenic tissue. The anechoic regions were thought to be either hemorrhage and/or necrosis. Sonographic diagnosis was acute pancreatitis. Medical therapy was instituted, and a recheck ultrasound 1 week later showed approximately 50% decrease in size with persistent nonhomogeneous echo pattern. The dog continued to improve with resolution of signs 2 weeks later.

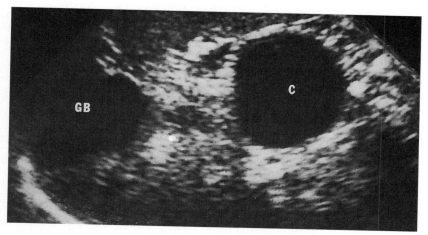

FIGURE 2-86 Sagittal liver scan of a mixed-breed dog presented with icterus and neurologic abnormalities. Gallbladder *(GB)* is distended. An anechoic cystic structure *(C)* is seen caudal to the gallbladder and liver. A pancreatic cyst was suspected. Laparotomy located a cystic bile-filled mass between the left and the right pancreatic limbs attached to omentum and an atrophic left pancreas. Diagnosis was a cystic structure with residual pancreatic tissue in the fibrous wall.

hepatic biliary duct obstruction may be observed. In the healing stage there may be homogeneous or irregular increased echogenicity, presumably due to fibrosis and/or calcification. Calcification may or may not show shadowing, depending on its thickness. Anechoic pseudocyst formation, either single or multiple, may occur (Figures 2-86 and 2-87). Nodular hyperplasia may develop in the pancreas (Figure 2-88), as well as diffuse pancreatic hyperplasia, which appears as a normal echogenicity but very enlarged with smooth borders, based on one case that was histologically confirmed.

FIGURE 2-87 Sagittal scan of the left pancreas *(arrows)* in a 12-year-old domestic short hair cat. Clinical signs were nonspecific anorexia and lethargy with normal results of blood tests. The pancreas is mildly enlarged, patchy hypoechoic, and irregular in shape and has a small anechoic structure that appears cystlike. Sonographic diagnosis was pancreatic inflammation with possible small cyst. The cat recovered with medical therapy.

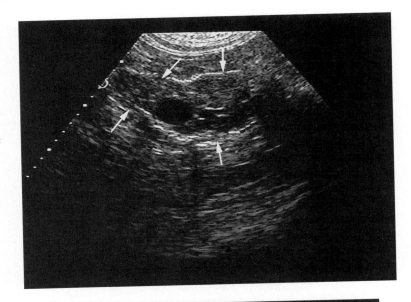

FIGURE 2-88 Images of the pancreas *(arrows)* in a 14-year-old domestic long hair cat with hematuria. The pancreas has several small **(A)** and large **(B)** hypoechoic nodules. At surgery for removal of cystic calculi, biopsy of a pancreatic nodule was performed, and the nodule was determined to be hyperplasia.

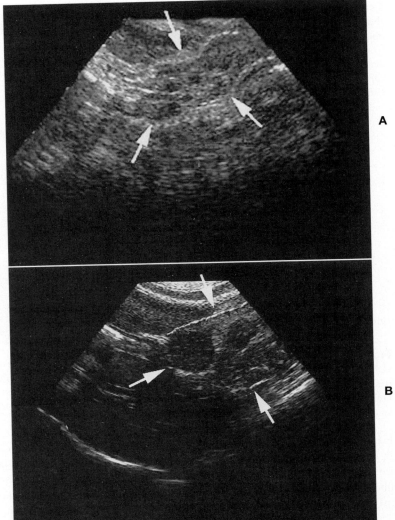

A

B

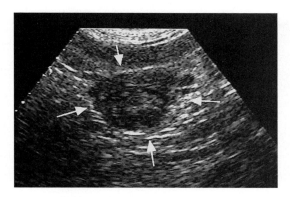

FIGURE 2-89 Scan of the pancreas *(arrows)* in a 10-year-old domestic medium hair cat with a history of weight loss and vomiting. There was a slight increase in lipase level, slight decrease in albumin level, and mild anemia. The pancreas has a circumscribed mixed hypoechogenic mass. Other areas of the pancreas imaged normally, but local lymph nodes were enlarged (not seen on this scan). Diagnosis was pancreatic andenocarcinoma.

Chronic Pancreatitis

The size of the pancreas may be normal or enlarged, with increased echogenicity or a mixed echo pattern. Calcification in pancreatic parenchyma may shadow. Biliary dilation may be observed, even when active obstruction no longer exists.

Pancreatic Masses

The pancreas is enlarged, and the mass may have well-defined borders. Masses may be hypoechoic or hyperechoic or have mixed echogenicity. Solid masses may be neoplasms, hematomas, granulomas, or abscesses (Figure 2-89). Large cystic lesions may occur in cystadenocarcinoma. Differentiation from pseudocyst is difficult; however, cystadenocarcinomas usually have an irregular wall thickness with small masses along at least one border of the cyst. Neoplastic processes may invade surrounding structures, especially adjacent vessels. Lymph node enlargement may be observed with neoplasia. Biliary obstruction may occur. Some tumors, such as insulinomas, are very small and difficult to identify.

REFERENCES

Agut A, Wood AKW, Martin CA: Sonographic observations of the gastroduodenal junction of dogs, *Am J Vet Res* 57:1266, 1996.

Baez JL et al.: Radiographic, ultrasonographic, and endoscopic findings in cats with inflammatory bowel disease of the stomach and small intestine: 33 cases (1990-1997), *J Am Vet Med Assoc* 215:349, 1999.

Biller DS, Kantrowitz B, Miyabayashi T: Ultrasonography of diffuse liver disease: a review, *J Vet Intern Med* 6:71, 1992.

Bostwick DR, Twedt DC: Intrahepatic and extrahepatic portal venous anomalies in dogs: 52 cases (1982-1993), *J Am Vet Med Assoc* 206:1181, 1995.

Delaney F, O'Brien RT, Waller K: Ultrasonographic small intestinal thickness in normal dogs, ACVR meeting, Nov-Dec 1999, Chicago (abstract).

Etue S et al.: Ultrasonography of the normal feline pancreas, ACVR meeting, Nov-Dec 1999, Chicago (abstract).

Farrar ET, Washabau RJ, Saunders HM: Hepatic abscesses in dogs: 14 cases (1982-1994), *J Am Vet Med Assoc* 208:243, 1996.

Gagne JM et al.: Clinical features of inflammatory liver disease in cats: 41 cases (1983-1993), *J Am Vet Med Assoc* 214:513, 1999.

Hess RS et al.: Clinical, clinicopathologic, radiographic, and ultrasonographic abnormalities in dogs with fatal acute pancreatitis: 70 cases (1986-1995), *J Am Vet Med Assoc* 213:665, 1998.

Holt DE, Schelling CG, Saunders HM: Correlation of ultrasonographic findings with surgical, portographic, and necropsy findings in dogs and cats with portosystemic shunts: 63 cases (1987-1993), *J Am Vet Med Assoc* 207:1190, 1995.

Hunt GB, Mahoney P, Bellenger CR: Successful management of an iatrogenic biliary pseudocyst in a dog, *J Am Anim Hosp Assoc* 33:166, 1997.

Jacobson LS, Kirberger RM, Nesbit JW: Hepatic ultrasonography and pathological findings in dogs with hepatocutaneous syndrome: new concepts, *J Vet Intern Med* 9:399, 1995.

Lamb CR: Abdominal ultrasonography in small animals: examination of the liver, spleen and pancreas, *J Small Anim Pract* 31:6, 1990.

Leveille R, Biller DS, Shiroma JT: Sonographic evaluation of the common bile duct in cats, *J Vet Intern Med* 10:296, 1996.

Morita Y et al.: Endoscopic ultrasonographic findings of the pancreas after pancreatic duct ligation in the dog, *Vet Radiol Ultrasound* 39:557, 1998.

Morita Y et al.: Endoscopic ultrasonography of the pancreas in the dog, *Vet Radiol Ultrasound* 39:552, 1998.

Newell SM et al.: Correlations between ultrasonographic findings and specific hepatic diseases in cats: 72 cases (1985-1997), *J Am Vet Med Assoc* 213:94, 1998.

Newell SM et al.: Sonography of the normal feline gastrointestinal tract, *Vet Radiol Ultrasound* 40:40, 1999.

Nyland TG, Koblik PD, Tellyer SE: Ultrasonographic evaluation of biliary cystadenomas in cats, *Vet Radiol Ultrasound* 40:300, 1999.

Penninck DG, Moore AS, Gliatto J: Ultrasonography of canine gastric epithelial neoplasia, *Vet Radiol Ultrasound* 39:342, 1998.

Rivers BJ et al.: Canine gastric neoplasia: utility of ultrasonography in diagnosis, *J Am Anim Hosp Assoc* 33:144, 1997.

Schwarz LA, Penninck DG, Leveille-Webster C: Hepatic abscesses in 13 dogs: a review of the ultrasonographic findings, clinical data and therapeutic options, *Vet Radiol Ultrasound* 39:357, 1998.

Weiss DJ, Gagne JM, Armstrong PJ: Relationship between inflammatory hepatic disease and inflamma-tory bowel disease, pancreatitis, and nephritis in cats, *J Am Vet Med Assoc* 209:1114, 1996.

Whiteley MB et al.: Ultrasonographic appearance of primary and metastatic canine hepatic tumors: a review of 48 cases, *J Ultrasound Med* 8:621, 1989.

Yeager AE, Mohammed H: Accuracy of ultrasonography in the detection of severe hepatic lipidosis in cats, *Am J Vet Res* 53:597, 1992.

ENDOSCOPY AND LAPAROSCOPY IN VETERINARY GASTROENTEROLOGY

Todd R. Tams

Biopsies of digestive system organs are commonly indicated in the practice of small animal medicine. Before the advent of endoscopy, laparoscopy, and ultrasonography in veterinary medicine, the routine method of obtaining tissue samples was by laparotomy. Liver samples were routinely obtained using either blind percutaneous or keyhole biopsy techniques, or wedge or needle samples were procured surgically.

The primary advantage of a surgical approach to organ biopsy is that, depending on the size of the incision, a large area of the digestive organs can be examined and palpated in conjunction with evaluation of other structures (e.g., lymph nodes, kidneys, ureters, prostate). Disadvantages of laparotomy include the invasive nature of the procedure when compared with endoscopy, laparoscopy, or ultrasonography; the longer periods of hospital-ization that are required for postoperative recovery; and an unwillingness on the part of many owners to subject their pets to any type of major procedure unless "it is really necessary."

Exploratory laparotomy has and always will be an excellent diagnostic procedure. The use of isoflurane anesthesia combined with our ever-increasing ability to provide better preoperative, intraoperative, and postoperative support for our animal patients, which includes more routine use of effective analgesic agents, has helped make exploratory laparotomy a safer procedure. However, the trend in human medicine over the last 20 years has moved strongly toward using the least invasive methods possible to examine and, when indicated, obtain biopsy samples from abdominal tissues. There has been a similar but more recent trend in veterinary medicine, beginning first in university and specialty practices and now encompassing many smaller practices. It is quite clear that, in situations in which it has been determined that biopsies are necessary, owners prefer and are more likely to allow procedures that are considered less invasive and as causing less overall discomfort to their pet. Indeed, most owners are aware of the tremendous advances in diagnostic technology in the human medical field, and they are often anxious to have these methods utilized in the diagnosis of their pet's disorder.

Endoscopy, laparoscopy, and ultrasonography have many applications in veterinary medicine. As awareness of the tremendous diagnostic potential of these procedures has increased among veterinarians, many clinicians are beginning to purchase equipment and learn these new techniques or are more readily making this technology available to their clients on a referral basis. Applications for use of ultrasonography for diagnosis of disorders of the digestive system, as well as many case examples, are presented in Chapter 2. Endoscopy and laparoscopy are discussed in this chapter, with emphasis on the clinical utility of these techniques.

ENDOSCOPY

Endoscopy is one of the best and yet most fundamental methods of examining the gastrointestinal (GI) tract. It is now a well-established procedure in veterinary medicine. The opportunity to directly examine and obtain tissue samples from the esophagus, stomach, and intestinal tract in a minimally invasive way has greatly altered the clinical approach to diagnosis and has made significantly more accurate the treatment of disorders of the digestive system. Despite the tremendous diagnostic advantages that endoscopy offers, it is still best used by the clinician as an adjunctive procedure in the evaluation of GI disease. A thorough review of the history, complete physical examination, and selected laboratory and radiographic examinations as appropriate for each individual case are still important for thorough patient evaluation. When used judiciously, endoscopy offers a valuable alternative to exploratory surgery for direct examination of tissues, procurement of biopsy samples, and retrieval of foreign bodies.

Selection of an Endoscope

Endoscopic equipment is no longer considered a luxury that only large referral centers or veterinar-

ians practicing in affluent areas can justify purchasing. An endoscope is one of the most versatile and diagnostically valuable pieces of equipment that a veterinary practice can have in its armamentarium. The selection of equipment to be used for performing endoscopy often depends on its versatility of application, durability, and expense. Many practices have been able to financially justify the purchase of high-quality endoscopic equipment. When consideration is given to the purchase of an endoscope, the most important factors to be reviewed should be the probable frequency of usage and versatility of the instrument rather than the purchase price.

Other important considerations are the quality of the optical system and ease of operating the endoscope. Significant differences exist, so equipment purchases should be made carefully! Too frequently veterinarians rank a lower purchase price as one of the most important factors. This can be a significant mistake because even the most skilled endoscopist may find performing a complete examination and making the correct diagnosis difficult while using an endoscope of poor quality.

My recommendation to veterinarians interested in purchasing their first endoscope is to buy a single high-quality endoscope that may be used for a variety of procedures (e.g., esophagogastroduodenoscopy, colonoscopy, bronchoscopy, and nasopharyngoscopy in dogs) in cats and small dogs, as well as in large dogs. A pediatric endoscope with *four-way* tip deflection capability meets these criteria well (Figure 3-1). Endoscopes

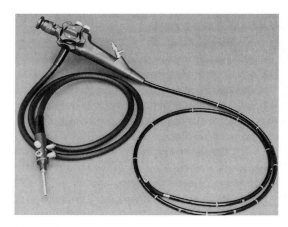

FIGURE 3-1 Storz pediatric veterinary endoscope. Specifications include 8.5mm–diameter insertion tube, 100-degrees forward-viewing field of view, 150-cm working length, 2.5mm–diameter accessory channel, and four-way tip deflection.

with two-way distal tip deflection capability have very limited use in GI endoscopy. Most of these endoscopes are relatively short (50 to 80 cm) and are intended to be used primarily as broncho-scopes. It is somewhat more difficult to maneuver an endoscope that is limited to two-way distal deflection through the antral canal, pylorus, and duodenum. The preferred insertion tube diameter should range from 7.8 to 9 mm. The major limitation of a large insertion tube (diameter of 9.8 mm or greater) is that there is more difficulty in passing it through the pyloric canal to the duodenum in cats and small dogs. *This is an important consideration because an effort should be made to examine the duodenum in all cases in which vomiting, diarrhea, or weight loss is part of the clinical presentation.* Larger endoscopes can be used quite effectively in many animal patients, but there are inherent difficulties in performing a complete examination in very small animals. This becomes an important factor for any urban practice in which many cats and small dogs are seen. A standard working length of 100 cm or more is adequate for performing a thorough examination in cats and most dogs. Unfortunately 100-cm endoscopes are occasionally not long enough to reach the duodenum in large breed dogs. Newer, more versatile pediatric veterinary endoscopes with an insertion tube length of 140 to 150 cm are now available. With these longer endoscopes it is possible to easily reach the duodenum in even the largest dogs.

In addition to the endoscope, other equipment that is needed includes a light source, a suction pump (any standard suction pump system can be used by attaching the tubing to the suction connector port on the endoscope), a biopsy instrument, and foreign body graspers. A number of different light source models are available that have a wide variety of features. There are two basic types of light sources. Smaller, lower-priced units that use a low-wattage (e.g., 150 watts) halogen lamp are quite adequate for most veterinary applications. Xenon lamps produce a brighter and whiter light than halogen lamps. Xenon light sources provide the best illumination for video documentation. If a light source is to be used for both flexible and rigid endoscopic applications, xenon is clearly preferred. Video cameras that can be attached to the eyepiece of the endoscope and high-resolution monitors are also available (Figure 3-2). Use of this equipment allows simultaneous viewing by any number of observers.

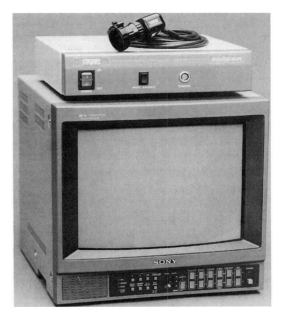

FIGURE 3-2 High-resolution endoscopic video camera and monitor. The camera (top) is attached to the eyepiece of the endoscope. The endoscopist performs the procedure while watching the image on the video monitor. The camera can be fully immersed and features automatic exposure control.

Learning Endoscopic Techniques

Once the decision is made to purchase an endoscope, whether new or used, every effort should be made to become proficient in its use. This is accomplished through attending one or several formal wet lab courses and then practicing the basic skills of maneuvering an endoscope and procuring biopsy samples. If proper skills of maneuvering and observation are not developed, even the most sophisticated endoscopes are of little value. Frustration resulting from unfamiliarity with proper instrument handling and unavailability of necessary ancillary equipment too often leads to disuse.

Indications for Gastrointestinal Endoscopy

During its early development, fiberoptic endoscopy was used primarily as an adjunct to other diagnostic methods, especially barium contrast x-ray examinations. However, in recent years many veterinary gastroenterologists have come to regard endoscopy as one of the most sensitive methods of evaluating GI tract symptoms. This has resulted in a substantial increase in the use of endoscopy in many veterinary hospitals, corresponding with a decrease in the number of barium series that are performed. This trend is expected to continue as more veterinarians become familiar with the distinct diagnostic advantages of endoscopy.

Most of the commonly encountered disorders of the GI tract involve either the mucosa of the organ in question or disrupted mucosal anatomy. Endoscopy offers the clear advantage of complete mucosal examination of the esophagus, stomach, descending duodenum (in cats and small dogs, the ascending duodenum and sometimes the proximal jejunum as well), terminal ileum in most dogs 10 lb or larger, and colon. Endoscopic biopsies provide rapid assessment and evaluation of many disorders. In addition, endoscopy plays an important therapeutic role in foreign body removal, guided bougienage or balloon dilation of esophageal and colonic strictures, and placement of gastric feeding tubes. Well-established indications for endoscopy are listed in Table 3-1. Disorders that can be reliably diagnosed via endoscopy are listed in Table 3-2.

Diagnosis of Esophageal Abnormalities

Esophagoscopy should be considered for any patient with signs of esophageal disease. The decision whether or not to actually perform an endoscopic examination of the esophagus is based on clinical impression and a review of any indicated laboratory tests and radiographic studies. Common signs of esophageal disease include regurgitation, dysphagia, excessive salivation, and change in appetite, which may be either increased or decreased.

In the esophagus, as elsewhere in the GI tract, endoscopy is most effective in diagnosis of disorders that affect the mucosa. Hence, it can be expected that diagnosis of inflammatory, neoplastic, and obstructive lesions (e.g., stricture, foreign body) will be relatively precise. Whereas survey or contrast radiography is useful for identifying an obstructive lesion, esophagoscopy provides a means of obtaining a definitive diagnosis and in some cases offers important therapeutic options. Esophageal foreign bodies (e.g., fishhooks, bones) can often be successfully removed using graspers that are passed through or alongside the endoscope. Any erosive damage to the esophagus can be assessed after a foreign body has been removed.

TABLE 3-1	Potential Indications for Gastrointestinal Endoscopy	
Initial	**Follow-up**
Regurgitation	Repeat esophageal stricture
Dysphagia	balloon dilation or bougienage
Retching	Follow-up biopsies in patients
Unexplained salivation	with moderate to severe gastritis, inflammatory bowel
Unexplained nausea	disease, colitis, neoplasia (i.e.,
Unexplained inappetence	assess progression of disease, efficacy of therapy)
Vomiting	
Hematemesis	
Diarrhea	Serial assessment during ulcer healing
Melena	
Dyschezia	Serial assessment of mucosal
Constipation	healing and examination for
Fecal incontinence	possible stricture formation following
Foreign body retrieval	esophageal mucosal damage from a foreign body
Feeding tube placement	
Guided stricture dilation	

Modified from Tams TR: Endoscopy. In Kirk RW, Bonagura JD, eds: *Current veterinary therapy X.* Philadelphia, 1989, WB Saunders.

Bougienage or balloon dilation procedures to dilate esophageal strictures are most safely performed under endoscopic visualization. Esophageal tumors can be diagnosed by guided biopsy. In human medicine, endoscopic laser therapy has been successfully used for ablation of neoplastic tissue. This is a palliative measure undertaken in esophageal cancer patients primarily to relieve luminal obstruction and hemorrhage.

Unexplained salivation is an important indication for esophagoscopy in animals because, in some cases of esophagitis or neoplasia, salivation may be the only prominent sign or one of several subtle signs that is exhibited early in the course of the disorder.

The diagnosis of reflux esophagitis cannot be made consistently solely on the basis of gross examination because in some cases changes are limited to microscopic inflammation. Certain endoscopic "clues" may be observed by an experienced endoscopist, however, that will suggest the

TABLE 3-2	Gastrointestinal Disorders Amenable to Diagnosis by Endoscopy			
Site of Disorder	**Type of Disorder**			
	Inflammatory	**Infectious/Parasitic**	**Anatomic**	**Neoplastic**
Esophagus	Esophagitis Chemical injuries (acid, alkali)		Strictures Foreign bodies Hiatal hernia Diverticula Megaesophagus (endoscopy rarely necessary for diagnosis)	Squamous cell carcinoma Adenocarcinoma Metastases Others
Stomach	Gastritis (e.g., lymphocytic- plasmacytic, eosinophilic, histiocytic) Chemical injuries Ulcer—benign and malignant	*Physaloptera*	Foreign bodies Hypertrophic gastropathies Polyps Extraluminal compressive masses	Lymphoma Adenocarcinoma Others
Duodenum	Inflammatory bowel disease	Giardiasis Histoplasmosis	Polyps (rare)	Lymphoma Adenocarcinoma Others
Colon	Colitis	Trichuriasis Cestodiasis Protozoal infections (examine mucosal brushings) Histoplasmosis	Polyps Strictures Cecal inversion Ileocolic intussus- ception	Lymphoma Adenocarcinoma Others

Modified from Tams TR: Endoscopy. In Kirk RW, Bonagura JD, eds: *Current veterinary therapy X*. Philadelphia, 1989, WB Saunders.

likelihood of reflux esophagitis (e.g., distal esophageal erythema, gastroesophageal sphincter dilation, pooling of fluid in the distal esophagus). Monitoring distal esophageal pH with a probe and performing a suction biopsy of the distal esophageal mucosa provide a more sensitive means of diagnosis of reflux esophagitis than visualization alone.

Esophageal motility disorders in which there is not easily detected radiographic evidence of marked esophageal dilation are best recognized by esophageal fluoroscopy and manometry studies. Endoscopic examination of the esophagus reveals certain appearances, however, that may suggest the possibility of a motor abnormality, and, in hospitals where fluoroscopy equipment is not available, esophagoscopy can still be useful as a diagnostic aid. Often a diagnosis of clinically significant decreased lower esophageal sphincter pressure can be inferred from the presence of grossly evident esophagitis lesions and variable degrees of dilation of the gastroesophageal junction.

In most patients with megaesophagus, endoscopic examination is not necessary for diagnosis and is rarely of benefit in determining a cause of the disorder. Megaesophagus is a specific syndrome characterized by generalized esophageal dilation and hypoperistalsis, and it is differentiated from other causes of esophageal dilation such as esophageal foreign body, vascular ring anomaly or other stricture disorders, and neoplasia. If pneumonia is ruled out in a megaesophagus patient that is anorexic, esophagoscopy may be indicated to examine for esophagitis.

Diagnosis of Gastric Abnormalities

Indications for gastroscopy include signs referable to gastric diseases, including nausea, salivation, vomiting, hematemesis, melena, and anorexia. Gastroscopy mainly defines abnormalities of the gastric mucosa, but it may also reveal distortion of the stomach's normal anatomic relationships by displacement or extrinsic compression as a result of a mass or enlargement of an adjacent organ structure. With proper technique the entire mucosal surface of the stomach and the antral-pyloric canal can be examined. The most common disorders diagnosed include chronic gastritis, gastric foreign bodies, and gastric motility disorders (Figure 3-3). Ulcers, neoplasia, and hypertrophic gastropathy can be readily diagnosed but are less commonly found (Figure 3-4). Special therapeutic considerations include foreign body

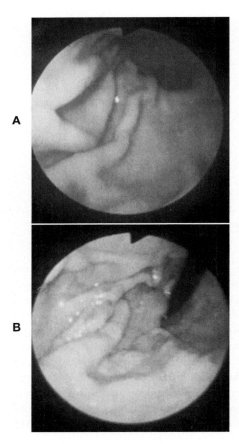

FIGURE 3-3 Endoscopic photos from feline stomach. **A,** Normal stomach of a cat, showing the midgastric and distal gastric body. Rugal folds are clearly in view, and the mucosa is smooth. **B,** Chronic gastritis in a cat. This is a retroversion view of the proximal stomach, with the endoscope in a curved position looking back on itself. The gastric mucosa is irregular throughout, and there are erosive changes on the rugal fold in the right field of view. Biopsies confirmed a diagnosis of chronic moderate lymphocytic-plasmacytic gastritis.

removal and endoscopy-guided percutaneous gastrostomy tube placement. Gastrostomy tube placement is a quick and simple procedure (see Chapter 12) and provides an excellent means of temporarily feeding an anorectic or debilitated patient.

In patients with chronic upper GI disorders, gastroscopy should be performed in conjunction with esophagoscopy and duodenoscopy. Important diagnostic clues may be evident in any or all of these areas during the course of an examination. Follow-up gastroscopy is a valuable aid in monitoring response to therapy in chronic gastritis and ulcer patients. Follow-up biopsies are especially important in patients with chronic severe histiocytic and granulomatous gastritis, chronic fibrosing gastritis, and gastric lymphoma. Important information that is useful in determining treatment protocol adjustments can often be obtained.

In evaluating a patient with signs suggestive of a gastric disorder, gastric mucosal biopsy samples should be obtained even if gross lesions are not present. It is common for a patient with chronic gastritis to have lesions identifiable only on microscopic examination. Different classifications of gastritis (e.g., lymphocytic-plasmacytic, eosinophilic, histiocytic) and degrees of involvement (e.g., mild, moderate, severe) can be determined from mucosal biopsy samples; these findings are extremely important in determining specific therapeutic regimens. If gross lesions are identified (e.g., localized hyperemic changes, nodules, or masses), forceps biopsies should be obtained from these areas, as well as from several normal areas. Six to eight biopsy samples are obtained from different areas of the gastric body and fundus if the stomach is grossly normal. Biopsy samples are best obtained from the surface of a gastric fold. The size of the tissue samples obtained may be inadequate if the stomach is too distended with air because the folds become too flattened. When the endoscope is first advanced to the stomach during the course of an examination, air is insufflated to distend the gastric walls so that thorough mucosal evaluation is enhanced. Suctioning some of the air out just before taking biopsy samples greatly increases the gastric fold surface area from which samples can be obtained. It is more difficult to obtain a tissue sample of adequate size from the gastric antrum than it is from other parts of the body unless there is hypertrophy or discrete raised or cratered lesions.

Clues that a gastric motility disorder may be present include pooling of bile or gastric fluid or finding undigested food in the stomach of a patient

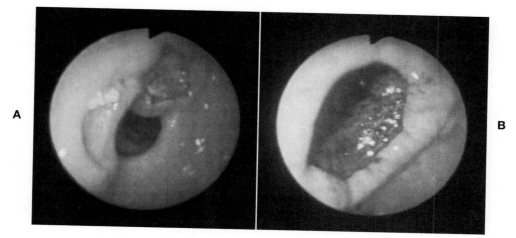

FIGURE 3-4 Gastric ulcers. **A,** Two peripyloric ulcers in a 14-year-old dog that was receiving nonsteroidal antiinflammatory drug (NSAID) therapy for severe osteoarthritis. The pyloric orifice *(center)* is open, and ulcers are seen to the left and above the pylorus. The dog had intermittent vomiting and inappetence. **B,** Large perforated gastric ulcer in an 8-year-old chow that had received naproxen (an NSAID) once daily for 7 days. On the sixth day vomiting and inappetence were first noted by the owner. Naproxen was discontinued on the seventh day, but the clinical signs persisted. Nine days after naproxen was discontinued, the dog was presented for endoscopy. The dog was bright and alert. The complete blood count (CBC) and biochemical profile were normal (packed cell volume [PCV] = 48%). On advancement into the gastric antrum the endoscope revealed a very deep ulcer with a thick rim *(entire upper left quadrant).* The pyloric orifice is at the lower left *(7 o'clock position).* The meshlike tissue seen through the ulcer crater is omentum (there was a complete omental seal). The ulcer area was subsequently resected surgically. (From Tams TR: Gastroscopy. In Tams TR, ed: *Small animal endoscopy,* St. Louis, 1999, Mosby.)

that has been fasted 8 to 10 hours or more. The stomach normally empties within 7 to 10 hours after a meal. There is often mucosal hyperemia caused by superficial irritation from bile, but, despite this gross abnormality, gastric biopsies in idiopathic gastric motility disorders are usually normal.

Because biopsy samples obtained from some masses with standard biopsy forceps are relatively small, sufficient tissue for definitive diagnosis is sometimes not obtained. Several biopsy samples from the same site of a mass should be taken, each time extending the biopsy forceps more deeply into the tissue (Figure 3-5). If tissue from only the surface of a neoplastic mass is obtained, a mistaken diagnosis of granulomatous or fibrous disease may be made. Samples from ulcerative lesions are best taken by grasping the wall or the junction of the wall and the gastric mucosa. Gastric polyps are reliably diagnosed on endoscopic biopsy in dogs and cats.

A major shortcoming of gastroscopy is that neoplastic diseases involving only the serosa or deep layers of the gastric wall cannot be identified or definitively diagnosed on mucosal biopsy. This pattern of tissue involvement is not commonly encountered, however. If endoscopic findings do not correlate with clinical signs, or if there is a poor response to therapy, exploratory surgery should be recommended.

Diagnosis of Duodenal Abnormalities

With a flexible pediatric endoscope (9-mm diameter or less), the duodenum can be directly examined in most cats and dogs. An endoscope with a diameter of 8.5 to 9 mm can consistently be advanced to the duodenum in cats and dogs weighing as little as 3 to 4 lb by an experienced endoscopist. The distal duodenum or proximal jejunum can often be reached in cats and small dogs (Figure 3-6). Certain portions of the duodenum, including the area immediately beyond the pylorus and the medial wall of the descending segment, are sometimes difficult to view other than tangentially, especially as the endoscope is initially advanced through this area. In small patients (especially cats) care must be taken not to be too forceful in advancing the endoscope through areas where there is increased resistance. It is possible to perforate the duodenum if too much force is applied in tight areas.

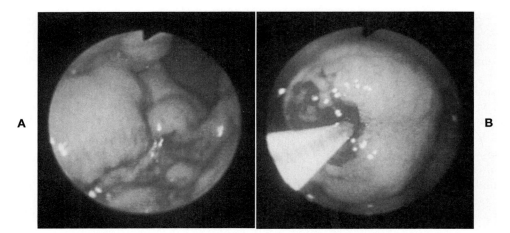

FIGURE 3-5 Gastric adenocarcinoma in a dog with chronic vomiting, weight loss, and recent anorexia. **A,** Marked proliferative changes in the lower gastric body, with complete loss of the normal rugal architecture. **B,** Close-up view of a mass in the midgastric body. The mass was rigid and had a very dense wall (suggestive of neoplasia). Masses such as this one should be biopsied as deeply as possible. If only superficial tissue is obtained, the endoscopist may fail to retrieve neoplastic cells. The first four attempts to biopsy the mass yielded only very small tissue samples, but on the fifth attempt the biopsy instrument advanced inside the mass. A number of large tissue samples were then obtained. (From Tams TR: Gastroscopy. In Tams TR, ed: *Small animal endoscopy,* St. Louis, 1999, Mosby.)

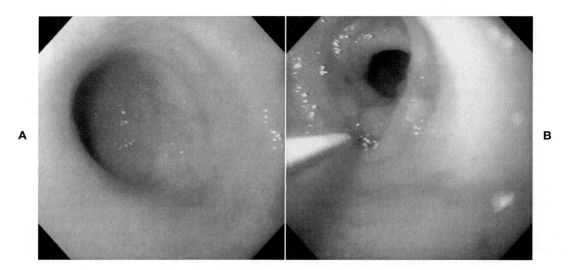

FIGURE 3-6 **A,** Grossly normal duodenum in a dog. **B,** Small intestine biopsy technique. Endoscopic forceps have been advanced into the duodenal mucosa.

Clinical signs of small intestinal disease include vomiting, diarrhea, melena, change in appetite, and weight loss. By far the greatest value of duodenoscopy is its capability of definitively diagnosing inflammatory small bowel disorders via biopsy. In fact, recognition that inflammatory bowel disease commonly occurs in dogs and cats became increasingly apparent as patients with various patterns of GI symptomatology began to be evaluated more thoroughly with endoscopic examination and biopsy. Frequently the only major sign in patients with inflammatory bowel disease is vomiting. If only gastric biopsies are performed in these patients, the diagnosis may be missed. In inflammatory disease the small bowel mucosa may appear normal or it may have varying degrees of irregularity, fissures, or follicular-like changes.

Endoscopy offers an alternative approach to obtaining small bowel biopsy samples in cases of protein-losing enteropathy when there is concern that full-thickness surgical biopsy sites may heal slowly. This is an especially important consideration in patients with a total protein level less than 3.5 g/dl. Multiple biopsy samples can be safely obtained using endoscopic biopsy forceps. In addition, the hospital stay is significantly shortened when endoscopy rather than surgery is performed, making this procedure more cost effective. The most common causes of protein-losing enteropathy in dogs are inflammatory bowel disease (by far the most common), lymphoma, and lymphangiectasia. Lymphangiectasia, a disorder of the intestinal lymphatics that results in malabsorption, has a characteristic histologic appearance, and in some cases pronounced gross changes can be seen at endoscopic examination. Often there is a characteristic patchy milky white appearance of the mucosa. In some patients, however, gross changes may be noted *only* at exploratory laparotomy. Occasionally the diagnosis will be missed if only the descending duodenum is examined and sampled. I have found this to be more of a problem in rottweilers than in other breeds.

Frequently biopsies reveal only mild lymphocytic-plasmacytic enteritis. In dogs that are markedly hypoproteinemic, as is often the case in those with lymphangiectasia, this degree of histologic change is not significant enough to substantiate a diagnosis of inflammatory bowel disease as the primary cause of the hypoproteinemia. Also, lymphangiectasia is often associated with mild lymphocytic-plasmacytic infiltrates in addition to its characteristic lesion of dilated lacteals. Therefore the clinician needs to be aware that enteroscopy limited to the upper small bowel may not establish the definitive diagnosis in some patients with lymphangiectasia. It is strongly recommended that both duodenoscopy and ileoscopy be performed in patients with chronic small bowel diarrhea, especially when hypoproteinemia is present. This approach provides the greatest opportunity for making the correct diagnosis when endoscopy rather than surgery is done to obtain biopsy samples.

Intestinal parasites (generally ascarids) are occasionally encountered on direct examination of the upper small intestine. These parasites can easily be snared with biopsy forceps or foreign body graspers and pulled up through the accessory channel. As is always done during endoscopy procedures, biopsy samples are still obtained even if

parasites are observed because the parasites could either represent an additional and unrelated problem regarding the primary disorder or might be a primary causative factor of the clinical signs. During duodenoscopy, saline lavage can be performed through polyethylene tubing advanced through the accessory channel of the endoscope in an effort to retrieve *Giardia* trophozoites. Direct smears of the aspirates should be examined within 20 minutes of collection with light microscopy at ×100 and ×400. Although endoscopy-guided duodenal lavage has been considered a very good test for diagnosing occult giardiasis, the availability of the fecal enzyme-linked immunosorbent assay (ELISA) for detecting *Giardia*-specific antigen, a very sensitive and practical test, now precludes the need for duodenal lavage in most diagnostically elusive cases of giardiasis.

Neoplasms that involve the small bowel mucosa can be reliably diagnosed on biopsy if a large enough sample of *representative* tissue is obtained. Any masses that are found should be sampled as deeply as possible. Lymphoma is the most common type of intestinal neoplasia in dogs and cats. GI lymphomas are believed to be less common in dogs than in cats. The diffuse type of lymphoma is the most amenable to diagnosis by endoscopy. Focal areas of lymphoma in the jejunum or proximal ileum may be missed because of insufficient endoscope length (most cases of GI lymphoma in dogs and cats involve diffuse rather than focal neoplastic infiltrates). Also, if lymphoma involvement is primarily in deeper muscle layers of the intestinal wall, mucosal biopsy samples as obtained with endoscopy forceps may not be deep enough to procure representative tissue. However, this problem is minimized by using proper instrumentation and technique and by routinely obtaining multiple samples (8 to 12) from the duodenum and, whenever possible, the ileum.

When lymphoma is present but not definitively diagnosed on the tissue submitted for examination, the mucosal tissue that is obtained is rarely normal. Usually moderate to severe lymphocytic-plasmacytic inflammatory infiltrates are present over or adjacent to neoplastic foci. A positive biopsy finding such as this may give the clinician false assurance that a definitive diagnosis has been reached. Poor or an only temporarily positive response to treatment that is initiated on the basis of biopsy results may then be an indication that some other, more significant disorder is present. Further biopsy samples should then be obtained, via either endoscopy or surgery. Surgery is generally the recommended procedure at this point because a much more extensive evaluation of the GI tract can be accomplished. *It should be emphasized that with proper instrumentation and technique, in conjunction with tissue examination by a pathologist experienced in evaluating the typically small tissue samples procured using endoscopic instrumentation, the correct diagnosis will be made in a great majority of animals that undergo endoscopy.*

Diagnosis of Abnormalities of the Ileum

As previously stated, examination and biopsy of the ileum are important in patients with chronic diarrhea or weight loss that is clinically consistent with a small intestinal disorder. Although it is not always possible to enter the ileum in dogs and is rarely accomplished in cats because of the narrow diameter of the ileocolic orifice, the ileocolic valve can be readily identified during complete colonoscopy as long as the ascending colon and ileocecocolic junction area are relatively clean (Figure 3-7). Biopsy samples can be blindly obtained from the ileum if the endoscope tip can be aligned with the ileocolic orifice so that the biopsy forceps can be passed through it and into the ileum. In dogs weighing more than 8 to 10 lb, I strongly prefer to obtain biopsy samples with the endoscope positioned in the ileum, whenever possible, so that any grossly abnormal areas can be pinpointed with the biopsy forceps.

The only disadvantage of ileoscopy compared with duodenoscopy is that the patient must be prepared for complete colonoscopy with a combination of fasting and colonic lavage. Ileoscopy done in conjunction with duodenoscopy also requires more anesthesia time and is therefore more expensive than if only one or the other is done. However, the great advantage of examining *both* the upper and the lower small bowel in patients with signs of chronic small intestinal disease is that a number of tissue samples can be obtained from a greater area of the intestinal tract. Histologic characteristics of the small intestine can then be more thoroughly evaluated. The large intestine is also routinely examined, and samples from it are obtained at the same time, even if there are no symptoms of colonic disease, because it has to be traversed to reach the ileum anyway. The thorough nature of this approach usually provides representative tissue for making an accurate diagnosis.

My experience to date has shown that in a majority of patients with inflammatory bowel disease, intestinal involvement is diffuse. Duodenal and jejunal changes are often similar in type and degree to those in the ileum. Sometimes a different cell type predominates in the ileum as compared with the duodenum, but usually no alteration in the treatment protocol is necessary. Occasionally, however, there are significant changes in the ileum when duodenal samples from the same patient are either normal or only mildly abnormal. I have examined several dogs with chronic diarrhea in which lymphoma was diagnosed on biopsies of the ileum, whereas duodenal samples revealed presence of only mildly abnormal inflammatory infiltrates. If ileoscopy had not been done in these patients, the diagnosis would have been missed! Also, the degree of inflammatory infiltrates is occasionally significantly more intense in the ileum than in the colon. Table 3-3 lists hematologic and histopathologic findings from a dog in which this was the case. I have also observed a patient with panhypoproteinemia that had mild lymphocytic-plasmacytic duodenitis. This degree of inflammatory disease is rarely significant enough to cause a protein-losing enteropathy. The patient did not respond to conventional therapy for inflammatory bowel disease. Subsequently, exploratory surgery identified adenocarcinoma in the terminal ileum, at a site where the diagnosis might have been made earlier if ileoscopy had been done.

These examples highlight the need to consider doing ileoscopy in patients with GI disorders characterized mostly by chronic diarrhea and weight loss. It is my impression that it is more important to recommend ileoscopy in dogs than in cats. Finally, if only colonoscopy is being done on a patient, using a flexible endoscope, it is wise to obtain ileum biopsy samples during the course of the procedure if access to the ileum can be gained. In this way, at least some information about the small intestine can be obtained. In my experience, most but not all patients with signs limited to large bowel diarrhea have normal ileum biopsies. If the ileum is abnormal, the treatment protocol might have to be altered.

Diagnosis of Large Intestinal Disorders

Flexible colonoscopy provides a means of thoroughly examining the entire colon to the level

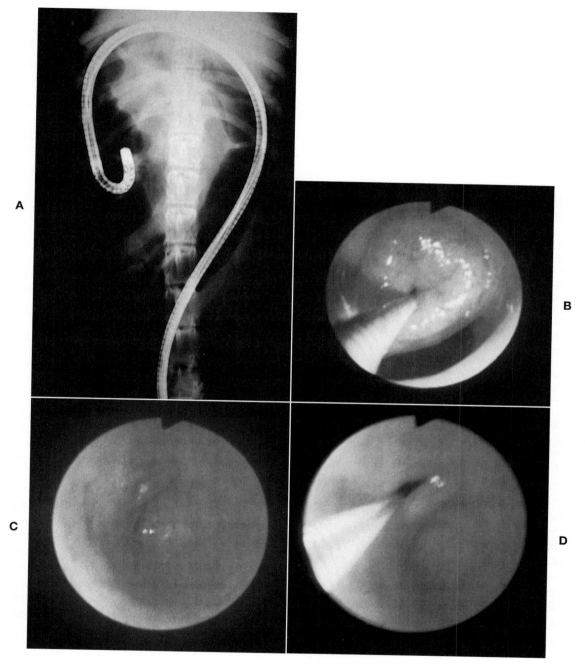

FIGURE 3-7 **A,** Radiograph showing the position of a flexible endoscope with the tip located close to the ileocecocolic area of a dog. With a flexible endoscope complete colonoscopy can be done, and in most dogs over 8 to 10 lb (and even in some smaller dogs when a pediatric endoscope is used) the endoscope can be passed into the ileum. **B,** Endoscopic view of the ileocolic orifice area in a dog. The ileocolic orifice in dogs usually appears as a broad, slightly raised papillary form. The cecal orifice is immediately below and is usually open. A biopsy forceps instrument has been advanced through the ileocolic orifice. **C** and **D,** Normal ileocolic orifice area of a cat. **C,** The ileocolic orifice appears as a very small opening (see **D**), and the cecum in the cat is simply a small blind pouch. **D,** An endoscopic biopsy instrument has been advanced through the ileocolic orifice. Since it is not usually possible to pass an endoscope into the ileum of most domestic cats, ileum biopsies are frequently obtained by passing a biopsy forceps into the ileum under endoscopic guidance.

TABLE 3-3	Hematologic and Histopathologic Findings in a 6½-Year-Old Spayed Female Shar-pei With a 2-Year History of Chronic, Unrelenting Diarrhea*			
PCV	31%	ALT (IU/L)		28
WBC	18,000	SAP (IU/L)		13
Neutrophils	12,960	Glucose		82
Lymphocytes	2,700	Cholesterol (n = 120-255 mg/dl)		96
Monocytes	2,340	TLI (n = 5-35 µg/L)		12
Total protein (n = 6-7.6 g/dl)	3.6	Cobalamin (n = 225-660 ng/L)		<27
Albumin (n = 2.8-3.8 g/dl)	1.8	Folate (n = 6.7-17.4 µg/L)		10.7
Globulin (n = 2.5-5.2 g/dl)	1.8			

BIOPSY RESULTS

Stomach: mild lymphocytic-plasmacytic gastritis
Duodenum: mild lymphocytic-plasmacytic duodenitis
Ileum: moderately severe atrophic lymphocytic-plasmacytic ileitis
Colon: moderate lymphocytic-plasmacytic-eosinophilic colitis

PCV, Packed cell volume; *WBC,* white blood cell count; *ALT,* alanine aminotransferase; *SAP,* serum alkaline phosphatase; *TLI,* trypsin-like immunoreactivity.
*Clinical signs were most consistent with a small bowel disorder. The dog had lost 18 lb in the last 3 months. Note the marked degree of panhypoproteinemia. The cobalamin level was quite low, whereas the folate level was normal. The subnormal cobalamin level was considered to be most consistent with intestinal bacterial overgrowth, which is common in shar-peis. It could also indicate significant disease in the ileum, although many dogs with ileal disease have a normal cobalamin level. Biopsies identified the most significant degree of disease to be in the ileum and colon. If only duodenal small bowel biopsies had been done, the true degree of small intestinal disease would have been misinterpreted, and treatment, especially drug doses prescribed, would most likely not have been aggressive enough. Also note the degree of histologic abnormality in the large intestine. This case example highlights the importance of doing ileoscopy and colonoscopy, as well as duodenoscopy, in dogs with chronic diarrhea.

of the ileocolic junction. The cecum in dogs can also be entered and examined. Indications for colonoscopy include signs of inflammatory disease (e.g., hematochezia, tenesmus, increased frequency of defecation), chronic diarrhea, constipation, fecal incontinence, and evaluation of a rectal or colonic mass. A second colonoscopy with follow-up biopsy is also useful as a means of monitoring response to therapy and in making decisions regarding treatment protocol adjustments in patients with inflammatory and neoplastic disorders. Colonoscopy is generally done only after dietary trials, therapeutic deworming either to treat known parasitism or to rule out the possibility of occult parasitism (especially whipworms), and empirical treatment for colitis have been tried and have proven ineffective in resolving symptoms. Colonoscopy should be done early in the course of symptoms that include hematochezia occurring with formed stools. The most common cause of this problem in dogs is rectal polyps. Abrasive material passing through the colon and chronic colitis

are the two most common causes of this problem in cats.

The most commonly diagnosed disorders include a variety of mucosal inflammatory disorders (lymphocytic-plasmacytic colitis is the most common) and rectal polyps. Colonic strictures, histoplasmosis, parasitic typhlitis, inverted cecum, ileocolic intussusception, and neoplasia are seen less commonly but can be reliably diagnosed by colonoscopy. Colonoscopy is much more accurate than contrast radiography in obtaining a definitive diagnosis of large intestinal disorders.

A majority of patients with idiopathic colitis have grossly normal mucosa. Confirmation of the diagnosis requires that the colon be properly prepared so that high-quality biopsy samples can be obtained from various levels of the colon. If the ileocolic area can be reached, an attempt should be made to obtain biopsy samples from the ileum as well. In patients with chronic diarrhea that is not clearly limited to large bowel signs, it is best to obtain biopsy samples from both the small and the large intestine.

Endoscopic Removal of Gastrointestinal Foreign Bodies

Many foreign objects can be successfully removed from the esophagus, stomach, and colon using endoscopic instrumentation. Rigid esophagoscopy under general anesthesia was the procedure of choice for removal of esophageal foreign bodies until the late 1970s. Even now it is occasionally used preferentially over flexible equipment in the retrieval of difficult-to-remove esophageal bone foreign bodies. Surgical removal via gastrotomy, enterotomy, and colotomy has long been the standard method of management for foreign bodies of the stomach, small intestine, and large intestine, respectively. Improvements in the optics and maneuverability of flexible fiberoptic endoscopes and development of foreign body grasping forceps, retrieval baskets, and polypectomy snares for use with endoscopes, however, have clearly made endoscopic retrieval the current procedure of choice for dealing with retained esophageal and gastric foreign bodies. The first reports of removal of GI foreign bodies with a flexible fiberoptic endoscope appeared in 1972. Since then physicians and veterinarians have become adept at retrieving objects of various sizes and shapes, and it is currently a very uncommon occurrence for a patient with a foreign body in the esophagus, stomach, or colon to have to undergo surgical removal. A majority of gastric foreign bodies can be successfully removed via endoscopy (85% success rate in my series in which endoscopy was attempted for foreign body retrieval). Case selection in regard to gastric foreign bodies is important; that is, a gastrotomy would be done without any attempt to do endoscopy if radiographs confirm the presence of a very large gastric foreign body.

There are numerous advantages to endoscopic foreign body removal when compared with other means of treatment. The procedure is minimally invasive and not appreciably time-consuming (average time in my series once anesthesia is induced is 5 to 15 minutes). Especially troublesome objects may require up to an hour, but endoscopy is still less expensive and less invasive than surgery. Patients are often discharged within 4 hours to 2 days of the procedure. Endoscopy allows for rapid intervention when sharp objects or valuable prized possessions such as jewelry or coins are ingested. Rather than rely on observation and radiographic surveillance in such clinical situations, endoscopic equipment can be used to quickly retrieve the object in question. The main limiting factor when considering endoscopy versus observation is the necessity for using general anesthesia for endoscopy.

Foreign objects that can be removed with a high rate of success include needles, coins, bottle caps, fruit pits, pieces of toys, cloth material, bone chips, rocks, food wrappers, narrow hairballs, and many others. The success rate for removal of fishhooks is variable (55% to 70%) and depends on how deeply the hook is imbedded in the mucosa before endoscopy. Frequently bones can be retrieved from the esophagus. If it is not possible to remove a bone through the mouth, attempts are made to advance it to the stomach. A decision is then made either to remove the bone via gastrotomy or, alternatively, to leave it in the stomach for digestion by gastric acid. Bones are usually decalcified by gastric juices, and the remaining fragments pass through the intestinal tract without incident. Foreign bodies that are not likely to be removed endoscopically include corn cobs, large rocks, and large hard rubber balls. Problems with retrieval of these objects are related to their size in relation to the width of the grasping range of pronged foreign body retrieval instruments and the likelihood that they can be positioned at an angle that will facilitate passage through the lower and upper esophageal sphincters. The weight and surface texture of the foreign body also must be taken into consideration. Smooth objects are sometimes difficult to grasp firmly enough for retrieval through the narrow areas of the lower and upper esophageal sphincters, especially when the object is heavily coated with gastric mucus.

A variety of instruments are available for foreign body retrieval. A laryngoscope and forceps (e.g., Kelly clamp, sponge forceps) are used for pharyngeal foreign bodies and for retrieval of any object that is difficult to pull through the upper esophageal sphincter with standard prong type of endoscopic grasping instruments. Two-, three-, and four-pronged grasping instruments are most commonly used with flexible endoscopes. The diameter of the working channel of the endoscope limits to some degree the type and size of grasping instruments that can be used. Larger, sturdier instruments made by some manufacturers require a 2.8-mm or larger working channel. Pediatric endoscopes that are less than 9 mm in diameter have a working channel diameter range of 2 to 2.5 mm,

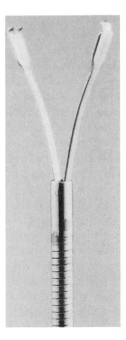

FIGURE 3-8 Two-pronged grasping forceps. Width between grasping teeth when fully separated is approximately 1.4 cm.

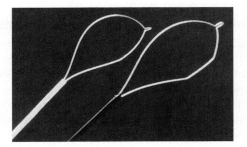

FIGURE 3-9 Oval *(left)* and crescent *(right)* grasping snares. Snares are the most versatile instruments for removal of foreign objects.

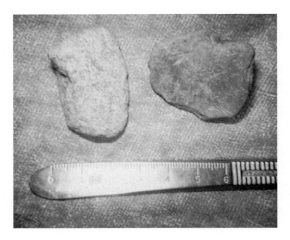

FIGURE 3-10 Two rocks retrieved with a two-pronged grasper (shown in Figure 3-8) from a golden retriever with a 6-day history of anorexia but no vomiting. A snare loop could also have been used. It is possible to retrieve fairly sizeable foreign objects with endoscopic instrumentation. (From Tams TR: Endoscopic removal of gastrointestinal foreign bodies. In Tams TR, ed: *Small animal endoscopy,* St. Louis, 1999, Mosby.)

depending on the manufacturer. In my experience, a majority of gastric and esophageal foreign bodies can be successfully retrieved with instrumentation that can be used through a 2-mm channel. A *sturdy* two-pronged instrument (Figure 3-8) is adequate for most foreign objects and can be used with pediatric endoscopes with a narrow working channel. Sheathed four-pronged graspers can be purchased for use through small working channels, but these instruments do not tend to be durable.

Polypectomy snares (Figure 3-9) are the most versatile instruments for removal of foreign objects. The snare loop can be extended around an object to provide a much stronger grasp than can sometimes be achieved by the single-end grasp applied by a pronged instrument. Basket retrievers can also be used for this purpose, but I have found snare instruments to be more versatile. The two instruments that I have used for virtually all of my foreign body cases are the two-pronged instrument and a polypectomy snare. Both of these instruments should be a part of standard instrumentation armamentarium since there are instances where each of the instruments will be superior to the other. Examples of successfully retrieved objects are shown in Figures 3-10 and 3-11.

LAPAROSCOPY

Laparoscopy is an operative procedure, performed through a keyhole opening with a rigid endoscope, that allows visual inspection and biopsy of the peritoneal cavity and its organs. Laparoscopy was first introduced in 1901 in human medicine, and it was quickly recognized in the early years as a valuable diagnostic procedure for diseases of the liver. With the laparoscopic instrumentation that is available today, bright, clear images of the peritoneal cavity are readily produced and laparoscopic photographs can be spectacular.

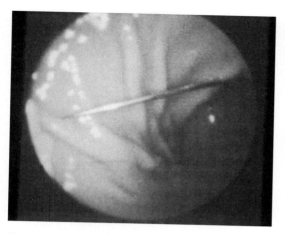

FIGURE 3-11 Needle foreign body in the stomach of a cat. Once grasped from either end, this foreign object can quickly and easily be removed via endoscopy. (From Tams TR: Endoscopic removal of gastrointestinal foreign bodies. In Tams TR, ed: *Small animal endoscopy,* St. Louis, 1999, Mosby.)

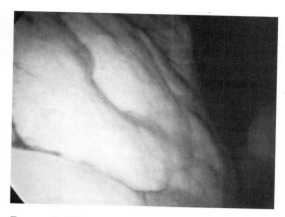

FIGURE 3-12 Laparoscopic view of normal canine pancreas (right limb). The examination was performed with a 5mm–diameter telescope.

Until fairly recently, the most common indications for laparoscopy in human clinical medicine included evaluation of liver disease, staging for cancer treatment (liver and peritoneal metastases), diagnosis of various peritoneal diseases (e.g., ascites of unknown etiology, fever of unknown origin, abdominal pain of unknown etiology, endometriosis, portal hypertension), and diagnosis of pelvic soft tissue disease, diseases of the spleen, and pancreatic disease. Laparoscopy has also been used extensively in recent years in evaluation of the female reproductive organs and for in vitro fertilization techniques. The list continues to grow! There have also been tremendous advances in laparoscopic surgical techniques over the last 10 years in human medicine. For example, it is now routine for cholecystectomy procedures to be done entirely via laparoscopy ("keyhole surgery"). Advantages of laparoscopic cholecystectomy in humans include significantly less postoperative pain and discomfort, short periods of hospitalization (most patients are discharged on the first postoperative day), and earlier feeding when compared with standard surgical cholecystectomy. Cholecystectomies done through a large abdominal incision (open cholecystectomy) have now become a rarity. Newer procedures that are now being done include laparoscopic removal of common bile duct stones through the cystic duct, management of hiatal hernias and recurrent or bilateral inguinal hernias, and left- or right-sided colectomies. Laparo-

scopic surgery is clearly one of the most exciting areas of study and new technology in the field of human surgery today.

Laparoscopy has been used in veterinary medicine with any degree of frequency only for the last 25 to 30 years. Its early use centered around reproductive function studies in food animals and equine, nonhuman primate, and various zoo and exotic species. Laparoscopy is most commonly used now in small animal medicine to examine and perform biopsies of the liver, kidneys, pancreas, and prostate. It provides an excellent means for visualizing the surface of the liver. Even subtle color and texture changes can be readily detected. The pancreas can usually be thoroughly examined (Figure 3-12). Pancreatic biopsy samples can be safely obtained, thus making laparoscopy a useful diagnostic procedure in evaluating patients for pancreatitis (Figure 3-13). Also, laparoscopic instrumentation is now used extensively in avian patients for examination of the abdominal and thoracic cavities. Panoramic views of both areas can be achieved through a single puncture site.

Most veterinarians have had little or no exposure to laparoscopy during their training in veterinary school. Ultrasonography has become the dominant procedure for imaging abdominal organs and for obtaining biopsy samples in a minimally invasive way. Laparoscopy still plays a major role in clinical practice for many veterinary gastroenterologists, however, and many small animal practitioners are now beginning to perform laparoscopy in their general practices. To see an organ clearly during biopsy, to obtain biopsy samples readily from even a small liver, to observe

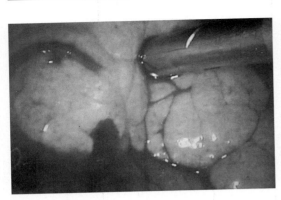

FIGURE 3-13 Pancreas biopsy site *(left of center near the bottom of the field of view)*. The closed spoon biopsy instrument is seen in the upper right, being used to hold the pancreas in position. A pancreatic vessel is observed in the upper left.

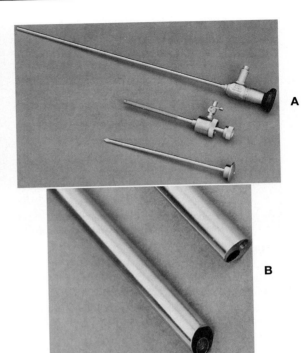

FIGURE 3-14 **A,** Laparoscopic instrumentation. Shown *(top to bottom)* are telescope (5 mm × 29 cm), insertion cannula (sleeve unit through which the telescope is passed to enter the abdomen), and trocar with pyramidal point. Abdominal puncture is made by advancing the trocar (placed inside the cannula unit) through a small incision, after a pneumoperitoneum has first been established. The insertion cannula is then advanced as the trocar unit is simultaneously backed out. **B,** Close-up view of laparoscope tips, with straight forward-viewing angle (0 degrees, *top*) and oblique forward-viewing angle (30 degrees, *bottom*).

directly the degree of hemorrhage associated with the biopsy, and to examine and obtain biopsy samples from the pancreas directly are major advantages of laparoscopy. Many veterinarians, once they observe the technique and see firsthand the sharp, clear views that can be achieved in the abdomen, express keen interest in learning more about laparoscopy and in purchasing equipment. Although the indications for laparoscopy may be far more extensive in human medicine, it still has many potential applications for use in veterinary medicine. It is a procedure that can be performed with a high degree of safety. Various minimally invasive surgical techniques (endosurgery) have now been developed for use in animals, and wet lab courses for training in these procedures are available. Although laparoscopy can be done in conjunction with local anesthesia and light sedation for minor procedures, I routinely do procedures under isoflurane general anesthesia while providing appropriate supportive care. This is well tolerated by a great majority of patients.

Instrumentation

The basic equipment needed to perform laparoscopy includes a telescope (laparoscope) and corresponding trocar-cannula unit (Figure 3-14), Veress (insufflation) needle, light source (Figure 3-15), gas insufflator unit, flexible fiberoptic light transmission cable, and tubing for transferring gas from the insufflation unit to the Veress cannula and the laparoscope cannula. A complete list of needed supplies appears in Box 3-1. If handled and cared for properly, laparoscopic instruments can last for

many years without need for repair. Many small animal practices could readily support the purchase of a set of instruments for performing laparoscopy.

It is beyond the scope of this chapter to provide a complete description of each instrument and technique for its use. One of the most important issues to discuss here involves which telescope diameter size is most suitable for use in cats and small dogs, as well as in large dogs. Laparoscopes applicable for use in small patients range from 1.7 to 10 mm in diameter. The 10-mm laparoscope requires a 2-cm incision for insertion of the cannula unit (the instrument through which the telescope is passed to enter the abdominal cavity). This size laparoscope is generally too large for use in cats and most small dogs. The smallest laparo-

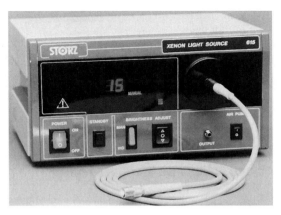

FIGURE 3-15 Endoscopic light source with automatic light intensity (175-watt Xenon). A fiberoptic light guide cable is attached. The same light source can also be used for other endoscope instruments (e.g., flexible endoscopes, bronchoscopes).

BOX 3-1	**Instrumentation for General Laparoscopy**

SUPPLIES FOR LOCAL ANESTHESIA, SKIN INCISION, AND CLOSURE

Syringes for anesthetic solutions
Lidocaine or Carbocaine (if general anesthesia is not used)
Towel pack and fenestrated drape
Towel clamps
Scalpel blades (no. 10, no. 15)
Thumb forceps
Gauze sponges
Bowl and sterile saline
Curved mosquito forceps (two)
Straight mosquito forceps (two)
Needle holder
Suture scissors
2-0 or 3-0 catgut or polydioxanone (PDS)
2-0 or 3-0 nylon

LAPAROSCOPIC INSTRUMENTATION

Veress needle
Laparoscope (telescope)
Fiberoptic light cable
Gas insufflation tubing
Laparoscope cannula (sleeve) with trocar
Second puncture cannula with trocar
Tactile (palpating-measuring) probe
Set of assorted rubber sealing caps
Tru-Cut biopsy needle
Biopsy forceps

Modified from Magne ML, Tams TR: Laparoscopy: instrumentation and technique. In Tams TR, ed: *Small animal endoscopy*, St. Louis, 1999, Mosby.

scope is used with a 2.2-mm cannula that can be advanced through a very small incision, thus making it useful for even very small patients. A major disadvantage of the smaller laparoscopes, however, is that they provide a limited field of vision. Also, a more powerful light source is required for good image quality because the smaller scopes contain fewer light bundles. A 5mm–diameter laparoscope is versatile and is the ideal size for use in dogs and cats. Many veterinarians experienced in performing laparoscopy recommend a 5-mm unit if only one scope is to be purchased.

For a thorough laparoscopic examination, it is essential that a pneumoperitoneum be established. This provides abdominal distention sufficient to maintain a workspace for the laparoscope and allows for greater range of visualization of abdominal organs. Various methods have been used to establish a pneumoperitoneum, including insufflation of room air by a syringe, three-way stopcock, and micropore air filter system, bulb pumps, gas tanks, and carbon dioxide dispensers. Although any of these methods can be used satisfactorily, use of an automatic insufflator unit for nitrous oxide or carbon dioxide is greatly preferred (Figure 3-16). These units have a self-contained internal tank that must be filled from an external tank. This provides for controlled insufflation and greater safety and convenience during the procedure.

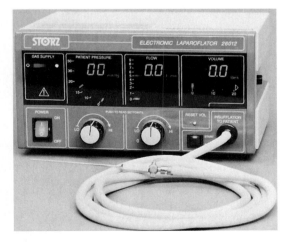

FIGURE 3-16 Gas insufflation unit for laparoscopy. Gauges that measure gas supply, intra-abdominal pressure, gas flow rate, and amount of gas insufflated are located on the front of the unit. A Veress needle is shown connected to the gas insufflation tubing by a Luer-Lok attachment.

Various ancillary instruments are available for use during laparoscopy (Figure 3-17). The most commonly used biopsy instrument is a double-spoon forceps (Figures 3-18 and 3-19). Although operating laparoscopes with a channel for insertion of accessory instruments are available, most veterinary laparoscopists prefer to use a double-puncture technique for biopsy. An accessory cannula is inserted to the abdomen through a second small incision. This technique allows greater mobility of accessory instruments (palpation probes, biopsy instruments). Alternatively, a biopsy needle can be inserted directly through the abdominal wall and then directed to the biopsy site under laparoscopic guidance.

Indications

The primary indications for laparoscopy in evaluation of diseases of the digestive system involve problems that necessitate examination and biopsy of the liver and/or pancreas.

Laparoscopy provides a superb view of the liver (Figure 3-20). Color, consistency, and contour of the liver are rapidly documented. A probe can be inserted through the second puncture cannula for the purpose of palpating the surfaces of the liver to evaluate for friability or excessive rigidity, to lift and separate the liver lobes in view so that the undersides can be examined, to palpate the gallbladder, and to displace omentum from a surface that must be examined (Figure 3-21). The liver is generally evaluated through a right lateral midabdominal approach. A significantly greater area of liver can be visualized from the right side compared with a ventral or left approach. The right lateral, right medial, and caudate lobes of the liver and the gallbladder and extrahepatic biliary tract can be thoroughly examined from the right side. A left approach is generally made only if disease

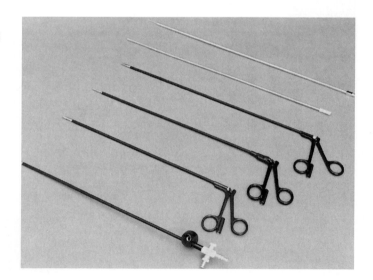

FIGURE 3-17 Assorted laparoscopic hand instruments. Included *(top to bottom)* are injection/aspiration needle, palpation probe, scissors, grasping forceps, biopsy forceps, and suction cannula.

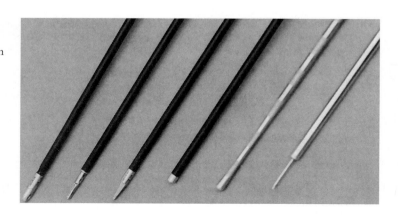

FIGURE 3-18 Close-up view of laparoscopic hand instrument tips. Shown *(left to right)* are double-spoon biopsy forceps, grasping forceps, scissors, suction cannula, palpation probe, and injection/aspiration needle.

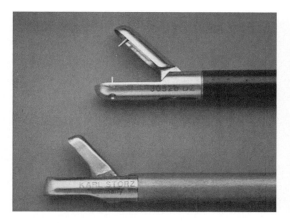

FIGURE 3-19 Close-up view of laparoscopic biopsy forceps: double-spoon grasping type of forceps *(top)* and cutting type of forceps *(bottom)*.

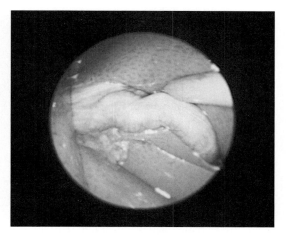

FIGURE 3-21 Normal gallbladder in a cat. A palpation probe is being used to lift liver away so that the gallbladder can be seen. The liver is paler than normal. Liver biopsy confirmed a diagnosis of hepatic lipidosis.

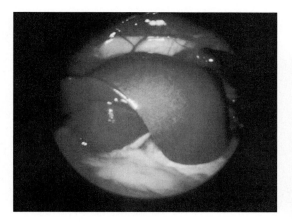

FIGURE 3-20 Normal canine liver viewed from a right lateral approach. The diaphragm is in the background.

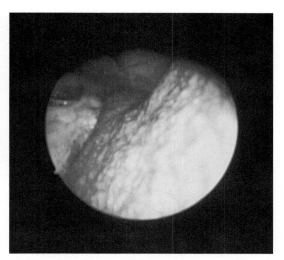

FIGURE 3-22 Marked diffuse granularity of the liver in a 4-year-old Maltese with chronic active hepatitis. This is an unusual appearance. The dog was clinically normal; however, screening laboratory tests done before a dental procedure suggested that the patient had a liver disorder, and both preprandial and postprandial serum bile acid levels were significantly elevated. Liver biopsies were obtained laparoscopically. (From Magne ML, Tams TR: Laparoscopy: instrumentation and technique. In Tams TR, ed: *Small animal endoscopy*, St. Louis, 1999, Mosby.)

involving the left lateral or medial lobe is suspected. Examination of the liver and surrounding structures usually takes only several minutes.

Abnormal gross liver changes that can be readily appreciated include hepatic lipidosis (the liver has a pale mustard color with friable texture), glycogen-laden liver, metastatic or multifocal neoplasia (raised and often discolored tumor nodules with central cavitations or depressions are seen), nodular hyperplasia (multiple raised nodules without central depressions, often with a yellow fatty appearance), cirrhosis, cholangiohepatitis, extrahepatic biliary tract obstruction, and others (Figure 3-22). Liver size and presence of any venous plexuses suggestive of acquired collateral shunting are readily appreciated.

A total of three to six or more liver biopsy samples, procured from any abnormal-appearing, as well as normal-appearing, areas, are usually obtained. Using grasping forceps advanced through the second puncture cannula, this can be done *quickly and safely*. One of the most significant advantages of laparoscopy-guided biopsy as compared with ultrasound-guided or blind percutaneous biopsy techniques is the direct visualization of the biopsy procedure itself. Once experience is gained, even biopsies of small livers can be rapidly performed (Figure 3-23). In cases in which extra tissue samples are needed for culture and/or quantitative copper analysis, the procedure can still be quickly completed. An additional advantage to direct visualization is that a gross description of the liver can be communicated to the pathologist. Finally, with use of spoon biopsy forceps sample size is somewhat larger than what is obtained with needle biopsy instruments, meaning that there is a greater certainty that representative liver tissue is being obtained for microscopic examination.

Indications for biopsy of the pancreas include ruling in or out acute pancreatitis when other tests have failed to establish clearly a diagnosis (i.e., obvious pancreatitis is not an indication for laparoscopy), identification of chronic recurring pancreatitis, and differentiation of pancreatic disease from liver disease. It is not uncommon for cats with chronic cholangitis or cholangiohepatitis to have concurrent chronic fibrosing pancreatitis. Simultaneous biopsy of liver and pancreatic tissue during laparoscopy aids in establishing extent of involvement in this syndrome.

The pancreas can usually be visualized through a right abdominal approach. It may be necessary to displace omentum from the pancreas in order to visualize it clearly. The right wing of the pancreas is found adjacent to the duodenum. Usually only a small portion of the left pancreatic lobe can be seen. In some obese patients it is difficult to find the pancreas. Biopsy samples of the pancreas are generally obtained only if the organ is grossly abnormal. The safest technique is to use grasping forceps to procure a small piece of the right pancreatic wing. The central duct area must be avoided. Parapancreatic fat nodules that represent either calcification, fibrosis, or necrotic tissue may be found. Great care in trocar placement must be exercised when performing laparoscopy in any patient that is likely to have acute pancreatitis.

Contraindications

Because laparoscopic procedures are generally short in duration (10 to 30 minutes when done by an experienced operator) and not considered significantly invasive, the risks are not as great as those that can be associated with exploratory laparotomy. By the time a decision to recommend laparoscopy is made, there has been ample opportunity for the clinician to evaluate the patient thoroughly through history, serial physical examinations, selected laboratory tests, and radiography. There are several absolute contraindications for performing laparoscopy. These include acute or unstable cardiopulmonary conditions, presence of an uncorrectable or severe coagulopathy, cases in which extensive intraabdominal adhesions could have developed, bowel obstruction, abdominal herniation (diaphragmatic or inguinal), and septic peritonitis.

A relative contraindication must be balanced against the need for diagnosis and risks of alternative methods of diagnosis. The latter options usually include either ultrasound-guided biopsy (sedation is still required) or general anesthesia and laparotomy. With administration of proper patient support and use of the safest possible sedation and anesthetic protocols (e.g., ketamine and diazepam or propofol and the general anesthetic agent isoflurane or sevoflurane), many elderly or compromised

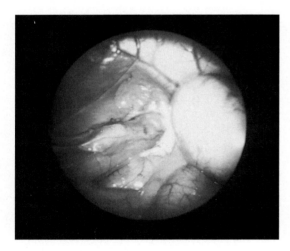

FIGURE 3-23 Microhepatia and cirrhosis in a 3-year-old cocker spaniel with a 3-week history of intermittent vomiting and anorexia. Liver enzyme levels were only mildly elevated, but both resting and postprandial bile acid values were markedly increased. Several small lobes of liver can be seen to the left of the gallbladder. The caudal vena cava is seen between two of the lobes *(8 o'clock position)*. The oval window of the diaphragm is in the background *(light area at the top of the field)*. The dog lived 15 months after the diagnosis of severe liver disease was made. NOTE: Laparoscopy is an ideal method for safely and quickly obtaining liver biopsies in patients with a small liver.

patients can tolerate laparoscopy with minimal or no problems. Ascites can complicate laparoscopy. The main problem involves clouding of the field of view. When ascites is present, it is usually best to remove as much of the fluid as possible before the procedure. This is best accomplished using either diuretics, if the ascites is mild and the procedure is not scheduled to be done for several days to a week, or centesis, on the day before or the day of the procedure if the ascites is moderate to severe.

Complications

The complication rate associated with laparoscopy depends on operator experience, accurate patient assessment and recognition by the clinician of appropriate indications and any possible contraindications, and quality of the laparoscopic equipment used. As an invasive procedure, laparoscopy is remarkably safe. Most surveys in human and veterinary medicine indicate that, as is the case with most procedures, errors and complications of laparoscopy are more common when the technique is still being learned. Complications during laparoscopy can be avoided with a high degree of success when the operator uses a systematic approach and careful attention to detail. Potential major complications that can occur include air embolism (related to abdominal insufflation), cardiopulmonary arrest, pneumothorax (from diaphragmatic puncture by a misguided instrument), damage to internal organs, bleeding, and infection. Because laceration of a major vessel can occur when attempting to obtain biopsy samples from a small liver with a needle instrument, it is recommended that grasping forceps be used instead in this situation (see Figure 3-19). In fact, this is the instrument that I routinely use to obtain liver samples in almost all liver biopsy cases. Patients with end-stage liver disease are at risk of decompensating at any time and in association with even minor procedures. Owners should be warned that this possibility exists before any type of procedure in a patient with severe liver disease. Minor complications include subcutaneous emphysema and subcutaneous leakage of ascites fluid around the puncture site. These are usually transient problems.

REFERENCES

Brady PG: Endoscopic removal of foreign bodies. In Silvis SE, ed: *Therapeutic gastrointestinal endoscopy*, New York, 1985, Igaku-Shoin.

Freeman LJ, Kolata RJ, Trostle S: Minimally invasive surgery of the gastrointestinal system. In Freeman LJ, ed: *Veterinary endosurgery*. St. Louis, 1999, Mosby.

Lightdale CJ: Indications, contraindications, and complications of laparoscopy. In Sivak MV, ed: *Gastroenterologic endoscopy*. Philadelphia, 1987, WB Saunders.

Magne ML, Tams TR: Laparoscopy: instrumentation and technique. In Tams TR, ed: *Small animal endoscopy*. St. Louis, 1999, Mosby, pp 397-408.

Morgenstern L: A new era of keyhole surgery, *Gastrointest Endosc Clin North Am* 3:183, 1993.

Nord HJ: Technique of laparoscopy. In Sivak MV, ed: *Gastroenterologic endoscopy*, Philadelphia, 1987, WB Saunders.

Quilici PJ: Laparoscopic cholecystectomy, *Gastrointest Endosc Clin North Am* 3:221, 1993.

Tams TR: Endoscopic examination of the small intestine. In Tams TR, ed: *Small animal endoscopy*, St. Louis, 1999, Mosby.

Tams TR: Endoscopic removal of gastrointestinal foreign bodies. In Tams TR, ed: *Small animal endoscopy*, St. Louis, 1999, Mosby.

Tams TR: Endoscopy, In Kirk RW, Bonagura JD, eds: *Current veterinary therapy X*. Philadelphia, 1989, WB Saunders.

Twedt DC: Laparoscopy of the liver and pancreas. In Tams TR, ed: *Small animal endoscopy*. St. Louis, 1999, Mosby.

Willard MD: Colonoscopy. In Tams TR, ed: *Small animal endoscopy*. St. Louis, 1999, Mosby, pp 217-245.

4

DISEASES OF THE ESOPHAGUS

Todd R. Tams

The esophagus is a muscular tube that transports ingested material from the pharynx to the stomach. In the resting state the esophagus is collapsed; however, it is capable of distending to accommodate passage of both fluid and solid materials. It is divided into three sections—the cervical, the thoracic, and the short abdominal portions—and it is bounded at each end by sphincters. The upper esophageal sphincter (UES) separates the cervical esophagus from the oropharynx. It is composed of fibers from the paired cricopharyngeus muscles and a portion of the thyropharyngeus muscle. Innervation of the muscles of the UES is involuntary and arises through the glossopharyngeal nerve and the pharyngeal branches of the vagus nerve.

The UES remains closed at all times, opening only to allow passage of a bolus. It closes promptly after the bolus is passed. The duration of opening of the UES is determined by a central neural mechanism that senses the volume of the bolus that is being propelled aborally by the pharynx. The state of consistent closure of the UES maintains a high-pressure zone that serves as an important defense mechanism, helping protect against esophagopharyngeal reflux and aspiration of ingesta.

The lower esophageal sphincter (LES) or gastroesophageal junction (GEJ) comprises the junction between the esophagus and stomach. The LES

functions as a physiologic sphincter. It acts as a zone of high resting pressure that promotes unidirectional flow from the esophagus to the stomach and helps prevent reflux of gastric contents into the esophagus. In dogs the LES consists of an outer layer of striated muscle and an inner layer of smooth muscle, whereas in cats the LES is composed entirely of smooth muscle. Mechanisms for prevention of gastroesophageal reflux include a variety of anatomic factors in addition to the LES itself. The entire abdominal segment of the esophagus, as well as the surrounding structures, plays a role. Gastric rugal folds, the diaphragmatic crus, the oblique angle of the distal esophagus as it enters the stomach, and compression of the intraabdominal esophagus by the fundus when the stomach is distended all contribute to LES integrity and help prevent gastric reflux.

The LES opens and closes in response to neural activity (vagal tone) associated with the swallowing mechanism. Its function can also be influenced, however, by hormones, by drugs (e.g., acepromazine, atropine, diazepam, propofol, xylazine, halothane, and isoflurane decrease LES pressure, whereas metoclopramide, cisapride, bethanechol, erythromycin, and domperidone increase LES pressure), and by local events such as inflammation. In response to esophageal peristaltic contractions, the LES undergoes a phase of initial relaxation that is followed by postdeglutition contraction. Initial relaxation begins when an esophageal peristaltic contraction occurs in the proximal esophagus. Postdeglutition contractions prevent reflux of a food bolus following its passage into the stomach.

Boluses are moved through the esophagus by a series of strong, well-coordinated contractions, which are produced by intense muscular activity. The esophagus of the dog is relatively longer than that of humans. Animals rely much more on propulsive esophageal activity than do humans, in whom gravity also plays a significant role in movement of material through the esophagus. In fact, it has been shown that the canine esophagus is able to develop 10 times the pressure that develops in the human esophagus.

The swallowing process has been divided into three major phases: oropharyngeal, esophageal, and gastroesophageal. Primary esophageal contractions are triggered by the oropharyngeal phase of swallowing. Secondary peristaltic waves occur in response to the effects of esophageal luminal distention and tactile stimuli. These waves begin proximal to the bolus. Progression of primary and secondary peristaltic waves depends on the size and the location of boluses present in the esophagus. Solids initiate stronger primary peristaltic contractions than do liquids. Secondary peristaltic contractions are more frequently required to clear liquids than to clear solids from the esophagus. The speed of esophageal peristalsis is much faster in dogs (75 to 100 cm/sec) than in cats (1 to 2 cm/sec). This is because striated muscles contract faster than smooth muscles. Among the most common clinical disorders of the esophagus observed in dogs are problems related to esophageal motility (e.g., variable degrees of esophageal hypomotility, megaesophagus). The primary symptom of these disorders is regurgitation, which results from an inability of the esophagus to transport ingested material to the stomach in a timely manner.

The esophagus has four distinct layers: the adventitia, the muscularis, the submucosa (which contains glands, nerves, and blood vessels), and the mucosa. With no serosal layer present, the submucosal layer of the esophagus is considered to have the greatest holding strength when sutured. In dogs, the muscle layer of the esophagus is composed entirely of striated muscle. In cats, the cranial two thirds of the esophagus is striated muscle, and the distal one third is smooth muscle. The only smooth muscle in the esophagus of a dog is the

muscularis mucosa. The muscularis mucosa has minimal contribution to peristaltic activity. The esophagus receives its innervation from the sympathetic and the vagus nerves, including the recurrent laryngeal branches. The vagal supply is the more important of the two. Branches of the thyroid arteries supply blood to the cervical esophagus; the bronchoesophageal arteries supply the cranial portions of the thoracic esophagus, and the branches of the aorta, the intercostals, and the gastric arteries supply the remaining portion of the esophagus.

The most common esophageal disorders that are seen in clinical practice are megaesophagus, esophagitis, esophageal strictures, and esophageal foreign bodies. These problems are discussed in detail in this chapter. Less common problems that are discussed include vascular ring anomalies, hiatal disorders, and esophageal neoplasia. A list of esophageal diseases based on signalment appears in Table 4-1.

█ MEGAESOPHAGUS

Megaesophagus is a syndrome characterized by *generalized* esophageal dilation and hypoperistalsis, which is often severe. It is differentiated from *localized* cases of esophageal dilation most of which are caused by mechanical problems with esophageal dilation occurring proximal to the site of obstruction (e.g., vascular ring anomalies, strictures, foreign bodies, neoplasia). There may or may not be abnormal peristalsis associated with these disorders. Clinicians should be aware that not all patients with esophageal motility disorders have megaesophagus. Some patients have various degrees of esophageal hypomotility (e.g., slow stimulation of secondary waves of esophageal contraction, or "sluggish motility") that may be segmental or diffuse. Survey thoracic radiographs are often normal in these patients. Mild to moderate esophageal hypomotility is best evaluated with fluoroscopic studies in which both liquid contrast alone and liquid with food are used to study the strength and coordination of esophageal peristalsis.

Megaesophagus may be congenital or acquired (adult onset). *In most clinical practices, adult-onset idiopathic megaesophagus is seen somewhat more commonly than congenital megaesophagus.* A familial predisposition for congenital megaesophagus has been identified for many breeds of dogs (Great Dane, German shepherd, Irish setter, golden retriever, Labrador retriever, greyhound, Newfoundland,

TABLE 4-1	Profiles for Esophageal Disease Based on Signalment
Parameter	**Clinical Association**
Age	
Young	Vascular ring anomaly; idiopathic megaesophagus; foreign body
Mature	Esophageal neoplasia
Breed	
Boston terrier	Vascular ring anomaly (PRAA)
Bouvier	Dysphagia caused by hereditary muscular dystrophy (oropharyngeal dysphagia and megaesophagus)
Cocker spaniel	Cricopharyngeal achalasia
Collie	Familial canine dermatomyositis (oropharyngeal dysphagia and megaesophagus)
English bulldog	Vascular ring anomaly (esophageal compression by left subclavian artery and brachiocephalic artery)
	Esophageal deviation cranial to the heart (normal variant)
German shepherd	Idiopathic megaesophagus
	Vascular ring anomaly (PRAA)
	Acquired myasthenia gravis
	Giant axonal neuropathy
Golden retriever	Idiopathic megaesophagus
	Acquired myasthenia gravis
Great Dane	Idiopathic megaesophagus
	Vascular ring anomaly (PRAA)
Greyhound	Idiopathic megaesophagus
Irish setter	Idiopathic megaesophagus
	Vascular ring anomaly (PRAA)
Jack Russell terrier	Congenital myasthenia gravis
Labrador retriever	Idiopathic megaesophagus
	Hereditary myopathy (megaesophagus)
Miniature schnauzer	Idiopathic megaesophagus
Newfoundland	Idiopathic megaesophagus
Rottweiler	Spinal muscular atrophy (megaesophagus)
Shar-pei	Idiopathic megaesophagus
	Hiatal hernia
	Esophageal deviation cranial to the heart (mild regurgitation)
Smooth fox terrier	Congenital myasthenia gravis
Springer spaniel	Cricopharyngeal achalasia
	Polymyopathy (megaesophagus)
	Congenital myasthenia gravis
Wirehaired fox terrier	Idiopathic megaesophagus
Siamese cat	Idiopathic megaesophagus

PRAA, Persistent right aortic arch.
From Johnson SE, Sherding RG: Diseases of the esophagus and disorders of swallowing. In Birchard SJ, Sherding RG, eds: *Manual of small animal practice,* ed 2, Philadelphia, 2000, WB Saunders.

shar-pei), as well as for Siamese cats (although megaesophagus rarely occurs in cats). Congenital megaesophagus is known to be inherited in wirehaired fox terriers and miniature schnauzers. It is transmitted in wirehaired fox terriers as a simple autosomal-recessive trait, whereas in miniature schnauzers it is transmitted as a simple autosomal-dominant or a 60% penetrance autosomal-recessive trait. The acquired form has been reported in many pure-breed dogs. Breeding of affected animals is not recommended.

Etiology

The pathogenesis of megaesophagus is poorly understood. Physiologic studies in dogs with megaesophagus suggest that a defect exists in the afferent neural pathway. Efferent neuromuscular pathways appear to be intact. It has been shown that dogs with idiopathic megaesophagus do have cyclical migrating motor complex activity and that the upper and lower esophageal sphincter responses to swallowing are intact and normal. Mechanisms may be similar for both congenital and acquired idiopathic megaesophagus. Diminished motor responses of the upper and lower esophageal sphincters to intraluminal stimuli have been identified.

Megaesophagus in dogs was previously incorrectly compared with a human esophageal disorder called achalasia, which is characterized by failure of the lower esophageal sphincter to relax properly and ineffective peristalsis of the esophageal body. Treatment of this human disorder involves cardiomyotomy. Achalasia has never been proven to occur in animals. Esophageal sphincter tone is normal, not increased, in dogs with megaesophagus. Cardiomyotomy is therefore clearly not indicated in dogs with megaesophagus.

Acquired megaesophagus occasionally occurs secondary to other disorders, especially diseases that can cause diffuse neuromuscular dysfunction (e.g., focal or generalized myasthenia gravis, hypoadrenocorticism, and dysautonomia in cats). Causes of megaesophagus are listed in Box 4-1. *Because appropriate management of some of these disorders may lead to resolution of megaesophagus, it is rec-* *ommended that patients with acquired megaesophagus be evaluated for the presence of a primary disorder. It is emphasized, however, that the majority of patients with megaesophagus have idiopathic disease, and treatment centers on general management principles.* Selected primary disorders are discussed in more detail later in this chapter.

Congenital Idiopathic Megaesophagus

Congenital idiopathic megaesophagus involves generalized esophageal dilation of unknown cause, with signs of regurgitation usually beginning at or shortly after weaning. Occasionally, regurgitation does not begin until 2 to 6 months after weaning. Congenital disease should be considered in any young patient with megaesophagus. The incidence is highest in Great Danes, German shepherds, golden retrievers, Shar-peis, Irish setters, wirehaired fox terriers, and miniature schnauzers, although many other breeds can be affected by the disease. A hereditary mechanism has also been suspected in young cats, especially Siamese cats. Multiple animals in a litter can be affected.

The most important differential diagnosis in young dogs and cats with regurgitation that occurs around the time of weaning is vascular ring anomaly. Vascular ring anomalies occur quite uncommonly. Differentiation can often be made on survey thoracic radiographs (generalized dilation of the *entire* esophageal body is usually readily identified with megaesophagus) (Figure 4-1). Contrast studies are done on patients with suspected vascular ring anomaly to highlight both the presence of an obstruction just cranial to the heart and the severity of dilation proximal to the obstruction. Other important differential diagnoses in young patients with regurgitation include esophageal stricture and foreign body.

Treatment for congenital megaesophagus primarily involves elevated feedings (45 to 90 degrees of upper body elevation). The consistency of the food that is fed depends entirely on what type is associated with the least postprandial regurgitation. Promotility therapy (cisapride) may also be attempted, although this drug is not expected to be useful in dogs because it is a smooth muscle prokinetic agent and the canine esophagus consists entirely of skeletal muscle. Treatment details for megaesophagus are discussed later in this chapter.

BOX 4-1	Causes of Megaesophagus

Idiopathic
   Congenital
   Acquired (adult onset)
Neuromuscular
   Myasthenia gravis (focal or generalized)
   Polymyositis and polymyopathy
   Systemic lupus erythematosus
   Dysautonomia (cats)
   Giant cell axonal neuropathy
   Polyradiculoneuritis
   Dermatomyositis
   Botulism
   Brainstem trauma or neoplasia
Toxic
   Lead
   Thallium
   Organophosphates
Endocrine
   Hypoadrenocorticism
   Hypothyroidism
Miscellaneous
   Pyloric stenosis (cats)
   Congenital lower esophageal stricture

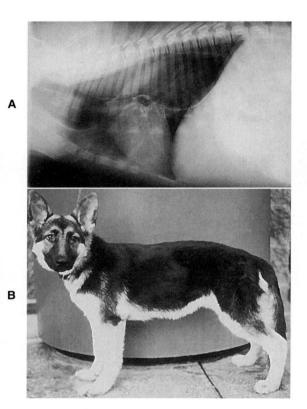

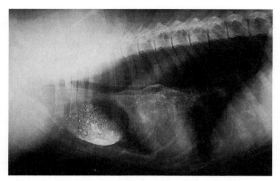

FIGURE 4-2 Severe congenital megaesophagus in a 6-month-old German shepherd. Note the marked ventral deviation of the esophagus cranial to the heart. There is an accumulation of foreign material in this large sacculated space. Esophagoscopy confirmed that the entire esophagus was dilated, with no evidence of a vascular ring anomaly. With diligent medical management, the dog lived an energetic life. However, because of increasingly frequent bouts of aspiration pneumonia, the dog was euthanized at 2 years of age.

FIGURE 4-1 Congenital megaesophagus in a 3-month-old German shepherd. There had been a recent onset of regurgitation. **A,** Lateral radiograph shows dilated, air-filled esophagus. Note that the entire esophagus is dilated, ruling out vascular ring anomaly. **B,** The puppy responded very well on an elevated feeding program. (This puppy is also shown in Figure 4-10, at 9 months of age.)

The prognosis for congenital megaesophagus is guarded. Although some patients can be successfully managed for many months to years, others suffer persistent regurgitation with frequent bouts of aspiration pneumonia, as well as wasting disease that results from the inability of the esophagus to transfer adequate amounts of nutrients to the stomach. Factors involved in determining prognosis include degree of dilation of the esophagus, especially that of the proximal thoracic esophagus, and degree of early response to positional feeding and dietary manipulation. Rarely some dogs may show spontaneous improvement. This may in part be due to the fact that the esophagus does not functionally mature until around 6 months of age. Dogs with severe esophageal dilation with pronounced sacculation proximal to the heart (Figure 4-2) often do more poorly over a period of time and have a shorter life span. Since esophageal function in patients with congenital megaesophagus does not commonly improve over time, owners must be counseled that long-term elevated feeding will be required to help control regurgitation. Breeding of affected patients is *not* recommended.

Acquired (Adult-Onset) Idiopathic Megaesophagus

Although acquired megaesophagus may occur secondary to many disorders, especially diseases causing diffuse neuromuscular dysfunction, the majority of affected patients have idiopathic megaesophagus. Despite this fact, successful treatment of an underlying cause may lead to complete resolution of the esophageal motility disorder. Therefore diagnostic tests are done to look for a primary cause. The extent of the diagnostic workup that is done in a patient with megaesophagus depends primarily on the signalment, the clinical signs, and the environment (e.g., toxicities such as lead poisoning and thallium and organophosphate intoxication can cause megaesophagus).

Signalment

Acquired megaesophagus has been reported in many pure- and mixed-breed animals. Although the age of onset of adult idiopathic megaesophagus is frequently 8 years or older, younger patients can be affected. There is no sex predilection.

Clinical Signs

The dominant clinical sign of megaesophagus is regurgitation. Regurgitation may occur minutes to hours after eating. Frequency varies from several episodes per week to many (10 to 20) episodes in a single day in some patients. Most affected dogs are initially presented with the chief complaint of what their owners describe as "vomiting" (which is actually regurgitation). It is up to the clinician to differentiate vomiting from regurgitation at the outset (see Chapter 1 for differentiation criteria).

It must be noted that the degree of esophageal dysfunction does not always correlate with the severity of clinical signs. Some dogs have megaesophagus for weeks to months before the onset of regurgitation episodes, or they regurgitate only infrequently despite the appearance of marked esophageal dilation on radiographs. Conversely, some dogs regurgitate frequently despite radiographic evidence of mild to moderate dilation.

Other clinical signs may include acute or chronic cough that may or may not be associated with dyspnea and fever. These signs are most consistent with aspiration pneumonia, which is the most common complication of megaesophagus. All patients with esophageal dysfunction are at risk for sudden death related to aspiration and subsequent upper airway obstruction. Coughing may also be related to compression of lung tissue and airways by the enlarged esophagus and its contents. Occasionally coughing is the *only* clinical sign demonstrated by a dog with megaesophagus. It may be weeks to months before regurgitation begins to occur in these cases.

Weight loss and emaciation occur secondary to inadequate food intake. Inappetence or salivation or both may result from discomfort caused by esophagitis.

In patients in which megaesophagus is associated with an underlying disorder, other clinical abnormalities that may be noted include generalized muscle weakness (myasthenia gravis, polymyopathy, hypoadrenocorticism), neurologic deficits (myasthenia gravis, central nervous system disease, polyneuropathy), generalized muscle atrophy or pain with polymyositis, vomiting (hypoadrenocorticism, lead poisoning, obesity and alopecia with hypothyroidism, and oropharyngeal dysphagia with generalized neuromuscular dysfunction).

Physical Examination

The most common physical finding in dogs with adult-onset idiopathic megaesophagus is loss of body condition. In some patients weight loss is pronounced by the time a definitive diagnosis is made (Figure 4-3). Mucopurulent nasal discharge and fever suggest aspiration pneumonia. Pulmonary crackles may be detected on auscultation. A Valsalva maneuver, in which the thorax and the mouth are occluded while the thorax is compressed to increase intrathoracic pressure, often results in a bulging on the left side of the neck caused by a dilated cervical esophagus. Oral examination may reveal the presence of accumulated food particles or thick saliva in the pharynx. The presence of muscle atrophy, weakness, or abnormal gait suggests the possibility of a neuromuscular disorder. A complete neurologic examination should

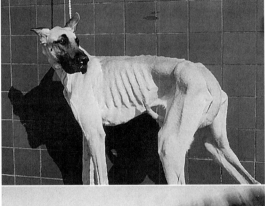

A

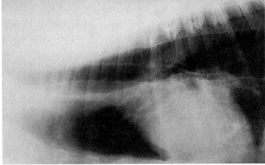

B

FIGURE 4-3 Adult-onset idiopathic megaesophagus in a 6-year-old Great Dane. Before referral the dog had undergone an extensive diagnostic work-up for vomiting. The primary problem, however, was actually regurgitation. **A,** Note the dog's obvious cachectic condition. **B,** A thoracic radiograph confirms a diagnosis of megaesophagus (note the dilated, air-filled esophagus).

be performed, with emphasis on cranial nerves IX (glossopharyngeal) and X (vagus).

Diagnosis

Acquired megaesophagus is most commonly diagnosed by the presence of generalized esophageal dilation on survey thoracic radiographs, without evidence of obstruction. If cervical radiographs are obtained, dilation of the cervical esophagus will usually be noted as well. Contrast studies (liquid barium) are occasionally necessary to confirm the presence of a dilated, hypoperistaltic esophagus. In many patients with obvious megaesophagus, it is unnecessary to perform contrast studies. The risk of aspiration of contrast material must always be considered. I most commonly perform a contrast study when I suspect an esophageal motility disorder and when the thoracic esophagus is not readily recognized on survey films. The technique for contrast radiography of the esophagus is discussed in Chapter 2.

Occasionally dogs with megaesophagus are first presented because of symptoms related to aspiration pneumonia. Therefore when evaluating thoracic radiographs from dogs with pneumonia, one must always look closely for any evidence of esophageal dilation.

Once the presence of megaesophagus is confirmed, appropriate ancillary tests should be performed. A complete blood count, a complete biochemical profile (including creatine kinase [CK]), and total serum thyroxine levels should be evaluated in all cases (TT_4). Leukocytosis (neutrophilia) with or without a left shift is consistent with aspiration pneumonia. Biochemical tests of particular interest include evaluations of sodium and potassium (hyponatremia and hyperkalemia are present in approximately 90% of dogs with hypoadrenocorticism); CK and aspartate transaminase (AST) (which may be elevated in patients with polymyositis); and cholesterol (hypercholesterolemia may suggest the possibility of hypothyroidism). In addition to baseline serum thyroxine level evaluation, free T_4 by equilibrium dialysis (fT_4ED) and a canine thyroid-stimulating hormone (cTSH) assay can also be done to more thoroughly examine for hypothyroidism. An **acetylcholine receptor antibody titer** should also be obtained in all adult dogs with megaesophagus to test for focal myasthenia gravis. *Focal myasthenia gravis occurs in the absence of muscle weakness. This is probably the second most common cause of acquired megaesophagus (a greater number of cases are idiopathic).* Megaesophagus secondary to acquired

myasthenia gravis is described in more detail later in this chapter.

Other tests that the clinician should consider in the evaluation of patients with megaesophagus, depending on clinical course and physical findings, include the following:

Adrenocorticotropic Hormone Stimulation Test for Hypoadrenocorticism. Hypoadrenocorticism is an uncommon cause of megaesophagus. Proposed causes of esophageal dilation include the effects of abnormal sodium and potassium concentrations on membrane potential and neuromuscular function, as well as a physiologic deficiency of cortisol, which may cause muscle weakness.

Hypoadrenocorticism has a predilection for young to middle-aged females. The most common clinical signs include anorexia, vomiting, lethargy, and weakness. Diarrhea also may occur. Most dogs that have megaesophagus associated with hypoadrenocorticism demonstrate one or all of these signs in addition to regurgitation. However, occasionally there may be only regurgitation. In addition, some of these dogs have atypical hypoadrenocorticism, in which sodium and potassium levels are normal. This complicates the diagnosis, so the clinician must maintain a high index of suspicion. An adrenocorticotropic hormone (ACTH) stimulation test is required for diagnosis. ACTH stimulation should also be performed to confirm the diagnosis in patients with characteristic hyponatremia and hyperkalemia. With proper treatment the megaesophagus will most likely resolve.

Tests for Hypothyroidism: fT_4ED and cTSH Assay. It has been proposed that megaesophagus may be associated with hypothyroidism. Very few dogs with hypothyroidism appear to develop megaesophagus. Tests including an fT_4ED and cTSH assay are warranted if baseline thyroid tests are subnormal. However, it is considered to be a rare occurrence for megaesophagus to resolve in response to treatment for hypothyroidism. Occasionally, a patient may have both hypothyroidism and focal myasthenia gravis. It is possible that the focal myasthenia gravis could resolve either spontaneously or as a result of treatment for hypothyroidism, with megaesophagus resolving as well.

Blood Lead Level for Lead Poisoning. Sources of lead include old paints, toys, lubricants, hobby materials, automotive materials, plaster board, roofing materials, fishing sinkers, and improperly glazed dishes. Young (less than 1 to 2 years), inquisitive patients are most commonly affected. Clinical signs of lead toxicity often include both gastrointestinal (GI) and neurologic abnormalities. Anorexia, vomiting, diarrhea, and/or abdominal pain are often demonstrated. Regurgitation occurs in patients that develop esophageal hypomotility and dilation secondary to lead toxicosis (a careful review of the history is necessary to determine that both regurgitation and vomiting, rather than vomiting alone, are occurring). Megaesophagus is not common in patients with lead toxicity. Neurologic abnormalities may range from sudden epileptic seizures to a variety of behavioral changes, including excitability, hysteria, continued barking or whining, dullness, and apparent blindness. A blood lead level of greater than 40 μg/dl is suggestive of lead poisoning, and a level of greater than 60 μg/dl is diagnostic. Abdominal radiographs may reveal radiopaque material in the GI tract, and there may be nucleated red blood cells and basophilic stippling on stained blood smears. In most cases administration of the antidote of choice (calcium ethylenediaminetetraacetic acid) is sufficient to correct the clinical manifestations of lead toxicity. If treated early enough, megaesophagus will resolve.

Antinuclear Antibody and Lupus Erythematosus Tests for Systemic Lupus Erythematosus. In my experience, systemic lupus erythematosus (SLE) is an uncommon cause of megaesophagus in patients. Antinuclear antibody (ANA) tests performed on patients with megaesophagus are rarely positive. Physical findings that should prompt the clinician to test for SLE as a cause of megaesophagus include gait abnormalities (e.g., stilted gait, shifting limb lameness), joint swelling or pain (polyarthritis), muscle pain (polymyositis), concurrent evidence of immune-mediated hemolytic anemia or immune-mediated thrombocytopenia, and skin lesions, which may include ulceration, erythema, crusting, and alopecia. Nonspecific signs of SLE may include weakness, lethargy, and anorexia.

Edrophonium Chloride (Tensilon) Challenge Test for Myasthenia Gravis. This test is used to detect generalized myasthenia gravis or, if a decreased or absent palpebral reflex is found on physical examination, focal myasthenia gravis. Most patients with generalized myasthenia gravis are thought to have at least some degree of esophageal dysfunction, ranging from mild hypomotility to megaesophagus. The most common

clinical signs of generalized myasthenia gravis are episodic weakness and decreased exercise tolerance. Difficulty with barking and with swallowing and prehending food also may be present. Mild cases may be difficult to differentiate from polymyositis, in which decreased exercise tolerance, dysphagia, and regurgitation associated with megaesophagus also may occur. Edrophonium chloride, a short-acting anticholinesterase drug, given at a dose of 0.05 to 0.1 mg/lb intravenously usually produces dramatic improvement in patients with myasthenia gravis that have collapsed or that are exercise intolerant. The response occurs within 1 to 2 minutes but lasts only for several minutes.

All dogs with myasthenia gravis should be tested for hypothyroidism, since it is estimated that 20% of dogs with myasthenia gravis will concurrently have hypothyroidism.

Electromyography. This study may be useful in the diagnosis and the differentiation of polymyopathy, polymyositis, myasthenia gravis, and polyneuropathy. For example, in myasthenia gravis, electromyography (EMG) and nerve conduction velocity studies are usually normal. On repetitive nerve stimulation, a decremental response is seen that is most characteristic of myasthenia gravis. The decremental response disappears when edrophonium chloride is given. EMG in patients with polymyositis may demonstrate positive sharp waves, fibrillation potentials, and bizarre high-frequency discharges. There is no decremental response to repetitive nerve stimulation, which differentiates polymyositis from myasthenia gravis.

In most patients with megaesophagus, endoscopic examination is not necessary for diagnosis and is rarely beneficial in determining a cause for the disorder. Patients with *mild* esophageal motility disorders may have a completely normal endoscopic examination; alternatively, there may be various degrees of fluid pooling. In contrast, patients with megaesophagus almost always demonstrate fluid retention and often small to moderate amounts of food residue. Many patients with megaesophagus have grossly normal esophageal mucosa. However, in some patients there may be evidence of esophagitis (e.g., mucosal erosions, patchy erythema, or focal hemorrhage occurring secondary to mucosal contact with the endoscope tip), which is most likely related to putrefaction of retained contents or reflux of gastric acid and activated enzymes. *The two primary rule-outs for patients with megaesophagus that become inappetent are pneumonia and esophagitis.*

Treatment

The main objectives of treatment for regurgitation disorders are to remove the initiating cause as early as possible, to minimize chances of aspiration of esophageal content, and to maximize nutrient intake to the GI tract. In most cases, idiopathic megaesophagus is incurable, and treatment involves an individually tailored feeding regimen, with the animal eating in an elevated position. Specific medical management is concurrently administered to patients with an associated disorder, such as myasthenia gravis, hypoadrenocorticism, SLE, polymyositis, and lead poisoning. Pneumonia is watched for carefully and treated aggressively if it occurs.

Patients with megaesophagus are best fed with the upper body in an elevated position of at least 45 degrees and, if possible, at a greater angle of elevation (Figure 4-4). Elevated feeding allows gravity to assist entry of food into the stomach. It is important that proper positioning be clearly demonstrated to the owner so that there is no misunderstanding about what has to be done. Otherwise, some owners will mistakenly think that elevated feeding simply means making sure that the head, rather than the entire upper body, is raised during feeding.

Significant difficulty may be experienced when one attempts to hold medium to large dogs with rear limb arthritis in a proper position. It is usually best to coax these dogs to sit down on their haunches while the owner stoops or kneels behind and helps hold the dog's body up by reaching around and supporting the sternum area. Food is placed on a table, a chair, or an elevated platform. The caregiver can reach around the dog to control the position of the food bowl if necessary. It is important to use a structure that is large enough for the patient to situate its front legs comfortably and strong enough to support its weight as it eats. *Attention must also be directed toward controlling joint pain associated with arthritis as completely as possible.* The more comfortable an arthritic patient is, the easier it will be for it to eat in the required position. *Dedicated animal owners can almost always find a way to get the job done properly.* Some owners build special platforms; others train their dogs to get into position with no assistance and stay until a command is given to get down. Giant-breed dogs such as Irish wolfhounds and Great Danes often do well when fed on indoor or outdoor house steps. Special "highchairs" have also been devised to aid in positioning and holding dogs upright (Figure 4-5). A shoulder harness can also be used for small dogs (Figure 4-6).

Cats rarely develop megaesophagus. Those that do often tolerate elevated feedings well. These feedings are accomplished either by holding the cat as demonstrated in Figure 4-7 or by supporting the animal from behind. I am also aware of cats that have been trained to eat in an elevated position (Figure 4-8).

The elevated position should be maintained for a full 10 minutes after food ingestion is completed. The importance of maintaining the elevated position for a sufficient time must be emphasized to the owner. Since the esophagus is virtually never completely empty in a patient with megaesophagus, it is often helpful to hold the patient in an elevated position for 5 to 10 minutes some time between meals and at bedtime. Nothing is fed at these times. I ask all my clients to do at least the bedtime elevation so that the esophagus will be as empty as possible before an expected period of prolonged recumbency. Some dogs regurgitate more during late evening and nighttime. This extra elevation maneuver often helps decrease the frequency of regurgitation significantly.

Patients with megaesophagus ideally are fed two to four times daily. This depends, of course, on the caregiver's time constraints. I have had the best success feeding soft-moist to solid (chopped) canned

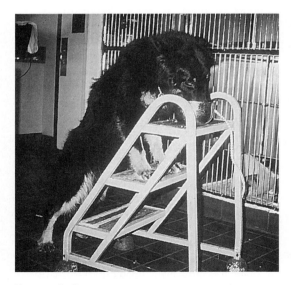

FIGURE 4-4 Ideal position for elevated feeding in a dog with megaesophagus. The dog was trained to remain on the ladder after it was finished eating until it was told to get down.

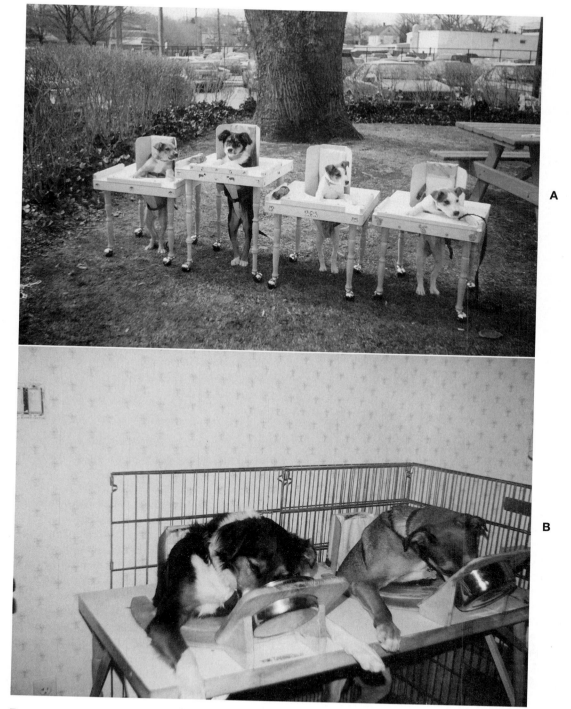

FIGURE 4-5 A, Specialized feeding chairs for dogs with megaesophagus. These chairs were designed by Donna Imhoff, a veterinary technician who has substantial experience in managing dogs with megaesophagus, and her husband. The chair provides full upright support for dogs to facilitate both feeding and holding them comfortably upright for the desired amount of time after they have eaten. The chair can be adjusted to accommodate patients of various sizes. Use of these chairs has the additional advantage of freeing the pet's owner from having to physically hold the patient in an upright position, and thus it is also more likely that the patient will be kept upright for the full recommended period of time. **B,** A tilt feature can be added to the highchairs to make it easier for the patient to reach the food bowl. (Courtesy Donna Imhoff, North Shore Animal League, Port Washington, NY.)

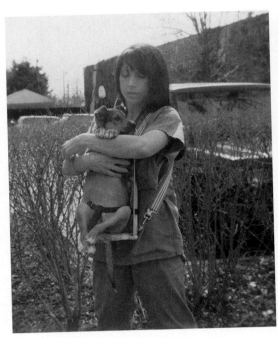

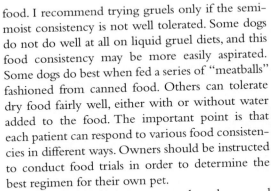

FIGURE 4-6 Use of a shoulder harness with a platform and restraint strap is another available means of feeding patients with megaesophagus. (Courtesy Donna Imhoff, North Shore Animal League, Port Washington, NY.)

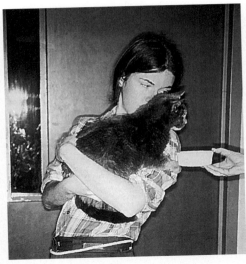

FIGURE 4-7 Elevated feeding position for a cat with megaesophagus. This 15-year-old cat had generalized gastrointestinal hypomotility. It had become hypothyroid after bilateral thyroidectomy for hyperthyroidism. The cat did not regurgitate as long as it ate in an elevated position. Thyroid supplementation did not improve gastrointestinal motility in this cat.

food. I recommend trying gruels only if the semi-moist consistency is not well tolerated. Some dogs do not do well at all on liquid gruel diets, and this food consistency may be more easily aspirated. Some dogs do best when fed a series of "meatballs" fashioned from canned food. Others can tolerate dry food fairly well, either with or without water added to the food. The important point is that each patient can respond to various food consistencies in different ways. Owners should be instructed to conduct food trials in order to determine the best regimen for their own pet.

Specific pharmacologic agents have been used in efforts to improve esophageal emptying. The promotility drug metoclopramide has been ineffective in my experience. Metoclopramide can increase lower esophageal contractions slightly in normal patients but does not improve contractile activity in patients with megaesophagus. Nifedipine is a calcium channel antagonist that promotes relaxation of the LES. It was tried with the thought that decreasing LES tone might make it easier for the esophagus to pass food into the stomach. Calcium channel antagonists, however, can cause serious side effects, and there is no

evidence that they are of any value in the treatment of megaesophagus. Their use is therefore not recommended.

The GI prokinetic drug cisapride is a benzamide derivative that promotes GI motility, increases antroduodenal coordination, and enhances LES tone. It has broader promotility effects than metoclopramide does. Cisapride has promotility effects in the esophagus of cats (distal esophagus where there is smooth muscle), the stomach, the small intestine, and the large intestine. It increases LES pressure, the amplitude of contractions in the distal esophagus, and the rate of gastric emptying. Cisapride, in theory, is likely to be of little benefit in dogs with megaesophagus because it stimulates smooth muscle motility and the canine esophagus is almost exclusively striated muscle. However, cisapride has been found to be helpful in decreasing significantly the frequency of regurgitation in several dogs with megaesophagus in our hospital series. These were cases that were being managed very diligently by their owners with elevated feeding programs but with poor responses (i.e., there was an ongoing high frequency of regurgitation). Concurrent with the institution of cisapride

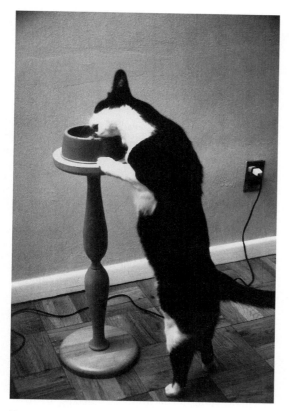

FIGURE 4-8 This cat had a regurgitation disorder and did quite well on an elevated feeding program. The cat learned to eat in a fully elevated position and regained lost weight rapidly once able to hold its food down. (Courtesy Dr. William Tepper.)

there was a dramatic decrease in the frequency of regurgitation. In one dog—a 14-year-old Labrador retriever cross with idiopathic megaesophagus, bilateral coxofemoral degenerative joint disease, and mild degenerative myelopathy—there was an ongoing high frequency of regurgitation (16 to 20 times per day despite a strict elevated feeding program). Once cisapride was instituted, the number of regurgitation episodes decreased to only one or two per day. This excellent response lasted 7 months, at which time the dog was euthanized because of its inability to walk due to severe degenerative myelopathy.

I am aware of anecdotal reports from academic institutions and private practices describing case histories in which cisapride has been effective in reducing the frequency of regurgitation in dogs with megaesophagus. In occasional cases the improvement has been dramatic. In other cases there has been minimal or no clinical improvement. In most cases it is not likely that the mega-

esophagus will be reduced with cisapride therapy. Presumably, the increase in motility in patients that have a positive response is, with elevated feedings, sufficient to improve esophageal emptying into the stomach.

The most common and severe complications of megaesophagus are aspiration pneumonia and significant weight loss. Most debilitated dogs with megaesophagus are quite hungry, but frequent regurgitation prevents them from being able to deliver enough food to their stomach. Another concern is that cachectic patients are immunocompromised and are unable to respond strongly to infection. *It is often best to begin feeding debilitated megaesophagus patients through a gastrostomy tube, unless there is a very good initial response to elevated feedings at the time the diagnosis is established.* Gastrostomy tube feeding bypasses the diseased esophagus and allows adequate caloric replacement. This is also an option in cases in which frequent regurgitation persists, with or without aspiration. Another advantage is that all required medications can be administered directly to the stomach through the tube. Gastrostomy tubes can be quickly placed under endoscopic guidance (e.g., percutaneous endoscopic gastrostomy, see Chapter 12). During tube placement, the esophageal mucosa can be concurrently evaluated for evidence of esophagitis. Surgical placement of a gastrostomy tube can also be done (see Chapter 12). The risks of general anesthesia must be considered. Precautions must always be taken in patients with megaesophagus to ensure that steps are taken to avoid aspiration during induction and recovery.

The length of time for which a feeding tube is left in place varies. Some dogs gain weight fairly quickly and respond well on an elevated feeding program with or without promotility therapy. In these cases the tube is often removed after 1 to 2 months. In other dogs tube feeding is the only possible way of successfully feeding on a long-term basis. Some large-breed dogs have been fed by gastrostomy tube for as long as 2 to 3 years. Periodic tube replacement is necessary in these dogs. The initial feeding tube is usually replaced with a "low profile" tube, which sits flush with the body wall (see Chapter 12). Complications related to gastrostomy tubes that could potentially cause significant problems in patients with megaesophagus include vomiting and gastroesophageal reflux. Many dogs with megaesophagus do well without ever having a gastrostomy tube placed. In summary, the two main indications for use of a gastrostomy tube are (1) significant weight loss with ongoing regurgitation despite elevated feedings and (2) aspiration pneumonia, in which it is best to avoid using the esophagus until the pneumonia is resolved and it is demonstrated that persistent regurgitation will not be a problem.

Treatment for aspiration pneumonia includes aggressive fluid therapy, antibiotics, coupage, nebulization, and nutritional support. Ideally, a tracheal wash should be done in patients with moderate to severe pneumonia as soon as the diagnosis is made. The initial choice of one or more antibiotics depends on cytologic studies and Gram stain results. The use of bactericidal antibiotics with a good gram-negative spectrum is recommended pending culture and sensitivity results. Trimethoprim-sulfonamide (Tribrissen) and enrofloxacin (Baytril) are good initial choices for mild pneumonia. Patients with mild pneumonia can often be treated with oral antibiotics on an outpatient basis.

If moderate to severe bacterial pneumonia is present and there is marked respiratory insufficiency, aggressive antimicrobial therapy should be instituted immediately. This usually involves combination therapy using cephalosporins (e.g., cefazolin [Kefzol], 10 to 15 mg/lb every 8 hours intravenously or intramuscularly, or cefoxitin [Mefoxin], 10 to 15 mg/lb every 6 to 8 hours intravenously) and aminoglycosides (gentamicin [Gentocin], 1 to 2 mg/lb intravenously or subcutaneously every 6 to 8 hours or 2.7 to 4.5 mg/lb intravenously or subcutaneously once every 24 hours, or amikacin [Amiglyde-V] 3 mg/lb every 8 hours or 9 mg/lb once every 24 hours intravenously, intramuscularly, or subcutaneously). Alternatively, imipenem (Primaxin) provides excellent four-quadrant coverage. Imipenem is administered as sole antimicrobial therapy at 2.5 to 5 mg/lb intravenously every 8 hours. Imipenem is a beta-lactam antibiotic. Beta-lactam agents have little if any dose-dependent toxicity. Imipenem has the same toxicity potential as that of other pencillins (e.g., ampicillin). The best use of this drug is in patients with renal compromise that cannot be given aminoglycosides safely. If the creatinine level is greater than 4 mg/dl, imipenem is administered at 12-hour, rather than 8-hour, intervals. Imipenem should be delivered over 30 minutes in the intravenous line.

Oral administration of antibiotics is contraindicated in seriously ill patients because of their low and erratic serum levels. There are also problems in ensuring that the medication is transported in a timely manner to the stomach in a patient with megaesophagus.

As previously mentioned, patients with megaesophagus occasionally develop esophagitis. The primary signs of esophagitis are decreased appetite and lethargy. Salivation also may be evident. Esophagitis should be suspected once pneumonia is ruled out. Treatment may include administration of a sucralfate (Carafate) suspension or H_2-receptor antagonist therapy to lower gastric acid levels or both. A proton pump inhibitor (e.g., omeprazole, lansoprazole, esomeprazole) is used to completely block acid release in patients with moderate to severe esophagitis, instead of an H_2-receptor antagonist. There is often rapid improvement once specific treatment is instituted. Duration of therapy depends on patient response. Management of esophagitis is discussed in more detail later in this chapter.

Dogs that seem to experience frequent bouts of mild pneumonia sometimes do best when maintained on long-term antibiotic therapy. In these cases, the antibiotics used are often rotated every 6 to 8 weeks. Likewise, an H_2-receptor antagonist or proton pump inhibitor is sometimes used on a long-term basis in dogs with chronic esophagitis.

Too often patients with megaesophagus are quickly assigned a poor prognosis. Granted, some patients do poorly on any form of therapy and euthanasia may unfortunately be inevitable. However, *many* patients with megaesophagus can be successfully managed for months to years. Owners who are willing to invest time and effort in the care of their pet with megaesophagus are often rewarded. To highlight this point, three cases of note are presented in Figures 4-9 and 4-10.

Megaesophagus Secondary to Acquired Myasthenia Gravis
Clinical Signs
Myasthenia gravis occurs both as an acquired autoimmune disorder and as a congenital, familial one. Acquired myasthenia gravis is an autoimmune disorder of neuromuscular transmission resulting from the actions of autoantibodies against nicotinic acetylcholine receptors at neuromuscular junctions. Conjointly there is complement medi-

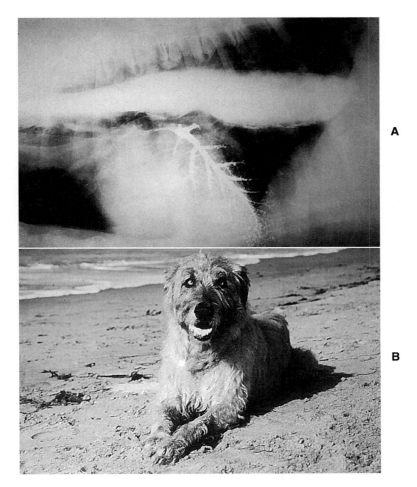

FIGURE 4-9 **A,** Contrast radiograph of an 8-year-old Irish wolfhound with adult-onset idiopathic megaesophagus. Note that there was aspiration of a small amount of barium into the airways. The dog was presented because of regurgitation. There was an excellent response to elevated feedings (the owner used a ladder and helped support the dog from the side). The diet consisted of kibble soaked in water. **B,** Photograph of the dog taken 5 months after the diagnosis was made. The dog regurgitated on average only two times per week.

ated destruction of the junction folds, altering the neuromuscular junction formation, or it may accelerate the internalization and the degradation of the acetylcholine receptor. Myasthenia gravis manifests itself in several clinical forms:

- Generalized myasthenia gravis: Manifests predominantly as tetraparesis, but there may be primarily pelvic limb paresis.
- Focal myasthenia gravis: Affects the cranial nerves mainly around the larynx and pharyngeal region.
- Acute fulminant myasthenia gravis: Flaccid tetraparesis, acute respiratory distress.

Megaesophagus associated with generalized myasthenia gravis has been well documented.

Clinical signs include premature fatigue during exercise (manifested by a spastic pelvic limb gait followed by tetraparesis and then collapse), tachypnea and dyspnea, and sialosis. More recently, a *focal form of myasthenia gravis,* in which megaesophagus occurs in the *absence* of detectable generalized weakness, has been recognized. The primary clinical sign is regurgitation. Other clinical signs that may occasionally be observed in focal myasthenia gravis include pharyngeal and laryngeal muscle weakness (dysphagia and dyspnea), weakness of the facial muscles, and a decreased palpebral reflex. In some dogs there is a change in the quality of the bark or an inability to bark. A myopathy or a neuropathy should always be considered as a differential diagnosis in laryngeal or pharyngeal problems.

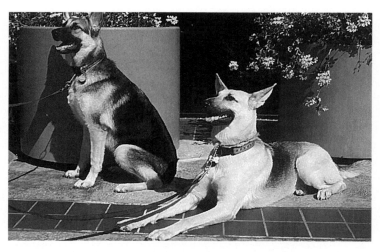

FIGURE 4-10 Two young German shepherd dogs with esophageal motility disorders. The dog on the left had congenital megaesophagus (also shown in Figure 4-1). Persistent right aortic arch was diagnosed in the dog on the right at 4 months of age. Surgery was successful in relieving the esophageal obstruction, but esophageal dilation persisted. The dogs are not related. Each of these dogs was adopted and cared for by a veterinarian on our staff. Note their excellent body condition. Long-term treatment for megaesophagus included twice daily elevated feedings. The diet consisted of a mixture of kibble, canned food, and water blenderized to an oatmeal consistency. Regurgitation rarely occurred, and both dogs remained highly energetic.

Diagnosis

Several large groups of affected dogs have been reported in the literature. In one group 40 of 152 dogs (26%) with megaesophagus were found to have elevated serum antibodies to acetylcholine receptors, diagnostic of acquired myasthenia gravis. Many breeds were affected, but Golden retrievers (7 of 20, 35%) and German shepherds (8 of 25, 32%) were the breeds most commonly involved.

A diagnosis of acquired myasthenia gravis is established by demonstration of circulating antibodies against canine acetylcholine receptors by immunoprecipitation radioimmunoassay. An antibody titer greater than 0.6 nmol/L is diagnostic for acquired myasthenia gravis in dogs, whereas a value of greater than 0.3 nmol/L is diagnostic in cats. *This test should be performed in all patients with acquired megaesophagus.* This assay is particularly valuable in cases of focal myasthenia in which muscle weakness is localized to esophageal or pharyngeal musculature and generalized weakness is not present. Serial serum antibody titers are also important in following a patient's clinical response to treatment.

The acetylcholine receptor antibody titer assay is available at the Comparative Neuromuscular Laboratory.* A blood sample is drawn into a red top tube and allowed to clot at room temperature. The sample is centrifuged as soon as possible after clotting has occurred. The serum is removed and refrigerated until the time of shipping. At least 1 ml (preferably 2 ml) of serum should be sent to the laboratory on a cold pack by an overnight mail service.

The edrophonium chloride challenge test may be useful in helping establish a presumptive diagnosis of focal myasthenia gravis in some dogs, especially those with a decreased or absent palpebral reflex. The administration of edrophonium chloride (0.05-0.1 mg/lb intravenously) may result in an improved blink reflex.

Treatment

Treatment includes drug therapy in conjunction with a standard elevated feeding program, as is done with any patient with megaesophagus. The cornerstone of treatment in generalized myasthenia gravis is anticholinesterase therapy. Pharmacologic management (anticholinesterase drugs or corticosteroids or both) may also be helpful in dogs with focal myasthenia gravis. Recent reports have highlighted azathioprine as

---

*Comparative Neuromuscular Laboratory, Basic Science Building Room 1057, University of California–San Diego, La Jolla, CA 90293-0612 (Phone: 619-534-1537).

an effective immunosuppressive drug for management of myasthenia gravis (see subsequent discussion).

In general, the following recommendations for pyridostigmine can be made. Careful monitoring is essential to the prevention of anticholinesterase overdose. Injectable neostigmine (Prostigmin) can be given at a dose of 0.2 mg/lb intramuscularly every 6 hours if administration by mouth or by gastrostomy tube is not possible or advisable (e.g., patients with frequent regurgitation should be treated initially with injectable medication because orally administered medication may not be transported to the stomach). Once oral medication can be tolerated, pyridostigmine bromide syrup or tablets (Mestinon) are administered at 0.25 to 1.5 mg/lb every 8 to 12 hours per os (start at the low end for focal myasthenia gravis patients because clinical response may be difficult to evaluate). Signs of overdose include muscle weakness, salivation, miosis, vomiting, and diarrhea. Administration of pyridostigmine may result in a decrease in clinical signs of regurgitation. Careful surveillance for the development of aspiration pneumonia is maintained at all times.

Corticosteroids may benefit some patients with myasthenia gravis. Corticosteroids alter macrophage function by inhibiting antigen processing and thus inhibiting interleukin-1 (IL-1) release. This alters B cell function. Corticosteroids also suppress interleukin-2 (IL-2) synthesis and thus alter T cell proliferation. Positive effects include enhanced presence of acetylcholine receptors, acetylcholine synthesis, and enhanced organization of the postsynaptic membrane.

Corticosteroids may cause some potentially negative effects in myasthenia patients, especially when used in high doses. Corticosteroids may actually antagonize acetylcholine and create a neuromuscular junction blockage effect of the acetylcholine receptor channel, which may then uncouple the excitatory processes. In some cases prednisone may actually create a fulminating myasthenic crisis.

Corticosteroids are instituted at immunosuppressive doses. It is recommended that steroids be started slowly, with an initial dose of 0.25 mg/lb of prednisone per day, divided BID. The dose is gradually increased over the next 5 days to 1 mg/lb per day. If aspiration pneumonia is present, administration of corticosteroids is avoided until the pneumonia has resolved. Caution must also be exercised when corticosteroids are used in conjunction with anticholinesterase drugs, since muscle weakness can be exacerbated by such treatment. It is difficult to assess

the effectiveness of corticosteroids accurately because many dogs with focal myasthenia gravis reportedly go into spontaneous remission in the absence of any drug treatment. Some clinicians, including myself, have observed dogs with focal myasthenia gravis that have demonstrated dramatic positive responses to corticosteroids. In some patients long-term, low-dose therapy has been required for control of symptoms, whereas in others medication has been successfully discontinued.

Recently there have been favorable reports about azathioprine as an effective form of therapy for myasthenia gravis. Azathioprine is an immunosuppressive drug that binds to and interferes with synthesis of ribonucleic acid (RNA) and deoxyribonucleic acid (DNA) and therefore alters T cell proliferation after antigenic stimulation. Azathioprine affects both cell mediated and humoral responses. It is thought to have more of an affect on the cell mediated side.

The recommended regimen is 0.5 mg/lb orally once daily for 14 days, followed by an increase to 1 mg/lb per day. The idea is to slowly suppress the immune response. Azathioprine has a delayed onset of action of 3 to 4 weeks or so. Pyridostigmine may be needed for a while to be used in conjunction with azathioprine. The acetylcholine receptor antibody (AcRAb) titer should be checked monthly during therapy. When clinical signs have resolved and there has been normalization of acetylcholine receptor antibody levels azathioprine is reduced to an every other day schedule. The titer should still be monitored once monthly.

Side effects to azathioprine are uncommon when it is used at the recommended dose. The major effect to watch for is bone marrow suppression. A baseline complete blood count (CBC) and platelet count are followed by recheck tests at 3 and 6 weeks, then every 2 months. Azathioprine is discontinued if the neutrophil count drops below 1,000/μl. Other uncommon but potential side effects include GI irritation, hepatotoxicity, drug induced pancreatitis, and slow hair growth.

Remission can be induced in most dogs, but relapses may occur. Three out of five patients in one report experienced complete remission of clinical signs within 3 months of therapy. Further studies to evaluate monotherapy with azathioprine and combination therapy with azathioprine and pyridostigmine or azathioprine, prednisone, and pyridostigmine are needed.

The course of focal myasthenia gravis is variable. Some affected dogs might progress to generalized myasthenia gravis, but if this is going to happen it generally occurs within the first few weeks after onset of clinical signs. Radiographs are also obtained periodically to monitor esophageal size. Esophageal function may return to normal, but remission may require days to months. Owners should also be warned that the disease may recur.

Several clinicians have reported seeing an occasional dog with both hypothyroidism (confirmed by a TSH response test) and focal myasthenia gravis. In some cases the myasthenic condition resolved after treatment for hypothyroidism was instituted.

VASCULAR RING ANOMALIES

Vascular ring anomalies are congenital malformations of the great vessels and their branches that entrap the intrathoracic esophagus and cause obstruction. Although a number of different congenital vascular ring anomalies can occur in dogs and cats, persistent right aortic arch (PRAA) is by far the most common (95%). Other anomalies that have been reported include persistent right ductus arteriosus, aberrant left or right subclavian arteries, double aortic arch, and esophageal compression by the left subclavian and brachiocephalic arteries (found in English bulldogs). Vascular rings are quite uncommon in cats.

In PRAA the right rather than the left fourth aortic arch forms the functional adult aorta. The esophagus becomes entrapped by the aorta on the right, by the pulmonary trunk on the left, by the ligamentum arteriosum dorsolaterally on the left, and by the base of the heart ventrally (Figure 4-11). This anatomic "ring" results in obstruction and progressive dilation of the esophagus cranial to the base of the heart.

Vascular ring anomalies are inherited. There is a breed predilection for German shepherds and Irish setters. There is also a higher than expected incidence among Boston terriers and English bulldogs. There is no reported breed predilection for cats. Multiple puppies in a litter may be affected. Breeding affected patients is not recommended.

Clinical Signs

The most common clinical sign in puppies and kittens is an acute onset of regurgitation at or shortly after the time of weaning to solid foods. In patients that do not show significant signs around the time of weaning, the diagnosis will almost always be made by 6 months of age. Rarely, significant clinical signs may not be apparent until later in life. As the proximal esophagus becomes more dilated, food may be retained for longer periods before regurgitation occurs. Affected patients become malnourished and weak and are smaller than their littermates. Coughing with respiratory distress is common and indicates a secondary aspiration pneumonia.

Diagnosis

The primary differential diagnosis for vascular ring anomaly is congenital megaesophagus. Foreign body obstruction also should be considered. Diagnosis is based on survey and contrast radiography of the thorax. Survey radiographs of vascular ring anomaly show esophageal dilation with food and air. The dilation tapers to normal at the base of the heart. With PRAA the normal opacity caused by the bulge of the aortic arch is absent. Contrast studies of vascular ring anomaly reveal a characteristic constricted appearance over the base of the heart, with variable degrees of esophageal dilation proximal to the site of obstruction. Fluoroscopy demonstrates a loss of motility of the proximal esophagus. Esophageal motility distal to the stricture is usually normal. In the rare instance that the diagnosis cannot be confirmed by radiography, esophagoscopy can provide useful information in differentiating a mural lesion from extraluminal compression. With extraluminal compression of the esophagus, a full circumference indentation may be seen from the lumen side. Endoscopy is also useful for ruling out esophageal foreign body and in removal if one is found. Foreign bodies can become lodged secondary to the PRAA.

Treatment

Definitive management of vascular ring anomaly is limited to surgical correction of the constricting band forming the vascular ring. For PRAA this involves ligation and transection of the ligamentum arteriosum.

It is best to stabilize and strengthen the patient as much as possible before subjecting it to a thoracotomy. Elevated feedings having a gruel consistency are given frequently and in small enough amounts to minimize regurgitation. A gastrostomy tube can be used if oral feeding is poorly tolerated. If pneumonia is present, it should be treated aggressively and resolved before surgery.

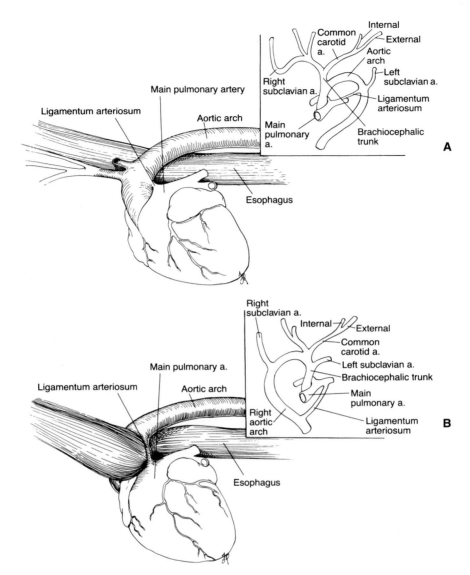

FIGURE 4-11 Persistent right aortic arch. **A,** Normal development of the aortic arch viewed from the patient's left side. Inset shows normal embryonic development of the great vessels from a dorsoventral view. **B,** When the embryonic right fourth aortic arch becomes the adult aorta, esophageal constriction occurs. Inset shows dorsoventral view of the vascular malformation. (From Birchard SJ, Sherding RG, eds: *Manual of small animal practice,* ed 2, Philadelphia, 2000, WB Saunders.)

The prognosis for *complete* recovery after surgery is guarded to poor. Regurgitation of some degree persists in most dogs that undergo surgical correction. The esophageal dilation that exists early in the course of the disease persists to some degree indefinitely in most patients. In addition, esophageal dilation caudal to the vascular ring site can occur, possibly due to neuromuscular disease. Recovery of normal esophageal function is more likely when surgery is performed at an early age.

Many patients significantly improve after surgery. If esophageal disease persists, an elevated feeding protocol should be followed. Surveillance for signs of aspiration pneumonia is always maintained.

A retrospective study examined whether the degree of esophageal dilation affects long-term outcome. Ten dogs and four cats with PRAA were studied through 6 months after surgery. Of all the animals, 35.7% (mean age 2.5 months) had a very good outcome, 42.9% (mean age 2.7

months) had a good outcome, and 21.4% (mean age 5.7 months, range 3 to 9 months) had a poor outcome. A measurement scheme was devised. After barium contrast esophagography the maximum diameter of the esophageal dilation cranial to the heart base (O_e) was compared with the height of the body of the 5th thoracic vertebra at its narrowest point (T_5). The degree of esophageal dilation was classified as mild, moderate, and severe on the basis of the ratio $O_e:T_5$. All measurements were made to the nearest millimeter. The ratio of $O_e:T_5$ for normal dogs and cats, based on esophageal contrast studies on 10 normal cats and 25 normal dogs, was considered to be less than or equal to 1. Mild dilation was considered to be less than or equal to 2.5, moderate less than or equal to 4, and severe greater than 4.

In this study a majority of the patients with a mild or moderate degree of dilation had a good to very good outcome after surgery. Of three patients that had a poor outcome (two cats and one dog), two had a severe degree of dilation (one cat and one dog), and one had a moderate degree of dilation. Although more animals must be evaluated using this scheme, it appears that the degree of preoperative esophageal dilation does affect the long-term outcome in patients with PRAA.

ESOPHAGITIS

Inflammatory diseases of the esophagus occur more commonly than they are recognized. The major causes of esophagitis are listed in Box 4-2.

BOX 4-2	Causes of Esophagitis

Gastroesophageal reflux (physiologic)
Anesthesia-related reflux
Foreign body passage or impaction
Food retention as that which may occur with megaesophagus
Any cause of persistent, severe vomiting: e.g., parvoviral enteritis, acute pancreatitis, renal failure, gastrinoma (vomited gastric content is very high in acid), gastric and intestinal foreign bodies
Caustic injury: e.g., toxic irritants, acids, alkalis, capsule or tablet medications that lodge in the esophagus
Infectious agents such as calicivirus, candida, phycomycosis in immunocompromised animals
Thermal injury: e.g., rapid ingestion of heated food
Radiation

Inflammatory changes can range from mild mucosal inflammation that may or may not be grossly evident, to moderate to severe ulceration and transmural involvement. Any disorder that causes acute or chronic frequent vomiting can potentially cause esophagitis. This especially includes causes of severe vomiting, such as intestinal foreign bodies, gastric foreign bodies, acute pancreatitis, parvoviral enteritis, and gastrinoma. Dogs with parvoviral enteritis that are debilitated and recumbent are especially at risk. Vomited fluid that is retained in the esophagus is not cleared adequately in weak and recumbent patients. As a result the esophageal mucosa is bathed with gastric acid and activated enzymes that will cause mucosal injury.

Other causes of esophagitis include esophageal foreign bodies (extent of injury depends on the size, texture, and duration of lodgment) and chemical and thermal injuries (e.g., ingestion of hot food). The latter two factors are uncommon causes of esophagitis. Chemical injury may result from ingestion of toxic chemicals or from failure of the esophagus to transport capsule or tablet medication completely to the stomach. It is not infrequent in humans for medications taken without water to become lodged somewhere in the esophagus. When certain medications dissolve there, mucosal irritation results. Medication associated esophagitis from caustic compounds such as NSAIDs and doxycycline have been associated with esophagitis or even stricture formation. Owing to anatomic and physiologic differences between the canine esophagus and the human esophagus (canine esophageal muscle is entirely striated; the human esophagus is mostly smooth muscle), this irritation is somewhat less likely to be a problem in dogs than in humans. However, it is likely to be more common in cats than in dogs. There have been reports of severe esophagitis occurring in patients secondary to injury from ingested capsule medication (e.g., doxycycline, chloramphenicol). There is also potential for a stricture to develop secondary to esophagitis. In fact, doxycycline-induced esophagitis with esophageal stricture formation has been reported in cats.

Gastroesophageal Reflux Disease

A study was reported recently on normal cats in which the passage of tablets and capsules when given alone (dry swallow) and when followed by a water bolus (wet swallow) was evaluated.

This investigation was undertaken as a result of experience with cats developing esophagitis and esophageal strictures subsequent to doxycycline tablet administration. Thirty healthy cats of various ages were used in this study. Each cat was given a 20-mg barium tablet and a 190-mg (size 4) capsule both as a dry and wet swallow. A wet swallow consisted of immediately following administration with 6.0 ml of water orally via syringe. Fluoroscopy was used to evaluate tablet or capsule passage at 30, 60, 90, 120, 180, 240, and 300 seconds following administration. Dry swallows and wet swallows were evaluated. Successful passage was defined as complete passage into the stomach at a given time interval.

The percentage of dry tablet swallows that successfully passed into the stomach was 0.0% at 30 and 60 seconds, 6.7% at 90 seconds, 13.3% at 120 seconds, 26.7% at 180 and 240 seconds, and 36.7% at 300 seconds. Wet tablet swallows successfully passed 90.0% of the time at 30 seconds, 93.3% at 60 seconds, and 100.0% of the time thereafter. The percentage of dry capsule swallows that successfully passed was 16.7% at each time interval. Wet capsule swallows successfully passed 96.7% of the time at 30 seconds and 100% of the time thereafter. For each time interval, wet swallows achieved significantly greater percentage passage into the stomach when compared with dry swallows.

The results of this study show that tablets or capsules given as a dry swallow in cats have prolonged retention in the esophagus. A water bolus following tablet or capsule administration results in significantly faster passage through the water bolus for cats receiving oral tablets or capsules to prevent possible medication associated esophagitis. *It is therefore now recommended that cats that receive oral tablet or capsule medications without food be given approximately 6 ml of water immediately after the medication to promote rapid clearing from the esophagus and transit to the stomach. It is also probably a good idea to do the same in dogs whenever medications are not given in food.*

Gastroesophageal reflux is the most common cause of esophagitis in animals and humans. This disorder is discussed in detail in this section. The term *reflux* refers to movement of gastric or duodenal contents into the esophagus without associated eructation or vomiting. As such this can be a "silent" disease. Reflux esophagitis is a disorder in which esophageal inflammation of variable degree occurs as a result of mucosal contact with gastric or duodenal fluid or ingesta. In many cases the inflammation may not be visible grossly. A variety of factors can contribute to its development in individual patients. It can be a particularly difficult diagnosis to make without special instrumentation (e.g., pH probe monitoring, endoscopy) because in many patients clinical signs are quite subtle. History and recognition of suggestive clinical signs constitute the basis for performing diagnostic procedures or instituting empirical therapy. *Because significant discomfort can result from reflux episodes, it is important that reflux esophagitis be diagnosed and treated in a timely manner.*

Gastroesophageal reflux disease in humans

Gastroesophageal reflux disease (GERD) is among the most common GI disorders that affect people. It is estimated that up to 50% of adults in the United States experience heartburn type of symptoms at least once a month. GERD is a very difficult diagnosis to establish in animals, largely because our patients are not able to describe for us the fact that they are experiencing the symptoms of this disorder and there are no hallmark signs, and it can also be difficult to diagnose definitively in humans. There is still no single test that can uniformly detect GERD. Of all the GI disorders that affect humans, the symptom pattern for GERD is among the most specific of any GI disorder. However, there are now well-recognized supraesophageal and extraesophageal reflux symptoms (e.g., laryngeal problems, cough) that will not be diagnosed with just a standard history. The tests used in human medicine to investigate for GERD are endoscopy, looking for esophagitis or other GERD complications, and 24-hour pH probe recording. Barium swallow is also performed in some cases, mostly to screen for other upper GI disorders. None of these tests is always diagnostic, however (e.g., it is known that 30% to 70% of patients undergoing endoscopy for GERD symptoms may have a grossly normal examination), and some gastroenterologists therefore use parallel tests to determine the presence of GERD. More recently another diagnostic approach in humans that has received attention is a therapeutic trial of high dose proton pump inhibitor (PPI) therapy. The basis for this test centers on the ability of the high dose PPI therapy to *completely* inhibit gastric acid secretion. If symptoms do not resolve on high-dose PPI therapy, they are not likely caused by GERD. There are sensitivity and specificity issues with this test as well, however.

Veterinarians should recognize that GERD is very common in people and that it likely occurs in animals much more commonly than we are able to recognize. Therefore we should maintain a high index of suspicion for this disorder when presented with patients that may be exhibiting any of the potential signs of esophagitis.

Pathophysiology

Normal LES function is essential to the prevention of gastroesophageal reflux and esophagitis. The LES is located at the GEJ and is a zone of high resting pressure that acts to prevent reflux of gastric contents into the esophagus. In response to esophageal peristaltic contractions, the LES undergoes a phase of initial relaxation that is followed by postdeglutition contraction. Initial relaxation begins when an esophageal peristaltic contraction is in the proximal esophagus. Postdeglutition contractions prevent reflux of a food bolus following its passage into the stomach.

Reflux of small amounts of fluid is considered a normal physiologic phenomenon in both animals and humans. Functional defense mechanisms prevent esophageal mucosal damage when these minor reflux episodes occur. These defenses include acid clearance by means of one or two esophageal peristaltic sequences that empty all or most of the acid from the esophagus, local mucosal protective factors, and neutralization of any postperistaltic residual acid by bicarbonate-rich saliva. It has been shown in humans that some individuals can experience significant reflux episodes without developing demonstrable esophageal mucosal changes. Although clinical signs of reflux may be experienced (heartburn, indigestion, dyspepsia), significant sequelae such as esophagitis, esophageal stricture, and chest pain often never develop.

Although the relationships and factors responsible for individual variations in response to reflux are unknown, a number of factors are probably involved in determining how significant a problem reflux episodes will be in an individual. These include volume and frequency of reflux, the duration of contact between the refluxate and the esophageal mucosa, character of the refluxed material, competency of esophageal clearing mechanisms, and gastric emptying patterns. It has been estimated that up to 7% of the general human population has symptoms of heartburn *daily*, and a much larger percentage experiences these symptoms *monthly* (approximately 50% as previously stated). Many humans never seek medical attention for what they consider a minor, normal physiologic event. The frequency in animals is unknown, since signs of mild reflux are extremely difficult to detect.

Manometric measurements of the LES have shown that a decrease in resting pressures is the major factor in the pathogenesis of gastroesophageal reflux. Reflux occurs primarily by one of three different mechanisms: transient complete relaxation of the LES, transient increase in intraabdominal pressure, or spontaneous free reflux associated with a low resting pressure of the LES. Human studies have shown that in normal individuals, reflux episodes are almost always caused by transient sphincter relaxation. The predominant reflux mechanism in reflux esophagitis patients varies, although transient LES relaxation seems to be most common. This transient relaxation mechanism may explain why some reflux esophagitis patients have resting LES pressure values that overlap those of normal controls.

Transient changes in intraabdominal pressure may intermittently overcome a hypotensive LES; however, complete sphincter relaxation alone does not guarantee that significant reflux will occur. Factors that may influence reflux in this situation include body position, intragastric volume, intragastric pressure, and relaxation of the diaphragmatic hiatus. Significant reflux can occur in animals that undergo general anesthesia, especially when there is ingesta or fluid retention in the stomach. Anesthetic agents promote relaxation of the LES, and any procedure that involves positioning the patient with the rear quarters elevated (e.g., tilting the surgery table so that the head and the upper body are below the lower body) can promote gravitational flow of gastric contents to the esophagus. Mild to severe esophagitis may result, and in some cases esophageal stricture formation occurs. Clinical situations in which a reflux episode may be exacerbated must be recognized, and preventive measures must be taken to decrease serious sequelae.

Mechanisms of Esophageal Mucosal Damage

Although both acid and pepsin were implicated in the past as the major injurious agents in reflux disease, it now appears that the importance of acid has been overemphasized and that of pepsin minimized. Animal studies have shown that pepsin, rather than acid, is a major causative agent of erosive esophagitis resulting from reflux of acid gastric contents.

Of the potentially injurious agents in *acid* gastric contents (e.g., acid, bile salts, pepsin, and trypsin), pepsin produces a mucosal injury consistent with both the macroscopic and the microscopic appearance of reflux esophagitis in symptomatic human patients. Hydrochloric acid (HCl) at physiologic pH values does not appear to break the esophageal squamous mucosal barrier to hydrogen ion back diffusion or to cause esophagitis. Pepsin, however, can cause mucosal permeability changes, resulting in severe hydrogen ion back diffusion. Rabbit esophageal perfusion studies have demonstrated that pepsin causes significantly more esophageal injury than does bile, trypsin, or acid alone. In these studies the extent of injury increased in a dose-dependent manner as pepsin concentration was increased. Pepsin injury was characterized by mucosal erosion and ulceration with submucosal hemorrhage. Acid, bile, and trypsin damage was generally limited to submucosal edema without mucosal disruption.

Excessive *alkaline* gastroesophageal reflux produces inflammatory changes comparable to those seen with excessive acid gastroesophageal reflux. The alkaline nature of refluxed material alone does not appear to produce mucosal damage. Rather, with alkaline reflux the pancreatic enzyme trypsin has been shown to be the factor that causes the most significant damage. Pepsin causes minimal esophageal changes in the presence of an alkaline environment. Trypsin is present in the gastric contents of patients with decreased pyloric tone and duodenogastric reflux. The pH of the refluxate appears to control which agent will be the most active in causing esophageal damage. Pepsin's optimal pH range for proteolytic activity is 2 to 4.5, and it is the most injurious agent when the refluxate is acid. Trypsin's optimal pH range for proteolytic activity is 5 to 8.

The bile salt taurodeoxycholate has been found to protect the esophageal mucosa from the injurious effects of acid and pepsin, but the effect of trypsin in the alkaline medium has been potentiated. Bile salts decrease pepsin's proteolytic activity, and the protective bile salt effect is dose related. The combination of bile, trypsin, and an alkaline refluxate could potentially cause the most severe degree of esophageal injury. Bile salts may play an important role in modulating the injurious effect of acid and pepsin in certain clinical settings. *The concentration of injurious agents in the refluxed gastric fluid and the duration of their contact with the esophageal mucosa are the major factors determining the likelihood and severity of mucosal injury.*

Etiology

Pharmacologic agents that have been associated with decreased LES pressure and reflux include atropine and other anticholinergic drugs, morphine, meperidine, diazepam, and pentobarbital. Phenothiazine-derivative tranquilizers also can decrease LES pressure. Glycopyrrolate does not cause as significant an effect on the LES as atropine does. For this reason, some clinicians use glycopyrrolate rather than atropine as their standard preanesthesia agent.

Pregnancy in humans is associated with an increased frequency of heartburn, a sensation of chest pain that is due to esophageal pain from mucosal contact with refluxate. This was originally thought to be due to reflux exacerbated by increased gastric pressure from an enlarging uterus. However, it is now recognized that elevated progesterone levels decrease LES pressure, increasing the likelihood of reflux. Reflux esophagitis in humans can also be predisposed by high-fat or spicy foods, chocolate, alcohol, and nicotine.

The most common causes of reflux esophagitis in dogs and cats are general anesthesia and persistent vomiting due to any cause (e.g., pancreatitis, gastric or intestinal foreign body, parvoviral enteritis). Hiatal hernia disorders, neuromuscular disorders (e.g., myasthenia gravis) that interfere with function of the esophagus and LES, delayed gastric emptying, and duodenogastric reflux are also important, but less common, disorders that are associated with reflux esophagitis episodes.

During anesthesia there is suppression of normal esophageal motility and decreased LES pressure. As a result, acid and other refluxed agents cannot be cleared as quickly as in an awake animal with normal esophageal defenses. Problems tend to occur more commonly in patients that have undergone prolonged surgical procedures; however, it has been shown that reflux can occur between 5 and 15 minutes after induction of anesthesia. Therefore reflux should be considered a possibility in any patient that undergoes anesthesia. In a study involving 100 dogs, it was found that the frequency of gastroesophageal reflux was 25% with regard to the type of surgery, 48% of the cases of reflux appeared during orthopedic surgery, 24% during abdominal surgery, and 28% during other types of surgery (e.g., skin, eyes). Consideration should be given to routinely treating these patients for reflux esophagitis for several days during the immediate postoperative period. It may also be beneficial to pretreat patients scheduled to undergo a prolonged (greater than 1 to 2 hours) surgical procedure with an H_2-receptor antagonist before induction of anesthesia (e.g., administer injectable famotidine or ranitidine 1 to 2 hours prior). As the duration of anesthesia increases, the risk of a significant reflux event also increases.

Some clinicians have also instituted a postoperative practice of lavaging the esophagus with saline or warm water after long surgical procedures, so as to dilute and remove offending substances before significant mucosal damage can occur. This can be done either under endoscopic guidance or simply by passing a tube blindly into the esophagus for lavage purposes, while the patient is still intubated. Use of an endoscope offers the advantage of lavage and suction under direct visualization. In addition to the anesthetic agents used, tilting of the surgery table so that the patient's abdomen is elevated relative to the thorax and improper preparation (e.g., incompletely evacuated stomach) also can play a major role in exacerbating reflux. Moderate to severe esophagitis can result in esophageal stricture formation (see later discussion).

Most hiatal hernia patients have some degree of reflux esophagitis. Decreased LES pressure leads to esophageal reflux in most patients with sliding hiatal hernias. Hiatal hernia patients are often presented for evaluation because of clinical signs that suggest a significant degree of esophagitis (e.g., salivation, inappetence, decreased activity, regurgitation). Treatment involves both management of esophagitis and medical management or surgical correction of the hiatal hernia.

Gastric emptying and gastric motility may be reduced in some patients with gastroesophageal reflux. Delayed emptying of liquids or solids would be expected to increase esophageal reflux. However, only a fraction of human patients with reflux esophagitis have delayed gastric emptying. Detailed studies have not been performed in animals, but clinical signs and endoscopic evidence of esophagitis have not been commonly observed in animals with gastric motility disorders. Probably the most important clinical situation regarding animals with gastric motility disorders involves general anesthesia. Every effort must be made to ensure that there is sufficient time for the stomach

to empty before anesthetic induction, since the combination of anesthesia and an incompletely evacuated stomach would increase the likelihood of a reflux episode and subsequent development of esophagitis.

Duodenogastric reflux may be damaging for two reasons: It increases gastric volume available for gastroesophageal reflux, and it adds bile and other potentially damaging duodenal fluid components to the gastric contents. Patients that have a chronic intermittent pattern of vomiting bile fluid may have duodenogastric reflux and should be watched carefully for signs of esophagitis.

Diagnosis of Esophagitis

The clinical signs of esophagitis vary considerably, depending on the degree of inflammation present. The clinician must maintain a high index of suspicion because in many cases only subtle clinical signs may be evident. With mild esophagitis there may be increased swallowing motions, salivation, and inappetence. In more severe cases there may be gulping, regurgitation, dysphagia due to pain, total anorexia, and signs that suggest esophageal pain, such as reluctance to move, standing with the head extended, reluctance to lie down, and trembling. Heartburn pain in humans can be quite intense, and it is suspected that a similar situation exists in animals. Esophageal hemorrhage may occur in severe cases.

The immediate past medical history must be reviewed carefully because it may provide important clues regarding both diagnosis and etiology. Signs such as increased attempts at swallowing, salivation, regurgitation, and inappetence that occur within 1 to 4 days of an anesthetic procedure strongly suggest reflux esophagitis. Coughing may indicate aspiration pneumonia. Patients with persistent vomiting should be observed carefully for signs of esophagitis. Severe esophagitis must be identified and treated early, since one of the potential sequelae is stricture formation.

Chronic reflux esophagitis occurs most commonly in patients with hiatal hernia disorders. Clinical signs include hypersalivation, regurgitation, and vomiting, which often are noted shortly after the patient eats. There also may be coughing, dyspnea, and exercise intolerance. Hiatal hernias are most commonly identified in immature patients.

Physical examination is usually unremarkable, but there may be physical evidence of glossitis or pharyngitis related to ingestion of a caustic substance. There may also be sensitivity on palpation of the cervical esophagus in animals with esophageal inflammation in that area.

Radiographic survey and contrast studies are often normal in patients with mild to moderate esophagitis. Survey films may show increased esophageal density in moderate to severe esophagitis. There also may be various degrees of esophageal dilation, since esophageal inflammation may inhibit motility. In fact, megaesophagus can occur secondary to inflammatory disease. Segmental narrowing and irregularity of luminal contour may occasionally be identified on contrast studies. Persistent contrast in the thoracic esophagus or esophageal dilation or both suggest the possibility of gastroesophageal reflux. In hiatal hernia the gastric cardia, the fundus, and the LES will be cranial to the esophageal hiatus. A definitive diagnosis may not always be possible in sliding hiatal hernia on spot films. Fluoroscopy may be needed to confirm the diagnosis.

A definitive diagnosis of esophagitis is most often made by endoscopic visualization of the esophageal mucosa. Variable degrees of mucosal erythema or isolated patches of eroded mucosa may be seen. Mucosal friability may be evidenced by bleeding caused by gentle manipulation with the endoscope tip or biopsy forceps. Fluid pooling in the esophagus or a markedly dilated gastroesophageal junction or both are not diagnostic, but these findings should alert the endoscopist to the possibility of a reflux disorder.

Numerous human studies have reported that 30% to 70% of patients with symptoms suggesting gastroesophageal reflux have an endoscopically normal esophagus. Symptom severity often does not predict the degree of endoscopic abnormality. When esophagitis is suspected in the absence of visible diagnostic changes in the mucosal surface, an esophageal mucosal biopsy specimen should be obtained from an area 2 to 5 cm proximal to the gastroesophageal junction. With proper technique, adequate mucosal biopsy specimens can be obtained with standard flexible forceps. Alternatively, specimens can be obtained with a suction biopsy instrument. Histologic changes appear before significant symptoms and endoscopically observable changes, and they persist after the endoscopic indicators have disappeared in response to therapy. An endoscopically demonstrable hiatal hernia is nearly always associated with reflux esophagitis.

Treatment

Because there are a variety of pathophysiologic mechanisms that contribute to reflux esophagitis, an individualized treatment program for each patient is often necessary. It is important to note that, although the esophagus is physically a very tough and resilient structure, once it is injured it does not always heal very quickly. For inflammatory disorders fairly aggressive combination drug therapy is often required. Treatment may include dietary modification, PPIs, H_2-receptor antagonists, GI promotility agents, anti-inflammatory drugs, and mucosal protectant therapy. Single or combination drug therapy may be required, depending on factors that include whether treatment is designed mostly for prevention, duration or severity of mucosal injury, and clinical signs. Most affected dogs and cats are managed with either an H_2-receptor antagonist or a PPI. Additionally, high-protein and low-fat diets, a promotility drug, and cytoprotective medication are indicated in some cases.

Mild reflux esophagitis is often asymptomatic and generally resolves without therapy. If clinical signs suggestive of reflux esophagitis occur within several days of an anesthetic procedure, treatment should be instituted, regardless of whether endoscopy is available for definitive diagnosis. Treatment in this situation usually includes an H_2-receptor antagonist or a PPI (e.g., omeprazole), the cytoprotective drug sucralfate, and a promotility drug (metoclopramide or cisapride). The duration of therapy will typically be 7 to 14 days. A longer duration will be required if clinical signs persist.

H_2-receptor antagonists such as cimetidine (Tagamet), ranitidine (Zantac), and famotidine (Pepcid) are used to decrease gastric acid production, thereby decreasing acid volume available for reflux. H_2-receptor antagonists also reduce the volume of gastric juice that is produced. There is no adverse effect on resting or stimulated LES pressure levels. Large multicenter human clinical trials have shown that H_2-receptor antagonist therapy results in consistent improvement in symptoms of reflux esophagitis. (However, as stated in the following discussion on PPIs, numerous studies on humans have documented the clinical superiority of PPIs relative to H_2-receptor antagonists in both relief of symptoms and healing of esophagitis). Cimetidine (2.5 to 5 mg/lb orally every 6 to 8 hours), ranitidine (1 mg/lb [dog], 1.5 mg/lb [cat] orally every 12 hours), or famotidine

(0.25 to 0.5 mg/lb orally every 24 hours, or every 12 hours if there is severe esophagitis) is generally used for 2 to 3 weeks in dogs and cats with acute reflux esophagitis. I prefer to use famotidine because of its long dosage interval and the fact that it is associated with fewer side effects. Another H_2-receptor antagonist that can be tried is nizatidine (Axid). The dosage is 1.25 to 2.5 mg/lb orally every 24 hours. Ranitidine and nizatidine also have a gastric prokinetic effect. Long-term therapy should be used in hiatal hernia patients with chronic reflux esophagitis if corrective surgery either is not performed or is unsuccessful.

PPIs are drugs that completely inhibit gastric acid secretion in response to all modes of stimulation. PPIs include omeprazole (Prilosec), lansoprazole (Prevacid), esomeprazole (Nexium, the S optical isomer of omeprazole), pantoprazole (Protonix), and rabeprazole (Aciphex). Omeprazole is the PPI that has been used most frequently in animal patients. PPIs decrease acid secretion by inhibiting H^+,K^+ATPase (commonly called the proton pump), thereby blocking the final, common step in the secretion of gastric acid. PPIs control both basal and meal-stimulated acid secretion. Therefore the acid suppression achieved by a PPI is more complete and longer lasting than can be attained with an H_2-receptor antagonist.

In humans, PPIs have now been shown to be superior to H_2-receptor antagonists in management of erosive esophagitis. Concurrently it is now also recommended in veterinary medicine that animals with esophagitis are better managed with a PPI than with an H_2-receptor antagonist. Although PPIs are more expensive, they produce quicker relief from symptoms in humans and total treatment time is also reduced in some patients. Results from human trials that investigated the use of PPIs in gastroesophageal reflux disease patients with nonerosive disease have demonstrated the superiority of PPI therapy over H_2-receptor antagonists. PPIs are now considered the most effective first-line treatment for nonerosive reflux esophagitis. More rapid responses have also been observed in animal patients treated with the PPI omeprazole. Therefore if esophagitis is judged to be greater than mild in degree, it is probably best to choose a PPI over an H_2-receptor antagonist as the primary therapy for controlling acid release. The recommended dosage for omeprazole is 0.3 mg/lb once daily.

Prokinetic drug therapy with metoclopramide or cisapride provides several beneficial effects.

Promotility drugs increase LES pressure, thereby decreasing reflux, and stimulate more rapid gastric emptying by increasing gastric contractions. They also enhance relaxation of the pylorus for more effective aboral movement of gastric contents and increase distal esophageal contractions. One problem with metoclopramide is that it may cause bothersome side effects such as restlessness, hyperactivity, and occasionally aggressive behavior. In my experience, these side effects are not common in dogs and cats, but owners should always be forewarned of the possibility that they may occur. If side effects occur, they usually will be noted within 1 hour of the first or second dose and subside within 3 to 4 hours. Unfortunately, lowering the dose does not usually alleviate side effects. The dosage of metoclopramide is 0.1 to 0.2 mg/lb (maximum starting dose, 10 mg) two to three times daily 30 to 45 minutes before feeding and at bedtime. Cimetidine or famotidine and metoclopramide are often used concurrently. Occasionally, the side effects of metoclopramide will be increased when it is used with cimetidine.

One significant advantage of cisapride is that, unlike metoclopramide, it is not associated with any significant side effects in animals. I have used cisapride in many patients that have experienced neurologic side effects from metoclopramide. I have observed no adverse reactions to cisapride in any of these patients, even in those whose side effects from metoclopramide included very bizarre behavior changes. The suggested dosage of cisapride is the same as that recommended for metoclopramide (see previous paragraph).

Early studies in humans showed promise for use of cisapride as primary therapy for reflux esophagitis. However, more recent studies have been disappointing. Cisapride provides symptomatic relief in less than half of patients with results comparable to those achieved with standard doses of an H_2-receptor antagonist. And cisapride used in combination with an H_2-receptor antagonist is less effective for symptomatic relief of esophagitis symptoms in humans than that achieved with a PPI. So cisapride and metoclopramide can play an important adjunctive role in management of reflux esophagitis, but prokinetic agents used alone are not likely to be very successful. Effective acid control is essential.

One of the most important forms of reflux esophagitis therapy involves use of sucralfate (Carafate) to provide an esophageal mucosal cytoprotective effect. Sucralfate is an aluminum salt that has been shown to bind selectively to areas of injured GI tract mucosa and to form a local protective layer that binds pepsin and bile and prevents them from causing further mucosal damage.

Sucralfate cytoprotection against pepsin-induced esophageal lesions has been demonstrated using a liquid preparation in short-term experiments in rabbits. A study in cats demonstrated a protective effect of liquid sucralfate against intermittent, repeated esophageal exposure to acid over a period of days. Sucralfate acts not only by adhering to damaged mucosa but also by enhancing normal mucosal defenses. Based on this information, it is recommended that administration of sucralfate in a liquid form be considered for patients with evidence of esophagitis. Its greatest value may be in treatment of acute reactions in the esophagus and in prevention of further damage. Sucralfate should also be considered for use as a preventive medication in situations in which a significant reflux episode could potentially occur (e.g., emergency surgery in a patient with an incompletely evacuated stomach). The recommended dosage is 1 g per 65 lb given orally every 6 to 8 hours. For treatment of esophageal disorders, a suspension form of sucralfate should be used. Sucralfate is now commercially available in suspension form. Alternatively, sucralfate tablets can be mixed into suspension. Sucralfate tablets readily dissolve in lukewarm water (10 to 15 ml). Once the suspension is thoroughly mixed, it is administered as a gavage.

A short course (several days to 2 weeks) of corticosteroid therapy (e.g., prednisone, 0.25 to 0.5 mg/lb orally every 12 hours) may be indicated in severe reflux esophagitis to minimize fibrosis and possible stricture formation. Corticosteroids are not indicated in mild cases of esophagitis.

Patients with moderate to severe esophagitis should be held nothing by mouth (NPO) for 24 to 72 hours. When food is resumed, a high-protein, low-fat diet is indicated. High-protein diets enhance LES function, whereas high-fat diets interfere with LES function. Patients that have been held NPO are generally started on a gruel-consistency diet for the first several days. Owners of overweight patients that are prone to developing esophagitis (e.g., due to hiatal hernia) should be encouraged to initiate weight reduction measures for their pet.

Animals with evidence of reflux esophagitis following anesthesia should be treated early and aggressively, since there is potential for esophageal stricture formation. Early recognition of esophagitis symptoms in clinical situations that can potentiate development of the disorder is very important. Early treatment often minimizes mucosal injury and in severe cases may help decrease the likelihood of stricture formation. One of the clinical situations in which early recognition is most important involves patients that have undergone general anesthesia, especially, but not exclusively, for a prolonged surgical procedure. Clinicians and nursing personnel should monitor for signs of esophageal reflux (e.g., salivation, pronounced gurgling, and regurgitation of fluid from the mouth or nostrils). Recommended early treatment measures include using low-grade suction attached to a feeding tube that has been passed into the esophagus in an attempt to remove retained fluid before its contents can cause mucosal injury. If there is concern that a significant amount of reflux has occurred, an endotracheal tube can be used to lavage the esophagus. Warm water is instilled as a diluting agent and then suctioned. Care must be taken to ensure that the endotracheal tube is cuffed adequately in order to prevent aspiration. The best method is to use an endoscope for direct visualization, lavage, and suction, following a prolonged anesthetic event. Any retained fluid can be quickly suctioned through the endoscope. The endoscope should be used to examine the stomach as well. Any fluid that is present should be suctioned; otherwise, it might be refluxed to the esophagus during the recovery period. Sucralfate or sucralfate and an H_2-receptor antagonist are then administered for 24 to 72 hours. This approach is very effective in helping prevent significant postoperative esophagitis and possibly later formation of esophageal strictures. If signs of esophagitis develop despite this therapy, a PPI such as omeprazole should be used and H_2-receptor antagonist therapy is discontinued.

Clinicians are also cautioned to be more attentive to patients that might have esophagitis secondary to frequent or severe vomiting (e.g., caused by GI foreign bodies, parvoviral enteritis, acute pancreatitis, or renal failure). Esophagitis can easily develop in these situations, and it no doubt adds significantly to the discomfort that the patient is already experiencing. In these cases, both sucralfate and an H_2-receptor antagonist are used to treat esophagitis. I use famotidine injectable at 0.25 mg/lb intravenously every 12 hours. An antiemetic drug such as chlorpromazine (Thorazine) is injected to help decrease the frequency of vomiting. Sucralfate is given orally, usually 30 to

60 minutes after antiemetic therapy has been administered.

The duration of therapy in patients with reflux esophagitis depends on the cause and degree of inflammation. For moderate to severe esophagitis, 4 to 8 weeks of therapy or more may be required to achieve full healing of the esophagus. For esophagitis related to frequent or severe vomiting (e.g., parvoviral enteritis, pancreatitis, toxic enteritis, linear foreign body), treatment is usually administered for 5 to 7 days, and only longer if clinical signs or endoscopic findings warrant. As discussed later in this chapter, patients with a hiatal hernia may require long-term therapy using either a PPI alone or a PPI with sucralfate. Patients should be monitored carefully for signs that can be associated with esophagitis, and use of endoscopy as both a diagnostic and a monitoring tool should be encouraged.

ESOPHAGEAL STRICTURES

Esophageal strictures occasionally occur in dogs and cats. Stricture usually occurs secondary to severe esophagitis that extends into deeper layers of the esophagus, inciting fibroblastic proliferation. Common causes of this degree of esophagitis in dogs and cats are reflux of gastric acid and enzymes during general anesthesia, persistent vomiting in patients that are also weak and recumbent (e.g., patients with parvoviral enteritis, pancreatitis), medications that induce esophagitis when they become lodged in the esophagus (e.g., that caused by NSAIDs in dogs, doxycyline tablets in cats), ingestion of strong acid or alkali, foreign body trauma, and thermal burns. Severe stricture may also occur in cats that develop esophagitis after a large hairball has been vomited or has become lodged in the esophagus. I have treated cats that developed a severe esophageal stricture within 7 to 14 days after vomiting a hairball as long as 12 to 15 cm. Presumably, the coarse texture of the hair significantly irritates the esophageal mucosa as it sits in and subsequently is ejected from the esophagus. Acid and enzymes that are mixed in the hair material add to the damage. Figure 4–12 illustrates a case in which a large hairball was lodged in the esophagus for approximately 36 hours before it was removed. Severe esophagitis resulted, and within 10 days there was a stricture, *despite* aggressive early medical management for esophagitis.

Anesthesia–related reflux is the most common cause of esophageal stricture. Stricture formation can occur after relatively short anesthetic procedures (e.g., for ovariohysterectomy), as well as after long procedures. It appears that prolonged anesthesia, especially when followed by inability of a patient to resume sternal or upright posture, promotes gastroesophageal reflux that may persist even beyond the duration of the anesthesia, and thereby initiating and perpetuating to some degree the transition from severe esophagitis to stricture formation.

Clinical signs of dysphagia and regurgitation are usually evident by 5 to 14 days after the anesthetic episode. Occasionally, significant clinical signs are not evident until 4 to 6 weeks later. Variable degrees of luminal narrowing can occur, and in some patients the lumen diameter at the stricture site is extremely narrow (sometimes as small as 1 to 2 mm) (Figure 4–13). Stricture length also varies. Occasionally, one or two additional strictures will develop at other sites in the esophagus.

Clinical Signs

Clinical signs generally progress over 5 to 14 days after their onset. The predominant sign is regurgitation of solid food. In some patients there initially is vomiting during the recovery phase after an anesthetic event that is followed by occasional vomiting over the ensuing several days. Regurgitation may then begin to occur. As a stricture worsens, only gruels can be successfully transported to the stomach. In strictures associated with a very narrow luminal diameter (1 to 2 mm), only water is likely to be retained. Affected patients typically remain active and alert and have excellent body condition. Signs of pain or discomfort are uncommon. The appetite is usually ravenous. Weight loss may occur over time as a result of decreased caloric intake associated with regurgitation.

Diagnosis

Esophageal strictures occur more commonly than many clinicians may recognize. A review of a patient's recent medical history is the first step in making an early diagnosis of esophageal stricture. Most patients with an esophageal stricture have undergone general anesthesia within the previous 2 to 3 weeks. Most patients that begin regurgitating shortly after an anesthetic event have an esophageal stricture. A recent history of frequent severe vomiting in dogs or cats, onset of regurgitation associ-

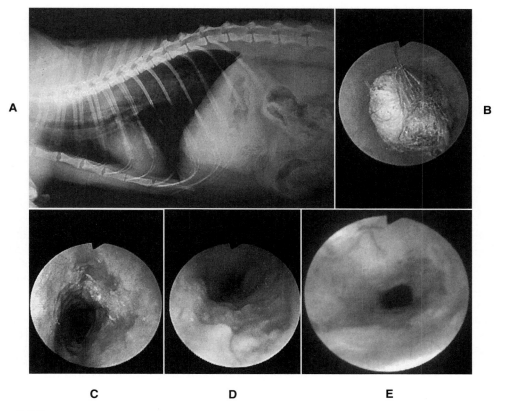

FIGURE 4-12 Esophageal foreign body in a cat with subsequent development of esophageal stricture. **A,** Note the long area of increased opacity in the dorsocaudal thorax (later confirmed to be a hairball). The history included salivation, increased respiratory rate, and anorexia. **B,** Esophagoscopy confirmed a diagnosis of esophageal foreign body (hairball). The hairball was very tightly wedged in the esophagus. It could be neither pulled orad nor pushed back into the stomach. A gastrotomy was done, and the hairball was pulled back to the stomach and removed. **C,** Immediate postoperative esophagoscopy, showing erosive damage of the esophagus (twelve o'clock and five o'clock positions). Sucralfate suspension, famotidine, metoclopramide, and corticosteroids were instituted for severe esophagitis. There was concern that an esophageal stricture might develop. **D,** Appearance of the esophagus 4 days after surgery. The mucosa was quite irregular and friable. There is evidence of esophageal narrowing and early stricture formation. **E,** Endoscopic appearance of an esophageal stricture identified at 10 days. Balloon dilation procedures were initiated.

ated with administration of NSAIDs to dogs, doxy-cycline tablets to cats, or other medications, or recent vomiting of a large hairball by a cat also should heighten suspicion of esophageal stricture.

A diagnosis is established either by endoscopy or by barium contrast radiography using a swallow of barium and either static radiographs or fluoroscopy (Figure 4-14). *In some cases barium liquid mixed with food is required to demonstrate an esophageal stricture, since liquid barium may pass easily through a stricture without delineating its presence.* Endoscopy allows evaluation of the appearance and pliability of the esophageal wall and luminal diameter. The endoscope is often too large to pass through the stricture area, so an assessment of stricture length often is not possible from direct examination alone. Stricture length can be assessed, however, by

advancing endoscopic biopsy forceps through the stricture and then opening the cups once the instrument has been passed. As the biopsy instrument is then retracted, the open cups will stop at the distal border of the stricture. A determination of stricture length also can be made by insufflating air into the esophagus, using the endoscope, and then making a lateral survey thoracic radiograph. There is an increased opacity at the stricture site as compared with the surrounding air.

Esophageal neoplasia occasionally causes intramural stricture formation, and there usually is an appearance of mucosal irregularity and intraluminal mass effect. However, rarely a malignant stricture will appear benign with no intraluminal mass effect typical of neoplasia. If any uncertainty exists regarding the cause of a stricture (e.g., no recent

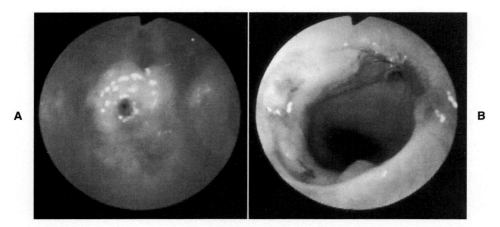

FIGURE 4-13 Severe cranial thoracic esophageal stricture in an 11-month-old cat that had been anesthetized 14 days before. There was a 5-day history of regurgitation that progressively worsened, resulting in referral for endoscopy. **A,** The extremely narrow esophageal lumen (approximately 1.5 mm) is visible just to the left of center. Note the white fibrous connective tissue around the lumen. Because the stricture was too narrow to attempt bougienage and balloon catheters had not yet been developed when this case was seen, stricture resection was performed through a right thoracotomy. Resection of 1.5 cm of esophagus was performed. **B,** Endoscopic examination 4 weeks after esophageal resection and anastomosis. Mild narrowing of the lumen remains, but the endoscope was easily advanced. Note the suture tags and the esophageal lumen beyond the anastomosis site. The cat was asymptomatic. (From Tams TR: Esophagoscopy. In Tams TR, ed: *Small animal endoscopy,* St. Louis, 1990, Mosby–Year Book.)

history of anesthesia to suggest a reflux episode), biopsies should be done to differentiate a truly benign stricture from a malignant one. Brushings for cytologic examination are useful for rapid assessment while one waits for biopsy results. If the lumen at the stricture site is extremely narrow, biopsy specimens should be taken before and after dilation. Also, a mass impinging on the outside of the esophagus may compress the esophageal lumen enough to cause a stricture effect. In this situation the esophageal mucosa will appear normal. The endoscopist will note that the esophageal walls do not readily distend in response to air insufflation. Additionally, it may not be possible to advance the endoscope through the narrowed area.

Treatment

Treatment options for benign esophageal stricture include surgical procedures such as resection and anastomosis or patch grafting, bougienage, and balloon catheter dilation. In humans laser therapy and prosthesis has also been utilized. The success rate in animals treated with surgical procedures has been reported as less than 50% and in those treated with bougienage techniques as 50% to 75%. Surgical resection may result in restricture at the site of the anastomosis. *Balloon catheter dilation is much more successful than either surgery or bougienage.*

The advantages of this technique over bougienage include decreased risk of esophageal perforation, longer symptom-free periods between procedures, and a smaller total number of procedures required to resolve the problem.

Bougienage

A wide variety of esophageal dilation devices whose diameters increase in stepwise fashion are available, including mercury-filled bougies and Pilling bougies. Bougies have either rounded tips or tapered ends with bases that are wider than the tips. The narrow tip is advanced to the stricture site under endoscopic guidance, and the wider area of the bougie dilates the stricture as the bougie is advanced through it. Care must be exercised to ensure that the bougie tip is directed into the stricture opening and not too far lateral to it. There is risk of perforation if the latter occurs. Other dilators that can be used in selected cases include endotracheal tubes (for cervical esophageal strictures in small patients) and the flexible endoscope itself.

The key to successful bougienage is to repeat the procedure as often as necessary to maintain improved luminal diameter. In many patients two to three bougienage procedures per week are necessary during the first several weeks of treatment before the desired effect is reached. After a stric-

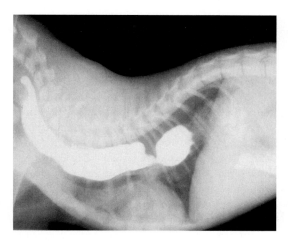

FIGURE 4-14 Barium liquid contrast radiograph from a 5-month-old kitten that had been regurgitating for 2 months. At the time the kitten was seen at a referral center, it was regurgitating solid food immediately after eating. The kitten had been anesthetized and neutered at a shelter at approximately 8 to 9 weeks of age. Note the proximal esophageal dilation and the narrowing of the dye column just caudal to the heart. Esophagoscopy confirmed a diagnosis of esophageal stricture, related to an internal fibrous band (i.e., there was no appearance of a narrowing due to external compression). Because of the kitten's poor body condition at the time of presentation at the referral center, a gastrostomy tube was placed surgically so that nutritional support could be provided immediately. The esophageal stricture was managed successfully through a total of four ballooning procedures performed under endoscopic guidance. At 2 years of age there had been no stricture recurrence, and the cat continues to do quite well. (Courtesy Dr. Susan Hackner.)

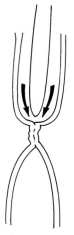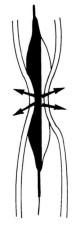

Bougienage
• Longitudinal shear
• Snowplow effect
• Risk of perforation

Balloon dilation
• Radial stretch
• Stationary force

FIGURE 4-15 A diagrammatic representation of the shearing forces associated with bougienage compared with the radial forces associated with balloon dilation. (From Dawson SI et al.: Severe esophageal strictures: indications for balloon catheter dilation. *Radiology* 153:631, 1984.)

ture has been forced open, the natural tendency is for it to narrow again as collagen is formed during epithelial healing.

Balloon Catheter Dilation

Balloon catheter dilation produces results superior to bougienage techniques. Advantages include a minimal chance of esophageal perforation, the ability to visualize more adequately the stricture dilation as the procedure progresses, and longer stricture-free intervals. A major advantage to balloon dilation is that it produces a radial stretch force rather than a longitudinal shearing force, as occurs with bougienage (Figure 4-15). In many patients only two to four balloon dilation procedures are required.

Balloon catheters are available commercially (Microvasive/Boston Scientific, Natick, MA 01760). The catheter is constructed of polyethylene, and

the balloon consists of a specially treated polyethylene located peripheral to the central tubing. There is a radiopaque visible metal band at each end of the balloon. Various size balloons are available. A full set of balloons for use in animals would include balloons of the following inflated diameters: 6, 8, 10, 12, 15, and 20 mm. 25 and 30 mm–diameter balloon catheters are available for use in large dogs.

Smaller balloon dilators can be passed through the instrument channel of an endoscope with a 2.6-mm or larger instrument channel. However, since pediatric size human and veterinary use flexible endoscopes have a channel size of 2.0 to 2.5 mm, most procedures are done in animals by passing the balloon dilator alongside the endoscope. The balloon can be inflated with dilute iodinated contrast material or water. With the patient under general anesthesia, the catheter is advanced under endoscopic guidance and positioned with the middle part of the catheter centered in the stricture. During the first procedure a lateral thoracic radiograph is usually made, especially in situations in which the stricture site is very narrow, to confirm whether or not the balloon positioning is correct. If fluoroscopy is used, the stricture and its response as the balloon is dilated can be observed directly. The stricture is apparent as a narrowing or waist in the balloon. Fluoroscopy is certainly not necessary to perform the procedure safely, however, and in most cases it is not used.

Once positioned, the balloon is distended with water or dilute contrast medium, and the luminal pressure is monitored with the pressure gauge. This increased pressure is associated with effacement of the waist, indicating dilation of the stricture (Figure 4-16). A dilation time of 2 to 4 minutes at 40 to 45 psi seems to be adequate for stricture dilation in dogs and cats (initially a time of 2 minutes is used so that initial response can be determined). After dilation, the balloon is deflated and the catheter removed. Immediate postdilation endoscopy is recommended to ensure resolution of the stricture. Dilation periods of 4 minutes are usually used in cases in which frequent procedures have not yet successfully solved the problem.

Mild to moderate hemorrhage around the stricture site is a normal postdilation finding. If there is no hemorrhage, the stricture was not dilated to any significant degree. With a very aggressive dilation, long and fairly deep longitudinal splits may occur in the esophageal wall. It is generally best to act a little conservatively during initial dilation procedures so as to minimize the likelihood of perforation that could result from using too large a balloon. Usually 2 to 3 progressively larger balloons are used in sequence during each individual anesthesia. *Because esophageal strictures tend to close down again fairly quickly after being dilated, two to three individual dilation procedures are routinely scheduled during the first 7 days. Subsequent procedures are scheduled based on patient response during the first 1 to 2 weeks.*

Factors that help determine the number of balloon dilation procedures that will be necessary

FIGURE 4-16 Radiographic appearance of a balloon catheter during an esophageal stricture dilation procedure. **A,** The balloon catheter is advanced under endoscopic guidance. The stricture is located over the base of the heart. The catheter's soft, flexible radiopaque guide tip is visible in the stomach and distal esophagus. The radiopaque wire in the catheter shaft is clearly visible in the cranial and middle thorax. **B,** A fully distended balloon catheter with a diameter of 20 mm. The stricture has been fully dilated.

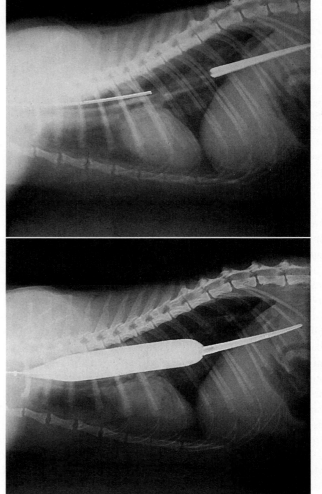

A

B

include severity and length of the stricture, number of strictures, and the ease of the initial stricture dilation. In general, tight strictures and those that were several millimeters long require more dilations than those of moderate severity and shorter length. Patients with multiple strictures tend to require more dilations than those with single strictures.

A stricture that has been present for longer than several months may become so fibrotic that it may not be possible to dilate the stricture with balloons. Therefore, once the presence of a stricture is confirmed, proper treatment should be instituted. A case in which an attempt to dilate a cervical esophageal stricture was not made until 9 months after it was diagnosed is illustrated in Figure 4-17. Surgery was required to remove the stricture.

After bougienage or balloon dilation is begun, intensive therapy for esophagitis is instituted. This includes H$_2$-receptor antagonist therapy, metoclopramide, sucralfate suspension, and prednisone (0.25 to 0.5 mg/lb/day). Food, usually chopped canned consistency, is usually resumed later on the same day or on the following day. If there is severe esophageal damage, it might be necessary to place a gastrostomy tube so that adequate nutritional support can be given. Most patients eat well very soon after a dilation procedure, even if there is significant esophageal mucosal tearing.

Prednisone is used to decrease fibroblastic activity. Whether or not it really helps to decrease or prevent further stricture formation is controversial. I have observed patients in which an esophageal stricture developed *despite* aggressive therapy (famotidine, sucralfate, metoclopramide, and prednisone) for acute moderate to severe esophagitis that was diagnosed early in its course via endoscopy. This therapeutic regimen is given both to treat the existing esophagitis and, it is hoped, to decrease the likelihood of stricture formation. Unfortunately, this approach does not always work. Some specialists have begun to take the additional step of injecting intralesional triamcinolone with a Wang needle, under endoscopic guidance, after dilating severe esophageal strictures in an effort to further decrease fibroblastic activity. Endoscopy guided laser treatment used as an adjunct to ballooning is also being investigated.

It is emphasized that careful surveillance for development of a stricture is warranted in animals that are most at risk (e.g., those with anesthesia-related esophagitis and those that have recently vomited a large hairball). Esophagoscopy is the ideal procedure to monitor for progression or regression of esophagitis. *Clinicians must recognize that once severe esophagitis is present, a stricture can form very rapidly.*

The prognosis for resolution of an esophageal stricture disorder is excellent when balloon dilation is used. Sometimes mild permanent narrowing remains at the stricture site, but this is usually clinically insignificant. Cats and small dogs can manage well with an esophageal diameter of 1 cm or less if food consistency is limited to soft meals. A diameter of 1 to 1.5 cm is necessary in medium to large dogs. Many patients are eventually able to eat foods of normal consistency.

▌HIATAL DISORDERS

The esophageal hiatus is the opening in the diaphragm through which the esophagus passes from the thorax into the abdominal cavity. Anatomic abnormalities of the hiatus may cause symptoms of esophageal disease. Hiatal lesions may allow hiatal hernia, paraesophageal hiatal hernia, gastroesophageal intussusception, or diaphragmatic hernia to occur. Hiatal hernias are protrusions of the abdominal esophagus, GES, and sometimes a portion of the gastric fundus through the esophageal hiatus into the caudal mediastinum cranial to the diaphragm. Hiatal hernias likely occur more commonly than they are recognized in dogs and cats.

Congenital or acquired enlargement of the esophageal hiatus or laxity of the surrounding phrenicoesophageal ligaments may predispose to hiatal hernias. Most hernias are probably congenital. Acquired hiatal hernias may occur secondary to high positive intraabdominal pressure (e.g., blunt abdominal trauma, vomiting) or very negative intrathoracic pressure associated with chronic upper airway obstruction (e.g., laryngeal collapse). Hiatal hernias are seen more commonly in brachycephalic breeds such as English bulldogs and in shar-peis. Although most symptomatic animals with congenital hiatal hernia demonstrate clinical signs by 1 year of age, significant signs may not occur until later. Patients with acquired hernias may develop signs at any age.

Clinical Signs

The most common clinical signs of hiatal hernia are regurgitation, dysphagia, hypersalivation, and vomiting. Hematemesis may occasionally occur.

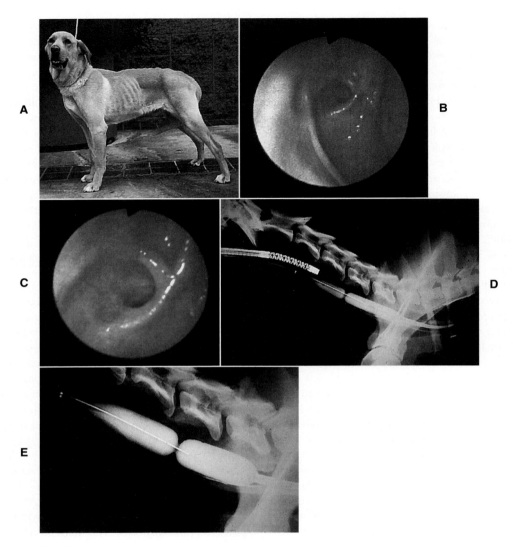

FIGURE 4-17 Chronic severe esophageal stricture that was not amenable to balloon dilation. **A,** A 6½-year-old male Labrador retriever that underwent a gastrotomy at an emergency clinic 10 months earlier for suspected foreign body removal. No foreign body was found. After the surgery there was intermittent vomiting. At 2 weeks the dog began to regurgitate solid food, and at 4 weeks esophagoscopy revealed a stricture in the cervical esophagus. Balloon dilation was recommended, but the dog's owner chose conservative management, which consisted of feeding a gruel diet. Nine months after the stricture was diagnosed, however, the owner decided to proceed with balloon dilation because he could not maintain the dog's weight. Weight loss totaled 33 lb since the initial diagnosis. **B,** Endoscopic photograph of the proximal cervical esophagus. Note the fibrotic band in the near field. An esophageal stricture is visible beyond the band. **C,** Close-up view of the stricture. There is a fibrotic ring around the stricture, and the narrowed lumen curves on the far side of the stricture. A 7.9-mm endoscope could not be advanced into or through the stricture. **D,** Under endoscopic guidance, a 15-mm balloon catheter was advanced through the stricture. In this radiograph both the endoscope and the dilated balloon are visible. The stricture is delineated by the narrowed waist in the balloon (just ventral to the proximal border of the fifth cervical vertebra). At 45 psi for 4 minutes the stricture did not dilate. **E,** The largest balloon available (20 mm dilated) was then used. At 45 psi for 9 minutes the stricture did not dilate because of severe fibrosis. The short stricture is clearly visible on this radiograph. Surgery was later done to resect the stricture, and the dog recovered uneventfully. During the following year the dog gained 33 lb. Histologic examination of the stricture revealed severe fibrosis. It is strongly recommended that balloon dilation be done on esophageal strictures early in their course.

Small hiatal hernias may be asymptomatic. Symptoms may be evident only occasionally in animals in which herniation occurs intermittently. In fact, the diagnosis is often difficult to prove in patients because many cases probably involve only sporadic movement. Most hiatal hernia cases are associated with some degree of reflux esophagitis. Malpositioning or a lack of support of the gastroesophageal sphincter reduces gastroesophageal pressure and leads to gastroesophageal reflux. Most of the clinical signs are related to esophagitis and altered esophageal motility.

Diagnosis

Various types of hiatal disorders have been described. These are depicted in Figure 4-18. The most common type of hiatal hernia in dogs and cats is a *sliding hiatal hernia* with cranial displacement of the abdominal esophagus, gastroesophageal junction, and a portion of the stomach through an enlarged and lax hiatus. *Paraesophageal hernias* are uncommon. In this type of hernia the gastroesophageal junction remains fixed in the intraabdominal location and the gastric fundus protrudes through a defect in the diaphragmatic hiatus parallel to the esophagus. Gastroesophageal reflux disease is less commonly associated with paraesophageal hernias because the LES remains functional and in a normal intraabdominal position.

Gastroesophageal intussusception is a rarely encountered syndrome. Gastroesophageal intussusception results when the gastric cardia invaginates into the terminal esophagus. The gastroesophageal sphincter does not move cranial into the thorax as occurs with a hiatal hernia. Entrapment of the stomach in the esophagus may result in acute esophageal obstruction.

Survey thoracic radiography may confirm the diagnosis in some cases. Findings include an increased opacity in the caudal dorsal mediastinum caused by presence of the stomach in the thoracic cavity. Positive contrast esophagrams may reveal displacement of a portion of the stomach into the thorax. Contrast radiography is used to determine the location of the GEJ and to evaluate the mucosal pattern of the lower esophagus. *Compressing the abdomen during radiography in patients with a suspected hernia may help force part of the stomach into the thorax and increase the likelihood of obtaining diagnostic films.*

Occasionally the diagnosis is made at endoscopy. Endoscopy may confirm gastroesophageal intussusception, in which gastric rugal folds are seen bulging into the lumen of the distal esophagus. A careful assessment of the esophageal mucosa, the GEJ, and the stomach is important in the determination of the treatment plan. Finding reflux esophagitis helps raise suspicions of a hiatal disorder. Endoscopic findings of cranial LES displacement and a large esophageal hiatus, in conjunction with appropriate clinical signs, is suggestive of a sliding hiatal hernia. When the endoscope is passed from the esophagus into the stomach, it should be retroflexed, after the stomach is insufflated with air, to view the LES from the gastric side. With gastric insufflation there may be cranial displacement of the LES and cardiac region of the stomach through a weakened or enlarged esophageal hiatus.

Treatment

Surgical correction is indicated in patients with a symptomatic hiatal hernia. Fundoplication procedures have been described. Other techniques include diaphragmatic hiatal reduction and plication, esophagopexy, and left-sided fundic gastropexy. Medical management for esophagitis is instituted as soon as the diagnosis is made. If surgery is not corrective, medication may have to be continued indefinitely in order to control symptoms of reflux esophagitis. Medical management (H_2-receptor antagonist, prokinetic therapy, and a low-fat diet) without surgery is often useful in patients with mild symptoms related to intermittent herniation. A PPI (e.g., omeprazole) is recommended over an H_2-receptor antagonist for moderate to severe esophagitis (see section earlier in this chapter on management of esophagitis).

ESOPHAGEAL FOREIGN BODIES

Dogs and cats occasionally experience lodgment of a foreign body in the esophagus. Although this problem occurs most commonly in young dogs and cats, older animals also may be affected. Because of their more indiscriminate eating habits, dogs tend to experience foreign body problems more commonly than cats do.

Major factors in determining whether a foreign body will pass uneventfully or be retained are its size and its configuration (e.g., rough versus smooth edges, presence or absence of projections, and width). There are four areas of physiologic narrowing in the esophagus: the UES, the thoracic inlet, the heart base area, and

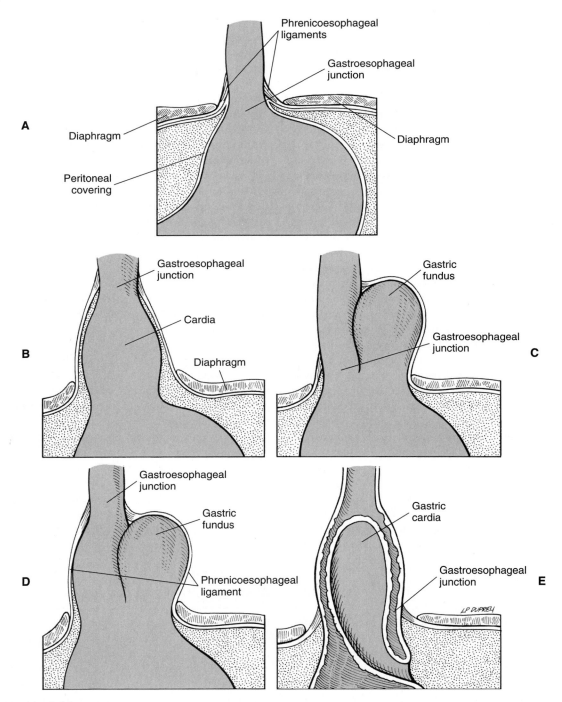

FIGURE 4-18 **A,** Diagram of a normal gastroesophageal junction. **B-E,** Diagrams of hiatal abnormalities: **B,** sliding or axial hiatal hernia, **C,** paraesophageal or rolling hiatal hernia, **D,** combination of sliding and paraesophageal hernia, and, **E,** gastroesophageal intussusception. (Hedlund CS: Surgery of the digestive system. In Fossum TW, ed: *Small animal surgery,* ed 2, St. Louis, 2002, Mosby).

the distal esophagus just proximal to the GEJ. Most foreign bodies become impacted in one of the latter three areas in dogs and cats. A variety of foreign bodies can be involved, but in my experi-

ence bones and fishhooks are the most common objects found in the esophagus. Needles are the most common foreign bodies found in cats. Although there is potential for a sharp object to perforate the aorta at the aortic arch or through the esophagus to cause a communication to the chest cavity, this is an extremely rare occurrence. Failure of blunt objects to pass through the esophagus spontaneously should raise suspicion that there is an esophageal motility disorder or a pathologic area of narrowing, such as a benign or malignant esophageal stricture.

Clinical signs

Clinical signs related to foreign body impaction in the esophagus are often acute and usually include salivation, which may become bloody, and regurgitation. There also may be odynophagia, dysphagia, forceful retching, lethargy or restlessness, and anorexia. Occasionally, a foreign body remains undetected in the esophagus for a number of days to even weeks. Chronic signs usually include depression, anorexia, salivation, and regurgitation. There also may be clinical evidence of an esophageal foreign body complication such as esophageal perforation with resultant pleuritis, mediastinitis, and pyothorax. Other potential sequelae include esophageal stricture, diverticula, and severe esophagitis.

Diagnosis

The diagnosis of a retained foreign body may be readily apparent from the history. For example, an owner may have observed the patient ingesting a bone found during a garbage foray, reported a missing section of a toy, or found a fishing line attached to a hook dangling from the pet's mouth. In other cases there is no specific relevant history, and in yet others the owner may deny any possibility of foreign body ingestion.

Survey radiographs of the cervical soft tissues and thorax should be the first studies performed because radiopaque objects can easily be localized in most cases. Lateral films of the neck are particularly important in recognizing bone fragments impacted in the cervical esophagus. There may be evidence of an esophageal foreign body. Thoracic radiographs should be carefully evaluated for any evidence of esophageal perforation, including pneumomediastinum and pleural effusion. Also, survey radiographs must be evaluated carefully for evidence of additional foreign bodies that may be less obvious than an easily recognized radiopaque object. Contrast radiography is occasionally necessary to identify radiolucent objects. An iodinated compound (e.g., Gastrografin) should be used instead of barium if there is a possibility of

esophageal perforation. Alternatively, esophagoscopy can be done to confirm or deny suspicions of an esophageal foreign body.

A complete blood count should be obtained if the patient is febrile, has aspiration pneumonia, or demonstrates evidence of esophageal perforation.

Treatment

Once a foreign body has been localized, a decision must be made whether to observe for its passage or to remove it endoscopically or surgically. Most esophageal foreign bodies are amenable to endoscopic retrieval. *As a rule, any foreign object retained in the esophagus should be removed as soon as possible or, if this cannot be done, at least advanced to the stomach.* Although uncommon, the risk of esophageal perforation always exists, especially when a sharp or pointed object is involved. Lodged esophageal foreign bodies can also cause significant pain. In most cases an esophageal foreign body does not have to be removed as a true "emergency" procedure. Exceptions include foreign body impaction in the proximal esophagus that is causing respiratory distress because of tracheal compression and a wedged sharp object such as a bone that is causing significant patient distress. This may be evidenced by groaning, copious salivation, or forceful gagging. If the situation does not require rapid intervention, the patient should be stabilized as needed with intravenous fluids, antibiotics, and pain relievers, and a thorough radiographic assessment should be completed. Ideally, endoscopy should be undertaken within 4 to 6 hours of presentation. Endoscopy is indicated as the initial procedure of choice for all esophageal foreign bodies. If endoscopic equipment is not available, the patient should be referred to an appropriate facility.

If pleural effusion is detected on thoracic radiographs, the chest should be tapped to obtain a sample for cytology, Gram stain, and culture and sensitivity. Pyothorax is best managed with placement of a chest tube for drainage and lavage. Once the patient is stabilized, a thoracotomy is done as soon as possible either alone or in conjunction with endoscopy to remove the foreign body and to evaluate and repair the esophageal wall. In my experience, it is rare for even bone foreign bodies that have been lodged in the esophagus for several days to weeks to cause complete esophageal perforation.

Safe extraction of an esophageal foreign body requires an adequate preliminary evaluation and the selection of proper equipment, including appropriate grasping forceps or snare. Although flexible endoscopes are used most commonly, rigid equipment is also excellent for esophageal foreign body retrieval. A laryngoscope and curved grasping forceps should also be readily available in case their use becomes necessary. As with any type of endoscopic procedure, the patient is maintained under general anesthesia in left lateral recumbency. The endotracheal tube is especially important in preventing tracheal compression as a large foreign body is pulled retrograde through the esophagus and in preventing aspiration of any object that might be inadvertently dropped in the pharynx during retrieval. The endoscope should be passed under direct visual guidance through the pharynx and the UES to avoid striking any foreign body material that may be present in the proximal esophagus and that consequently has the potential for causing mucosal damage. The esophageal mucosa should be carefully evaluated for any foreign body–related damage as the endoscope is advanced. Air should be insufflated to distend the esophageal walls so that visualization is enhanced, but the patient's respiratory status must be monitored while this is being done. Air may be forced around an impacted foreign body and into the stomach, which can lead to significant gastric distention. The distention should be relieved as quickly as possible. In most cases, this can be done by periodically passing the endoscope around the foreign body and into the stomach so that the air can be suctioned. *Air insufflation to a perforated esophagus can result in acute respiratory signs and death. The anesthetist is advised to monitor both respiratory character and degree of gastric distention during the procedure.*

Successful extraction of a foreign body requires adequate visualization, a firm grasp of the object, and removal with minimal force to avoid further damage. The tip of a flexible endoscope should not be used as a "ramming rod" to dislodge or advance an object because such action could cause significant damage to the endoscope. Once freed, most objects can be pulled back to the tip of the endoscope, and the endoscope and foreign body can then be gently removed simultaneously. *Undue force should not be exerted. Gentle manipulation is the rule.* If at all possible, pointed objects such as bones and needles should be withdrawn with the pointed end trailing. If there is a sharp-ended object (e.g., toothpick or needle) positioned proximally, the grasping prongs can sometimes be used to cover it so that the esophageal mucosa is protected, or the object can

be advanced to the stomach and repositioned so that the sharp end trails. This technique works well when irregular pieces of material such as plastic are involved. Alternatively, objects with sharp or irregular edges can be removed with the aid of an overtube to prevent mucosal damage. After the esophageal foreign body is removed, the entire esophagus should be inspected for damage, and the stomach also should be examined for the presence of any foreign material. There is usually some degree of mucosal laceration at the site of bone impaction in the esophagus. The extent of damage should be carefully evaluated and appropriate medication instituted after the procedure.

If the foreign body cannot be retrieved in a retrograde manner, an attempt should be made to advance it to the stomach. Bones are usually rapidly decalcified by gastric juices, and the remaining fragments will pass through the intestinal tract without incident. If a bone is firmly wedged in the distal esophagus at the time of presentation, it may be best to direct all efforts to advancing it to the stomach rather than risking any problems by pulling it retrograde. Foreign bodies other than bones that are advanced to the stomach are removed via gastrotomy. If the foreign body cannot be removed endoscopically and cannot be advanced into the stomach, an esophagotomy should be done. With availability of either rigid or flexible endoscopic equipment, this is rarely necessary.

The esophageal wall is invariably damaged by impaction by a bone or another sharp object and subsequent retrieval efforts (Figure 4-19). Most lacerations heal uneventfully, however, and when careful endoscopic techniques are used, surgical intervention is rarely necessary. The mucosa should be carefully inspected once the bone is removed. The degree of damage is usually directly related to the length of time the foreign body was lodged and can be worsened by retrieval efforts. If there is significant erosive damage, treatment for severe esophagitis should be administered as described earlier in this chapter. Pain relief medication also should be given as needed. Effective analgesia may include fentanyl CRI, morphine administered SQ or IM q6h, oxymorphone or hydromorphone, or a fentanyl patch with an injectable opioid administered in conjunction until the patch has been in place long enough for effective blood levels of fentanyl to be reached.

Water is generally offered 12 hours after bone removal, and soft food can be offered at 18 to 24 hours. If there is any concern about esophageal

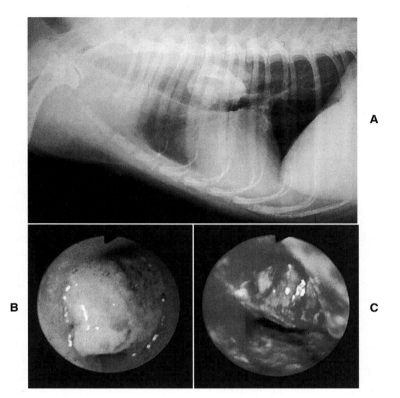

FIGURE 4-19 Esophageal foreign body (pork bone) in a 4-year-old 14-lb mixed-breed dog. The owner had given the bone to the dog as a treat and observed frequent gagging episodes 1 hour later. Radiographs were not obtained at the referring hospital until 3 days after bone ingestion. Clinical signs included intermittent gagging, salivation, nausea, and regurgitation shortly after eating. **A,** Lateral thoracic radiograph showing a large irregular bone lodged in the esophagus at the heart base. **B,** Endoscopic appearance of the bone. The bone had been lodged for 3 days before examination. **C,** The bone was successfully retrieved. Severe esophageal trauma resulted from lodgment of the bone and efforts to remove it. Postendoscopy treatment included sucralfate suspension, intravenous famotidine, subcutaneous amoxicillin, butorphanol for pain, intravenous fluids, and NPO for 36 hours. Several follow-up endoscopies were done over the following 2 weeks to examine for stricture formation. No stricture developed, and the esophagus was grossly normal at 2 weeks. (From Tams TR: Endoscopic removal of gastrointestinal foreign bodies. In Tams TR, ed: *Small animal endoscopy,* St. Louis, 1990, Mosby–Year Book.)

perforation, thoracic radiographs should be obtained immediately and at 12 and 24 hours after bone removal and compared with preprocedure films. Pneumomediastinum, pneumothorax, or pleural fluid may be present if there has been a perforation. Most patients are discharged from the hospital 1 to 4 days after the foreign body has been removed.

If there has been severe esophageal mucosal damage, periodic endoscopic surveillance during the first 1 to 3 weeks after a bone has been removed is recommended to evaluate for stricture formation. Once-weekly examination is usually adequate. If damage has been particularly severe, the first examination should be done at 3 to 5 days.

ESOPHAGEAL NEOPLASIA AND PERIESOPHAGEAL MASSES

Esophageal neoplasia occurs uncommonly in dogs and cats. Malignant tumors of the esophagus include squamous cell carcinoma, osteosarcoma, fibrosarcoma, and undifferentiated carcinoma. Primary esophageal sarcomas are often associated with *Spirocerca lupi* infections. Benign tumors are occasionally detected, commonly as incidental findings at endoscopy or necropsy, and are usually leiomyomas. In cats, squamous cell carcinoma is by far the most common primary esophageal tumor. Metastatic neoplasms to the esophagus that have been reported include pulmonary alveolar carcinoma, gastric carcinoma, thyroid carcinoma, mammary adenocarcinoma, and squamous cell carcinoma.

Esophageal neoplasia is discussed in detail in Chapter 11. *Spirocerca lupi* will be described in this section. Mass lesions arising from the periesophageal tissues may cause esophageal obstruction by compressing the walls of the esophagus. This type of obstruction is somewhat more common in cats than in dogs. Anterior mediastinal lymphoma is most common. Other causes include thymic masses, lymphadenopathy, and lung masses. I have observed a cat with a periesophageal stricture and pleural effusion that had an undifferentiated sarcoma (based on cytologic analysis of the effusion).

The endoscopic appearance associated with periesophageal compression includes normal mucosa and collapsed walls. The characteristic sign is an inability to dilate the esophagus with air. It is often also difficult to advance the endoscope through the narrowed esophageal lumen.

Clinical Signs

Esophageal tumors usually occur in older patients. *Many dogs and cats with primary esophageal tumors are asymptomatic until quite late in the course of the disease.* The diagnosis is often initially made as an incidental finding on survey thoracic radiographs that are made for some other reason. When clinical signs do develop, they primarily include slowly progressive regurgitation and inappetence. There also may be salivation, dysphagia, fetid breath, and weight loss.

Mediastinal lymphoma occurs most commonly in young cats. Regurgitation occurs when the mass becomes large enough to compress the esophagus. Other potential signs include dyspnea from pleural effusion, a noncompressible cranial thorax, and Horner's syndrome. Diagnosis and treatment are discussed in Chapter 11.

Spirocerca Lupi

S. lupi is a nematode parasite of dogs in the southern United States. There is a developmental period of 6 months. The parasite lives in the wall of the esophagus. The parasite lays eggs that pass into the lumen of the esophagus and subsequently pass through the GI tract and out of the body in the feces. Coprophagic beetles ingest eggs, which then hatch and encyst in the beetle. This stage is infective for dogs. Birds and rodents may act as transport hosts. Following ingestion, the encysted larvae are freed and migrate through the wall of the stomach and the aorta to the esophagus, where they mature.

Larval migration and worm nodules in the esophagus can cause aortic aneurysms, spondylosis in adjacent vertebral bodies, esophageal granulomas, and esophageal neoplasia. Fibrosarcoma and osteosarcoma of the esophagus are often associated with *S. lupi*. An interesting feature of the spondylosis is that it forms immediately below vertebral bodies, with no bridging to another vertebral body until the disease is very advanced. Hypertrophic osteopathy has been reported in cases of esophageal fibrosarcoma with and without pulmonary metastasis.

Diagnosis of *S. lupi* esophageal granulomas may be made by lesion appearance and location. Ova may occasionally be identified in the feces. In one recent report of seven cases, ova were found in the feces of only two of the dogs. Six dogs had signs of esophageal disease, and one dog did not. Four dogs had evidence on thoracic radiographs of a caudodorsal mediastinal mass. Two of these dogs had spondylitis of midthoracic vertebrae. Endoscopy identified a single esophageal nodule in five dogs, three nodules in one dog, and six nodules in the other.

Disophenol had been the only anthelmintic proven effective against the adult stage of *S. lupi*. It is not effective against larval stages. Further, it is no longer available. Doramectin (Dectomax, Pfizer Animal Health) has now been shown to be effective in treatment of *S. lupi*. Treatment before doramectin became available was limited to surgical excision of the esophageal granulomas.

In the study cited here, doramectin was administered at a dosage of 90 µg/lb SQ every 2 weeks for three treatments. Endoscopy was then performed at 2, 4, and 6 weeks after treatment. Six weeks after treatment, clinical signs had resolved in six dogs. The esophageal lesions were completely resolved in four of the dogs and reduced in size in the other three dogs. Two dogs with incomplete resolution were subsequently treated with doramectin administered orally at 225 µg/lb daily for 6 weeks. Esophageal nodules resolved in all dogs, as confirmed by endoscopy, and there was no recurrence at 3 years. No adverse clinical signs were noted.

ESOPHAGEAL DISORDERS OF CHINESE SHAR-PEIS

Shar-peis have a high incidence of disorders of the GI tract. These include abnormal esophageal motility, hiatal hernias, inflammatory bowel disease, and small intestinal bacterial overgrowth.

Detailed radiographic studies on shar-peis have shown that either segmental or generalized esophageal hypomotility and esophageal redundancy are commonly present. These signs are not uncommon in clinically normal shar-peis, so they may represent incidental findings in many cases. In one study 29 puppies were evaluated over 15 months, beginning when they were 3 months old. Of this group 69% had relatively slow stimulation of secondary waves of esophageal contraction, 48% had generalized poor esophageal tone or motility, and 38% had esophageal redundancy. Esophageal redundancy appeared as a prominent ventral deviation of the esophagus in the cranial portion of the mediastinum. Sequential studies revealed apparent improvement with age in clinically normal puppies in which slow motility, in the absence of redundancy, was recognized on initial studies done at a young age. This study also evaluated nine shar-pei puppies with histories of either vomiting or regurgitation. Five of the nine puppies had a hiatal hernia, and two had megaesophagus.

These findings indicate that shar-peis with signs consistent with upper GI dysfunction (e.g., regurgitation, dysphagia, salivation, vomiting) should be thoroughly evaluated for anatomic abnormalities *early* in the course of the development of clinical signs, rather than receiving conservative symptomatic therapy for more than several days to a few weeks. Initial diagnostic evaluation should include survey radiographs of the neck and thorax. If megaesophagus is present, there is little need to perform contrast studies. If megaesophagus is not readily apparent, one should perform barium swallows, looking for evidence of esophageal hypomotility and hiatal hernia. As previously described, it may be useful to apply abdominal pressure in order to enhance movement of the stomach into the thorax so that a hernia can be identified on spot films. Barium meals are used to evaluate esophageal motility further. If available either in-house or on a referral basis, fluoroscopic studies are recommended. Endoscopy also should be performed to evaluate for esophagitis, to detect evidence of esophageal motility (pooling of fluid in the esophagus), and to assess the appearance of the GEJ area and the stomach.

REFERENCES

Bartges JW, Nielson DL: Reversible megaesophagus associated with atypical primary hypoadrenocorticism in a dog. *J Am Vet Med Assoc* 201:889, 1992.

Berry WL: *Spirocerca lupi* esophageal granulomas in 7 dogs: resolution after treatment with doramectin, *J Vet Intern Med* 14:609, 2000.

Chacon MB, Uson JM, Vives MA, et al.: Gastroesophageal reflux in canine clinical practice. *Eur J Compar Gastroent* 4(1): 25-29, 1999.

Geldof H, Hazelhaff B, Otten MH: Two different dose regimens of cisapride in the treatment of reflux esophagitis: a double-blind comparison with ranitidine, *Aliment Pharmacol Ther* 7:409, 1993.

Guilford WG, Strombeck DR: Diseases of swallowing. In Guilford WG, et al., eds: *Strombeck's small animal gastroenterology,* Philadelphia, 1996, WB Saunders.

Guilford WG, Strombeck DR: Diseases of swallowing. In Strombeck DR, Guilford WG, eds: *Small animal gastroenterology,* Davis, Calif, 1990, Stonegate.

Hedlund CS: Surgery of the esophagus. In Fossum TW, ed: *Small animal surgery,* St. Louis, 1997, Mosby.

Johnson SE, Sherding RG: Diseases of the esophagus and disorders of swallowing. In Birchard SJ, Sherding RG, eds: *Manual of small animal practice,* ed 2, Philadelphia, 2000, WB Saunders.

Melendez LD, Twedt DC, Wright M: Suspected doxycycline-induced esophagitis with esophageal stricture formation in three cats, *Fel Pract* 28(2):10, 2000.

Overholt BF: Photodynamic therapy and thermal treatment of esophageal cancer, *Gastrointest Endosc Clin North Am* 2:433, 1992.

Rallis T et al.: Persistent right aortic arch: does the degree of esophageal dilatation affect long-term outcome? A retrospective study in 10 dogs and 4 cats, *Eur J Compar Gastroent* 5(1):29, 2000.

Shelton GD: Disorders of muscle and neuromuscular junction. In Birchard SJ, Sherding RG, eds: *Saunders manual of small animal practice,* ed 2, Philadelphia, 2000, WB Saunders.

Shelton GD, Schule A, Kass PH: Risk factors for acquired myasthenia gravis in dogs: 1, 154 cases (1991-1995), *J Am Vet Med Assoc* 211(11):1428, 1997.

Shelton GD et al.: Acquired myasthenia gravis: selective involvement of esophageal, pharyngeal, and facial muscles, *J Vet Intern Med* 4:281, 1990.

Sherding RG, Johnson SE, Tams TR: Esophagoscopy. Tams TR, ed: *Small animal endoscopy.* St. Louis, 1999, Mosby.

Spielman BL, Shaker EH, Garvey MS: Esophageal foreign bodies in dogs: a retrospective study of 23 cases, *J Am Anim Hosp Assoc* 28:570, 1992.

Stickle R et al.: Radiographic evaluation of esophageal function in Chinese Shar Pei pups, *J Am Vet Med Assoc* 201:81, 1992.

Tams TR: Endoscopic removal of gastrointestinal foreign bodies. In Tams TR, ed: *Small animal endoscopy,* ed 2, St. Louis, 1999, Mosby.

Tams TR: Reflux esophagitis. In Kirk RW, ed: *Current veterinary therapy X*, Philadelphia, 1989, WB Saunders.

Vigneri S et al.: A comparison of five maintenance therapies for reflux esophagitis, *N Engl J Med* 333:1106, 1995.

Willard MD: Disorders of the oral cavity, pharynx, and esophagus. In Nelson RW, Couto CG, eds: *Essentials of small animal internal medicine,* ed 2, St. Louis, 1998, Mosby.

DISEASES OF THE STOMACH

Robert C. DeNovo

FUNCTIONAL ANATOMY

The stomach is a pouch-shaped organ positioned transversely between the lower esophageal sphincter (LES) and the pylorus. The stomach has four functionally distinct anatomic and functional regions (Figure 5-1). The cardia, fundus, and body are located to the left of midline, whereas the antrum lies mostly in a transverse position to the right of midline. Convergence of muscles of the esophagus and stomach forms the gastric inlet or cardia. The main function of the LES and cardia is to allow entry of ingesta into the stomach while preventing reflux of gastric contents into the esophagus. The fundus is the dome-shaped portion of the stomach located left and dorsal to the cardia. The fundus dilates during gastric filling to accommodate a volume of ingesta without increasing intragastric pressure. The body is the large middle portion of the stomach extending from the cardia and fundus to the antrum. The body stores ingesta and secretes hydrochloric acid, pepsin, and lipase for the initial phase of digestion. The distal third of the stomach is the tubular-shaped antrum, which extends from the incisura angularis of the lesser curvature to the pylorus. The pylorus is the most distal and narrowly tubular part of the stomach. The pylorus is composed of a thick muscular wall to form the small-lumen

pyloric sphincter, which connects to the duodenum. The primary function of the antrum is to grind food into smaller particles, whereas the pylorus limits the size of food particles that pass into the duodenum and prevents reflux of duodenal contents into the stomach.

The stomach wall has three layers: the mucosa, the muscularis, and the serosa. The mucosa consists of the surface epithelium, the glandular lamina propria, and the muscularis layer. Columnar surface epithelial cells of the mucosa secrete copious amounts of mucus and bicarbonate that protect the underlying tissue from the damaging effects of luminal acid and proteolytic pepsin. The lamina propria contains glands composed of columnar epithelial cells that are functionally different in each part of the stomach. Glands in the cardia secrete mucus and pepsinogens, whereas glands in the fundus and body have parietal cells that secrete hydrochloric acid and chief cells that secrete pepsinogens. These chemicals hydrolyze dietary proteins and inactivate ingested microbes. Glands in the antrum also secrete pepsinogens and mucus and contain specialized G cells that secrete gastrin, which is a potent secretagogue for acid production. The muscularis consists of an inner circular and an outer longitudinal layer of smooth muscle, with a thin oblique muscle layer in between. The thickness of the muscular coat increases distally through

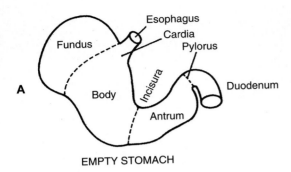

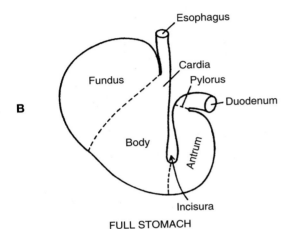

FIGURE 5-1 Diagram of cross section of stomach showing anatomic and functional regions. **A,** Empty stomach. **B,** Full stomach, showing that increase in size is due to changes in the proximal part of the stomach. (From Guilford WG, Strombeck DR: Gastric structure and function. In Guilford WG et al., eds: *Strombeck's Small Animal Gastroenterology*, ed 3, Philadelphia, 1996, WB Saunders.)

the stomach, reaching maximum thickness at the pylorus. The serosa is the outer layer of the stomach.

The blood supply to the stomach is from the celiac, hepatic, and splenic arteries. Venous return to the hepatic portal vein is through the gastrosplenic and gastroduodenal veins. Gastric lymph empties into the cisterna chyli via the hepatic and mesenteric lymph nodes. Extrinsic autonomic innervation consists of sympathetic afferent and efferent fibers from the celiac plexus and parasympathetic efferent fibers from the vagus nerves. The intrinsic myenteric plexus innervates the muscular and submucosal layers and functions to control mucosal secretion.

GASTRIC MOTILITY

Normal passage of ingesta into the stomach and duodenum requires coordination of esophageal, gastric, and duodenal motility. Esophagogastric and gastroduodenal motility is coordinated by the esophageal myenteric plexus, which is continuous with the gastric myenteric plexus, which is continuous with that of the pylorus and small intestine. Gastric storage, mixing, grinding, and transport functions all require different types of motility. Gastric filling stimulates stretch receptors in the fundus and body to cause gastric relaxation, facilitating reservoir function without causing increased intragastric pressure. Mixing and grinding of food and transport of liquid and small food particles to the pylorus occur as several peristaltic contractions per minute travel from the gastric body to the antrum. As a peristaltic wave approaches the pylorus, small amounts of liquid chyme pass into the duodenum. The pylorus then closes, and larger particles remain in the antrum and gastric body for additional digestion. High concentration of carbohydrate, protein, or fat entering the duodenum stimulates pyloric closure to slow gastric emptying and prevent small intestinal overload.

THE GASTRIC MUCOSAL BARRIER

The stomach is well protected from the damaging effects of gastric acid, pepsin, bile acids, and other digestive enzymes by a complex of physical and chemical components known as the gastric mucosal barrier (GMB). The most superficial component of the GMB is a thick mucus-bicarbonate layer secreted by gastric epithelial cells. Surface mucus acts as a lubricant to prevent mechanical damage. An underlying glycoprotein gel adheres to the mucosa and traps bicarbonate secreted by epithelial cells to maintain surface mucosal pH above 6. This layer provides an electrical-chemical barrier to impede diffusion of luminal acid and pepsin into the epithelium. Gastric epithelial cells have low permeability to water and ions and have tight intercellular junctions, features that also inhibit diffusion of luminal chemicals into the epithelium. Another important feature of the GMB is the ability of gastric epithelial cells to continually and rapidly repair injured cells, a characteristic known as epithelial restitution. In the event of superficial mucosal injury, cells at the edge of the damaged area migrate over the defect within a few hours to prevent deeper damage to the mucosa. A dense network of submucosal capillaries supplies oxygen and nutrients to meet the high metabolic demands of mucus and bicarbonate secretion and of rapid cellular renewal. Perhaps the most important component of the GMB is prostaglandin produced by the GI mucosa. Prostaglandin E increases mucus and bicarbonate secretion, regulates mucosal blood flow, stimulates epithelial cell growth, and inhibits acid secretion. The collective effect is to enhance rapid epithelial restitution, to prevent damage to the surface mucosa, and to prevent progression of damage deeper into the submucosa.

DIAGNOSIS OF GASTRIC DISEASE

History and Physical Examination

Vomiting is the predominant and most consistent sign of the patient with gastric disease; however, the vomiting patient is a diagnostic and therapeutic challenge. Many nongastric disorders cause vomiting (Boxes 5-1 and 5-2), and not all patients with gastric disease are observed to vomit. Vomiting does not always indicate presence of a serious problem, but it is often the first sign of many life-threatening diseases such as parvovirus, hemorrhagic gastroenteritis (HGE), pancreatitis, intussusception, hypoadrenocorticism, and acute renal failure. For these reasons, a detailed history and thorough physical examination are essential to determine if a serious problem exists and to formulate a logical and economical diagnostic plan.

Clinical abnormalities in patients with primary gastric disease are usually nonspecific. Vomiting, hematemesis, melena, anorexia, abdominal pain, and distention are the predominant signs of gastric disease, whereas diarrhea and weight loss occur less frequently. Vomiting is considered to be the hallmark of gastric disease. Unfortunately, most owners do not distinguish between vomiting and regurgitation when describing the problem and will also confuse vomiting with dysphagia, gagging, or coughing. Most patients that are diagnosed with esophageal disease at the University of Tennessee Veterinary Teaching Hospital initially have vomiting instead of regurgitation as the pri-

---

BOX 5-1 Causes of Acute Vomiting

NON–LIFE-THREATENING
Acute gastritis
  Dietary indiscretion
  Abrupt dietary change
  Ingested foreign material
  Drugs (antibiotics, nonsteroidal antiinflammatory drugs [NSAIDs])
  Ingested chemicals
Ascaris infection (puppies)
Giardia
Motion sickness

POTENTIALLY LIFE-THREATENING
Gastric-duodenal foreign body
Gastric-duodenal ulcer
Intussusception
Canine parvovirus enteritis
Canine distemper virus enteritis
Infectious canine hepatitis
Leptospirosis
Hemorrhagic gastroenteritis
Acute gastric dilatation-volvulus
Acute pancreatitis
Acute renal failure
Acute hepatic failure
Hypoadrenocorticism
Pyometra
Peritonitis
Sepsis
Salmon poisoning *(Neorickettsia helminthoeca)*

---

mary owner complaint. To avoid misinterpretation of clinical signs, the owner must be questioned carefully to distinguish between what has been observed versus the owner's interpretation of those observations. Characteristics helpful in differentiating among vomiting, regurgitation, and dysphagia are listed in Table 5-1.

Hematemesis and melena are commonly caused by gastric bleeding from erosive or ulcerative gastric disease (Box 5-3) but can also be caused by esophageal or small intestinal bleeding. Digested blood in the vomitus is typical of gastric bleeding, whereas fresh blood is more likely to be of oral or esophageal origin. Black stool can result from bleeding from any portion of the upper GI tract; however, gastric bleeding is the most common cause of melena. Coagulopathy should always be ruled out in any patient with hematemesis or melena.

Abdominal distention is a less common but important sign of gastric disease. Acute abdominal

BOX 5-2 Causes of Chronic Vomiting

METABOLIC DISEASE
Renal disease
Pancreatitis
Hepatic disease
Biliary disease
Hypoadrenocorticism
Diabetic ketoacidosis
Hypercalcemia
Hypokalemia
Heartworm disease (cats)

GASTRIC DISEASE
Partial obstruction
  Foreign body
  Mucosal hypertrophy
Chronic nonspecific gastritis
  Superficial, hypertrophic, atrophic
Helicobacter-associated gastritis
Mycotic gastritis
  Phycomycosis
  Histoplasmosis
Parasites
  Physaloptera spp.
  Ollulanus spp.
Neoplasia
  Lymphosarcoma
  Adenocarcinoma
Benign gastric polyps
Gastric hypomotility

Enterogastric reflux
Gastric dilatation

ESOPHAGEAL DISEASE
Hiatal hernia
Gastroesophageal reflux
Distal esophagitis

SMALL INTESTINAL DISEASE
Parasites
  Giardia
  Nematodes
Inflammatory bowel disease
Obstruction
  Foreign body
  Neoplasia
Diffuse neoplasia
Fungal disease
Ileus

LARGE INTESTINAL DISEASE
Chronic colitis
Obstipation

NEUROLOGIC DISEASE
Vestibular disease
Autonomic epilepsy
Neoplasia

TABLE 5-1 Features of Dysphagia, Regurgitation, and Vomiting

Symptom	Characteristics	Significance
Dysphagia	Difficult swallowing Repeated swallowing Drooling	Localizes disease to oral cavity or pharynx
Regurgitation	Passive expulsion of nondigested food and fluid Occurs soon after meal No prodromal nausea or retching	Localizes disease to esophagus
Vomiting	Forceful expulsion of ingesta and/or fluid Preceded by salivation, retching, abdominal contractions No consistent temporal relation to eating	Localizes disease to stomach or proximal intestine or caused by metabolic disease

distention accompanied by unproductive retching, particularly in larger-breed dogs, are cardinal signs of gastric dilatation-volvulus (GDV). In this instance distention is primarily caused by air in the stomach. Delayed gastric emptying, caused either by pyloric outflow obstruction or by abnormal gastric motility, is often characterized by postprandial distention from retention of fluid and ingesta in the stomach. Nongastric causes of abdominal distention occur more gradually and include ascites, peritonitis, organomegaly, tumor, Cushing's syndrome, and obesity.

Laboratory Evaluation

Laboratory tests help to distinguish primary GI causes of vomiting from metabolic causes and to assess patient status for complications. Complete

BOX 5-3 Predisposing Causes of Gastric Erosive-Ulcerative Disease

NONSTEROIDAL ANTIINFLAMMATORY DRUGS

Aspirin	Piroxicam
Phenylbutazone	Naproxen
Indomethacin	Ibuprofen
Ketoprofen	Indoprofen
Meclofenamic acid	Flunixin meglumine

CORTICOSTEROIDS

High dose, long duration
Associated with other risk factors

METABOLIC DISEASES

Liver failure	Renal failure
Hypoadrenocorticism	Acute pancreatitis
Neurologic disease	Inflammatory bowel disease

ALTERED GASTRIC BLOOD FLOW—STRESS-RELATED FACTORS

Hypotension	Surgery
Shock	Spinal cord disease
Sepsis	Gastric dilatation-volvulus

INCREASED SECRETION OF GASTRIC ACID

Gastrin-secreting tumor
Mast cell tumor
Pyloric outflow obstruction—chronic gastric distention

TOXIC-TRAUMATIC AGENTS

Bile salts	Foreign bodies
Pancreatic enzymes	Alcohol
Lead	Corrosive compounds

GASTRIC NEOPLASIA

blood counts (CBCs) are often normal in patients with primary gastric disease; however, a CBC can provide clues to the cause of vomiting. Chronic gastric bleeding can result in nonregenerative anemia, often with characteristics of iron deficiency (microcytosis, hypochromasia, thrombocytosis). Acute gastric hemorrhage can cause either a regenerative or nonregenerative anemia, depending on severity and duration of bleeding. Parvovirus usually causes profound neutropenia, whereas other enteric viruses cause no characteristic changes in the CBC. Acute pancreatitis, bacterial enterocolitis, and inflammatory bowel disease (IBD) can cause a neutrophilic leukocytosis. Eosinophilia in the vomiting patient can occur from parasitism, eosinophilic gastroenteritis, and adrenocortical insufficiency.

Biochemical tests provide important diagnostic and therapeutic information in the vomiting patient. Normal biochemical test results eliminate most metabolic causes of vomiting. One exception is cortisol-dependent hypoadrenocorticism, in which electrolyte concentrations are normal despite the patient having clinical signs typical of Addison's disease. In this instance an adrenocorticotropic hormone (ACTH) stimulation test is needed to rule out hypoadrenocorticism as a cause of vomiting. Hypoproteinemia occurs infrequently as a result of chronic infiltrative or granulomatous disease such as gastric lymphoma, carcinoma, or infection with *Pythium* spp. Urinalysis is useful to rule out nongastrointestinal causes of vomiting such as renal failure and diabetic ketoacidosis.

Vomiting of short duration does not change fluid, electrolyte, or acid-base balance, whereas pro-

fuse or protracted vomiting can cause significant abnormalities. These changes, however, do not reliably indicate the cause of the problem. Dehydration is the most common problem caused by vomiting. Hypokalemia frequently occurs as a result of loss of potassium both in the vomitus and urine, coupled with lack of dietary intake. Hypochloremia occurs from loss of chloride-rich gastric secretions and from reduction of chloride reabsorption in the distal nephron that occurs when the patient is hypokalemic. The acid-base status of the vomiting patient can be acidotic, alkalotic, or normal depending on the composition of the vomitus and the presence of dehydration, lactic acidosis, or metabolic disease such as renal insufficiency. Many vomiting patients have normal acid-base status because of simultaneous loss of gastric hydrochloric acid and bicarbonate-rich duodenal juice. Others will have metabolic acidosis caused by dehydration, prerenal azotemia, and lactic acidosis from decreased tissue perfusion. Hypochloremic metabolic alkalosis indicates that loss of a substantial amount of gastric contents has occurred and is most indicative of gastric outflow obstruction. Duodenal or biliary obstruction, acute pancreatitis, or renal failure can cause similar imbalances from loss of large quantities of gastric juice. If the vomiting patient is hyperkalemic, hypoadrenocorticism and oliguric or anuric renal failure are the most likely causes of the vomiting. Occasionally, severe intestinal disease caused by trichuriasis or by bacterial enterocolitis will mimic hypoadrenocorticism, causing a syndrome of vomiting and diarrhea and hyponatremia-hyperkalemia that is typical of hypoadrenocorticism.

Imaging

Survey and contrast radiographs are valuable when evaluating the patient with suspected gastric disease. Survey radiographs identify foreign bodies and gastric distention, displacement, or malposition. Gastric distention with gas is common in an excited or struggling patient due to aerophagia or in patients with dyspnea, but it can also occur with GDV. Simple aerophagia causes a large but normally positioned and nontympanic stomach. GDV causes a tense and malpositioned stomach in a patient with signs of retching and vomiting. The major radiographic feature of GDV is gas and fluid distention of the stomach, with displacement of the pylorus dorsally and to the left. *Radiographic determination of the location of the pylorus is the essential differentiating feature between simple gastric*

dilation and GDV. This is best accomplished by comparing left and right lateral recumbent views (Figure 5-2, *A* and *B*). A stomach distended with fluid or ingesta in a patient that has been fasted overnight is indicative of delayed gastric emptying. Gastric wall thickness, gastric ulcers, and gastric masses are very difficult to accurately identify using survey radiographs unless outlined by intraluminal air. Pneumoperitoneum indicates rupture of a viscus such as a penetrating gastric or intestinal ulcer, abdominal infection with gas-forming bacteria, or less commonly from perforation of the vagina or uterus.

Contrast radiographs of the stomach and duodenum can be helpful when laboratory data and survey radiographs have not revealed the cause of vomiting. Gastric or intestinal foreign bodies,

FIGURE 5-2 Gastric dilatation-volvulus. **A,** Left lateral recumbent view of an 8-year-old German shepherd with gastric dilatation-volvulus. The stomach is very distended with gas in the fundus and the body. The pyloric portion is fluid filled and not well visualized. **B,** Right lateral recumbent view of the same dog. The stomach is distended with gas. A fold of soft tissue *(arrows)* separates the dorsally displaced, gas-filled tubular pylorus *(P)* from the dilated fundus of the stomach, key findings that confirm the presence of volvulus. The bowel is displaced caudally and ventrally, and the spleen is not identified because of gastric malposition. (Courtesy Dr. William Adams.)

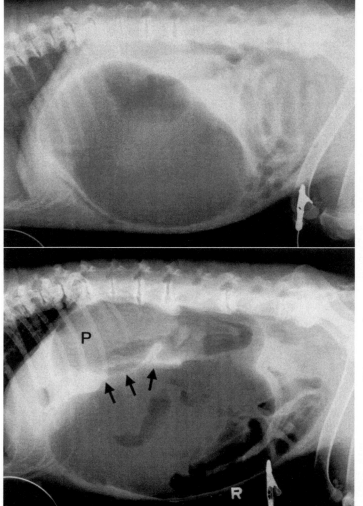

masses, ulceration, or evidence of delayed gastric emptying can usually be identified. Filling the stomach with air to provide negative contrast can help to identify foreign bodies, gastric wall masses, or deep ulcers. Positive contrast gastrography using premixed barium sulfate is more reliable. Barium should be given by stomach tube to the fasted patient; recommended doses are 4 to 6 ml/lb for small dogs and cats and 2 to 4 ml/lb for large dogs. Ventrodorsal, right lateral, and left lateral radiographs should be taken within 5 minutes of giving the barium and repeated in 20 to 30 minutes. Liquid barium should be observed in the duodenum within 5 to 20 minutes, and the stomach should be nearly empty within 3 hours. If barium does not enter the duodenum within 30 minutes, or if the stomach remains barium filled with no evidence of peristalsis, a gastric motility disorder or gastric outflow obstruction should be suspected (Figure 5-3, A). The presence of a persistently narrowed stream of barium at the pylorus is suggestive of pyloric obstruction from hypertrophy, neoplasia, or inflammatory disease (Figure 5-3, B and C). Atropine, aminopentamide, ketamine, and xylazine will significantly slow gastric emptying, giving the false impression of gastric outlet obstruction. If a tranquilizer is needed, acepromazine is recommended. (See Chapter 2 for details on GI contrast radiography.)

Liquid barium contrast radiographs are most useful to detect gross abnormalities of the gastric mucosa. This technique, however, is an insensitive indicator of gastric emptying of a meal when a functional gastric motility disorder or partial obstruction in the stomach or bowel is suspected. This limitation, in addition to the difficulty encountered in administering barium by orogastric tube, the need for multiple radiographs to be taken at specific times, the risk of barium aspiration, and the inaccuracies in interpretation of results have led to the development of a new method to evaluate GI motility.

Barium-impregnated polyethylene spheres (BIPS)* are commercially available radiopaque markers that are given orally to quantitatively measure the gastric emptying rate and intestinal transit time of food. Diagnostic sets of BIPS consist of multiple (30 1.5-mm spheres and 10 5.0-mm spheres) contained within gelatin capsules that dissolve in the stomach and release the spheres. The primary function of the large spheres is to detect GI tract obstruction, whereas the smaller spheres provide a quantitative measure of gastric emptying rate and intestinal transit time of food. The rate of gastric emptying is calculated by determining the percentage of markers that remain in the stomach after a standard period of time and comparing that percentage with reference ranges provided by the manufacturer. Various radiographic patterns showing selective movement or retention of small versus large spheres or patterns that show a bunching of spheres are also used to identify and localize specific problems such as partial obstruction. Use of these spheres is a practical diagnostic tool to evaluate gastric emptying of solids in dogs and cats. Patients with chronic vomiting, particularly those with chronic postprandial vomiting, recurrent bloating, or suspected radiolucent foreign body, or patients with anorexia of unknown cause are good candidates for a gastric motility study using BIPS.

Gastric emptying of solids can also be evaluated using fluoroscopy to observe movement of barium mixed with food into the duodenum. Nuclear scintigraphy is used to evaluate gastric emptying of liquids versus solids. These techniques are obviously limited in availability to referral institutions, whereas use of BIPS is practical for most veterinary practices. Ultrasonography has limited use in evaluating the stomach wall for abnormalities because of interference from air in the gastric lumen. Filling the stomach with water via gastric tube helps to eliminate this problem and improves sonographic visualization of the gastric wall. (See Chapter 2 for a discussion on GI ultrasonography.)

Endoscopy

Gastroduodenoscopy (Figure 5-4, A and B; see color plate) is the most useful method available for the diagnosis of gastric disease because it allows direct visualization and biopsy of the surface of the stomach and duodenum. Small lesions not detected by radiographs can usually be seen with an endoscope, foreign bodies can be removed, and biopsy specimens can be obtained. Because histologic lesions can be present in a normal-appearing stomach or duodenum, multiple biopsy specimens should always be obtained, even if the gross appearance is normal. If endoscopy is not available, exploratory surgery must be done to remove foreign bodies and to obtain biopsy specimens.

*Medical ID Systems Inc., Grand Rapids, MI, 49512.

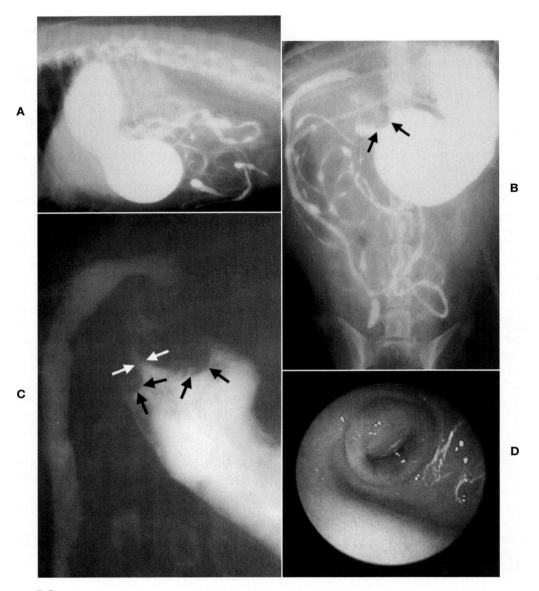

FIGURE 5-3 Delayed gastric emptying. **A,** Right lateral recumbent radiograph of a 5-year-old, 16-lb female/spayed (F/S) Chihuahua-mix with chronic intermittent vomiting caused by antral pyloric hypertrophy. The stomach is distended with liquid barium, most of which is retained in the stomach 5 hours after administration. **B,** Ventrodorsal radiograph showing a narrowed pyloric antrum. Filling defects *(arrows)* caused by antral hypertrophy were consistent throughout the series of radiographs. **C,** Close-up ventrodorsal view of the pyloric region. Hemispheric filling defects *(black arrows)* protruding into the lumen cause an annular stricture of the pyloric sphincter. A faint narrow stream of barium (beak sign) *(white arrows)* can be seen passing through the partially obstructed pylorus into the duodenum. **D,** Endoscopic appearance of the pylorus showing circumferential thickening and bulging of a masslike lesion of the pylorus. The pylorus was rigid, and the endoscope could not be passed into the duodenum. Endoscopic biopsy revealed mild lymphocytic-plasmacytic gastritis and mucosal hyperplasia. A Y-U antral advancement flap pyloroplasty was done, and excisional biopsy confirmed the presence of hypertrophic gastropathy.

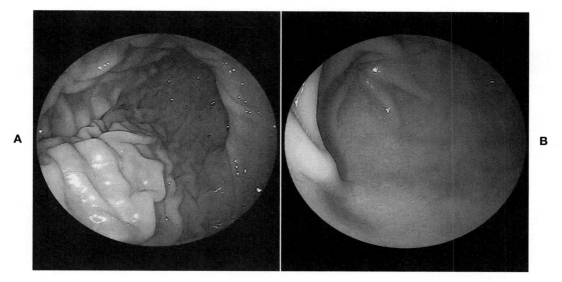

FIGURE 5-4 Normal stomach. **A,** Endoscopic appearance of a normal stomach. The smooth, pale-pink rugal folds of the greater curvature of the gastric body gradually become more linear distally at the junction with the pyloric antrum. The incisura angularis appears as a curved fold located at the 12 to 3 o'clock position. **B,** Appearance of a normal pyloric antrum *(foreground)* and pylorus *(upper left)*. The antral mucosa is smooth, pale pink, and without rugal folds. The closed pyloric orifice is located at the center of the converging mucosal folds. (See color plate.)

BOX 5-4	Causes of Acute Gastritis

DIETARY
Spoiled foods
Food sensitivity
Foreign body

INFECTIOUS
Viral
  Parvovirus
  Distemper
  Infectious hepatitis
  Coronavirus
Bacterial
  Helicobacter spp.★
Parasitic
  Physaloptera spp.★
  Ollulanus spp.★

DRUGS
Nonsteroidal antiinflammatory drugs (NSAIDs)★
Corticosteroids★

CHEMICALS/TOXINS
Cleaning products
Ethylene glycol
Herbicides
Fertilizers
Petroleum distillates
Organophosphates
Heavy metals
Plant toxins

★Can cause chronic gastritis.

ACUTE GASTRITIS AND GASTRIC EROSIVE-ULCERATIVE DISEASE

Causes

Acute gastritis occurs commonly in dogs and cats and is caused by numerous factors that result in gastric mucosal injury and inflammation. Dietary indiscretion, food intolerance, or allergy; ingestion of foreign material, chemicals, and plant irritants; viral and parasitic infections; and drugs are causes of acute gastritis (Box 5-4). Many patients, however, respond to symptomatic treatment, and a definitive cause of the acute gastritis is not identified. Repeated exposure to dietary antigens, drugs, chemicals, toxins, or infectious agents is thought to initiate an allergic or immune-mediated response, ultimately causing chronic gastritis. Diagnostic features of acute nonspecific gastritis and gastric ulceration are listed in Tables 5-2 and 5-3, respectively.

There are many causes of gastric erosion-ulcer (GEU) (see Box 5-3), and the signs can be acute or chronic. Nonsteroidal antiinflammatory drugs (NSAIDs) continue to be one of the most common causes of GEU, particularly in dogs. Mucosal damage caused by NSAIDs is primarily the consequence of two effects: NSAIDs cause direct damage to the gastric mucosa, and more importantly

TABLE 5-2	Diagnostic Features of Acute Gastritis
History	Acute onset of vomiting, often exacerbated by eating or drinking; diarrhea may be present
Physical examination	Usually normal findings; may be dehydrated or febrile
Laboratory	Usually normal results; may reveal systemic disease, metabolic disease, electrolyte or acid-base imbalance
Recovery	Rapid response to symptomatic treatment (nothing by mouth [NPO], fluids, antiemetics); often spontaneous recovery
Biopsy*	Normal to mild inflammation (neutrophilic or lymphocytic); erosion or ulceration in some

*Biopsy is seldom necessary for the diagnosis of acute gastritis.

TABLE 5-3	Diagnostic Features of Gastric Erosion–Ulceration
History	Intermittent vomiting; variable hematemesis or melena; acute onset of weakness or collapse; recent nonsteroidal antiinflammatory drug (NSAID) and/or corticosteroid treatment.
Physical examination	Often normal findings; may have signs of anemia, abdominal pain, melena noted on digital rectal examination.
Laboratory	Anemia is common, ranging from regenerative to nonregenerative hypochromic microcytic.
	Biochemistry studies may reveal systemic disease such as renal failure, liver disease, hypoadrenocorticism.
Radiography	Survey radiographs are usually normal.
	Peritonitis or pneumoperitoneum is indicative of perforation.
Endoscopy	Appearance of benign ulcers varies from punctate superficial erosions to deep ulcer crater with smooth margins. Malignant ulcers have thickened and irregular margins, often associated with mass lesions. Biopsy deep into ulcer margin is needed to differentiate benign from neoplastic lesions.

NSAIDs inhibit synthesis of gastroprotective prostaglandins. All commonly used NSAIDs, especially ibuprofen, piroxicam, and flunixin, have the potential to cause GEU. *Ibuprofen, which owners frequently give to their pets thinking it is safe, is particularly dangerous because it undergoes enterohepatic circulation, which significantly prolongs the half-life of the drug compared with humans; the same is true for piroxicam.* Flunixin has strong antiprostaglandin potency and is often used in combination with corticosteroids and/or in conditions where there is hypoperfusion of the GI tract such as occurs with parvoviral enteritis and HGE and in the postoperative patient. Such patients are predisposed to GEU because of the effects of mucosal hypoperfusion, and the use of flunixin or corticosteroids compounds the risk of severe gastric ulceration and possible perforation. Most dogs treated with

combinations of NSAIDs and corticosteroids develop endoscopically visible gastroduodenal hemorrhages, erosions, or ulcers (Figures 5-5 and 5-6; see color plate). Because these lesions are often clinically silent, the potential for severe and sometimes fatal GI hemorrhage or perforation is frequently overlooked. Even the selective cyclooxygenase-2 (COX-2) inhibitors have been associated with GEU in dogs, although much less frequently than with the nonselective NSAIDs.

Corticosteroids are another important category of drugs that increase the risk of GEU. Corticosteroids decrease mucosal cell growth and mucus production and increase gastric acid secretion. *Use of corticosteroids alone is not usually ulcerogenic; however, corticosteroids do enhance the damaging effects of NSAIDs, hypotension, refluxed bile acids, and other factors of mucosal damage.* Prednisolone is usu-

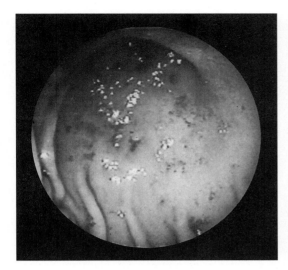

FIGURE 5-5 NSAID-induced ulcerative gastritis. Diffuse ulcerative gastritis in a 9-year-old German shepherd–mix with degenerative joint disease. The dog was being treated with aspirin (325 mg 2 times a day). Treatment began 2 months before presentation, but clinical signs of weakness, vomiting, melena caused by acute gastrointestinal blood loss, and anemia did not occur until the day of presentation. (See color plate.)

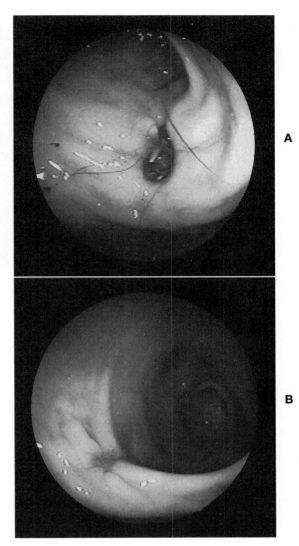

FIGURE 5-6 NSAID-induced gastric ulcer. **A,** Gastric ulcer in pyloric antrum of a 5-year-old Welsh corgi that had been treated for back pain with ibuprofen (325 mg every day for 5 days). The dog had an acute onset of vomiting and an episode of melena on the day of presentation. **B,** Healing gastric ulcer in the same patient after 7 days of treatment with omeprazole (0.3 mg/lb every day). (See color plate.)

ally not a problem unless used in very high dosages (e.g., greater than 2 mg/lb/day) for more than a few days. There is no doubt, however, that high dosages of dexamethasone can cause significant GEU, especially if other factors of mucosal damage are present.

Many metabolic diseases predispose to GEU, especially chronic liver disease, renal disease, and hypoadrenocorticism. Liver insufficiency results in decreased gastric mucus production, decreased gastric epithelial cell renewal, and decreased gastric blood flow. These factors, coupled with an increase in serum bile acid concentration that stimulates gastrin and gastric acid secretion, can cause significant GEU. Injury to gastric epithelial cells and submucosal vessels by uremic toxins and by decreased renal metabolism of gastrin account for GEU that occurs in acute and chronic renal failure. Adrenocortical insufficiency, in which mucosal damage is likely caused by hypotension and loss of vascular tone, is an infrequent cause of GEU. Although most dogs with hypoadrenocorticism do not have signs of GEU, this disorder should be considered in dogs that have hematemesis or melena if drug therapy and liver

or renal disease have been eliminated as causes of the clinical signs.

Hypotension from shock, sepsis, hypovolemia, spinal trauma, and surgery are common but frequently unrecognized causes of GEU. The fundus and body of the stomach are very dependent on a rich submucosal blood supply to maintain mucosal barrier function. Reduced blood flow to the gastric mucosa impairs epithelial cell renewal. Endogenous vasoconstrictive catecholamines and corticosteroids that are secreted in response to hypotension further potentiate ulcer formation, as will the administration of exogenous corticosteroids. *All critically ill patients, especially those with severe trauma, major surgery, organ failure, or sepsis, should be considered likely candidates for development of ulcers.*

Mast cell tumors (MCT), pancreatic gastrin-secreting tumors (gastrinomas), and pancreatic polypeptide-secreting tumors can cause severe gastritis and significant GEU. MCTs, even those benign-looking subcutaneous lumps that at first glance appear to be nothing more than a lipoma, can release excessive amounts of histamine that stimulate hypersecretion of gastric acid, which subsequently damages the gastric and duodenal mucosa. Most dogs with MCT do not have clinical signs of GEU at the time of diagnosis. However, surgical manipulation or aggressive palpation can cause massive mast cell degranulation and release of histamine. Corticosteroids, which are sometimes used to treat MCT, can further predispose to GEU and occasionally cause gastric perforation.

Gastrinomas are small pancreatic tumors that secrete large amounts of gastrin, a trophic hormone that stimulates growth of gastric mucosa and secretion of excessive gastric acid. Severe gastroesophageal reflux, esophagitis, esophageal ulceration, chronic gastritis, duodenitis, and proximal duodenal ulceration will typically occur. Gastrinoma should be considered in any adult dog that has chronic vomiting, weight loss, diarrhea, melena, and/or signs of esophagitis. Increased fasting concentration of serum gastrin is diagnostic. Other causes of increased gastrin concentration that must be considered when interpreting serum gastrin results include renal failure and conditions that cause chronic gastric distention. In addition, treatment with proton pump inhibitors (e.g., omeprazole, lansoprazole) that have potent acid-suppressing effects will cause increased gastrin production because of the lack of negative feedback of acid on gastrin-secreting cells in the pyloric antrum. Treatment for gastrinoma requires tumor removal (partial pancreatectomy), which can be curative if no metastasis has occurred. Medical management requires use of the proton pump inhibitors such as omeprazole to maximally suppress acid secretion and control symptoms. Therapy is indefinite. Patients with metastatic disease and those not controlled with acid-suppressing drugs alone can be treated with octreotide (Sandostatin), an antisecretory drug that inhibits gastrin secretion.

Medical Management

Treatment of acute gastritis, erosions, and ulceration requires elimination of predisposing causes and symptomatic-supportive therapy to enhance mucosal defenses (Box 5-5). In general, fluids are given to prevent dehydration and to maintain mucosal perfusion. Oral intake should be stopped until vomiting resolves. Parenteral or enteral nutrition should be given to patients in poor nutritional condition (see Chapter 12), and blood transfusion is given to patients with severe anemia and evidence of ongoing GI bleeding. Surgical treatment is indicated when uncontrolled hemorrhage or perforation is suspected.

Drugs used for nonspecific medical management of gastritis and GEU include H_2-receptor antagonists, proton pump inhibitors, cytoprotective agents, and prostaglandin analogues (Table 5-4) and antiemetics (Table 5-5). The drugs listed in Table 5-4 were developed primarily for the treatment of gastric ulcer disease. However, they are very useful to treat a broad variety of disorders, including esophagitis, gastritis, and GI bleeding, as well as GEU. Suppression of gastric acid promotes healing of damaged mucosa and diminishes the proteolytic effects of gastric pepsin, which is most active in an acid environment. Cytoprotectants and prostaglandin analogues strengthen mucosal defenses. Promotility drugs reduce gastroesophageal and enterogastric reflux and help to control vomiting. Antiemetic therapies are designed to diminish either the humoral or neural pathways of the vomiting and are recommended for short-term use to provide patient comfort and to reduce fluid and electrolyte losses.

Antisecretory Drugs. Histamine, gastrin, and acetylcholine stimulate the gastric parietal cell to secrete acid; simultaneous stimulation by all three causes maximal acid secretion. H_2-receptor antagonists competitively and reversibly bind to H_2-receptors on acid-producing gastric parietal cells to block the acid-stimulating effects of histamine and to render the cell less responsive to stimulation by acetylcholine and gastrin. Because these drugs are competitive inhibitors, they suppress but do not eliminate gastric secretion. The H_2-receptor antagonists cimetidine, ranitidine, nizatidine, and

BOX 5-5   Symptomatic Management for Acute Gastritis and Gastric Erosive-Ulcerative Disease

DIETARY

Nothing by mouth (NPO) for 24 to 48 hours.

Feed small portions of a low-fat, single-source protein diet starting 6 to 12 hours after vomiting has ceased.

FLUIDS

Deficits, maintenance, and ongoing losses must be provided parenterally:

If dehydration is less than 5%, subcutaneous route is adequate.

If dehydration is greater than 5%, or if vomiting is persistent, intravenous route is recommended.

Normal saline if electrolyte and acid-base status are unknown.

POTASSIUM

Supplementation is not necessary unless vomiting is frequent and persists for more than 24 hours.

If serum potassium is not known, 20 mEq KCl added to 1 L of 0.9% saline can be used for replacement and maintenance fluid therapy.

If serum potassium is known, supplement according to:

Serum Potassium (mEq/L)	Potassium Added per Liter (mEq/L KCl)
<2.0	80
2.0–2.5	60
2.5–3.0	40
3.0–3.5	30

Do not exceed 0.23 mEq potassium/lb/hr intravenously.

ANTIEMETICS

(See Table 5-5.)

Phenothiazines for 24 to 36 hours if vomiting is severe or persistent. Do not use until dehydration is corrected.

Metoclopramide may be more effective if gastric stasis or ileus is suspected. Do not use if gastrointestinal (GI) obstruction is suspected.

ANTACIDS

(See Table 5-4.)

H_2-receptor antagonists for 7 to 10 days, particularly if hematemesis or melena is present.

Omeprazole if severe erosive-ulcerative gastritis or esophagitis is suspected or if response to histamine H_2-receptor antagonist therapy has been unsatisfactory.

PROTECTIVES

(See Table 5-4.)

Sucralfate if oral medication does not stimulate vomiting.

Misoprostol is indicated for patients with suspected nonsteroidal antiinflammatory drug (NSAID)-induced gastritis.

---

famotidine are useful to treat gastritis and GEU in dogs and cats. All are effective and differ primarily in acid-suppressing potency, frequency of dosing, and in prokinetic effects. Cimetidine is the least potent and must be given three to four times daily to achieve adequate acid suppression. Ranitidine and nizatidine both have about 5 times the potency of cimetidine. Ranitidine must be given twice daily, whereas nizatidine needs to be given only once daily. Famotidine is the most potent H_2-receptor antagonist, being approximately 20 times more potent that cimetidine, and requires only once-daily dosing.

In addition to blocking acid secretion, ranitidine and nizatidine have a prokinetic effect on the GI tract. Both drugs increase acetylcholine, the primary stimulatory neurotransmitter of GI smooth muscle, by inhibiting acetylcholinesterase. The effects are to

promote gastric emptying, which is helpful in controlling vomiting for patients with gastritis, and to decrease gastroesophageal and enterogastric reflux. Because of the dual prokinetic and acid suppression effects of ranitidine, this drug is a good first-choice H_2-receptor antagonist. The reported incidence of side effects from H_2-receptor antagonists is low, and use of these drugs is safe in both dogs and cats. Cimetidine can cause vomiting, diarrhea, and depression in dogs and cats. Because cimetidine and ranitidine inhibit the same hepatic enzymes that metabolize drugs such as theophylline and warfarin, these drugs should not be given concurrently.

Proton Pump Inhibitors

Benzimidazole drugs such as omeprazole and lansoprazole block the hydrogen-potassium adenosine-triphosphatase (ATPase) enzyme of the gastric

TABLE 5-4	Drugs Used in the Treatment of Gastritis and Gastrointestinal Ulcer Disease			
Generic Name	Mechanism	Product (Mfr)	Suggested Dosage	How Supplied	Side Effects
H₂ Receptor Antagonists	Decrease acid secretion				
Cimetidine		Tagamet (GlaxoSmithKline)	2.5–5.0 mg/lb q6h PO, IV, IM	Tablet 200 mg / 300 mg / 400 mg / 800 mg Liquid 60 mg/ml Injection 150 mg/ml	Inhibition of hepatic microsomal enzymes; may cause drug interactions; mental depression
Ranitidine		Zantac (GlaxoSmithKline)	1.0 mg/lb q8–12h PO, IV, IM, SQ	Tablet 150 mg / 300 mg Liquid 15 mg/ml Injection 25 mg/ml	Similar to cimetidine, but to lesser extent
Nizatidine		Axid (Lilly)	2.5 mg/lb qd PO	Capsule 150 mg / 300 mg	None reported
Famotidine		Pepcid (Merck)	0.25 mg/lb qd PO, IV	Tablet 10 mg / 20 mg / 40 mg Liquid 8 mg/ml Injection 10 mg/ml	Similar to ranitidine
Proton Pump Inhibitor	Blocks acid secretion				
Omeprazole		Prilosec (AstraZeneca)	20 mg qd PO (>45 lb) 10 mg PO (11–45 lb) 5 mg PO (<11 lb)	Capsule 10 mg / 20 mg / 40 mg	Prolonged use can cause reversible gastric mucosal hypertrophy No clinically significant side effects reported with short-term (2–4 weeks) use

Drug	Brand (Manufacturer)	Action	Dosage	Supply	Side Effects
Mucosal Protectant					
Sucralfate	Carafate (Hoechst Marion Roussel)	Forms protective barrier / Inactivates pepsin / Adsorbs bile acids / Stimulates prostaglandins	1 g/15 lb q6-8h PO	Tablet 1 g	Constipation
Prostaglandin Analogue					
Misoprostol	Cytotec (Searle)	Cytoprotective: Increases mucus and bicarbonate secretion / Enhances mucosal blood flow / Decreases acid secretion	1-2.5 µg/lb q8h PO	Tablet 100 µg, 200 µg	Diarrhea / Abdominal cramps / Vomiting / Abortion
Prokinetic Drugs					
Metoclopramide	Reglan (Robins)	Enhances gastric emptying; antiemetic	0.15-0.25 mg/lb q8h PO, SQ / 0.5-1 mg/lb q24h IV	Tablet 5 mg, 10 mg / Liquid 1 mg/ml / Injection 5 mg/ml	Hyperactivity, constipation
Erythromycin	Erythromycin	Accelerates gastric emptying of solids	0.25-0.5 mg/lb q8h PO		
H_2-receptor antagonist	Zantac (Glaxo SmithKline) Axid (Lilly)	Enhances gastric emptying and duodenal motility	0.25-0.5 mg/lb q8h PO		

PO, Orally; IV, intravenously; IM, intramuscularly; SQ, subcutaneously.

TABLE 5-5 Antiemetic Drugs and Dosages

Drug	Primary Site of Action	Dosage	Side Effects
Prochlorperazine (Compazine, GlaxoSmithKline)	CRTZ Vomiting center	0.25 mg/lb q8h SQ, IM	Hypotension Sedation
Chlorpromazine (Thorazine, GlaxoSmithKline)	CRTZ Vomiting center	0.15-0.25 mg/lb q8h SQ	Hypotension Sedation
Yohimbine (Yobine, Lloyd Labs)	CRTZ Vomiting center	0.15-0.25 mg/lb q12h SQ, IM	Hypotension Sedation
Diphenhydramine (Benadryl, Parke-Davis)	CRTZ	1-2 mg/lb q8h PO, IM	Sedation
Dimenhydrinate (Dramamine, Searle)	CRTZ	2-4 mg/lb q8h PO	Sedation
Haloperidol (Haldol, Ortho-McNeil)	CRTZ	0.01 mg/lb q12h	Sedation
Metoclopramide (Reglan, Robins)	CRTZ GI smooth muscle (facilitates gastric emptying)	0.15-0.2 mg/lb q6h PO, SQ, IM 0.5-1 mg/lb/day as continuous IV infusion	Extrapyramidal signs
Domperidone (Motilium, Janssen)	GI smooth muscle cells (facilitates gastric emptying)	0.05-0.15 mg/lb q12h IM, IV	None reported
Cisapride (Propulsid, Janssen)	GI smooth muscle Myenteric neurons (facilitates gastric emptying)	0.05-0.25 mg/lb q8h PO	None reported
Scopolamine (Hyoscine, Fujisawa)	Vestibular system CRTZ	0.02 mg/lb q6h SQ, IM	Ileus Xerostomia Sedation
Ondansetron (Zofran, GlaxoSmithKline)	CRTZ Blocks vagal afferent neurons	0.05-0.15 mg/lb slow IV q8-24h or 30 minutes before chemotherapy PO	Sedation Head shaking

CRTZ, Chemoreceptor trigger zone; *SQ,* subcutaneously; *IM,* intramuscularly; *PO,* orally; *IV,* intravenously.

parietal cell to profoundly and irreversibly inhibit gastric acid secretion. Because these drugs block the final step of hydrogen ion secretion, they prevent secretion of gastric acid stimulated by histamine, acetylcholine, and gastrin. These drugs noncompetitively block the proton pump and therefore are much more potent than the H_2-receptor antagonists. Proton pump inhibitors accumulate in the parietal cell and increase with each dose until acid secretion is almost totally inhibited after the fifth dose. Because of this delay in gastric acid suppression, H_2-receptor antagonists should be used concurrently with proton pump inhibitors for the first 3 to 4 days of treatment in patients where rapid acid suppression is needed.

Proton pump inhibitors are recommended for the treatment of severe esophagitis and GEU that has not responded to therapy with H_2-receptor antagonists and sucralfate. They are recommended as the drugs of choice for treatment of patients with hypersecretion of gastric acid that occurs with MCT and gastrinoma. Omeprazole and lansoprazole are similar in potency, are given once daily, cause no clinical, hematologic, or biochemical abnormalities, and are safe to use in cats and dogs.

Sucralfate
Sucralfate is a sulfated disaccharide—aluminum hydroxide complex that accelerates gastric mucosal healing by adhering to mucosal erosions

and ulcers to provide a barrier to acid penetration. Sucralfate inactivates pepsin and adsorbs gastric-damaging bile acids refluxed from the duodenum. Sucralfate also stimulates endogenous prostaglandin synthesis in the gastric mucosa, resulting in increased secretion of mucus and bicarbonate and accelerated ulcer healing. Sucralfate is effective at acidic to near neutral pH and can therefore be used concurrently with antisecretory drugs such as H_2-receptor antagonists or proton pump inhibitors. However, because sucralfate can adsorb other orally administered drugs, it should not be given within 2 hours of other oral drugs. Sucralfate is recommended for the treatment of esophagitis, gastritis, and gastric ulcer of any cause in dogs and cats. Its safety is well established, with constipation being the only reported side effect.

Synthetic Prostaglandins

Synthetic prostaglandin analogues such as misoprostol have been developed that impart protection to gastric mucosa in a manner similar to endogenous prostaglandins. Misoprostol stimulates gastric mucus secretion, increases bicarbonate secretion, increases gastric mucosal blood flow, and inhibits gastric acid secretion. Because most NSAIDs inhibit the production of endogenous prostaglandins, treatment with misoprostol helps to prevent gastric ulceration in patients in which chronic NSAIDs are used to control inflammation and pain from degenerative joint disease. Clinical studies of human and canine arthritic patients have shown misoprostol to be effective in preventing NSAID-induced gastric hemorrhage, erosion, or ulceration. Diarrhea, vomiting, and transient abdominal discomfort are potential side effects, particularly if used above the recommended dosage range of 1 to 1.5 µg/lb every 12 hours. No adverse hematologic or biochemical effects have been reported with the use of misoprostol in dogs; similar information in cats is lacking. *Misoprostol will cause abortions and should not be used in pregnant patients.*

Prokinetic Drugs

Prokinetic drugs have no direct healing effect on gastric erosion or ulcer. However, these drugs improve gastric emptying and decrease enterogastric reflux, thereby helping to prevent damage to the gastric mucosa from refluxed bile acids and pancreatic enzymes. Metoclopramide is especially effective because it has both central antiemetic and peripheral gastric prokinetic effects. The antiemetic effect is mediated through antagonism of dopaminergic D_2

receptors in the chemoreceptor trigger zone (CRTZ) of the medulla to inhibit vomiting induced by drugs, toxins, metabolic disease, and acid-base imbalances. Because serotonin receptors predominate in the CRTZ of the cat, metoclopramide does not appear to be as effective as a centrally acting antiemetic in the cat as in the dog. The prokinetic effect of metoclopramide is mediated through stimulation of serotonergic $5\text{-}HT_4$ receptors on GI smooth muscle to improve coordination of antral, pyloric, and duodenal contractions. The primary prokinetic effects are to accelerate gastric emptying of liquids and to decrease duodenogastric reflux, whereas gastric emptying time of solids does not appear to be shortened.

Metoclopramide is more effective as a centrally acting antiemetic than it is as a prokinetic drug. It is best used to control vomiting caused by nonspecific gastritis, uremia, and chemotherapy. The peripheral effects of metoclopramide to prevent gastric stasis and duodenogastric reflux, and to inhibit retrograde peristalsis that precedes vomiting, further help to diminish the severity of vomiting. Metoclopramide is administered parenterally to the vomiting patient at 0.1 to 0.25 mg/lb body weight every 8 hours. Constant intravenous infusion of 0.5 to 1.0 mg/lb body weight per 24 hours is usually more effective to initially control vomiting, particularly in patients with severe vomiting. Metoclopramide should not be used if gastric outlet obstruction or GI perforation is suspected or if the patient has a seizure disorder. Some patients are very sensitive to the effects of this drug and will actually have increased vomiting, presumably caused by excessive gastric contractions. *Central effects of metoclopramide can also cause behavioral changes in some patients, ranging from lethargy in some to hyperactivity and agitated behavior in others.* These effects can occur at recommended dosages and occur most frequently in cats. Pacing, vocalization, aggressive or agitated behavior, chewing at an intravenous catheter, and excessive panting are signs that should alert the clinician to sensitivity to or overdosage of metoclopramide. Side effects usually resolve when the drug is discontinued. However, if central nervous system (CNS) signs are severe, treatment with diphenhydramine (Benadryl) at 1 to 2 mg/lb intravenously will effectively reverse the side effects without altering promotility effects of the drug. Because metoclopramide is excreted by the kidneys, the dosage should be reduced by 50% in patients with renal failure.

Cisapride is a serotonergic agonist that binds to $5\text{-}HT_4$ receptors on enteric postganglionic cholinergic neurons to increase release of acetyl-choline and stimulate GI smooth muscle contraction. Unfortunately, cisapride has been taken off the market in the United States because of an association with fatal arrhythmias in humans. No reports of similar complications occurring in the dog or cat exist. The future availability of this drug for veterinary use is uncertain, which is unfortunate because cisapride does have distinct advantages compared with metoclopramide. However, it is currently readily available through compounding pharmacies. Cisapride does not cross the blood–brain barrier; therefore it does not have the central antiemetic properties or CNS side effects of metoclopramide. Consequently, animals that experience metoclopramide-associated CNS side effects can be switched to cisapride without concern that the same side effects will occur. Cisapride accelerates gastric emptying by stimulating both pyloric and duodenal motor activity, by enhancing antropyloroduodenal coordination, and by increasing the propagation distance of duodenal contractions. As a result, this drug is much more effective than metoclopramide in enhancing gastric emptying, particularly that of solids. In addition, cisapride stimulates smooth muscle contraction throughout the GI tract, from the distal esophagus to the colon. In species such as the cat that have a smooth muscle component to the distal esophagus, distal esophageal contraction and gastroesophageal sphincter tone are enhanced. The effect of stimulating motility in the small intestine and colon has made this drug especially useful for the treatment of constipation and megacolon.

Erythromycin is a macrolide antibiotic that also generates prokinetic effects on the GI tract by stimulation of motilin receptors in GI smooth muscle. The primary effect is to stimulate gastric antral contractions similar to those that occur during phase III of the migrating myoelectric complex (MMC). Normally phase III contractions occur during the interdigestive phase rather than in the fed phase and act primarily to empty the stomach of larger indigestible solids. As a result, erythromycin accelerates gastric emptying of solids. Because of this action, it should be given during the fasted state and not until several hours after a meal has been eaten. The prokinetic dose for erythromycin (0.25 to 0.5 mg/lb orally every 8 hours for dogs and cats) is much lower than the antimicrobial dose, so side effects such as vomiting are uncommon.

Summary

In general, H_2-receptor antagonists and/or sucralfate are effective first-choice drugs in treating gastritis, erosions, and ulcers. Although the effectiveness of these drugs in preventing GEU in the dog and cat is not known, treatment with these drugs should be considered for patients with disorders such as immune hemolytic anemia or immune thrombocytopenia that require treatment with high-dose and/or potent corticosteroids. Omeprazole should be considered for those patients not responding to first-line treatment and for those patients with hypersecretory disorders such as gastrinoma. Misoprostol is indicated for patients that require chronic NSAID treatment and possibly for the critically ill patient where endogenous prostaglandin production might be impaired. The duration of treatment with these drugs varies depending on the underlying cause. In most patients, treatment with antiulcer medications for 2 to 3 weeks is adequate, providing that predisposing causes of GEU have been eliminated.

Chronic Gastritis

Chronic gastritis appears to occur frequently in the dog and cat; however, the true prevalence is unknown. More frequent use of endoscopy has led to a significant increase in the diagnosis of chronic gastritis, the causes of which include food allergy, chronic NSAID therapy, and bacterial, parasitic, or fungal infection. Infection with gastric spiral bacteria (*Helicobacter* spp.) in particular appears to be a common cause of chronic gastritis in dogs and cats. In general the causes of chronic gastritis are similar to those of acute gastritis. In many instances, gastric inflammation is confirmed with biopsy; however, a specific cause cannot be identified. In this circumstance the histologic findings, although nonspecific, might point to an etiologic diagnosis and assist in making therapeutic and prognostic decisions (Table 5-6).

Chronic gastritis is characterized clinically by intermittent episodes of vomiting, sometimes with acute episodes, that have not responded to symptomatic treatment. Other signs are nonspecific and include inappetence, anorexia, weight loss, and abdominal pain. Hematemesis and melena occur if GEU or neoplasia is present. Diarrhea is uncommon unless the patient has inflammatory bowel disease. Diagnosis is based on laboratory tests to exclude metabolic causes of chronic vomiting, radiography, sonography, and endoscopic or surgi-

TABLE 5-6	Histologic Classification of Chronic Gastritis
Predominant Histologic Type*	**Possible Causes to Consider**
Eosinophilic	Immune response to dietary antigens, parasites, foreign material
	Idiopathic eosinophilic gastroenteritis
	Mast cell tumor
	Pythiosis
Granulomatous	Chronic infections
	Histoplasmosis
	Phycomycosis
	Mycobacteria
	Parasitic
	Immune response to foreign material
	Neoplasia
	Chronic nonsteroidal antiinflammatory drug (NSAID) therapy
Lymphocytic-plasmacytic	*Helicobacter* (lymphoid nodules in some)
	Immune response to dietary antigens
	Idiopathic lymphocytic-plasmacytic gastroenteritis
	Lymphosarcoma

*Many gastric diseases cause mixed inflammatory cell reaction.

cal biopsy. Laboratory abnormalities that might occur are nonspecific and include anemia, leukocytosis, eosinophilia, and hypoproteinemia. Survey radiographs help to identify gastric foreign bodies but seldom identify primary gastric lesions. Contrast radiographs may show a thickened gastric wall, mucosal ulceration, mass lesions, or evidence of delayed gastric emptying.

Specific Causes of Chronic Gastritis

Helicobacter-associated Gastritis

Spiral bacteria of the genus *Helicobacter* infect the stomachs of many mammalian hosts, including humans, dogs, and cats. These gram-negative spiral organisms characteristically produce urease, an enzyme that helps these organisms to adapt to the gastric environment and can be used diagnostically to confirm infection. In humans, infection with *Helicobacter pylori* has been shown to be the primary cause of chronic gastritis and of gastric and duodenal ulcer disease and has been identified as a predisposing cause of gastric carcinoma and mucosal lymphoma. Several species of *Helicobacter* are commonly found in the stomachs of dogs and cats, and although the entire clinical significance of *Helicobacter* infection in these species is not known, evidence indicates that infection is a cause of chronic gastritis in dogs and cats.

Helicobacter heilmannii, Helicobacter felis, Helicobacter bizzozeronii, and *Helicobacter salomonis* are the most common types found in dogs, having been identified in clinically normal dogs, as well as in dogs with clinical signs of chronic gastritis and with histologic

findings of gastritis. *H. felis, H. heilmannii,* and *H. pylori* are the most common types found in cats. The reported prevalence of gastric *Helicobacter* infection is high in clinically normal dogs and cats, as well as in dogs and cats with signs of gastritis. In our hospital approximately 50% of dogs and cats that have had gastroscopy to determine the cause of chronic vomiting are infected with *Helicobacter.*

Despite the high incidence of infection, most dogs and cats infected with *Helicobacter* are not symptomatic for gastritis. However, some infected animals are symptomatic, a situation similar to that observed in humans. These observations pose the obvious question, *Does infection cause disease?* Most evidence indicates that certain *Helicobacter* spp. do cause disease, although the incidence of disease is much lower than the incidence of infection. A few anecdotal reports exist that describe resolution of *Helicobacter*-associated clinical gastritis following treatment with various combinations of antimicrobial-antacid therapy. These reports are limited by having small numbers of patients, by lack of biopsy-confirmed resolution of gastritis, and by lack of clinical controls. Perhaps the most compelling evidence of cause and effect is in a study of 100 animals (62 dogs and 38 cats) with clinical signs of gastritis. *Helicobacter* spp. were found in 63 animals (43 dogs and 20 cats), 62 of which had histologically confirmed gastritis. Treatment of infected animals with antibiotics plus antacids was associated with resolution of clinical signs in more than 90% of the affected animals. Of 19 animals in which biopsy was performed after treatment, 14 were negative for organisms and histologic gastritis had resolved in all. Other studies of experimental infection in dogs and cats have confirmed that *Helicobacter* spp. can induce a lymphocytic gastritis in these species. In our hospital, many patients evaluated for clinical signs of gastritis have biopsy-confirmed *Helicobacter* infection associated with lymphocytic gastritis, where no other cause for the gastritis or clinical signs can be found. Symptoms and histologic disease have resolved in most, but not all, following combination antibiotic–antacid therapy.

Diagnosis of Helicobacter *infection is confirmed by gastric cytologic findings or results of biopsy.* Cytologic analysis of gastric mucosal biopsy impression smears stained with new methylene blue is a sensitive test to confirm presence of *Helicobacter* organisms. Cytologic findings obtained by endoscopic brush of the gastric mucosa are less sensitive. Routine hematoxylin and eosin (H&E) stain histopathologic study is usually adequate to identify the organisms in gastric biopsy specimens. Use of a silver stain (e.g., Warthin-Starry stain) is best, especially to identify organisms located in the deeper areas in the gastric glands and mucosa.

Biopsy specimens obtained by endoscopy can be rapidly tested for urease production by placing the biopsy sample in a medium containing urea and a pH indicator. Urease-producing *Helicobacter* organisms in the specimen convert urea to ammonia, causing a color change in the medium. Commercial test kits are used routinely in humans to rapidly screen endoscopic biopsy samples for *Helicobacter* (CLO Test*). These tests are sensitive and specific for *Helicobacter* and work well to detect infection in dogs and cats. In our hospital, gastric biopsy specimens from all dogs and cats undergoing gastroscopic examination for vomiting are screened for the presence of urea-producing organisms using this type of test, in addition to doing cytologic studies of gastric biopsy specimens or mucosal brushings. If cytologic examination reveals the presence of spiral organisms and the urea test is positive, treatment for *Helicobacter* is started pending histopathologic results. If no other cause of vomiting is revealed by histopathologic studies, treatment for *Helicobacter* is continued for at least 14 days. (See the following discussion.)

Urease production by *Helicobacter* spp. is also the basis for the carbon-14 breath test, which was designed to noninvasively detect infected patients and to monitor treatment efficacy. Limited clinical application indicates that this test might eventually be useful in dogs and cats. Measurement of humoral IgG to *H. pylori* is a sensitive, specific, and noninvasive method of diagnosis in humans. Naturally and experimentally infected dogs and cats also produce antibody titers; however, a serologic test has not been available for use in dogs and cats. Most species of *Helicobacter* are very difficult to culture, and this method is not recommended for diagnosis. Electron microscopy, polymerase chain reaction, and in situ hybridization are techniques used to identify species and subspecies.

Endoscopic appearance of suspected *Helicobacter*-associated gastritis is variable, ranging from a normal-appearing mucosa to mucosal hyperemia to punctate erosions. Some patients will have a diffuse nodular gastritis with a raised follicular appearance (Figure 5-7; see color plate) caused by accumulations of lymphocytes. Histologic findings associated with *Helicobacter* in humans, dogs, and cats vary in severity from mild vacuolization of surface epithelium to lymphocytic-plasmacytic or neutrophilic mucosal inflammation. Lymphoid nodules occur in more severely affected patients. Infected dogs and cats that have mild histologic gastritis are often nonsymptomatic, whereas those with moderate to severe histologic gastritis are symptomatic.

Uncertainty regarding the pathogenicity of *Helicobacter* infection in dogs and cats raises another fundamental question for the clinician: *Should* Helicobacter *infection be treated?* Based on current information and clinical experience, a logical approach to this question is to first rule out other causes of chronic vomiting. Anthelmintic treatment for gastric nematodes (refer to the discussion of parasitic gastritis), followed by a complete blood count (CBC), biochemical profile, urinalysis, and abdominal radiographs, should be done initially. Endoscopic biopsy to confirm the presence of both *Helicobacter* infection and gastritis should then be considered. In our hospital, treatment for *Helicobacter* is recommended for dogs and cats in which biopsy has confirmed the presence of *Helicobacter*-associated gastritis for which no other cause of the clinical signs can be identified. For symptomatic patients in which endoscopy is not an option, the question that frequently arises is, *Should the patient be treated empirically for* Helicobacter-*associated gastritis?* This issue is debatable. If the patient is not systemically ill and is not losing weight, and if metabolic causes of chronic

---

*Trimed Specialties, Lenexa, Kan.

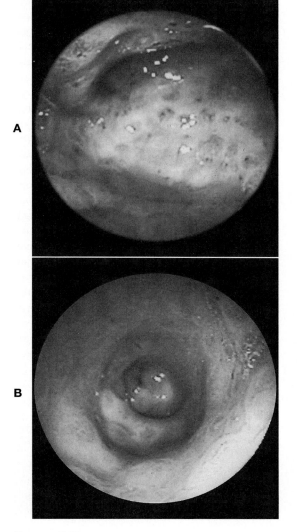

FIGURE 5-7 *Helicobacter* gastritis. **A,** Endoscopic view of the gastric body and incisura in a 3-year-old English bulldog with chronic intermittent vomiting. Raised nodules, some with a central reddened craterlike appearance, were present throughout the body and antrum. **B,** Endoscopic view of the pyloric antrum from the same dog showing a diffusely nodular mucosa. The pylorus is seen distally in the center of the image. Biopsy revealed the nodules to be accumulations of lymphocytes. Urease-positive *Helicobacter* organisms were present on the surface musosa and extending into the gastric pits. Clinical signs resolved after treatment with omeprazole (0.3 mg/lb every day) in combination with amoxicillin (10 mg/lb 2 times a day) for 14 days. (See color plate.)

vomiting and GI foreign body have been ruled out, a 14-day therapeutic trial for *Helicobacter*-associated gastritis is a therapeutically and economically reasonable approach.

Treatment of *Helicobacter* is difficult because the organism quickly develops resistance to most antibiotics when used as a single-drug treatment. Many regimens have been developed to treat *Helicobacter* gastritis in humans, using one to three antibiotics in combination with an antisecretory drug and/or a bismuth-containing compound. Acid suppression renders the organism more susceptible to the effects of antibiotics, and bismuth has antimicrobial activity against *Helicobacter*. Multiple-drug therapy using various combinations of metronidazole or bismuth with an antibiotic (tetracycline, amoxicillin, or azithromycin) and an antisecretory drug (H_2-receptor antagonist or omeprazole), given for 10 to 14 days, is considered to be the most effective treatment in humans. However, compliance and side effects are limitations to these multidrug treatments. Dual-therapy protocols using amoxicillin-omeprazole or azithromycin-omeprazole for 10 to 14 days are similar in efficacy to the three- or four-drug protocols in humans. Several two-, three-, and four-drug protocols have been extrapolated for use in dogs and cats. In my experience, dual therapy using amoxicillin or azithromycin in combination with omeprazole for 14 days is effective, well tolerated, and economical. The following is a suggested protocol for treatment of dogs and cats:

- Amoxicillin (10 mg/lb every 8 hours) plus omeprazole (0.35 mg/lb every 24 hours) is given for 14 days.
- Azithromycin (2.5 mg/lb every 24 hours for cats, 5 mg/lb every 24 hours for dogs) can be substituted for amoxicillin if incomplete response or relapse appears to have occurred.
- Metronidazole (5 mg/lb every 8 hours) can be added to either of the above treatments to treat suspected relapse for an additional 7 to 14 days.

Parasitic Gastritis

Gastric parasites have generally been regarded to be an infrequent cause of clinical disease in dogs and cats. Infrequency of diagnosis might be explained in part by difficulty finding the ova or adult parasites. Diagnosis of *Physaloptera rara* in the dog by fecal flotation is difficult because few ova are shed. Diagnosis of *Ollulanus tricuspis,* the gastric nematode of cats, is also difficult and requires examination of the vomitus for adult parasites. The increased use of endoscopy in chronically vomiting animals has revealed that gastric nematodes might be a more common cause of chronic gastritis than was once thought. In our hospital, gastric parasites have been diagnosed via endoscopy in several dogs and cats with chronic vomiting where the only abnormality found was a single parasite attached to the gastric mucosa. Treatment for these parasites has resolved the clinical signs. Adult worms are easily identified as 1- to 4-cm-long nematodes in the fundus or antrum, but the smaller larvae are difficult to visualize. Some parasitized animals have gastric erosions and moderate lymphocytic-plasmacytic or eosinophilic gastritis. Because nonendoscopic diagnosis is difficult, it is advisable to treat chronically vomiting dogs and cats that are not systemically ill for gastric parasites before recommending extensive diagnostic tests and endoscopy. Treatment with a single dose of pyrantel pamoate (2.3 mg/lb orally) eliminates *Physaloptera* from dogs, whereas cats require two doses (2.3 mg/lb) given 3 weeks apart. Treatment for *Ollulanus* is uncertain; however, fenbendazole (4.5 mg/lb every 24 hours for 2 days) appears to be effective in cats.

Chronic Gastritis of Unknown Cause

Lymphocytic-plasmacytic gastritis is a common histologic diagnosis characterized by gastric mucosal infiltrate with lymphocytes and plasma cells, but without evidence of an underlying cause. Three types have been described based on histologic appearance. *Diffuse superficial gastritis* is characterized by mucosal infiltrate with lymphocytes and plasma cells, often involving full thickness of the mucosa. *Atrophic gastritis* is characterized by severe inflammatory infiltrate with reduced mucosal parenchyma and loss of gastric glands and prominent fibrosis. *Hypertrophic gastritis* is characterized by diffuse or focal mucosal hypertrophy with variable inflammatory infiltrate and fibrosis (see discussion of pyloric mucosal hypertrophy). Plasmacytic-lymphocytic gastritis usually occurs as part of the more diffuse syndrome of IBD and likely has a similar etiopathogenesis. A permeability defect in the gastric mucosal barrier, possibly caused by dietary sensitivity, drug-induced damage, or infection, might allow abnormal absorption of luminal antigens into the mucosa, thereby initiating an immune-mediated response. Clinical, laboratory, and radiographic findings are nonspecific, and diagnosis is based on results of biopsy. Severe lymphocytic infiltrate can sometimes be difficult to distinguish from gastric lymphoma, particularly when evaluating small endoscopic biopsy specimens. Treatment is essentially symptomatic, centering on dietary protein change coupled with immunosuppressive therapy (Box 5-6).

BOX 5-6 | **Symptomatic Management of Chronic Gastritis of Unknown Cause**

DIETARY

Feed diet containing a protein novel for that patient (e.g., fish, venison, rabbit) for 2 to 4 weeks. Depending on response, continue or change to another diet with a different protein source.

ANTACIDS

H_2-receptor antagonist or omeprazole for 2 to 4 weeks, especially if hematemesis or melena is observed.

PROTECTANTS

Sucralfate is well tolerated long term and enhances healing of gastric mucosa; it should be used whenever hematemesis or melena is observed.

PROKINETICS

Metoclopramide or cisapride may be helpful in decreasing chronic vomiting and can be used indefinitely.

ANTIBIOTICS

If *Helicobacter*-associated gastritis is suspected.

Corticosteroids

Generally not used unless histologic diagnosis has confirmed lymphocytic-plasmacytic or eosinophilic

gastritis of unknown etiology; or if no response to controlled diets, protectants, and antibiotics.

Prednisone dose: 0.5-1.0 mg/lb q12h for 1 to 2 weeks.

Decrease dose by 50% every 2 weeks during next 2 months to the lowest alternate-day dose that controls the clinical signs.

Steroids can be discontinued in many patients that are then managed long term with dietary control.

AZATHIOPRINE

Use if response to steroids is inadequate or as adjunct to steroids in severe lymphocytic-plasmacytic disease; rarely needed to control eosinophilic gastroenteritis.

Dose: 0.5 mg/lb once daily for 2 weeks, followed by alternate-day therapy.

Alternate-day treatment with azathioprine-prednisone for long-term maintenance.

Monitor CBC for neutropenia or thrombocytopenia every 2 weeks for first month of therapy and monthly thereafter. Decrease dose or discontinue drug if evidence of bone marrow suppression occurs.

Eosinophilic gastritis is characterized by diffuse mucosal infiltration predominantly with eosinophils; discrete granulomatous masses with ulceration and necrosis occur rarely. The etiology and pathogenesis are unknown, but hypersensitivity to dietary antigens is a likely cause in some; an immune response to migrating parasites or microbial antigens is another suggested but unproven cause. Many but not all animals with eosinophilic gastritis have peripheral eosinophilia. Diagnosis is based on gastric biopsy results obtained after other causes of vomiting in patients with eosinophilia, such as GI parasitism, hypoadrenocorticism, mastocytosis, and heartworm disease in cats, have been ruled out.

Treatment of lymphocytic-plasmacytic and eosinophilic gastritis in most instances is based on dietary change and immunosuppressive therapy. Dietary change using a diet consisting of a novel protein that has not been part of that animal's previous diet (e.g., fish, venison, rabbit, cottage cheese) may help control the disease but is seldom effective as the sole treatment. Most patients require initial treatment with corticosteroids, and sometimes with azathioprine, to gain clinical remission. Much individual variation in response to treatment occurs. For dogs, initial treatment with prednisone, 0.5 mg/lb every 12 hours orally for 7 to 10 days, followed by an additional 7 to 10 days at 0.5 mg/lb every 24 hours orally is usually effective to induce a remission of clinical signs. The dose should then tapered to an alternate-day treatment for the next several weeks. Depending on the clinical response, prednisone dosage is further tapered by 50% decrements until it can be discontinued without recurrence of clinical signs. Cats tend to require a higher initial dosage, usually 1 to 2 mg/lb every 12 hours orally for 10 to 14 days, followed by gradually tapering doses for the next several months. Occasionally some patients do not respond well to corticosteroids or will require unacceptably high dosages to maintain remission. In this instance azathioprine is a good alternative or can be used as an adjunct to corticosteroids. In dogs azathioprine can be started at a dose of 0.45 mg/lb every 24 hours orally for 10 to 14 days. At the same time the daily dose of corticosteroid is decreased by 50%. Azathioprine and prednisone are then alternated on a daily basis. Depending on the response, the corticosteroid dose can gradually be tapered and eventually eliminated. Remission may require continued alternate-day treatment with azathioprine. Cats are very sensitive to myelotoxic and hepatotoxic effects of azathioprine; a low dose of 0.1 to 0.2 mg/lb every 48 hours is usually safe in cats. Reversible bone marrow suppression, usually occurring within the first 2 to 6 weeks of therapy, is the most common side effect of azathiaprine. A CBC should be done every 14 days during the first 2 months of therapy and at monthly intervals thereafter. If neutropenia or thrombocytopenia occurs, the drug should be stopped. Less frequent side effects are vomiting, hepatopathy, and rarely pancreatitis. The long-term prognosis for most patients with lymphocytic-plasmacytic and eosinophilic gastritis is good. Most respond well to corticosteroids and dietary changes, although some cats do not respond to even aggressive treatment. Remission can often be maintained with carefully controlled diets; however, long-term low-dose corticosteroid or azathioprine therapy is necessary in some. Rarely some patients have large eosinophilic granulomatous masses that initially require surgical resection to relieve partial luminal obstruction. These patients respond surprisingly well postoperatively but still require dietary and immunosuppressive treatment.

DELAYED GASTRIC EMPTYING AND GASTRIC MOTILITY DISORDERS

Delayed gastric emptying can be caused by mechanical obstruction of gastric outflow, by functional gastric motility disorders, or by a combination of both. Causes of mechanical outflow obstruction include gastric foreign bodies, pyloric mucosal hyperplasia or muscular hypertrophy, antral polyps, neoplasia, eosinophilic granuloma, or fungal granuloma. Duodenal neoplasia and pancreatic inflammation or abscess also impair gastric emptying, as will external compression on the pylorus from intraabdominal tumors.

Functional gastric motility disorders occur secondary to inflammatory, infiltrative, or ulcerative disease of the upper GI tract, electrolyte imbalances (hypokalemia), metabolic diseases (hypoadrenocorticism, diabetes mellitus, uremia, hypergastrinemia), drugs (anticholinergics, β-adrenergic agonists, opiates), and peritonitis. Gastric hypomotility often occurs postoperatively, particularly following GDV or spinal injury. If delayed gastric emptying is observed in a patient with chronic vomiting and an underlying cause such as mechanical or metabolic disease is not found, a functional motility disorder should be considered as the cause of the clinical signs. Several types of motility disorders occur in the dog, including retrograde transit (duodenogastric reflux), delayed gastric emptying, and accelerated gastric emptying that infrequently occurs secondary to gastroduodenal surgery. Similar functional motility disorders have not been described in cats. Delayed gastric emptying and retrograde transit are probably caused by a functional abnormality of the gastric myenteric plexus or gastric smooth muscle and are referred to as primary or idiopathic delayed gastric emptying. Specific causes of delayed gastric emptying are listed in Box 5-7.

Clinical signs of mechanical gastric-outlet obstruction and functional gastric motility disorders are similar but vary according to the underlying cause. Onset of signs is usually gradual, with intermittent vomiting of large amounts of partially digested food and fluid occurring several hours after eating. Vomiting progresses to a more predictable postprandial vomiting, especially if partial obstruction is present. Abrupt vomiting of nondigested food without retching will sometimes be described by the owner and incorrectly interpreted by the clinician to be regurgitation rather than vomiting. Gastric foreign bodies are an exception, usually causing acute and persistent vomiting. Postprandial abdominal distention and discomfort that are relieved by vomiting might be observed, particularly in dogs with chronic hypertrophic pyloric gastropathy. Between episodes of vomiting, most dogs will appear to be normal, with no physical or predictable laboratory abnormalities occurring unless metabolic complications such as electrolyte imbalance or dehydration occur. With time, moderate weight loss and abdominal distention may occur. If an inflammatory or neoplastic disease is the underlying cause, signs such as anorexia, weight loss, hematemesis, and melena might be observed.

Diagnosis of delayed gastric emptying is made on the basis of history, physical examination, exclusion of metabolic diseases that cause chronic vomiting, and radiographic studies (Table 5-7). In general, laboratory changes caused by delayed gastric emptying are minimal and nonspecific. Anemia, often with iron deficiency, may occur with ulcerative malignancy such as gastric carcinoma. Electrolyte and acid-base imbalances are uncommon unless significant obstruction to gastric outflow has occurred, in

---

BOX 5-7 Causes of Delayed Gastric Emptying

GASTRIC OUTLET OBSTRUCTION
Chronic hypertrophic pyloric gastropathy
Chronic hypertrophic gastritis
Gastric ulcer
Gastric neoplasia
Gastric foreign body
Gastric antral polyps
Granulomatous gastritis/granuloma
  Pythium
  Eosinophilic
  Idiopathic
External compression
  Pancreatitis
  Pancreatic abscess/tumor
  Abdominal mass

GASTRIC MOTILITY DISORDERS
Subacute

Gastroenteritis	Hypercalcemia
Pancreatitis	Hypocalcemia
Peritonitis	Hypokalemia
Abdominal pain	Drugs
Trauma/stress	Anticholinergics
	Narcotics
	β-adrenergic agonists

Chronic

Dysautonomia	Hypothyroidism
Post–gastric	Diabetes mellitus
dilatation–volvulus	Hypoadrenocorticism
(Post-GDV)	Uremia
Chronic gastritis	Liver failure
Gastric ulcer	Inflammatory bowel disease
Gastric neoplasia	Constipation
Gastric arrhythmia	
Idiopathic	

---

which instance hypochloremic alkalosis might develop. Hypokalemia can result from chronic vomiting; however, it can also be a cause of gastric hypomotility.

Survey abdominal radiographs can be normal or might reveal an enlarged stomach, depending on the cause, duration, and severity of delayed emptying. Survey abdominal radiographs are usually normal with functional gastric motility disorders, whereas obstructive lesions often cause a fluid-filled and distended stomach. Contrast radiographs using barium sulfate liquid can be used to outline the lumen of the stomach and to subjectively evaluate gastric emptying (see Figure 5-3). Food mixed with bar-

TABLE 5-7	Diagnostic Features of Delayed Gastric Emptying
History	Vomiting of partially digested food at times more than 8 hours after eating; vomiting large volumes of liquified food or fluid without usual prodromal signs of vomiting; postprandial abdominal distention and discomfort
Physical examination	Normal or nonspecific findings such as dehydration or abdominal discomfort; abdominal distention or tympany may be present
Laboratory	Often normal results; gastric outflow obstruction may cause hypochloremic metabolic alkalosis
Radiography	Fluid-distended stomach on survey radiographs; contrast studies confirm abnormal gastric emptying and may identify narrowed pyloric lumen or obstructing mass
Endoscopy or celiotomy	Confirms presence of gastric outflow obstruction; if no obstructing lesion is identified, a primary gastric motility disorder is likely

ium more accurately estimates gastric emptying time of solids. Interpretation of both types of contrast studies is subjective, and results of both can vary significantly in normal animals. Fluoroscopic examination improves accuracy of interpretation by allowing visualization of sequential changes in the shape of the stomach and pylorus and of movement of contrast through the pylorus. Liquid barium should begin to enter the duodenum within 15 minutes after administration, and gastric emptying of liquid should be complete within 1 to 4 hours. Complete gastric emptying of a barium meal should occur within 8 hours but might not be complete in some normal dogs until 15 hours after feeding. If most of the liquid barium is retained in the stomach after 4 hours, if liquid barium is present in the stomach longer than 12 hours, or if a large amount of a barium meal is retained longer than 8 to 10 hours, delayed gastric emptying is present.

An alternative method to barium studies for evaluation of gastric emptying is the use of radiopaque BIPS. BIPS are given with a canned-food meal consisting of approximately 25% of the daily caloric intake. Abdominal radiographs should then be taken at 4- to 6-hour intervals over the next 12 to 24 hours. The percentage of BIPS that have left the patient's stomach is compared with a standard curve for normal gastric emptying that is provided by the manufacturer. When radiographic gastric-emptying studies are done, it is important to remember that fear and anxiety from physical restraint often cause a transient delay of gastric emptying. More importantly, potent anticholinergic drugs such as aminopentamide (Centrine) can delay gastric emptying for several hours. *Because aminopentamide can cause profound and prolonged gastric stasis and ileus, which sometimes worsens the emesis and diarrhea that it was intended to resolve, it is not recommended for antiemetic therapy.*

More accurate techniques to evaluate gastric motility are limited to hospitals with nuclear medicine and GI motility laboratory facilities. Scintigraphic studies using radioactive tracers mixed with food is the method of choice for measuring gastric emptying time. Electrogastrograms can also be done and are useful to detect abnormal patterns of gastric motility such as tachygastria and bradygastria.

Functional gastric motility disorders are characterized by delayed gastric emptying in the absence of morphologic lesions. Partial obstruction caused by restrictive or infiltrating mural diseases of the pylorus, such as muscular hypertrophy, neoplasia, or granulomatous diseases, produces annular narrowing of the pyloric canal. Barium may only fill the narrow entrance to the pylorus, resulting in a thin stream of barium often referred to as having a "beaklike" appearance (see Figure 5-3, C); this is a common finding with antral pyloric hypertrophy. Polyplike filling defects can be caused by mucosal hypertrophy, inflammatory granuloma, neoplasia, or foreign body.

Once delayed gastric emptying has been confirmed, additional diagnostic procedures such as ultrasonography, endoscopy, or exploratory surgery are necessary to determine if an obstructive lesion is present. Ultrasonography is useful to detect foreign bodies, mural thickening, and masses not detected by radiographs. Endoscopy and mucosal biopsies are useful in diagnosing chronic gastritis, IBD, neoplasia, or foreign body. Surgical examination and biopsy should be considered if the cause of delayed gastric emptying is uncertain. Full-thickness gastric biopsy allows examination of muscle and nerve plexuses not included in endoscopic pinch biopsy specimens that usually extend only into the submucosa. Surgery provides an opportunity for resection of masses and for procedures to relieve gastric outlet obstruction.

Specific Syndromes of Delayed Gastric Emptying

Antral pyloric hypertrophy syndrome, also referred to as pyloric stenosis and chronic hypertrophic pyloric gastropathy (CHPG), occurs either as a congenital condition or more frequently as an acquired disorder (Table 5-8). Young to middle-age male brachycephalic breeds, particularly boxers, Boston terriers, Lhasa apsos, and Maltese, Pekingese, and shih tzu dogs, are most commonly affected. Clinical and radiographic signs of delayed gastric emptying with intermittent gastric dilatation and episodes of projectile vomiting are often observed. Physical examination and laboratory findings are usually normal. Contrast radiographs often reveal a distended stomach with delayed gastric emptying of contrast material and an abrupt narrowing of the pyloric canal with only a narrow stream of barium passing through (see Figure 5-3, C). Endoscopic examination usually reveals a thickened pyloric mucosa that sometimes appears as a protuberant mass, often with mucosal erosions (see Figure 5-3, D). Histologically the mucosa is thickened with edema and hyperplasia, and the muscularis is usually hypertrophied.

Treatment requires pyloroplasty with submucosal resection to remove thickened mucosal folds to reestablish gastric outflow. Y-U antral advancement flap pyloroplasty is the most effective method of reestablishing gastric outflow while preserving normal pyloric function. Prognosis is generally good following pyloroplasty, although

some patients require a feeding schedule of small frequent meals and treatment with metoclopramide to enhance gastric emptying.

Primary Gastric Motility Disorders

Delayed gastric emptying can be caused by abnormally slow gastric contraction (bradygastria), rapid rhythm (tachygastria), or irregular rhythm (dysrhythmia), conditions thought to be caused by abnormal gastric pacemaker activity. Bradygastria causes infrequent gastric contraction, whereas tachygastria can cause reversed propagation of motor activity, which prevents normal emptying. Gastric dysrhythmias have been observed to occur normally in healthy dogs during fasting, whereas feeding will abolish the dysrhythmia. Animals symptomatic for gastric dysrhythmias are presented for signs of post prandial abdominal discomfort, bloating, or chronic vomiting. Diagnosis requires documentation of gastric retention and elimination of obstructive and metabolic causes of delayed gastric emptying (Figure 5-8; see color plate). Measurement of gastric electrical activity is diagnostic but is limited to referral institutions.

Treatment relies on a combination of dietary changes and prokinetic drugs to improve gastric emptying (Box 5-8). Surgical procedures are generally not successful to improve gastric emptying for patients with primary functional gastric motility disorders. Liquified or blenderized diets are useful to try because liquids empty from the stomach more rapidly than solids. Because fats and proteins delay gastric emptying, diets low in fat and protein and high in carbohydrates should be tried

TABLE 5-8	Diagnostic Features of Chronic Antral Pyloric Hypertrophy Syndrome
History	Chronic vomiting, especially in small-breed and brachycephalic-breed dogs
	Postprandial abdominal distention and discomfort, often relieved by vomiting
	Normal to increased appetite
Physical examination	Usually normal findings
	Weight loss occurs infrequently
Laboratory	Usually normal results
Radiography	Fluid-filled distended stomach
	Contrast study reveals gastric outlet obstruction; narrowed pyloric lumen has typical "beaklike" appearance
Endoscopy	Thickened pyloric mucosal folds, sometimes with punctate erosions or ulcers
	Protuberant pylorus that is difficult to intubate with the endoscope
Celiotomy	Pylorus feels stiff and thickened
	Gastrotomy reveals thickened mucosal and/or muscular layers

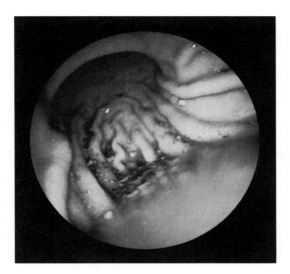

Figure 5-8 Gastric retention of food particles and bile-colored fluid in a 12-year-old miniature poodle with clinical signs of intermittent vomiting, regurgitation, inappetence, and bloating. The dog had no food or water for 14 hours before endoscopy. Results of gastric mucosal biopsies were normal, and the dog was diagnosed with primary (idiopathic) gastric motility disorder. Clinical signs improved, but did not resolve, when the dog was treated with cisapride and dietary management (small meals, fat-restricted food). (See color plate.)

initially for patients with suspected functionally delayed gastric emptying. If dietary changes are unsuccessful, gastric prokinetic drugs should be added to the therapeutic plan.

Different prokinetic drugs have different modes of action and therefore have different effects on gastric, pyloric, and duodenal contractions. For that reason, whether a particular drug is effective in improving motility depends on both the specific effects of that drug and how the underlying abnormality is affecting gastric motility. In general, cisapride has been considered to be the most effective prokinetic drug because it accelerates gastric emptying in dogs by stimulating both pyloric and duodenal motor activity, by improving coordination among antral, pyloric, and duodenal contractions, and by increasing propagation distance of duodenal contractions. The result is a predictable promotility effect, particularly in the upper GI tract, with no significant adverse effects being reported in dogs or cats. Because of the uncertain availability of cisapride, other drugs, including metoclopramide, erythromycin, and ranitidine, are alternatives to consider for treatment of delayed gastric emptying. Metoclopramide is not as effective as cisapride in accelerating gastric emptying. However, it does enhance coordination of gastro-pyloroduodenal contractions to improve gastric emptying of liquids and to prevent gastric stasis and enterogastric reflux. Metoclopramide also inhibits dopaminergic D_2 receptors in the CRTZ to diminish central stimulation of nausea and vomiting that can occur from delayed gastric emptying. Another alternative is erythromycin, which at low dosages will induce antral contractions and accelerate gastric emptying of solids. The contractions stimulated by erythromycin are similar to those that normally occur in the fasting state to empty the stomach of nondigestible solids. As a result, treatment with erythromycin might result in larger than normal and less-digested food particles being expelled into the duodenum, which could possibly cause worsening of the GI signs. The H_2-receptor antagonists ranitidine and nizatidine are

---

BOX 5-8	**Management of Delayed Gastric Emptying**

DIETARY
Frequent feeding of small meals
Low-fat, limited-protein, high-carbohydrate (fiber) diets
Blenderized diets
 	
PROKINETIC*
Metoclopramide
   Dopamine antagonist at CRTZ (central antiemetic) and at gastrointestinal (GI) receptors (stimulates GI motility)
   Potential for CNS side effects
   0.1-0.25 mg/lb q8h PO, SQ, IM
	Cisapride
	   Stimulates enteric cholinergic transmission[†]
	   No adverse effects
	   0.1-0.25 mg/lb q8h PO
	Erythromycin
	   Stimulates GI smooth muscle motilin receptors
	   Stimulates GI cholinergic receptors
	   2.5 mg/lb q8h PO[†]
	
	SURGICAL
	Various pyloroplasty and pyloromyotomy procedures indicated for pyloric outflow obstruction

CRTZ, Chemoreceptor trigger zone; *CNS,* central nervous system; *PO,* orally; *SQ,* subcutaneously; *IM,* intramuscularly.
*Contraindicated in gastric outlet obstruction.
[†]May be more effective than metoclopramide to enhance gastric emptying of solids.

used primarily to inhibit gastric acid secretion. These drugs also stimulate GI motility by inhibiting acetylcholinesterase activity, thereby increasing the amount of acetylcholine available to bind to smooth muscle muscarinic receptors. The result is primarily stimulation of gastric emptying, with some increase in small intestinal and colonic motility.

The choice of which prokinetic drug to use first depends in part on whether an underlying cause has been identified. For example, ranitidine and nizatidine are useful in the treatment of gastric motility disorders associated with gastric ulcerative or inflammatory diseases where both acid suppression and stimulation of gastric emptying are beneficial. Metabolic causes of delayed gastric emptying such as uremia or diabetic ketoacidosis, where central stimulation of vomiting might also occur, and gastric hypomotility following surgery for GDV tend to respond well to treatment with metoclopramide. If an underlying abnormality cannot be identified, the choice of treatment is trial and error. In general, cisapride (if available) should be tried initially, with erythromycin being a second choice. Metoclopramide and ranitidine or nizatidine are considered if inadequate response is achieved with the initial treatment.

Clinical experience indicates that several days of treatment are often required before a clinical response is observed. Some patients with functional dysrhythmias that respond to prokinetic drugs may require treatment indefinitely, perhaps at lower or less frequent dosing than the standard recommendations, whereas other patients might eventually be weaned off therapy. To determine if a lower drug dose is adequate requires individualized treatment for each patient. A suggested protocol is to first decrease the frequency of dosing (e.g., if a drug is being given three times a day, decrease to two times a day; if being given two times a day, decrease to every day). If clinical signs are adequately controlled for several days, alternate-day treatment can then be tried. If signs are still controlled, discontinuing the drug should be considered. If the signs reoccur, treatment must be resumed, and the lowest possible effective dose is used on a longer-term basis.

GASTRIC DILATATION-VOLVULUS SYNDROME

Acute GDV occurs most frequently in large-breed dogs, particularly Great Danes, German shepherds, Irish setters, Saint Bernards, and Doberman pinschers. Occasionally smaller-breed dogs such as bassets, bulldogs, miniature poodles, dachshunds, and Pekingese are affected. GDV is rare in cats. GDV occurs in animals ranging in age from 2 months to 15 years, with a mean of about 6 years. No sex predilection has been identified.

No single cause of GDV has been identified; however, several risk factors are thought to be of importance for the development of this condition. Deep-chested breeds of dogs appear to have an increased potential for rotational instability of the stomach, in part because of laxity of hepatoduodenal and hepatogastric ligaments. Large-volume intake of food and water causes chronic gastric distention that can potentially impair gastric emptying. Exercise with a distended stomach, particularly in deep-chested dogs, might subsequently cause the stomach to become displaced and result in volvulus. Dietary composition, particularly feeding dry-food diets, has also been suggested as a contributing factor to GDV; however, a direct relationship has not been established. The incidence of GDV was reported to decline when dry food was dampened before feeding, presumably preventing swelling of dry food with water in the stomach. Aerophagia from rapid eating, hyperventilation, and esophageal motility abnormalities have also been associated with recurrent GDV. Impaired eructation may result from an anatomically or functionally abnormal gastroesophageal junction (GEJ) in deep-chested dogs. The oblique angle of the GEJ may become exaggerated, especially if the stomach is distended following a large meal, preventing normal eructation.

Pathophysiology of Gastric Dilatation-Volvulus

GDV traps ingesta, fluid, and gas in the stomach, which rapidly causes extreme increase of intragastric pressure. A cascade of life-threatening effects develops that, if not corrected rapidly and aggressively, will cause death. The most immediate effect is impedance of gastric blood flow by increased intragastric pressure, gastric wall edema, vasoconstriction, and thrombosis. Gastric ulceration, necrosis, and perforation develop rapidly. As the stomach enlarges, respiratory tidal volume and cardiac venous return from the viscera decrease, resulting in impaired respiration, acidosis, and decreased cardiac output. Malposition of the spleen results in splenic congestion, thrombosis, and necrosis. Ischemic viscera release endotoxins that further contribute to hepatic, renal, pancreatic, and cardiac damage.

Vascular collapse, disseminated intravascular coagulation (DIC), and sepsis occur. Treatment by gastric deflation and derotation and by the rapid administration of fluids, although very necessary, can have further detrimental effects on the patient. Reperfusion injury and release of endotoxins and cardiodepressant factors, hemodilution, and metabolic acidosis further contribute to metabolic dysfunction and cardiovascular compromise.

The metabolic consequences of GDV are variable but can be severe, depending on the duration of the problem. Acid-base and electrolyte imbalances may initially be absent but usually develop during treatment. Frequent monitoring of these parameters is necessary until the patient is stabilized. Metabolic acidosis occurs commonly in the GDV patient from decreased circulating blood volume, arterial hypoxemia, and lactic acidosis. Metabolic alkalosis, caused by fluid sequestration in the stomach and by loss of gastric H^+, Cl^-, and K^+, occurs less frequently. Hyperventilation can cause respiratory alkalosis, whereas hypoventilation from gastric distention can interfere with diaphragmatic function and cause respiratory acidosis. Electrolyte abnormalities occur less frequently than acid-base imbalances, with hypokalemia being the most common.

Presumptive diagnosis of GDV is made on the basis of clinical findings and is confirmed by radio-graphic findings and gastric decompression. Clinical features of GDV are listed in Table 5-9. The most characteristic clinical signs are an acute onset of retching, but without vomiting, rapidly developing abdominal distention and tympany, and depression. Some animals are reluctant to stand, whereas others are recumbent. Rapid and weak pulses, prolonged capillary refill time, and pale, congested, or cyanotic mucous membranes are indicative of cardiovascular failure. Cardiac arrhythmia is usually present or develops soon after presentation. Arrhythmias are usually ventricular in origin and range from intermittent ventricular premature conductions to ventricular tachycardia; supraventricular arrhythmias such as atrial fibrillation occur occasionally.

Radiographs taken following initiation of fluid therapy and decompression are necessary to determine if volvulus is present. Radiographic determination of the location of the pylorus is the key feature to differentiate gastric dilation from gastric volvulus. This is best accomplished by comparing left and right lateral recumbent views (see Figure 5-2). Gastric volvulus usually results in displacement of the pylorus dorsally and to the left, creating a shelflike partition of soft tissue that appears to compartmentalize the stomach. With the pylorus shifted to the left and the patient in left lateral recumbency, the pylorus fills with fluid and gas fills the rest of the stomach. However, when the patient

TABLE 5-9	Clinical Features of Gastric Dilatation-Volvulus
History	Acute onset of nonproductive retching without vomiting
	Acute onset of abdominal distention
Physical examination	Severe depression to collapse and shock
	Reluctant to stand or walk
	Severe abdominal tympany
	Cardiovascular failure characterized by the following:
	Rapid, weak pulse or arrhythmia
	Pale mucous membranes
	Prolonged capillary refill time
	Rapid and shallow respirations
Laboratory	Hemoconcentration
	Metabolic acidosis most common
	May see hypochloremic metabolic alkalosis, respiratory acidosis, or respiratory alkalosis
	Variable hypokalemia, hypernatremia, and hypochloremia
	Variable increases in blood urea nitrogen (BUN), creatinine, and alanine aminotransferase (ALT)
Radiography	Right and left lateral recumbent positions
	Large gas- and fluid-distended stomach
	Soft tissue fold compartmentalizes the stomach
	Gas-filled pylorus located dorsal to fundus
	Esophagus dilated with air or fluid

is in right recumbency, gas fills the pyloric portion and fluid shifts to the fundus or body of the stomach. The finding that the pylorus fills with fluid when in the left lateral recumbent position and fills with gas when in the right lateral recumbent position indicates that the pylorus has rotated to the left. The presence of abdominal fluid is suggestive of peritonitis or hemorrhage, and air in the abdominal space indicates that perforation has occurred. Megaesophagus is a common finding.

Treatment

Successful treatment begins with rapid fluid therapy and gastric decompression, followed by surgical repositioning of the stomach and gastropexy. Concurrent therapy for electrolyte imbalances, arrhythmias, and DIC are necessary. Box 5-9 provides guidelines for the emergency treatment of the patient with GDV.

Initial Stabilization

Fluid therapy should be started immediately. A balanced crystalloid such as lactated Ringer's solution should be given intravenously (25 ml/lb) within the first 15 minutes to reestablish cardiac output; an additional 25 ml/lb is then given over the next 30 to 45 minutes. After this initial bolus, a colloid such as hetastarch should be given at a dose of 5 ml/lb as a slow intravenous bolus over

---

BOX 5-9   Emergency Treatment of Acute Gastric Dilatation-Volvulus

TREAT HYPOVOLEMIA AND SHOCK

1. **Aseptically place intravenous catheter** (16 to 18 gauge) and collect samples for CBC, serum electrolyte concentrations, blood chemistry studies, and coagulation tests.
2. **Circulatory resuscitation:**
   Balanced electrolyte solution at 25 ml/lb for the first 15 minutes, then 25 ml/lb for the next 30 minutes.
   Next give hetastarch at 5 ml/lb over the next 10 to 15 minutes. Hypertonic saline-dextran (7% NaCl in 6% dextran-70) at 2.5 ml/lb slow bolus is a good alternative.
3. **Maintenance fluids:**
   Balanced electrolyte solution at 10 to 20 ml/lb/h until stable.
   Colloids or blood products may be needed to maintain circulatory stability.
   PCV, TP, CVP, BP, and urine output monitored every 30 to 60 minutes. Modify fluid type, amount, and rate to maintain mean arterial BP greater than 65 mm Hg and hematocrit greater than 30%.
4. **Corticosteroids** initially for shock
   Prednisolone sodium succinate (20 mg/lb IV, q1-3h prn) or dexamethasone sodium phosphate (5 mg/lb IV, q3-6h prn).

GASTRIC DECOMPRESSION

1. **Sedate** with oxymorphone (0.05 mg/lb IV) followed by diazepam (0.1 to 0.25 mg/lb IV) sedation.

2. **Decompress** by positioning in sternal recumbency; using a large diameter nasogastric tube with large side and end holes, measure length from the external nares to last rib; advance tube the measured distance.
3. **If unable to pass the tube:**
   Withdraw tube a few centimeters, rotate in counterclockwise direction, and readvance using gentle forward pressure.
   Place dog in upright sitting position or hold dog in a vertical position, and attempt to pass tube.
   Do a gastrocentesis using a 14 to 16 gauge needle or catheter placed in the right paracostal space at the point of greatest tympany to decompress the stomach enough to allow intubation.
   Anesthetize the sedated patient (see Box 5-10) and advance a gastroscope into the stomach to facilitate decompression and passage of the stomach tube.

CONFIRM GASTRIC VOLVULUS

1. **Right lateral** recumbent abdominal radiograph; if inconclusive, left lateral and ventrodorsal position should be done.
2. Features of GDV include a dilated, gas-filled stomach divided into a dorsal compartment (dorsally positioned pylorus) and ventral compartment (fundus and corpus) by the soft tissue of the lesser curvature of stomach wall; splenic enlargement and malposition may be present.

CBC, Complete blood count; *PCV,* packed cell volume; *TP,* total plasma protein; *CVP,* central venous pressure; *BP,* blood pressure; *IV,* intravenously; *prn,* as needed; *GDV,* gastric dilatation-volvulus.

10 to 15 minutes. Depending on patient response, crystalloid fluid should be resumed at a rate of 10 to 20 ml/lb/hr for the next 2 hours and then decreased to 5 to 10 ml/lb/hr. Pulse quality, capillary refill, central venous pressure, and urinary output should be used as a guide for continued fluid needs. The packed cell volume and plasma total protein concentration should be monitored hourly to avoid hemodilution (total plasma protein concentration should not decrease to less than 3.5 g/dl). Following gastric decompression, the fluid rate can usually be decreased to 5 ml/lb/hr, depending on patient stability. Hetastarch can be repeated within 6 to 12 hours if needed to maintain perfusion. If the plasma protein concentration decreases to less than 3.5 g/dl, a plasma transfusion (10 ml/lb) should be given.

Gastric decompression must be accomplished immediately, occurring as soon as intravenous fluid therapy has begun. Decompression is achieved either by passage of a stomach tube or by gastric trocarization. Trocarization is easier and better tolerated by the patient than gastric intubation; rarely does it cause peritonitis. A 16-gauge 2-inch needle or 14- to 16-gauge over-the-needle catheter is used to trocarize the stomach on the left side at the site of maximal distention. Partial decompression in this manner often facilitates passage of a large-bore orogastric tube for more complete decompression and for gastric lavage. Once a gastric tube is passed, gastric contents should be removed. If possible, the tube should be left in place while radiographs are taken. If the stomach tube is difficult to pass, attempts should be made to pass the tube while holding the patient in an upright or sitting position. Gently shaking the patient while in the upright position may help. Forcing the tube can cause esophageal or gastric perforation. *Inability to pass the tube does not necessarily mean that volvulus is present, nor does the ability to pass the tube mean that volvulus is not present.* Gastric decompression can also be achieved by gastrostomy, usually done under sedation and local anesthesia. This is a temporary procedure that fixes the stomach caudal to the right costal arch but does not return the stomach to normal position. It is indicated for patient stabilization if a gastric tube cannot be placed or if the patient needs several days of stabilization before surgical repositioning and gastropexy. As an alternative, gastric decompression can be done using an endoscope if passage of an orogastric tube has not been successful. The patient must be anesthetized for this procedure; either mask induction using an inhalant anesthetic or use of a short-acting injectable anesthetic is sufficient. Once decompression has been achieved, an *oral-gastric* tube can usually be placed to facilitate ongoing patient stabilization.

Surgical Correction

As soon as the clinical condition has been stabilized, surgery should be done to reposition and stabilize the stomach (Box 5-10). The optimal time for surgery to occur is variable, depending on patient condition and response to initial therapy. In general, surgery should not be delayed beyond the initial period of time required for stabilization. If gastric contents are noted to contain digested blood suggestive of gastric ulceration and/or necrosis, if there is radiographic evidence of perforation or peritonitis, if decompression cannot be achieved, or if decompression is difficult to maintain, surgery should not be delayed for more than 1 or 2 hours. If the patient responds well to initial therapy and decompression is sustained, surgery can be delayed for 12 to 24 hours if necessary. In this circumstance decompression must be maintained by nasogastric or pharyngostomy tubes, gastrostomy, or repeated orogastric intubation. Spontaneous repositioning of the stomach occurs infrequently following decompression. In this circumstance surgery can be delayed or may not be necessary.

A gastropexy should be done to prevent recurrence of volvulus. A recent study determined that 55% of dogs that did not have gastropexy following surgery had a recurrence, compared with 4% recurrence for dogs that did have gastropexy. Median survival time was 188 days for dogs not having gastropexy, compared with 547 days for dogs that did have a gastropexy. Several types of gastropexy done through laparotomy have been described and include incisional gastropexy, circumcostal gastropexy, belt-loop gastropexy, and tube gastropexy. The benefit of doing a prophylactic gastropexy to prevent GDV in a dog that is conformationally or genetically predisposed has not been scientifically proven. It is logical, however, that gastropexy would be of benefit to prevent a first episode of GDV in such patients, as well as for patients in which an episode of GDV was managed medically. A rapid laparoscopic gastropexy technique that provides a strong fibrous adhesion between the stomach and abdominal wall has recently been described that could be used for this purpose, thereby eliminating the need for laparotomy.

BOX 5-10	Surgical Correction of Volvulus

1. **Anesthetic induction**: Repeat intravenous oxymorphone-diazepam combination used for sedation (see Box 5-9).

   Lidocaine (1 mg/lb IV) to facilitate intubation and decrease cardiac arrhythmia.

2. **Anesthetic maintenance**: Halothane, isoflurane, or sevoflurane and oxygen; *nitrous oxide should not be used until permanent gastric decompression is achieved.*

3. **Monitor** continuous ECG, BP, and urine output. Maintain mean arterial BP greater than 65 mm Hg and a urine output greater than 1 ml/lb/hr.

4. **Reposition stomach**, and evaluate stomach and spleen for vascular compromise; remove necrotic portions. A gastropexy should then be performed to prevent recurrence of the volvulus. Basic details are given below; refer to surgical text for description of surgical procedure.

   Ventral midline laparotomy incision; an omentum-covered stomach is usually the first structure visible when a clockwise volvulus has occurred.

   Decompress stomach by gastrocentesis or by orogastric intubation.

   Retract pylorus in the counterclockwise direction; downward pressure on the right side of the visible portion of stomach will facilitate repositioning of the stomach and spleen.

   Examine stomach and spleen for signs of irreversible vascular compromise. Palpate gastric and splenic vessels for pulse.

   If organs look grossly normal, lavage stomach with warm water via orogastric tube.

   Ligate sites of active hemorrhage; hemoperitoneum usually occurs from avulsion of short gastric branches of splenic arteries.

   If gastric serosal surface is dark purple to green-black after 10 minutes of normal gastric position, irreversible ischemic damage has likely occurred and resection of that portion of stomach should be performed.

5. **Gastropexy** should then be performed to prevent recurrence of the volvulus. Refer to surgical texts for detailed description of various procedures.

IV, Intravenously; *ECG,* electrocardiogram; *BP,* blood pressure.

Medical Management (Box 5-11)

Antibiotics should be given to dogs with GDV because shock, mucosal damage, and portal hypertension predispose to sepsis. Antibiotics should be effective against gram-positive, gram-negative, and anaerobic organisms. A combination of ampicillin (10 mg/lb intravenously) and enrofloxacin (2.5 mg/lb intramuscularly) is a good choice. Second-generation cephalosporins (e.g., cefoxitin 10 mg/lb every 8 hours intravenously) or trimethroprim-sulfa antibiotics are reasonable alternatives. Corticosteroids may be beneficial for the initial management of shock to improve capillary blood flow, to decrease capillary permeability, to reduce intestinal absorption of endotoxin, and to inhibit tissue-damaging phospholipases. Short-term, high-dose therapy is recommended; prednisolone sodium succinate (20 mg/lb intravenously, given every 1 to 3 hours as needed) or dexamethasone sodium phosphate (5 mg/lb intravenously, given every 3 to 6 hours as needed) is recommended to treat shock. H_2-receptor antagonists can be given to help diminish gastric ulceration. This therapy can be started during initial therapy and continued for 7 to 10 days. If gastric mucosal damage has been severe, omeprazole should be used as soon as oral medication can be tolerated because it is a more potent gastric antisecretory drug.

Management of Complications

Cardiac arrhythmias, DIC, and GI motility disorders are common complications occurring during the acute and convalescent phases of disease. Cardiac arrhythmias can occur at the time of presentation but may not develop until as long as 72 hours after onset of GDV. Continuous electrocardiographic (ECG) monitoring is required from presentation until the dog is discharged from the hospital. Ventricular premature contractions (VPCs), paroxysmal ventricular contractions, and ventricular tachycardia are common. Correction of acid-base, electrolyte (especially potassium), and fluid balance is the first step in control of arrhythmias. Antiarrhythmic therapy is indicated if ventricular tachycardia with a heart rate of 150 beats

BOX 5-11	Postoperative Treatment of the GDV Patient

1. **Monitoring**

    CBC, serum electrolyte levels, acid-base and coagulation tests every 12 to 24 hours until stable.

    Pulse, respiration, and temperature, blood pressure, urine production, and continuous ECG monitoring are necessary to detect hypoperfusion, electrolyte and acid-base imbalances, infection, DIC, and aspiration pneumonia.

2. **Maintain Perfusion**

    Fluid therapy with a balanced electrolyte solution at a rate of 3 to 5 ml/lb/hr for 24 hours.

    If PCV and TP are low and the patient is hypotensive, blood products or colloids should be given to correct the deficits.

    If perfusion is good and the patient is stable 24 hours postoperatively, IV fluids can be decreased to 2 ml/lb/hr for the next 24 hours.

    If the patient is stable, small amounts of water and food can be offered 48 to 72 hours postoperatively.

3. **Analgesia**

    Systemic opioids such as morphine at 0.2 mg/lb IM given every 4 to 6 hours for 12 to 24 hours postoperatively will relieve pain and improve recovery.

    Butorphanol tartrate at 0.1 mg/lb IV or 0.2 mg/lb IM every 4 to 6 hours can be used as an alternative for mild pain and for longer-term analgesia.

    NSAIDs should be avoided because of potential to cause GI ulceration.

4. **Treat Cardiac Arrhythmias**

    Correct acid-base and electrolyte imbalances and fluid deficits.

    If cardiac function is poor (hypotension, sustained ventricular tachycardia),

attempt should be made to abolish the arrhythmia with lidocaine infusion at a rate of 10 to 20 µg/lb/min.

5. **Postoperative Complications**

    Esophagitis, gastric hypomotility, aspiration pneumonia. Metoclopramide is effective in restoring gastric motility, diminishing gastroesophageal reflux, and controlling vomiting.

    Ranitidine or omeprazole help reduce gastritis and enhance gastric mucosal healing.

    Aspiration pneumonia is treated with broad-spectrum antibiotics and pulmonary therapy with nebulization, coupage, and supplemental oxygen.

    DIC is treated with fresh frozen plasma (10 ml/lb) and heparin (100 units/lb every 8 hours) until platelet count and coagulation times begin to normalize.

    Local cellulitis and peritonitis around the tube gastropexy site occur from leakage of gastric contents.

    If this occurs within 2 to 3 days postoperatively, replace the tube under anesthesia.

    If this occurs 5 to 7 days postoperatively, the tube can usually be left in place.

    Thrombosis or avulsion of splenic vessels, or splenic infarction is indication for partial or complete splenectomy. If splenic torsion has occurred, splenectomy should be done before reducing the twist to lessen the release of thromboemboli and toxins to the circulation.

    A three-layer closure of the stomach using polypropylene suture or surgical stapling should be done following partial gastric resection.

CBC, Complete blood count; *ECG,* electrocardiogram; *DIC,* disseminated intravascular coagulation; *PCV,* packed cell volume; *TP,* total plasma protein; *IV,* intravenous; *IM,* intramuscularly; *NSAID,* nonsteroidal antiinflammatory drug; *GI,* gastrointestinal.

per minute or greater is present or if multifocal VPCs are occurring. Ventricular arrhythmias are initially managed using lidocaine (1 to 2 mg/lb as a slow intravenous bolus followed by infusion of 25 to 40 µg/lb/min). *Lidocaine infusion can also be used as an excellent adjunct to other analgesics for the control of postoperative pain.* Procainamide is used as a supplement to lidocaine if the arrhythmia is

refractory to lidocaine, or as longer-term maintenance therapy (5 to 10 mg/lb intramuscularly or orally every 6 hours). DIC is a frequent complication of GDV and is detected initially by presence of progressively worsening thrombocytopenia and prolonged coagulation times. If DIC is suspected, treatment with plasma (10 ml/lb) in combination with heparin (45 units/lb every 8 hours subcutaneously) should be initiated. Heparin is continued until platelets begin to increase and other coagulation parameters stabilize; plasma transfusions should be repeated if the platelet count continues to decline or if coagulation times become more prolonged. When platelet counts and coagulation times normalize, heparin should be decreased gradually by giving doses every 12 hours for 24 hours and then every 24 hours for the next day to avoid rebound hypercoagulation.

Gastric atony, delayed gastric emptying, and ileus frequently occur following GDV; in most instances these are transient. If intermittent vomiting persists, therapy with promotility drugs (metoclopramide or erythromycin) is helpful to reestablish gastric emptying. Treatment with antisecretory drugs and sucralfate may also be beneficial.

The prognosis for GDV is guarded, especially if gastric damage is severe and requires gastrectomy. Mortality is reported to be from 23% to 60%. Poor prognostic signs at presentation include a pulse rate greater than 180 beats per minute, arrhythmia, cyanotic mucous membranes, prolonged capillary refill time, and severe coagulopathy.

GASTRIC NEOPLASIA

The incidence of gastric neoplasia in the dog and cat is low, and clinical signs are insidious in onset. Often the only signs observed are inappetence, which can be present for months before other symptoms develop, and subtle weight loss. Partial obstruction of pyloric outflow and abnormal motility cause progressively worsening vomiting, anorexia, and weight loss. Ulceration and chronic blood loss causes hematemesis and melena. Gastric neoplasia is summarized here. A more detailed discussion is included in Chapter 11.

Adenocarcinoma is the most common gastric malignancy in dogs, followed by lymphosarcoma, leiomyosarcoma, fibroma, squamous cell carcinoma, and plasmacytoma. Adenocarcinoma occurs more frequently in males, with an average age of 8 years at the time of diagnosis. Lymphosarcoma is the most common gastric tumor of cats but does not have breed or gender predisposition. Diagnosis of gastric tumors is based on radiographic, endoscopic, or surgical findings. Contrast radiographs may reveal a thickened and ulcerated gastric wall. Endoscopic findings often reveal discolored and thickened mucosa, raised plaques with large central ulceration and thick raised margins (Figure 5-9; see color plate), or polypoid lesions. Diffuse

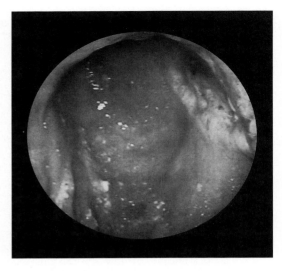

FIGURE 5-9 Malignant gastric ulcer located on the incisura angularis (1 to 3 o'clock position in the field of view) in a 13-year-old weimaraner with a 2-month history of chronic vomiting and weight loss. The dog had hypochromic microcytic anemia. The raised edges and central crater of the ulcer were very firm and required that multiple biopsy specimens be obtained from each of several sites to ensure adequate depth of tissue was obtained. Histopathologic findings confirmed gastric adenocarcinoma. (See color plate.)

thickening of the gastric wall, referred to as *scirrhous carcinoma,* also occurs. More than half of tumors occur in the pyloric antrum, often near the incisura. Lymphosarcomas can appear as raised nodular masses anywhere in the gastric wall (Figure 5-10; see color plate) or as diffuse mucosal thickening, often with erosion or ulceration. Leiomyoma is the most common benign tumor and the second most common gastric tumor in dogs but is rare in cats. Leiomyomas are often asymptomatic unless pyloric outflow is obstructed. Benign polyps appear as pedunculated or polypoid nodules that protrude from the mucosal surface. Their cause is unknown, and they seldom cause problems unless they are large enough to cause delayed gastric emptying.

Focal gastric carcinomas are best treated by surgical resection, whereas diffuse or extensive lesions are not usually resectable. Metastasis of carcinomas to lymph nodes, liver, or lungs has often occurred by the time of diagnosis, and adjunctive chemotherapy is not effective in improving survival. Lymphosarcoma is treated with chemotherapy, although the prognosis is guarded. Benign tumors and adenomatous and hyperplastic polyps causing partial outflow

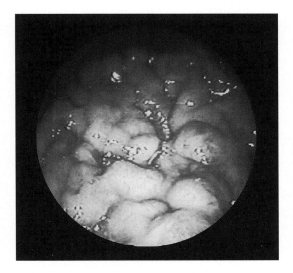

FIGURE 5-10 Diffuse nodular gastric lymphosarcoma in a 9-year-old beagle with intermittent vomiting of 2 weeks' duration and weight loss. Clinical signs resolved with chemotherapy (Adriamycin and L-asparaginase). After 6 months of remission, clinical signs reoccurred and the dog was euthanized. (See color plate.)

obstruction can successfully be resected with a good long-term prognosis.

REFERENCES

Albibi R, McCallum RW: Metoclopramide: pharmacology and clinical application, *Ann Intern Med* 98:86, 1983.

Allan DA et al.: Hypertonic saline/dextran resuscitation of dogs with experimentally induced gastric dilatation-volvulus shock, *Am J Vet Res* 52:92, 1991.

Allen FJ, Guilford WG: Radiopaque markers: preliminary clinical observations *J Vet Intern Med* 8:151J, 1984 (abstract).

Arnbjerg J: Gastric emptying time in the dog and cat, *J Am Anim Hosp Assoc* 28(1):77, 1992.

Barber DL, Mahaffey MB: The Stomach. In Thrall DE, ed: *Textbook of veterinary diagnostic radiology*, ed 3, Philadelphia, 1998, WB Saunders.

Bayerdorffer E et al.: High dose omeprazole treatment combined with amoxicillin eradicates *H. pylori*, *Gastroenterology* 102:A38, 1992.

Brockman DJ, Holt DE, Washabau R: Pathogenesis of acute canine gastric dilitation-volvulus syndrome: is there a unifying hypothesis? *Compend Contin Educ Pract Vet* 22(12):1108, 2000.

Burns J, Fox SM: The use of a barium meal to evaluate total gastric emptying time in the dog, *Vet Radiol Ultrasound* 27:169, 1986.

Carrig CB, Seawright AA: Mastocytosis with gastrointestinal ulceration in a dog, *Aust Vet J* 44:503, 1968.

Cheville NF: Uremic gastropathy in the dog, *Vet Pathol* 16:292, 1979.

Couto CG: Gastrointestinal neoplasia in dogs and cats. In Kirk RW, ed: *Current veterinary therapy XI*, Philadelphia, 1993, WB Saunders.

DeNovo RC, Magne M: Current concepts in the management of *Helicobacter* gastritis. Proceedings, American College of Veterinary Internal Medicine Forum, Orlando, Fla, 1995.

Dewey CW et al.: Azathioprine therapy for acquired myasthenia gravis in five dogs, *J Am Anim Hosp Assoc* 35:396, 1999.

DiBartola SP et al.: Clinicopathologic findings resembling hypoadrenocorticism in dogs with primary gastrointestinal disease, *J Am Vet Med Assoc* 187:60, 1985.

Editorial: antibacterial therapy of *Helicobacter pylori*–associated peptic ulcer disease: a new strategy, *J Clin Gastroenterol* 19(1):6, 1994.

Ellison GW: Gastric dilatation volvulus: surgical prevention, *Vet Clin North Am Small Anim Pract* 23:513, 1993.

Feldman M, Burton ME: Histamine$_2$-receptor antagonists: standard therapy for acid-peptic diseases, *N Engl J Med* 323:1672, 1990.

Flemstrom G: Gastric and duodenal mucosal bicarbonate secretion. In Johnson LR, ed: *Physiology of the gastrointestinal tract*, New York, 1987, Raven Press.

Freston JW: Overview of medical therapy of peptic ulcer disease, *Gastroenterol Clin North Am* 19:121, 1990.

Glickman LT et al.: A prospective study of survival and recurrence following the acute gastric dilatation-volvulus syndrome in 136 dogs, *J Am Anim Hosp Assoc* 34:253, 1998.

Graham DY: The relationship between nonsteroidal anti-inflammatory drug use and peptic ulcer disease, *Gastroenterol Clin North Am* 19:171, 1990.

Guilford GW, Strombeck DR: Chronic gastric diseases. In Guilford GW et al., eds: *Strombeck's small animal gastroenterology*, ed 3, Philadelphia, 1996, WB Saunders.

Guilford WG, Strombeck DR: Gastric structure and function. In Guilford WG et al., eds: *Strombeck's small animal gastroenterology*, ed 3, Philadelphia, 1996, WB Saunders.

Hall JA, Twedt DC, Burrows CF: Gastric motility in dogs. II. Disorders of gastric motility, *Compend Contin Educ Pract Vet* 12:247, 1990.

Hall JA et al.: Gastric motility in dogs. I. Normal gastric function, *Compend Contin Educ Pract Vet* 10(11):1282, 1988.

Handt LK, Fox JG, Dewhrist FD: *Helicobacter pylori* isolated from the domestic cat: public health implications, *Infect Immun* 62:2367, 1994.

Hayden DW, Fleischman RW: Scirrhous eosinophilic gastritis in dogs with gastric arteritis, *Vet Pathol* 14:441, 1977.

Horne WA et al.: Effects of gastric distension-volvulus on coronary blood flow and myocardial oxygen consumption in the dog, *Am J Vet Res* 46:98, 1985.

Hosgood G: Gastric dilatation-volvulus in dogs, *J Am Vet Med Assoc* 204:1742, 1994.

Jenkins CC, DeNovo RC: Omeprazole: a potent antiulcer drug, *Compend Contin Educ Pract Vet Ed* 13:1579, 1991.

Johnson SA et al.: The effect of misoprostol on aspirin-induced gastroduodenal lesions in dogs, *J Vet Intern Med* 9(1):32, 1995.

Johnson SE: Fluid therapy for gastrointestinal, pancreatic and hepatic disease. In DiBartola SP, ed: *Fluid therapy in small animal practice,* Philadelphia, 1992, WB Saunders.

Kim CH, Azpiroz F, Malagelada JR: Characteristics of spontaneous and drug-induced gastric dysrhythmias in a chronic canine model, *Gastroenterology* 90:421, 1986.

Konturek SJ, Pawlik W: Physiology and pharmacology of prostaglandins, *Dig Dis Sci* 31:6S, 1986.

Lee A et al.: Role of *Helicobacter felis* in chronic canine gastritis, *Vet Pathol* 29:487, 1992.

Miller ME, Christenson GC, Evans HE: The digestive system and abdomen. In *Anatomy of the dog,* Philadelphia, 1964, WB Saunders.

Miyabayshi T, Morgan JP: Gastric emptying in the normal dog, *Vet Radiol Ultrasound* 25:187, 1984.

Muir WW: Acid-base and electrolyte disturbances in dogs with gastric dilatation-volvulus, *J Am Vet Med Assoc* 181:229, 1982.

Murray M et al.: Primary gastric neoplasia in the dog: a clinicopathologic study, *Vet Rec* 91:474, 1972.

Murtaugh RJ et al.: The use of misoprostol for prevention of gastroduodenal hemorrhage and ulceration associated with aspirin therapy, *J Vet Intern Med* 6(2):129, 1992.

Neiger R, Simpson K: *Helicobacter* infection in dogs and cats: facts and fiction, *J Vet Intern Med* 14(2):125, 2000.

Orton EC, Muir WW: Hemodynamics in experimental gastric dilatation-volvulus in dogs, *Am J Vet Res* 44:1512, 1983.

Patnaik AK, Hurvitz AL, Johnson GV: Canine gastrointestinal neoplasms, *Vet Pathol* 14:447, 1997.

Pennick DG et al.: Ultrasonographic evaluation of gastrointestinal diseases in small animals, *Vet Radiol Ultrasound* 31(30):134, 1990.

Rawlings CA et al.: A rapid and strong laparoscopic-assisted gastropexy in dogs, *Am J Vet Res* 62(6):871, 2001.

Robert A: Cytoprotection by prostaglandins, *Gastroenterology* 77:761, 1979.

Sikes RI et al.: Chronic hypertrophic gastropathy: a review of 16 cases, *J Am Anim Hosp Assoc* 22:99, 1986.

Silen W, Ito S: Mechanisms for rapid re-epithelialization of the gastric mucosal surface, *Ann Rev Physiol* 47:217, 1985.

Simpson K et al.: The relationship of *Heilcobacter* spp. infection to gastric disease in dogs and cats, *J Vet Intern Med* 14(2):223, 2000.

Skirrow MB: Diseases due to *Campylobacter, Helicobacter* and related bacteria, *J Comp Pathol* 111:113, 1994.

Smout AJ, Akkermans LM: *Normal and disturbed motility of the gastrointestinal tract,* Petersfield, UK, 1992, Wrightson Biomedical.

Sorjonen DC et al.: Effects of dexamethasone and surgical hypotension on the stomach of dogs: clinical, endoscopic, and pathologic evaluations, *Am J Vet Res* 44:1233, 1983.

Stanton ME, Bright RM: Gastroduodenal ulceration in dogs, *J Vet Intern Med* 3:238, 1989.

Tarnawski A, Hollander D, Gergely H: The mechanism of protective, therapeutic and prophylactic actions of sucralfate, *Scand J Gastroenterol* 22(suppl 140):7, 1987.

Twedt DC: Cirrhosis: a consequence of chronic liver disease, *Vet Clin North Am* 15:151, 1985.

Van den Brom WE, Happe RP: Gastric emptying of a radionuclide-labeled test meal in healthy dogs: a new mathematical analysis and reference values, *Am J Vet Res* 47:2170, 1986.

Wallace JL, Bell CJ: Gastroduodenal mucosal defense, *Curr Opin Gastroenterol* 8:911, 1992.

Wallmark B, Lorentzon P, Lorsson H: The mechanism of action of omeprazole: a survey of its inhibitory actions in vitro, *Scand J Gastroenterol* 20(suppl 108):37, 1985.

Walter MC, Matthiesen DT: Acquired antral pyloric hypertrophy in the dog, *Vet Clin North Am* 23:547, 1993.

Zerbe CA et al.: Pancreatic polypeptide and insulin-secreting tumor in a dog with duodenal ulcers and hypertrophic gastritis, *J Vet Intern Med* 3:178, 1989.

ACUTE MEDICAL DISEASES OF THE SMALL INTESTINE

Andrew Triolo
Michael R. Lappin

PATHOPHYSIOLOGY OF ACUTE SMALL INTESTINAL DISEASE

Normal physiologic functions of the small intestine include **motility** (propulsion and mixing of food), **secretion** (fluids of differing electrolyte concentrations added to intestinal contents), **digestion** (physicochemical reactions breaking down ingesta into simpler compounds that can be absorbed), and **absorption** (selective uptake of products of digestion along with water and electrolytes). Very large quantities of water and electrolytes, relative to total body stores, are cycled through the gastrointestinal (GI) tract daily. For example, nearly half the total volume of extracellular fluid is secreted into the upper GI tract each day, an amount greatly exceeding oral intake. Under normal conditions fecal losses of water and electrolytes amount to only approximately 0.1% of the total amount cycled through the GI tract. However, when normal small intestinal absorptive or secretory function is disrupted acutely, massive fluid and electrolyte losses may ensue.

Absorption of most important nutrients occurs by active mechanisms that require specific mucosal carriers. Mucosal villi are the primary site of absorption, whereas intestinal crypts are largely responsible for secretion. Passive transport of ions is determined largely by relative transmucosal concentration and electrical potential differences. Absorption may also be modified by incorporation of solute into bulk flow of water (solvent drag). Absorption of sodium, mediated by energy-requiring active transport processes in both the large and the small intestine, is crucial to the absorption of water, electrolytes, and certain nutrients.

Within the jejunum, glucose, other actively absorbed monosaccharides, amino acids, and bicarbonate all enhance sodium absorption. Sodium resorption in turn enhances absorption of glucose and amino acids. Therefore fluids administered for purposes of oral rehydration should contain both glucose and sodium, because absorption of sodium is necessary for passive absorption of water. Potassium moves inward across the intestinal mucosa along its concentration gradient.

Chloride follows passively inward along an electrical gradient established by inward sodium transport. Bicarbonate is rapidly absorbed in the jejunum by active transport or is neutralized by hydrogen ions, generating water and carbon dioxide. In the ileum, chloride absorption and bicarbonate absorption are coupled, such that bicarbonate moves out in exchange for inward transport of chloride. As a result, pH and bicarbonate concentration increase in the distal small bowel; fluid losses originating there are more likely to cause metabolic acidosis than are losses from the proximal small intestine.

Intestinal **secretion** involves the net efflux of an isotonic solution of water and electrolytes. This is an important mechanism of fluid loss and may induce severe diarrhea. Intestinal secretion can be triggered by a number of stimuli, including bacterial enterotoxins, malabsorbed substances such as unconjugated bile acids and fatty acids, certain drugs, and mechanical obstruction of the small bowel.

Abnormal intestinal motility also may induce diarrhea and fluid losses, although the relationships between intestinal motility, secretion, and absorption are generally poorly understood.

Diarrhea results from either impaired absorption or excessive solute (including exudation) secretion. Increased osmolality within the intestinal lumen results in net water loss as well. Diarrhea usually results in loss of fluids isotonic to plasma. The major solutes in diarrhea fluid are sodium, chloride, organic anions, and potassium. In most instances the primary body deficits due to diarrhea are in sodium and water. Loss of isotonic fluid decreases circulating plasma volume and may in severe instances (e.g., parvoviral enteritis) precipitate hypovolemic shock. Because isotonic fluids are lost, serum electrolyte concentrations usually remain normal initially. During diarrheal diseases the most important source of potassium loss is via urine, mediated by aldosterone released in response to extracellular fluid volume depletion. When diarrhea is severe and/or prolonged, significant amounts of potassium also may be lost via feces. Mild metabolic acidosis and hypokalemia are the most common acid-base and electrolyte alterations observed in patients with acute small intestinal disease and diarrhea.

Causes of Diarrhea

Acute diarrheas can be grouped by mechanism or disease. The most common mechanisms include *abnormal fluid secretion* (primarily sodium), *malab-sorption,* and *abnormal intestinal motility*. The best understood stimuli in humans are bacterial enterotoxins resulting in secretory diarrhea. Bacteria such as *Escherichia coli* and *Vibrio, Clostridium,* and *Staphylococcus* spp. induce intestinal secretion by increasing intracellular concentrations of cyclic adenosine nucleotides. Acute diarrhea in patients that eat spoiled food (garbage enteritis) may be from ingestion of preformed enterotoxins. Dietary fatty acids and bile acids also stimulate intestinal secretion, as do certain GI hormones and intestinal obstruction.

Malabsorptive diarrhea results from mucosal or submucosal diseases that impair absorption by either the small or the large intestine. Diseases of the intestinal mucosa may directly impair sodium resorption, thereby inhibiting water resorption and inducing diarrhea. Poorly absorbed dietary substances (e.g., complex carbohydrates such as sucralfate) also may interfere with water resorption by altering osmotic gradients. Some products of maldigestion, such as bile acids, may directly inhibit sodium transport in the colon and also induce diarrhea.

Intestinal mucosal damage results in generalized transudation of water and electrolytes, as well as plasma proteins and blood, when injury is severe. Normal mechanisms for sodium transport also are disrupted. These mechanisms (combined secretory and malabsorptive diarrhea) are thought to be largely responsible for diarrhea that develops in acute small intestinal diseases characterized by severe, bloody diarrhea. Examples include acute viral enteritis and canine hemorrhagic gastroenteritis.

It is likely that altered intestinal motility plays a role in the pathogenesis of acute diarrhea, although the mechanisms and prevalence in animals are poorly understood. Segmental contractions of the intestines are reduced with most causes of diarrhea, leading to hypomotile gut. For this reason, drugs that reduce intestinal motility, such as anticholinergic agents, are not recommended for symptomatic treatment of acute diarrhea.

Diseases resulting in acute diarrhea can be grouped into primary (diseases of the intestine) or secondary (diseases outside the intestine with diarrhea as a sequela) causes (Box 6-1). *The most common primary diseases are parasites, infectious diseases, ingestion of toxins, and obstruction.* Secondary diarrheas are less common causes of acute diarrhea and are discussed in other chapters.

BOX 6-1	Differential Diagnoses for Vomiting and Diarrhea in Dogs and Cats

PRIMARY GI DISEASES

Obstruction: masses, foreign body, intussusception, hiatal hernia
Dietary intolerance
Drugs/toxins
Inflammatory gastric and bowel diseases
Neoplasia
Infectious diseases (viral, bacterial, fungal)
Parasites

SECONDARY GI DISEASES

Renal disease
Hepatic disease
Pancreatitis
Hypoadrenocorticism (rare in cats)
Diabetes mellitus with ketoacidosis
Peritonitis
Central nervous system/vestibular disease
Pancreatic exocrine insufficiency (diarrhea only; rare in cats)

DIAGNOSTIC CONSIDERATIONS

Optimal management of patients with acute intestinal disease hinges on a specific diagnosis if possible. This is particularly true for patients with enteritis caused by an infectious agent that may have a specific treatment (Box 6-2). Although initial treatment in most cases varies little (fluid administration, correction of volume and electrolyte disturbances), specific treatment is preferred to more general, nonspecific measures such as indiscriminate administration of antibiotics, motility modifiers, adsorbents, and intestinal protectants. For these reasons, diagnostic tests should be done *early,* before administering treatments that may interfere with test results.

Physical examination allows immediate assessment of hydration status, severity of volume depletion, and initial fluid replacement needs. Careful abdominal palpation may reveal evidence of intestinal obstruction. Viral gastroenteritis is more likely in young and in febrile patients, especially those without adequate vaccinations. Rectal examination may often provide early evidence of impending diarrhea and allow assessment of stool characteristics (presence of blood or mucus, odor,

BOX 6-2	INFECTIOUS DISEASE DIFFERENTIAL DIAGNOSES FOR VOMITING AND DIARRHEA IN DOGS AND CATS

VIRUSES

Astrovirus (S)
Canine and feline coronaviruses (S)
Canine parvovirus (S)
Canine distemper virus (S)
Feline leukemia virus–associated lymphoma (S, M)
Feline immunodeficiency virus (S)
Feline panleukopenia (S)
Rotavirus (S)

BACTERIA

Bacterial cholangiohepatitis (S)
Bacterial overgrowth (S)
Bacterial peritonitis (S)
Campylobacter jejuni (S, M, L)
Clostridium perfringens (M, L)
Enterotoxigenic *E. coli* (S, M)
Helicobacter spp. (V)
Salmonella spp. (S, M, L)

HELMINTHS

Ancylostoma/Uncinaria (S, M, L)
Dirofilaria immitis (V only; mainly cats)
Ollulanus tricuspis (V only; cats only)
Physaloptera (V only)
Strongyloides spp. (S)
Toxascaris (V mainly)
Toxocara spp. (V mainly)
Trichuris vulpis (dog, L)

PROTOZOANS

Balantidium coli (ciliate; L)
Cryptosporidium spp. (coccidian; S)
Giardia spp. (flagellate; S)
Isospora spp. (coccidian; L)
Entamoeba (amoeba; L)
Pentatrichomonas (flagellate; L)

MISCELLANEOUS

Prototheca (algae; L)
Histoplasma (fungal; L)
Neorickettsia spp. (rickettsia; S)

S, Small bowel; *L,* large bowel; *M,* mixed; *V,* vomiting.

color, consistency). Occasionally parasites may be noted.

Due to the high prevalence of parasitic and infectious diseases associated with acute diarrhea, fecal testing is mandatory. To adequately assess patients for infectious causes of diarrhea, a direct smear, fecal flotation, fecal cytologic study, and *Cryptosporidium parvum* screening test should be performed.

Direct Smear. Liquid feces or feces that contains large quantities of mucus should be microscopically examined immediately for the presence of protozoal trophozoites, including those of *Giardia* spp., *Pentatrichomonas hominis,* *Balantidium coli,* and *Entamoeba histolytica.* A direct saline smear can be made to potentiate observation of these motile organisms. The amount of mucus and feces required to cover the head of a pin is mixed thoroughly with one drop of 0.9% NaCl. Following application of a coverslip, the smear is evaluated for motile organisms by examining it under × 100 magnification. Use of fresh feces gives the highest yield of positive results.

Fecal Flotation. Cysts, oocysts, and ova in feces can be concentrated to increase sensitivity of detection. Most ova, oocysts, and cysts are easily identified after zinc sulfate centrifugal flotation. This procedure is considered by many to be optimal for the demonstration of protozoan cysts, in particular *Giardia* spp., and so is a good choice for a routine flotation technique in practice (Figure 6-1). Sugar centrifugation can be used for routine parasite evaluation and may be superior to many techniques for the demonstration of oocysts

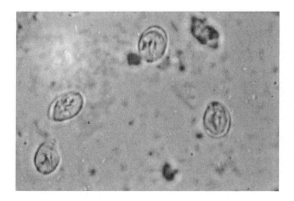

FIGURE 6-1 *Giardia* cysts.

of *Toxoplasma gondii* and *C. parvum.* *Giardia* cysts are distorted by sugar centrifugation but can still be easily identified. Fecal sedimentation will recover most cysts and ova but will also contain debris. This technique is superior to flotation procedures for the documentation of fluke eggs. Some parasites such as *Trichuris* spp. and *Giardia* spp. are shed intermittently and so can be occult. Performing two to three fecal flotations over 5 to 7 days will increase sensitivity of detection of these parasites. Feces should be refrigerated, not frozen, until assayed for parasites. If a fecal sample is to be sent to a diagnostic laboratory for further analysis and will not be evaluated for parasites within 48 hours, it should be preserved. Polyvinyl alcohol, Merthiolate-iodine-formalin, and 10% formalin preservation can be used. Because of routine availability, 10% formalin is commonly used; add 1 part feces to 9 parts formalin and mix well.

Stained Smear. A thin smear of feces should be made from all dogs or cats with large or small bowel diarrhea. Material should be collected by rectal swab if possible to increase chances of finding white blood cells. A cotton swab is gently introduced 3 to 4 cm through the anus into the terminal rectum, directed to the wall of the rectum, and gently rotated several times. Placing a drop of 0.9% NaCl on the cotton swab will facilitate passage through the anus of cats but not adversely affect cell structure. The cotton swab is gently rolled on a microscope slide multiple times to give areas with varying thickness. Following air drying, a slide should be stained with Diff-Quik or Wright's or Giemsa stain. The slide should be examined for white blood cells and bacteria morphologically consistent with *Campylobacter jejuni* or *Clostridium perfringens* (Figure 6-2). Presence of neutrophils on rectal cytologic examination can suggest inflammation induced by *Salmonella* spp., *Ca. jejuni,* or *C. perfringens;* fecal culture is indicated in these cases (see the following section). *Histoplasma capsulatum* or *Prototheca* may be observed in the cytoplasm of mononuclear cells. Methylene blue in acetate buffer (pH 3.6) stains trophozoites of the enteric protozoans. Iodine stains and acid methyl green are also used for the demonstration of protozoans. Acid-fast staining of a fecal smear is one of the *C. parvum* screening procedures that should be performed in dogs or cats with diarrhea. *C. parvum* is the only enteric organism of approximately 4 to 6 μm in diameter

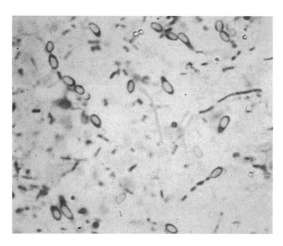

FIGURE 6-2 *Clostridium perfringens* spore-forming rods.

that will stain pink to red with acid-fast stain (Figure 6-3). Alternatively, antigen testing is available for this organism (see the following section).

Immunologic Techniques. Parvovirus, *C. parvum, Giardia* spp., and *C. perfringens* enterotoxin detection procedures are available as point-of-care tests for use with feces. Parvovirus assays detect both vaccine and field strains of canine parvovirus, and so results should be interpreted cautiously (see the viral diseases section). Recently, human *C. parvum* and *Giardia* spp. antigen assays have been applied to feces from small animals.* Minimal sensitivity and specificity results are currently available. For example, it is not known if the assays detect the canine and feline genetic variants of *C. parvum*. If used, results of these assays should be interpreted in

conjunction with results from fecal examination techniques. *C. perfringens* enterotoxin can be detected in both healthy and diseased animals, and so positive test results do not confirm disease due to this organism (see bacterial diseases section).

Culture. Culture of feces for *Salmonella* spp., *Campylobacter* spp., and *Cl. perfringens* is occasionally indicated in small animal practice. Approximately 2 to 3 g of fresh feces should be submitted to the laboratory immediately for optimal results; however, *Salmonella* and *Campylobacter* are usually viable in refrigerated fecal specimens for 3 to 7 days. The laboratory should be notified of the suspected pathogen so appropriate culture media can be used. If a delay in sample submission is expected or to increase yield of positive results, a transport medium such as Cary-Blair† medium should be used.

Electron Microscopy. Electron microscopy can be used to detect viral particles in feces of dogs and cats with GI signs of disease. Approximately 1 to 3 g of feces without fixative should be transported to the laboratory‡ by overnight mail on cold packs for performance of this assay.

MANAGEMENT OF ACUTE DIARRHEA
General Considerations
Clinically, most acute medical diseases of the small intestine in dogs and cats are characterized by watery diarrhea generally passed two to four times daily. Vomiting results from vagal afferent input into the emetic center and is present in many cases. Depending on the cause, abdominal pain and signs of systemic illness (fever, leukogram abnormalities) can occur. Rarely can the exact cause of acute small intestinal disease be determined by the results of patient history and

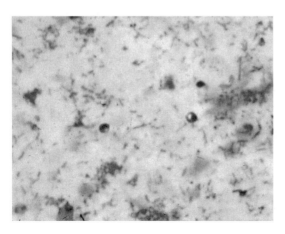

FIGURE 6-3 *Cryptosporidium parvum* oocysts.

---

*Remel, Lenexa, Kan.
†Becton Dickinson Microbiology Systems, Franklin Lakes, N.J.
‡Diagnostic Laboratory, Colorado State University, College of Veterinary Medicine and Biomedical Sciences, Fort Collins, Colo.

physical examination findings. However, history and signalment can help aid in ranking differential diagnoses. For example, viral enteritis and diarrhea due to parasitism is most common in puppies and kittens from crowded environments. Diagnostic testing is usually necessary to make a definitive diagnosis. In most cases the therapeutic plan for many patients with acute medical diseases of the small intestine and severe diarrhea is initially handled in a similar manner.

Fluid and Electrolyte Imbalances

In cases with acute GI disturbances, of immediate concern is correction of fluid and electrolyte imbalances. In most instances patients are presumed to have lost sufficient isotonic fluids to become dehydrated. Restoration of normal circulating fluid volume is an immediate priority, both to prevent renal functional impairment and to minimize further GI injury. Even if clinical evidence of dehydration is not apparent, patients are assumed to be at least 5% dehydrated. Fluid administration is calculated on the basis of the formula in Box 6-3.

In dehydrated patients fluids should always be administered intravenously. If dehydration is so severe that an intravenous catheter cannot be placed, fluids should be given initially using intraosseous administration. Subcutaneous administration of fluids has unpredictable absorption and is too slow to be useful in replacing large-volume deficits in hypovolemic, hypotensive patients. Jugular catheters are preferred over peripheral catheters in most cases; blood samples can be drawn, the catheters can be maintained for up to 5 days, the catheters are rarely affected by position changes, there is reduced risk for phlebitis, and there is the potential to measure central venous pressure to aid in monitoring fluid therapy.

Fluids are initially administered rapidly (approximately 5 to 10 ml/lb over 30 to 60 minutes, then the infusion rate is slowed) in patients with clinical hypovolemic shock (weak femoral pulse pressure, tachycardia, delayed capillary refill time, tacky mucous membranes). For more prolonged fluid administration, fluid needs for 24 hours are calculated, and the total volume is divided into three equal amounts, each to be administered every 8 hours. An infusion pump is optimal for constant-rate fluid infusion to patients of any size to avoid overhydration.

The fluid of choice for initial volume replacement is either a buffered crystalloid solution such as lactated Ringer's solution or Normosol-R or 0.9% saline solution. Both supply sodium and chloride in adequate amounts. Also, lactated Ringer's solution and Normosol-R are mildly alkalinizing (the buffer supplies bicarbonate) and may be beneficial in patients with metabolic acidosis, especially patients with severe diarrhea. The buffer sources in Normosol-R are acetate and gluconate. There has been a trend toward using gluconate and acetate because they do not require hepatic metabolism and they do not contribute to lactate levels. Administration of hypertonic solutions (e.g., 5% dextrose in lactated Ringer's solution) has been advocated because hypertonic fluids, by shifting water from the intracellular to the extracellular compartment, may expand the extravascular fluid compartment more than do isotonic fluids. Fluids without high sodium concentrations (e.g., 2.5% dextrose in water or 2.5% dextrose in 0.45% saline) should be avoided because of the failure to replenish the sodium deficit, which may decrease circulating fluid volume.

Adequacy of fluid replacement therapy can be easily and accurately evaluated by serial measurement of body weight relative to body weight on

---

BOX 6-3	**Fluid Calculations for Use With Acute Gastrointestinal Diseases**

REPLACEMENT OF LOSSES

Dehydration (%) × body weight (kg) × 10 = ml fluid to be administered over 18 to 24 hours

MAINTENANCE NEEDS

30 ml/lb/day

ONGOING LOSSES

Estimate continuing losses via vomiting and/or diarrhea (overestimate if in doubt) and replace every 8 hours

SAMPLE CALCULATION

25-kg dog, 5% dehydrated, losing 200 ml of stool every 8 hours

Replacement of losses: 1250 ml

Maintenance needs: 1500 ml

Ongoing losses: 600 ml

Total volume to be administered over 24 hours: 3350 ml, or 1117 ml every 8 hours entry. Body weight should increase over the first 24 hours by at least the calculated fluid deficit (dehydration); 500 ml of water weighs 1 lb. Fluid administration rate should be increased if body weight begins to drop and should be decreased if body weight increases excessively (more than 5% to 10% of calculated normal weight). Other parameters for assessing adequacy of fluid replacement therapy include serial measurement of hematocrit and plasma protein concentration, estimation of pulse pressure, capillary refill time, and mucous membrane texture.

Early potassium supplementation is critical for optimum management of dogs and cats with severe gastroenteritis and volume depletion, because depletion of body potassium stores develops rapidly. Routine potassium supplementation should begin before hypokalemia is detected because serum potassium content represents only a small fraction of total body potassium stores. Adverse consequences of hypokalemia are numerous and include decreased GI motility, decreased cardiac output, hypotension, skeletal muscle weakness, and general malaise and inappetence. Cats seem particularly likely to develop hypokalemia during periods of GI fluid loss and fluid replacement therapy, and they should be supplemented early and aggressively. Empirical supplementation of potassium is begun at 20 to 40 mEq/L of fluids administered; cats should receive at least 40 mEq/L. Daily measurement of serum potassium is recommended to facilitate maintenance of normal concentration. If at all possible, serum potassium concentration should be determined *before* initiating supplementation. For example, although patients with adrenocortical insufficiency and advanced oliguric renal failure often develop GI disease, they should *not* receive potassium because they are often hyperkalemic. These two important disorders may be detected, and inappropriate potassium supplementation avoided, by determination of serum electrolyte and urea nitrogen levels. A rapid and reasonably reliable screening test for identifying life-threatening hyperkalemia early is an electrocardiogram. Typical early electrocardiographic changes include tall, peaked T waves, loss of P waves, and wide QRS complexes.

Glucose administration is particularly beneficial in treating septic patients, especially dogs with parvoviral enteritis and severe diarrhea. Sepsis results in a number of disturbances in glucose metabolism that are often manifested clinically by development of hypoglycemia. Hypoglycemia also develops more readily in young patients because of their small hepatic glucose reserves. In these patients, glucose administration (typically as a 5% solution) may produce a dramatic response. The caloric content of a 5% dextrose solution is far less than the patient's requirements but nonetheless seems to be helpful in alleviating some of the adverse effects of sepsis. Glucose supplementation is begun either at the outset or early in the course of fluid therapy in patients with severe enteritis. It is recommended that glucose levels be evaluated every 8 to 12 hours during the period of intensive therapy. Blood glucose levels in normal patients on a 5% dextrose drip should range from approximately 130 to 180 mg/dl. A patient on a 5% dextrose infusion with a low-normal glucose level is probably significantly hypoglycemic and may be septic. Additional glucose (e.g., 7.5% infusion or intravenous bolus [0.5 ml of 25% dextrose per pound]) and other treatments for sepsis (see later section in this chapter on acute viral enteritis) may be indicated. Bicarbonate administration is rarely indicated and in most instances is contraindicated by the added risks of iatrogenic hypernatremia, hyperosmolality, and alkalosis. Metabolic acidosis usually corrects rapidly after volume deficit replacement.

Nonspecific Treatment of Diarrhea

Many episodes of acute diarrhea are of viral or bacterial origin, are self-limiting, and generally do not require specific therapy. Patients should not receive solid foods for at least 24 to 48 hours but should still be allowed access to liquids, because intestinal absorptive functions are usually intact. Electrolyte-containing solutions may be useful as sources for oral fluid replacement in patients without severe GI disease and large fluid losses. Suitable electrolyte replacement solutions include Enterolyte or Gatorade. Alternatively, a replacement solution can be formulated using guidelines developed by the World Health Organization: each liter of replacement solution should contain 120 mEq sodium, 25 mEq potassium, 48 mEq sodium bicarbonate, and 1.1 g glucose.

Antidiarrheal agents are occasionally indicated for the treatment of idiopathic, acute diarrhea of nonbacterial origin (fecal cytologic findings are noninflammatory; see earlier section on diagnostic considerations), especially diarrhea caused by dietary changes. Narcotics, generally considered the most effective antidiarrheal agents, act by increasing segmental contractions of the small and large intestine. Recommended narcotics for short-term treatment of acute diarrhea (Table 6-1) include paregoric, diphenoxylate (Lomotil), or loperamide (Imodium). Diphenoxylate is contraindicated in patients with severe underlying hepatic disease. Neither diphenoxylate nor loperamide should be used in patients with viral enteritis, because delayed intestinal motility may predispose to the development of sepsis. In addition, these agents have been shown to prolong illness in humans with salmonellosis, shigellosis, and campylobacteriosis by interfering with normal immune clearance mechanisms.

Salicylate-containing drugs, such as bismuth subsalicylate (Pepto-Bismol), may be beneficial for treatment of prostaglandin-mediated diarrhea. Intestinal adsorbents such as kaolin pectate are generally of limited usefulness and must be administered in high doses.

Antiemetic medication may be indicated for treatment of patients with persistent vomiting. However, these agents should not be administered to patients that are vomiting as a result of intestinal obstruction or before completing an adequate diagnostic work-up. Injectable drugs are usually needed, and their use is therefore restricted to in-hospital patients.

Chlorpromazine (Thorazine) is preferred as the initial agent because it has a wide safety margin and is a potent antiemetic, acting on the emetic center, chemoreceptor trigger zone, and peripheral chemoreceptors (see Table 6-1). In addition, chlorpromazine is thought to function as a calcium channel antagonist, thereby decreasing cyclic adenosine monophosphate concentration in intestinal epithelial cells. The result is decreased intestinal epithelial cell secretion, especially when excess secretion is mediated by enterotoxins. Chlorpromazine is also excellent for alleviating some of the discomfort caused by nausea. Chlorpromazine may precipitate hypotension in dehydrated patients and should therefore not be given before fluid replacement in volume-depleted patients.

Metoclopramide (Reglan) given subcutaneously or as a constant intravenous infusion (see Table 6-1) exerts antiemetic activity in the chemoreceptor trigger zone of the dog and increases gastric emptying in dogs and cats. Adverse effects from metoclopramide in dogs and cats are uncommon, consisting largely of excessive excitement. Severe,

TABLE 6-1	Drugs Commonly Used in the Management of Acute Gastrointestinal Diseases
Drug	**Regimen**
Amikacin	7-9 mg/lb IV one time a day
Ampicillin	7-9 mg/lb IV three to four times a day
Bismuth subsalicylate	0.5-1 mg/lb PO three to four times a day
Cefazolin	9-15 mg/lb IV three times a day
Cetoxitin	9-15 mg/lb IV three times a day
Chlorpromazine	0.1-0.3 mg/lb IM three to four times a day
Diphenoxylate*	0.028 mg/lb PO three times a day
Enrofloxacin†	1.1-3 mg/lb IV two times a day
Flunixin meglumine*	0.45 mg/lb IV once
Hetastarch	10-20 ml/lb IV over 24 hours
Imipenem‡	2.2-4.5 mg/lb IV three times a day
Loperamide*	0.04 mg/lb PO three times a day
Metoclopramide	Constant infusion; 0.02-0.04 mg/lb/hr IV
	0.1-0.3 mg/lb SQ three to four times a day
Metronidazole‡	5-7 mg/lb IV two to three times a day
Ondansetron	0.05-0.1 mg/lb slow IV two to three times a day
Paregoric*	1-2 ml PO four times a day or as needed
Plasma (immunotherapy)	0.45 ml/lb IV, SQ, IM
Plasma (oncotic pressure)	2.3-5 ml/lb IV

IV, Intravenously; *PO,* orally; *IM,* intramuscularly; *SQ,* subcutaneously.

*Dogs only.

†Extralabel use, give as slow bolus.

‡Administer over 20 to 30 minutes.

protracted vomiting that does not respond well to either chlorpromazine or metoclopramide should prompt consideration of possible intestinal obstruction or pancreatitis and additional diagnostic evaluation before continuing prolonged antiemetic therapy.

Ondansetron (Zofran) is a potent antiemetic drug that is frequently effective in reducing severe and frequent vomiting. It has been used in human cancer patients undergoing therapy with cisplatin, a drug that frequently causes nausea and severe vomiting. Ondansetron acts as a selective antagonist of serotonin $5HT_3$ receptors (a principal mediator of the emetic reflex). It is also effective in decreasing the frequency of vomiting in patients with severe parvoviral enteritis and should be used when chlorpromazine and metoclopramide do not provide adequate control. As the nausea and vomiting are controlled, a state of increased comfort seems to prevail. At this time the primary limitation for ondansetron is expense. It is strongly recommended, however, that all hospitals that treat dogs and cats stock at least one bottle of ondansetron so that it will be readily available for use in patients that have intractable vomiting.

MANAGEMENT OF SPECIFIC ACUTE SMALL INTESTINAL DISEASES

Acute Viral Enteritis

General Considerations. The viral causes of acute small intestinal disease in dogs include parvoviruses 1 and 2, canine distemper virus, coronavirus, astrovirus, and rotavirus (see Box 6-2). Disease due to coronavirus, astrovirus, and rotavirus infection is rare. The disease caused by parvovirus in dogs (destruction of intestinal crypt epithelium, lymphocyte depletion, neutropenia) is much more severe that that caused by coronavirus (destruction of tips of intestinal villi). The severity of disease associated with parvovirus infection of dogs is subjectively greater in some breeds, such as Doberman pinschers, rottweilers, and pit bull terriers. These breeds may have an inherited immunodeficiency, but this has not been proved conclusively to date. Coronavirus is generally associated with disease only in very young puppies.

In cats, panleukopenia virus and enteric coronavirus are the two most common viral causes of intestinal disease. However, the panleukopenia-like syndrome associated with feline leukemia virus (FeLV) and feline immunodeficiency virus (FIV) enteritis cause acute diarrhea in some cats. Feline panleukopenia is caused by a parvovirus closely related to canine parvovirus, and the intestinal lesions are similar. In contrast to dogs, many parvovirus-infected cats have vomiting without diarrhea.

Clinical outcome following exposure to parvoviruses depends largely on the degree of prior maternal immunity, virus strain, host immune responses, and infecting dose of virus. Onset of signs is usually within 3 to 5 days of exposure. Small intestinal disease results from intestinal mucosal injury that induces a combination of secretory and malabsorptive diarrhea. Sepsis occurs commonly in both dogs and cats with parvoviral enteritis as a result of absorption of preformed bacterial toxins, as well as intact bacteria, across the damaged intestinal epithelium. Bacteremia is more likely to occur in severely leukopenic patients.

Diagnosis. Acute onset of vomiting, fever, diarrhea (often bloody), and leukopenia (variable finding) in a previously unvaccinated dog is consistent with parvovirus infection. Parvovirus antigen can be detected in feces by enzyme-linked immunosorbent assay (ELISA),[*] but results can be falsely negative based on timing of the infection or can be falsely positive due to modified live vaccine administration. Coronavirus usually induces milder disease, and leukopenia, if present, is generally less severe than in parvovirus infection. Diagnosis of viral enteritis from organisms other than parvovirus can be confirmed by fecal electron microscopy.

Feline panleukopenia is tentatively diagnosed in a young, previously unvaccinated cat with initial acute onset of vomiting and fever that progresses to bloody diarrhea and leukopenia (especially neutropenia) within 24 to 48 hours. Diagnosis is confirmed by fecal electron microscopy or paired serology. *A primary differential diagnosis for dogs and cats exhibiting findings consistent with parvoviral infection is salmonellosis.*

Treatment. Fluid losses, potassium deficits, and hypoglycemia should be corrected as described. In patients with signs of advanced sepsis, short-term administration of a glucose-insulin-potassium mixture (3 g glucose/1 unit regular insulin/0.5 mEq

---

[*]Synbiotics and IDEXX.

potassium chloride/kg, to be infused over 4 to 5 hours) may be warranted. If possible, once-daily measurement of serum electrolyte concentrations and blood glucose monitoring at least twice daily are recommended while the patient remains critically ill. Both food and water are withheld for at least the first 48 to 72 hours of treatment and are usually not reinstituted until vomiting and diarrhea have subsided. Small amounts of water (or water plus electrolytes) are offered first over a 24-hour period and, if well tolerated, are followed by small meals of solid, easily digestible, bland food over the next several days.

Broad-spectrum antibiotics are indicated for treatment of dogs and cats with severe gastroenteritis (especially those with hemorrhagic diarrhea), particularly if clinical findings consistent with sepsis are detected. However, routine use of antimicrobial therapy in all patients with acute viral enteritis is not indicated, because many with milder disease can be effectively managed without antibiotics, thus avoiding the unnecessary expense and risk their use entails. Studies have shown that bacteremia is most likely to occur in patients with enteritis and concurrent severe leukopenia, and it is these patients that are most likely to benefit from antimicrobial therapy. Bacteremia occurs uncommonly in patients with acute enteritis and normal white blood cell counts.

The GI tract has a rich normal flora, and so broad-spectrum coverage is necessary to cover for both aerobic bacteria (especially *E. coli*) and facultative anaerobic bacteria (especially *Bacteroides* and *Clostridium*). Adequate coverage for both types of bacteria can usually be attained by administration of a penicillin or first-generation cephalosporin parenterally. Addition of an aminoglycoside or quinolone is indicated for treatment of severely septic patients. Maintenance of normal blood volume is essential when using aminoglycoside antibiotics, and patients should be monitored carefully by means of a daily urinalysis for signs of possible aminoglycoside-induced nephrotoxicity. Once-daily aminoglycoside protocols should be used, and this drug class should not be administered until hypovolemia and hypokalemia have been resolved. Development of proteinuria or urine casts is often the first warning of renal injury; aminoglycoside treatment should be discontinued at this point. Cefoxitin, a second-generation cephalosporin, provides single-agent broad-spectrum coverage for patients with severe sepsis and avoids the potential toxicity of aminoglycocides. In general, antibiotic

treatment is administered for short periods of time (usually until the white blood cell count returns to normal); follow-up treatment with orally administered antibiotics is not indicated. Leukocyte rebound is a favorable sign and usually indicates that the patient will recover.

Flunixin meglumine (Banamine) has been shown experimentally to increase survival of dogs after endotoxin administration and has been recommended for treatment of dogs with sepsis due to parvoviral enteritis. Because of potential for gastric injury, only a single dose for emergency management of sepsis in dogs should be used.

In some parvovirus patients with severe leukopenia, recombinant granulocyte colony-stimulating factor (Neupogen) has been shown to be effective in increasing white blood cell counts. However, use of these products has not correlated to increased survival or decreased morbidity. Thus granulocyte colony-stimulating factor may not be indicated for treatment of parvoviral enteritis.

Passive immunotherapy with serum or plasma from hyperimmune dogs or cats may lessen the morbidity of acute viral enteritis, especially parvovirus. Administration of antiparvovirus antibody in this fashion may lessen viremia. Use of fresh plasma has the added advantage of potentiating opsonization of bacteria by fibronectin. On day 1 of hospitalization, 0.5 ml/lb of hyperimmune serum or plasma should be given intravenously, subcutaneously, or intramuscularly. Vaccinated blood donor animals or survivors of parvovirus infection are excellent donors. Red blood cells should not be administered unless needed.

Hypoproteinemia often develops rapidly in patients with severe diarrhea and serious small intestinal injury. As a consequence, plasma oncotic pressure drops and fluid losses via the bowel are accelerated. Plasma or hetastarch should be used to help restore normal oncotic pressure (see Table 6-1). Plasma has the advantage of supplying passive immunotherapy. Sufficient plasma is administered to increase total protein concentration to at least the low-normal range. An in-line filter is used to remove particulate material during plasma infusion.

Sequelae. Intestinal intussusception is the most serious sequela that may develop during treatment for viral gastroenteritis. Altered intestinal motility is implicated. Careful abdominal palpation for the presence of an abdominal mass should be performed daily. Persistent vomiting after apparent clinical recovery should prompt a careful search for intussusception. Abdominal radiographs, ultrasound, or contrast studies may be necessary to diagnose intussusception. Other potential complications include bacterial embolization and metastatic abscessation (joints, subcutis, kidney) and intravenous catheter infection. Catheters should be maintained in a sterile manner under a bandage that completely covers the catheter, and catheters should be rotated to a different vein every 72 hours (up to 5 days for jugular catheters).

Gastrointestinal Parasitism

General Considerations. Parasitism is common in dogs and cats, and, depending on the parasite, can occur regardless of age, breed, or sex. Although outdoor animals are more likely to be parasitized than indoor animals, indoor animals can be exposed to some parasites from transmission by transport hosts such as rodents, flies, and cockroaches. Predominant clinical signs of disease vary by the parasite (see Box 6-2), but most can induce vomiting and diarrhea.

The most common helminth parasites causing GI tract disease in dogs and cats are listed in Box 6-2. *Toxocara* spp., *Toxascaris leonina, Ollulanus tricuspis,* and *Physaloptera* are generally found in the upper GI tract and are commonly associated with vomiting. The hookworms *Ancylostoma* spp. and *Uncinaria stenocephala* are found in the intestines and cause diarrhea and significant blood loss, particularly in small dogs or cats. *Trichuris* spp. live in the large intestine and cecum and can result in large bowel diarrhea. *Dipylidium caninum, Taenia* spp., and *Echinococcus* spp. are the most common cestodes that infect small animals. Dogs and cats are infected with *D. caninum* after ingesting infected fleas and with *Taenia* spp. and *Echinococcus* spp. by carnivorism. Clinical signs are minimal but may include failure to thrive.

The most common protozoal agents potentially causing GI tract disease in dogs and cats are *Giardia* spp., *Cryptosporidium* spp., *Isospora* spp., and *Pentatrichomonas* (see Box 6-2). Giardiasis and cryptosporidiosis most commonly induce small bowel diarrhea; *Isospora* spp. and *P. hominis* are most commonly associated with mixed or large bowel diarrhea. *Isospora* spp. infection usually causes disease only in puppies and kittens. Only cats complete the coccidian life cycle of *T. gondii;* oocysts in dog feces are from the ingestion of cat feces. This parasite rarely induces diarrhea and is only associated

with the short-term oocyst shedding period (generally less than 14 days).

Diagnosis. All dogs and cats with acute vomiting or diarrhea should be evaluated for parasites (see diagnosis section). Diagnosis of helminth infections is based on demonstration of ova after fecal flotation. Ova detection can be used to document cestode infection, but proglottid detection occurs most commonly (*D. caninum* and *Taenia* spp.). Trophozoites of protozoans are best demonstrated by wet mounts performed on fresh feces. For parasites that are commonly occult, such as *Trichuris vulpis, Giardia,* and *Cryptosporidium* spp., performance of multiple fecal evaluations improves sensitivity. *Physaloptera* and *Ollulanus* rarely shed eggs in feces and frequently are diagnosed only by endoscopy or therapeutic trials. *Giardia* can be found in duodenal aspirates of dogs but lives in the distal small intestine of cats. Antigen ELISA is being assessed as a diagnostic aid for giardiasis and cryptosporidiosis (see diagnosis section).

Treatment. There are multiple antiparasite drugs that can be effective (Table 6-2). Anthelmintics such as pyrantel pamoate should be routinely administered to all puppies and kittens on initial examination and again 2 to 3 weeks later because of zoonotic health risks. In heartworm endemic areas, use of preventatives that also control helminths is indicated. Because *T. vulpis* infection is commonly occult, all dogs with large bowel diarrhea with no obvious cause should be given fenbendazole or other anthelmintic with activity against *T. vulpis.* Praziquantel is one drug with activity against the three major canine tapeworms. Fenbendazole can be effective for the treatment of *Taenia* spp. infection. *Entamoeba, Giardia, Balantidium,* and *Pentatrichomonas* generally respond clinically to metronidazole, but *Pentatrichomonas* and *Giardia* may not be cleared from the GI tract. Fenbendazole, albendazole, paromomycin, and febantel-pyrantel-praziquantel (dogs) are alternate anti-*Giardia* drugs. If *Giardia* infection alone is suspected, fenbendazole is superior to metronidazole. Albendazole has been associated with neutropenia in dogs and cats, and so fenbendazole appears to be safer. Addition of insoluble fiber to the diet may aid in the control of giardiasis. Sequential administration of clindamycin followed by tylosin blocked oocyst shedding and resolved diarrhea in one cat with chronic, clinical cryptosporidiosis. Tylosin alone was apparently successful in blocking

TABLE 6-2   Drugs Commonly Used in the Management of Parasitic Diseases Associated With Acute Gastrointestinal Disease

Organism/Generic Drug Name	Common Canine Dosage	Common Feline Dosage
Balantidium coli		
Metronidazole	4.5-11 mg/lb PO q12h for 8 days	NA
Tetracycline	11 mg/lb PO q8h for 7-10 days	NA
Cryptosporidium parvum		
Azithromycin	2.5-5 mg/lb PO q12h for 5-7 days	3-7 mg/lb PO q12h for 5-7 days
Paromomycin	75 mg/lb PO q12h for 5 days	75 mg/lb PO q12h for 5 days
Tylosin	4.5 mg/lb PO q8-12h for 21 days	4.5 mg/lb PO q8-12h for 21 days (administer in capsules for cats)
Isospora spp.		
Trimethoprim-sulfonamide	6-13 mg/lb PO q12h for 5 days	6 mg/lb PO q12h for 5 days
Sulfadimethoxine	22-25 mg/lb PO daily for 5-20 days	22-25 mg/lb PO daily for 5-20 days
Furazolidone	3-9 mg/lb PO q12-24h for 5 days	3-9 mg/lb PO q12-24h for 5 days
Amprolium	300-400 mg PO daily for 5 days	60-100 mg daily for 5 days
Paromomycin	75 mg/lb PO q12h for 5 days	75 mg/lb PO q12h for 5 days
Giardia		
Metronidazole	4.5-11 mg/lb PO q12h for 8 days	4.5-11 mg/lb PO q12h for 8 days
Fenbendazole	22 mg/lb PO q24h for 3-7 days	22 mg/lb PO q24h for 3-7 days
Furazolidone	1.8 mg/lb PO q12h for 7 days	1.8 mg/lb PO q12h for 7 days
Paromomycin	75 mg/lb PO q12h for 5 days	75 mg/lb PO q12h for 5 days
Praziquantel, pyrantel, and febantel	PO daily for 3 days	NA
Pentatrichomonas hominis		
Metronidazole	4.5-11 mg/lb PO q12h for 8 days	4.5-11 mg/lb PO q12h for 8 days
Paromomycin	75 mg/lb PO q12h for 5 days	75 mg/lb PO q12h for 5 days
Toxoplasma gondii		
Azithromycin	2.5-5 mg/lb PO q12h for 5-7 days	3-7 mg/lb PO q12h for 5-7 days
Clindamycin hydrochloride	5.5 mg/lb PO, IM q12h for 28 days	5.5 mg/lb PO, IM q12h for 28 days
Clarithromycin	2.5-5 mg/lb PO q12h for 7 days	2.5-5 mg/lb PO q12h for 7 days
Pyrimethamine	0.1-0.25 mg/lb PO q24h for 28 days	Usually not used due to toxicity
Trimethoprim-sulfonamide	6.5 mg/lb PO q12h for 28 days	6.5 mg/lb PO q12h for 28 days
Doxycycline	2.5-5 mg/lb PO q12h for 4 weeks	2.5-5 mg/lb q12h PO for 4 weeks (caution regarding potential for esophageal stricture formation in cats, see Chapter 4)
Ascarids		
Dichlorvos	5 mg/lb PO once	5 mg/lb PO once
Febantel	5 mg/lb PO q24h for 3 days	5 mg/lb PO q24h for 3 days
Pyrantel pamoate	2.2 mg/lb PO once	2-7 mg/lb PO once
Fenbendazole	25 mg/lb PO once	NA
Hookworms		
Dichlorvos	5 mg/lb PO once	5 mg/lb PO once
Febantel	5 mg/lb PO q24h for 3 days	5 mg/lb PO q24h for 3 days
Pyrantel pamoate	2.2 mg/lb PO once	2-7 mg/lb PO once
Fenbendazole	25 mg/lb PO once	NA
Dipylidium caninum		
Epsiprantel	2.5 mg/lb PO, repeat in 3 weeks	1.25 mg/lb PO, repeat in 3 weeks
Praziquantel	2-6 mg/lb PO, SQ, repeat in 3 weeks	2-6 mg/lb PO, SQ, repeat in 3 weeks
Taenia pisiformis		
Epsiprantel	2.5 mg/lb PO, repeat in 3 weeks	1.25 mg/lb PO, repeat in 3 weeks
Praziquantel	2-6 mg/lb PO, SQ, repeat in 3 weeks	2-6 mg/lb PO, SQ, repeat in 3 weeks
Echinococcus		
Epsiprantel	2.5 mg/lb PO, repeat in 3 weeks	1.25 mg/lb PO, repeat in 3 weeks
Praziquantel	2-6 mg/lb PO, SQ, repeat in 3 weeks	2-6 mg/lb PO, SQ, repeat in 3 weeks

PO, Orally; *NA,* not applicable; *IM,* intramuscularly; *SQ,* subcutaneously.

oocyst shedding in 12 other dogs or cats with diarrhea. Paromomycin,* an orally administered aminoglycoside, has effect against *Pentatrichomonas, Cryptosporidium,* and *Giardia* but has been associated with acute renal failure in cats with hemorrhagic diarrhea. The *T. gondii* oocyst shedding period in cats can be shortened by administration of clindamycin. Clinical signs from *Isospora* spp. generally respond to the administration of sulfadimethoxine; alternatives include other sulfas, clindamycin, and paromomycin. Drugs used to treat *Isospora* spp. are static, and so cysts may still be seen after treatment.

Sequelae. Severe blood loss anemia may occur from hookworm infestation. Some intestinal parasites such as *Giardia* or *Cryptosporidium* may be difficult to clear. In addition, chronic vomiting or diarrhea from secondary inflammatory cell infiltrates into the GI tract may occur (see other sections). Some parasitic infections are zoonotic. Visceral larva migrans can occur in humans following infection by *Toxocara* spp. eggs. Following human ingestion of infectious eggs, larvae penetrate the intestinal wall and migrate through the tissues, leading to eosinophilic granulomatous reactions involving the skin, lungs, central nervous system, and eyes. Ocular larva migrans most commonly involves the retina and can cause reduced vision, strabismus, uveitis, and endophthalmitis. Cutaneous larva migrans in humans can be induced with infection by all three species of hookworms infecting dogs and cats in the United States. Larvae are released from eggs passed into the environment in feces; infectious larvae infect humans by skin penetration. Larval migration results in the development of an erythematous, pruritic cutaneous tunnel. Occasionally larvae will reach the lungs and cornea. *Ancylostoma caninum* also causes eosinophilic enteritis in humans. Transmission of small animal cestodes to humans occurs following ingestion of the intermediate host (flea, *Dipylidium*) or by the ingestion of eggs *(Echinococcus)*. *Dipylidium* infection is most common in children and can lead to diarrhea and pruritus ani. Following human ingestion of eggs, *Echinococcus* enters the portal circulation and spreads throughout the liver and other tissues, causing hydatid disease. Prevention and/or control is primarily by use of taeniacides and sanitation procedures. To lessen human risks, dogs and cats should not be allowed to hunt and flea control

should be maintained. *Giardia, Cryptosporidium, Entamoeba, Balantidium,* and *Pentatrichomonas* should be considered potentially zoonotic. Not all *Giardia* or *C. parvum* isolates cross-infect other species, but this cannot be determined by microscopic examination. Cats have not been shown to be infected by *Balantidium* and are unlikely to give *Entamoeba* to people because it is rare in cats and cats are unlikely to form cysts.

Acute Bacterial Gastroenteritis
General Considerations. The most commonly recognized primary bacterial pathogens of the GI tract of dogs and cats include *Salmonella* spp., *C. jejuni, C. perfringens, Helicobacter* spp., and enterotoxigenic *E. coli.* Each agent can cause vomiting; all but *Helicobacter* spp. are commonly associated with the clinical signs of large, small, or mixed bowel diarrhea. *C. perfringens*–associated disease appears to be less common in cats than in dogs. Each of the bacterial infections can be associated with contaminated environments, direct contact with infected animals, or potentially ingestion of infected prey species. Salmonellosis and campylobacteriosis are commonly associated with ingestion of undercooked poultry products. It is also possible that each of the organisms could be carried by healthy animals only to overgrow and induce disease because of other stimuli such as stress, diet change, or antimicrobial therapy. Salmonellosis is commonly associated with polysystemic clinical signs such as fever, as well as neutropenia, in the sepsis stage of infection. Approximately 50% of the cats with salmonellosis are seen for evaluation of fever without GI tract disease signs; the owner may report a recent history of songbird ingestion. Campylobacteriosis is most common in puppies and kittens, and the organism is less likely to cause polysystemic signs than salmonellosis. Small animals can also be infected by other potential bacterial pathogens such as *Shigella* and *Yersinia enterocolitica* but seem to be relatively resistant to disease induced by these organisms.

Diagnosis. Helicobacteriosis is diagnosed clinically by the combination of demonstration of spirochetes by cytologic or histologic studies, positive urease test results, presence of inflammation, exclusion of other causes of inflammation, and response to treatment (see Chapter 5). Presence of large numbers of neutrophils on rectal cytologic

---

*Parke-Davis, Morris Plains, N.J.

examination suggests but does not prove bacterial disease induced by *Campylobacter* spp., *Salmonella* spp., or *C. perfringens* enterotoxin production but is a relative indication for fecal culture (see diagnosis section). *C. perfringens* are large rod-form bacteria; pathogenic strains generally have an unstained spore. A positive *C. perfringens* culture or presence of large, spore-forming rods does not prove enterotoxin production; enterotoxin measurement in feces is available at most large commercial laboratories. Because *C. perfringens* enterotoxin can be detected in healthy patients, as well as those that are clinically ill, positive results cannot be used to definitely confirm a disease association. *Campylobacter* spp. are spirochetes but are small and so difficult to identify cytologically; definitive diagnosis is based on culture.

Treatment. Supportive care and nonspecific therapy as discussed for acute viral diseases should be given as indicated. Holding the patient off food for 24 hours may speed resolution of clinical disease. *C. perfringens* generally responds to treatment with ampicillin, amoxicillin, tylosin, or metronidazole. The drug of choice for campylobacteriosis is erythromycin; alternative drugs are tetracyclines, chloramphenicol, and potentially tylosin. Salmonellosis should be treated only parenterally because of rapid resistance that occurs following oral administration of antibiotics. Appropriate antibiotics for the treatment of salmonellosis include chloramphenicol, trimethoprimsulfonamide, and amoxicillin; quinolones are effective but should be reserved for resistant infections. *Helicobacter* spp. infection is usually treated with the combination of metronidazole and tetracycline or amoxicillin and metronidazole with acid reduction therapy (e.g., omeprazole, famotidine). Clarithromycin can be effective and can be used once daily in cats.

Sequelae. Chronic gastritis is associated with *Helicobacter* spp. infection in some cases. It is possible that some chronic diarrheas are associated with bacterial infections. There *appears* to be minimal zoonotic risk associated with *Helicobacter* infections of small animals. However, dogs and cats infected with *Salmonella* and *Campylobacter* will shed the organisms into the human environment for a period of time after acute infection. Thus feces of these patients should be handled carefully.

Acute Hemorrhagic Gastroenteritis

General Considerations. Hemorrhagic gastroenteritis (HGE) is a disease of unknown cause that occurs most often in small-breed dogs. The pathophysiology of the disease most closely resembles that of acute hemorrhagic enteritis of humans induced by certain enterotoxigenic strains of *E. coli*. Anaphylactic reaction to as yet undetermined toxins also has been implicated. The clinical course of the disease is frequently peracute, progressing rapidly to death if not treated aggressively and promptly. Early signs are vomiting and depression, progressing to hematemesis and copious, malodorous, bloody diarrhea, often of currant-jelly consistency. Recovery after treatment is usually equally rapid.

Diagnosis. Diagnosis is based on the presence of significant hemoconcentration (packed cell volume may approach 70% to 80%), with little to no increase in total protein concentration, in a small dog with typical clinical signs. Hypovolemia is thought to account for the increase in hematocrit, whereas gut losses of serum proteins serve to prevent a corresponding increase in serum total protein concentration.

Treatment. Early, aggressive replacement of fluid volume deficits is critical to successful management of dogs with HGE. Either normal saline or lactated Ringer's solution (9 to 18 ml/lb) is infused rapidly intravenously over 1 to 2 hours, followed by slower infusion of a sufficient volume of fluids to correct dehydration, replace ongoing losses, and provide for maintenance needs (see previous discussion of fluid therapy) over the next 24 hours. Electrolyte concentration and body weight should be monitored closely during treatment. To date, evidence has not been presented to indicate that administration of antibiotics is beneficial, although patients with evidence of severe leukopenia or presence of a left shift on complete blood count should probably receive antibiotic treatment. Antiemetic drugs may be warranted if vomiting is severe or prolonged.

Sequelae. Coagulation abnormalities, especially thrombocytopenia, may develop but are usually reversed once fluid deficits are corrected. Recovery typically occurs rapidly over 24 to 48 hours, and residual effects from HGE are rare.

Acute Gastrointestinal Disease Resulting From Ingestion of Garbage and Intoxicants

General Considerations. Development of acute GI disease after ingestion of garbage or decayed organic matter occurs commonly in dogs. In most instances illness is manifested by acute onset of vomiting, often accompanied by profuse, watery diarrhea. Animals are rarely febrile, and significant leukogram abnormalities are uncommon. Illness is thought to result either from osmotic overload with nondigestible substances or from ingestion of preformed bacterial toxins. There are multiple drugs associated with vomiting.

Diagnosis. Occasionally the toxicant ingested is known, especially if iatrogenic. Definitive diagnosis of food poisoning requires laboratory identification of the offending enterotoxin. Because this is rarely performed, most cases are presumptively diagnosed by history and physical examination findings and treated nonspecifically.

Treatment. Supportive care designed primarily to prevent dehydration is generally the mainstay of treatment for acute garbage enteritis in dogs. Food and water are withheld for 12 hours, and then only water (or water plus electrolytes) is given for the next 12 to 24 hours, depending on the course of the disease. If vomiting and/or diarrhea persist for longer than 24 hours, more serious GI disease is likely. Antidiarrheal drugs should be administered cautiously if the source of intoxication is unknown, because they may potentially worsen, by slowing elimination, disease caused by bacterial enterotoxins. Antiemetic drugs can be given by injection to control severe vomiting, provided clinical evidence of dehydration or hypovolemia is not present. Intestinal protectants (kaolin, activated charcoal) are likely to be of little benefit.

Sequelae. For most cases, clinical signs resolve quickly, without sequelae. Some intoxicants cause severe gastric ulcers (glucocorticoids, aspirin) or disease of other organ systems such as the kidneys or liver (nonsteroidal antiinflammatory agents).

Acute Small Intestinal Obstruction

General Considerations. Causes of acute mechanical small bowel obstruction in dogs and cats include bowel impaction by foreign bodies, bowel-constricting lesions (volvulus, hernias), and lesions that compress the bowel lumen (tumors). Signs are variable, depending on the location of the obstruction: proximal obstruction is more likely to cause vomiting, whereas more distal obstruction is most likely to cause diarrhea or constipation. Intussusception should be considered in any young dog with acute onset of bloody diarrhea and a firm, tubular abdominal mass. Mechanical small intestinal obstruction has several important consequences. Experimentally, 6 to 12 hours of small bowel obstruction in dogs results in distention and decreased absorption from the bowel proximal to the lesion. If obstruction persists, net secretion of sodium and water quickly ensues. These changes are thought to occur as a consequence of increased intraluminal pressure, increased portal venous and lymphatic pressures, and liberation of toxins by bacteria that rapidly proliferate in the obstructed bowel. Bacteria figure prominently in the pathogenesis of changes occurring in bowel obstruction, because mortality is greatly reduced and survival prolonged in newborn or gnotobiotic dogs with experimental intestinal obstruction. If obstruction persists, blood supply to the obstructed bowel is compromised and edema, hemorrhage, and eventually necrosis of the bowel wall develop. Intestinal mucosal permeability increases, allowing plasma proteins to leak into the bowel lumen and at the same time promoting uptake of bacteria and bacterial toxins into the portal circulation. Bacterial peritonitis frequently accompanies untreated, complicated small bowel obstruction.

Metabolic complications of prolonged small bowel obstruction include hypovolemia, hyponatremia, and hypochloridemia. Significant hypovolemia may develop rapidly in distal small bowel obstruction, because fluid is sequestered within the bowel lumen. Within 24 hours of obstruction, 50% or more of total plasma volume may be lost; additional fluid also may accumulate within the peritoneal cavity. These losses may be sufficient to precipitate hypovolemic shock. Because fluid losses are isotonic, plasma electrolyte concentrations may initially be normal. Hyponatremia may, however, become apparent when a patient drinks water in an attempt to replace volume losses. Chloride loss occurs through vomiting, although vomiting occurs in only approximately 10% of dogs with complete proximal small bowel obstruction. Mild metabolic acidosis may develop as a result of bicarbonate loss (vomiting) and renal functional impairment (hypovolemia). Outcome after correction of bowel obstruction depends largely on whether complications occur (sepsis, peritonitis, bowel perforation, and acute renal failure).

Diagnosis. Abdominal palpation and radiographic evaluation are the two primary methods of diagnosis of obstruction. Survey abdominal radiographs are obtained first, and if evidence of obstruction is observed (see Chapter 2), contrast material (e.g., liquid barium or barium-impregnated polyethylene spheres [BIPS]) may be administered to enhance visualization of possible obstructive lesions and to evaluate intestinal motility. Abdominocentesis and cytologic evaluation of any fluid obtained also may be helpful in determining whether bowel leakage and subsequent peritonitis have occurred.

Treatment. *If acute small intestinal obstruction is diagnosed, immediate surgery is nearly always indicated,* because delay in surgical correction of an obstructing lesion may lead to further ischemic injury and possible intestinal necrosis and perforation. Thorough abdominal exploration is done at the time of surgery, even if an obvious lesion is initially identified. If a lesion cannot be identified grossly, intestinal biopsy (at least jejunum and ileum) is warranted, because certain intestinal infectious or inflammatory diseases may induce signs that mimic intestinal obstruction. If bowel perforation with severe peritonitis has developed, delayed body wall closure with sterile open packing of the abdomen may be used to facilitate drainage. The abdomen is closed after several cycles of abdominal lavage and when the infection appears to be under control (usually 1 to 2 days). If there is any question as to bowel viability at the time of initial exploratory laparotomy, a second laparotomy 24 hours later may be indicated to better assess intestinal viability. Serosal patching of bowel segments (especially colon) that

have perforated or that have undergone ischemic injury may be helpful in enhancing intestinal healing and guarding against bowel leakage.

Sequelae. Complications after intestinal surgery, although generally uncommon, include peritonitis, stricture formation, abscessation, formation of adhesions, and malabsorption syndromes following resection of large segments of small bowel.

REFERENCES

Bornay-Llinares FJ et al.: Identification of *Cryptosporidium felis* in a cow by morphologic and molecular methods, *Appl Environ Microbiol* 65:1455, 1999.

Cubeddu LX et al.: Efficacy of ondansetron and the role of serotonin in cisplatin-induced nausea and vomiting, *N Engl J Med* 322:810, 1990.

Hill S et al.: Prevalence of enteric zoonoses in cats, *J Am Vet Med Assoc* 216:687, 2000.

Lappin MR, Calpin JP: Laboratory diagnosis of protozoal infections. In Greene CE, ed: *Infectious diseases of the dog and cat,* ed 2, Philadelphia, 1998, WB Saunders.

Marks SL et al.: Evaluation of methods to diagnose *Clostridium perfringens*–associated diarrhea in dogs, *J Am Vet Med Assoc* 214(3):357, 1999.

Macintire DK et al.: Treatment of dogs naturally infected with canine parvovirus with lyophilized canine IgG. ACVIM Proceedings, June 10, 1999, Chicago.

Obradovich JE et al.: Evaluation of recombinant canine granulocyte colony-stimulating factor as an inducer of granulopoeisis, *J Vet Intern Med* 5:75, 1991.

Pieniazek NJ et al.: New *Cryptosporidium* genotypes in HIV-infected persons, *Emerg Infect Dis* 5:444, 1999.

Rewerts JM et al.: Recombinant human granulocyte colony-stimulating factor for treatment of puppies with neutropenia secondary to canine parvovirus infection [see comments], *J Am Vet Med Assoc* 213:991, 1998.

Sargent KD et al.: Morphological and genetic characterisation of *Cryptosporidium* oocysts from domestic cats, *Vet Parasitol* 77:221, 1998.

Triolo AJ: Clinical use of hypertonic saline. ACVIM Proceedings, June 10, 1999, Chicago.

CHRONIC DISEASES OF THE SMALL INTESTINE

Todd R. Tams

Chronic disorders of the small intestine in dogs and cats are frequently encountered in clinical practice. A majority of these disorders can be successfully managed. It is urged, however, that clinicians pursue *early* meaningful diagnostic evaluation on patients that have chronic symptoms (lasting more than 2 to 4 weeks) because some disorders, if not treated appropriately, can result in severe malabsorptive disease and death. In the interim some patients with chronic disorders are lethargic, inappetent, and sometimes uncomfortable (e.g., intestinal cramping and pain may be present). Owner frustration also escalates when symptoms persist with little or no improvement. Early diagnostic evaluation and correct therapeutic intervention alleviate many problems.

In the dog and cat the primary function of the small intestine is to assimilate nutrients by the processes of digestion and absorption. Important motility functions include rhythmic segmentation to slow the passage of contents through the tube and peristalsis to move contents continuously in an aboral direction. The movement of contents through the small intestine is the net effect of these two important types of motility. Intestinal disease usually disrupts normal function of the small intestine and results in vomiting and/or diarrhea, and weight loss.

CLINICAL SIGNS OF SMALL INTESTINAL DISEASE

The most common clinical signs associated with chronic small intestinal disease are diarrhea and weight loss. Vomiting is common in inflammatory disorders, and intermittent inappetence, listlessness, borborygmus, flatulence, trembling, and signs of abdominal pain are also important symptoms. Signs of abdominal pain may be subtle and not obvious to the owner. In association with marked hypoproteinemia resulting from infiltrative intestinal diseases (protein-losing enteropathy), signs may include pitting subcutaneous edema, ascites, or dyspnea associated with hydrothorax.

Colonic disorders are a common cause of diarrhea. Diarrhea of large intestinal origin should be differentiated clinically from small intestinal causes

211

because work-up and treatment often differ (see Chapter 8).

CLASSIFICATION

Malabsorption syndrome includes chronic enteropathies that cause a generalized failure of digestion and absorption, resulting in diarrhea and weight loss. Some common causes include diffuse chronic inflammatory bowel disease (IBD) (lymphocytic-plasmacytic enteritis, eosinophilic enteritis, granulomatous enteritis), lymphangiectasia, lymphosarcoma, idiopathic villous atrophy, and histoplasmosis. Malabsorption may occur secondary to bacterial overgrowth, parasitic infections such as giardiasis, and massive bowel resection.

Protein-losing enteropathy refers to a group of disorders characterized by excessive loss of serum proteins into the intestinal tract. Blood chemistry profiles reveal proportionately equal depressions of albumin and globulin concentrations, often with a total protein of less than 5.5 g/dl. Hypoproteinemia results from either decreased production or increased loss of protein. Hypoproteinemia due to chronic liver disease is characterized by primary hypoalbuminemia, resulting from decreased production of albumin. In protein-losing nephropathies there is a primary hypoalbuminemia, due to increased loss of albumin. Macroglobulins are generally not lost until disease is severe and glomerular membranes become porous. In contrast, protein loss from the GI tract generally involves loss of all fractions at an equal rate, regardless of molecular size.

The most common causes of protein-losing enteropathy (PLE) in the dog include moderate to severe lymphocytic-plasmacytic enteritis, lymphangiectasia, diffuse intestinal lymphosarcoma, and histoplasmosis. Pythiosis causes severe intestinal inflammation and protein loss and is generally seen in dogs living in the Gulf Coast states, although it has been recognized in other southern states as well (see later discussion on pythiosis). Chronic parasitism, including giardiasis, can also result in intestinal protein loss. Subnormal protein levels in cats due to GI disease are not commonly recognized. Among this group, lymphosarcoma and severe IBD are the most common causes.

This chapter presents diagnostic and detailed treatment information for some of the most important and challenging chronic small intestinal disorders seen in clinical practice. These include chronic giardiasis, IBD, intestinal bacterial overgrowth, lymphangiectasia, pythiosis, short bowel syndrome, and intestinal neoplasia. The diagnostic approach to the problem of chronic diarrhea was reviewed in Chapter 1. The diagnosis and treatment of each individual disorder are presented here.

CHRONIC GIARDIASIS

Giardia as a cause of acute diarrhea was discussed in Chapter 6. Diarrhea is the most common clinical sign in symptomatic dogs and cats. Until a diagnosis is made and adequate therapy instituted, *Giardia* may cause intermittent or chronic ongoing diarrhea. In some practice areas *Giardia* is the most common parasitic cause of diarrhea. Other signs may include weight loss and unthriftiness. Occasionally vomiting may be the predominant sign.

Giardia has proven to be a difficult problem both to diagnose definitively and to treat successfully. For example, despite adequate treatment regimens using both metronidazole (Flagyl) and quinacrine (Atabrine) in the past, some dogs in our practice remained infected and symptomatic. It should be recognized that there may be one or several concurrent intestinal disorders (e.g., intestinal bacterial overgrowth, IBD) that complicate resolution of clinical signs. In some cases, even though *Giardia* is present, it may not be a significant pathogen. Some other process then may be responsible for the clinical abnormalities.

Individual host immunity factors also play an important role in infection control. Deficiency of secretory IgA has been shown to be a factor in persistent *Giardia* infection in humans, and the same may be true for animals. A competent cell-mediated immune system is required to resist infection. Also, immunosuppressive doses of corticosteroids can cause recrudescence of *Giardia* infections in dogs and other species. Noting the prevalence of IBD in dogs and cats and the frequent use of corticosteroids to treat the syndrome, every effort should be made to identify the presence of *Giardia* and to ensure that adequate treatment be administered in patients that are also being treated for IBD (either empirically or because a definitive diagnosis has been made).

In dogs, diarrhea may begin as early as 5 days after exposure to infection. The life cycle of *Giardia* is direct, and the prepatent period lasts between 1 and 2 weeks. *Giardia* occurs in both trophozoite and cyst forms. Trophozoites attach to the brush border of the villous epithelium of the small intestine. The cyst form is infective. Trophozoites may also be passed, especially with diarrheic stools, but they are incapable of causing infection and soon die.

Diagnosis

As described in Chapter 6, standard diagnostic tests used in any practice setting should include fresh saline fecal smears and zinc sulfate flotation. Trophozoites are more likely to be found in loose stools, whereas cysts are more often found in semi-formed or formed stools.

A fresh saline smear is made by mixing a drop of feces with a drop of saline on a glass slide. A coverslip is applied, and the preparation is examined immediately under ×40 magnification. Trophozoites are pear shaped and have a characteristic concave ventral disk. They demonstrate wobbly motion, similar to a falling leaf. A drop of Lugol's solution of iodine on the edge of the coverslip enhances the morphologic features of the organisms and makes them easier to find. The iodine kills the parasite, so its motion is no longer seen if this procedure is used. Differentiation of trichomonads from *Giardia* is based on a different motion pattern (more forward motion with trichomonads), the

absence of a concave disk, a single nucleus, and the presence of an undulating membrane. Identification of *Giardia* trophozoites is diagnostic, but their absence in fecal samples does not rule out giardiasis.

Many studies have now shown that zinc sulfate concentration, with centrifugation is the most reliable test available for demonstration of *Giardia* cysts in a fecal sample. The test can be done in any practice setting, or fecal samples can be submitted to a commercial laboratory for detailed evaluation. The technique is described in Box 7-1. Zinc sulfate concentration is also a very effective method for identifying nematode eggs in feces. It is therefore now used as the standard test for screening for intestinal parasites in some academic and private practices. Studies have shown that approximately 70% of *Giardia*-positive dogs can be identified on a single zinc sulfate centrifugal flotation test (as opposed to approximately 40% of dogs after three separate saline smear preparations).

Slides should be examined within 10 minutes of preparation because the cysts may begin to shrink. Because animals shed *Giardia* on an intermittent basis, it is recommended that a series of zinc sulfate concentration tests be run over 3 to 5 days to maximize chances of accurately diagnosing

---

BOX 7-1 | Zinc Sulfate Flotation Technique

1. Thoroughly mix approximately 2 g of feces with approximately 15 ml of 33% zinc sulfate solution (33 g zinc sulfate made up to 100 ml with distilled water; specific gravity 1.18).
2. Strain the solution through cheesecloth or a tea strainer.
3. Pour the strained suspension into the 15-ml centrifuge tube; polypropylene tubes are preferable to polystyrene tubes.
4. Place the tube in a centrifuge (a standard bench-top centrifuge can be used). If the tubes hang vertically in the centrifuge, flotation solution can be added until a reverse meniscus forms. A coverslip is added and spun in place on top of the tube. If the tubes are placed in the centrifuge at an angle, the surface layer is harvested after spinning.
5. Spin the tube at approximately 1500 rpm for 3 to 5 min.
6. Remove the coverslip and the adhering drop of fluid and place them on a microscope slide. When a coverslip is not used, collect the surface layer of fluid by touching a glass rod (a 3-ml blood collection tube makes a convenient substitute) or bacteriologic loop to the surface of the centrifuge tube. Deposit the collected fluid on a slide, add a coverslip, and examine. Lugol's iodine may be added, if desired, to stain organisms.

Some of the debris in the fecal sample can be removed by initially mixing the sample with water and centrifuging it. Resultant supernatant is discarded, and zinc sulfate solution is added to the pellet and centrifuged as described above. This initial water wash is not necessary on a routine basis. When steatorrhea is present, large amounts of fat float with the Giardia cysts and may complicate reading of the slide. In these situations, an ethyl acetate sedimentation technique can be used; the sample is mixed with water, filtered, and placed in a centrifuge tube with 2 to 3 ml of ethyl acetate or ether. After centrifuging, the supernatant, including a distinct layer containing the organic solvent and fat, is discarded. The pellet is then resuspended, and a drop is stained with Lugol's iodine and examined.

From Barr SC, Bowman DD: Giardiasis in dogs and cats, *Compend Contin Educ Pract Vet* 16:605, 1994; from Zajac AM: Giardiasis, *Compend Contin Educ Pract Vet* 14:606, 1992.

or ruling out *Giardia* in patients with chronic diarrhea. Diagnostic efficiency increases to 95% when three zinc sulfate examinations are conducted over 3 to 5 days. A positive result on any of the tests warrants treatment for *Giardia*.

Whether or not any other diagnostic work-up is suspended until a therapeutic response is determined depends on the patient's clinical situation. If it is likely that some other disorder is more responsible for the patient's overall condition (e.g., severe protein-losing enteropathy and significant weight loss that would be highly unlikely to occur solely from a *Giardia* infection), *Giardia* might be considered a concurrent but less important problem. When evaluating a patient for a chronic GI disorder, the clinician must focus on finding the most significant problem. Sometimes a particular diagnostic "lead" is pursued too long while the patient's overall condition continues to decline.

Other diagnostic tests for *Giardia* include an enzyme-linked immunosorbent assay (ELISA) for *Giardia* antigen in feces, a direct immunofluorescent assay, duodenal aspiration under endoscopic guidance, and the peroral string test.

The fecal ELISA detects *Giardia* antigen that is produced by dividing trophozoites. The test is very sensitive in humans and reportedly detects 30% more cases of *Giardia* than does zinc sulfate. Studies in dogs, however, have shown that the ELISA appears to be less sensitive than a series of zinc sulfate centrifugal flotation tests. It may be a little more sensitive than a single zinc sulfate test. Keep in mind, however, the quality of the test being run and the accuracy of microscopic interpretation in the hands of an inexperienced observer. This is a common problem area in small animal hospital laboratories. One advantage of the ELISA is that, because it detects antigen in the feces, it avoids the problem of intermittent cyst excretion in the feces. This test can be run either in-house or at a commercial laboratory. In human medicine the recognized "gold standard" for diagnosis of *Giardia* is to run both a *Giardia* antigen test and a zinc sulfate assay. This is now a commonly used approach in veterinary medicine as well.

Treatment

For many years the primary treatment for *Giardia* in dogs and cats involved metronidazole. For dogs in which metronidazole proved ineffective,

quinacrine was often used. It was also used in cats. Although quinacrine has been shown to be more effective than metronidazole, it frequently causes side effects, including lethargy, anorexia, and vomiting. Quinacrine is no longer available. More recently it was shown that albendazole (Valbazen) is highly effective in controlling *Giardia* and that it has a high safety factor. However, it was later found that albendazole can cause leukopenia and lethargy, and so its use in dogs and cats is no longer recommended. Fenbendazole (Panacur), well known for its effectiveness against a variety of intestinal parasites, is very effective, as is febantel (in the combination product Drontal Plus, which includes febantel, praziquantel, and pyrantel pamoate).

Metronidazole is still a useful drug for treating *Giardia,* and it has the added advantage of having antibacterial as well as antiinflammatory properties. In situations in which it is unclear whether diarrhea is due to giardiasis, bacterial overgrowth, or mild IBD, metronidazole is an excellent choice, especially when an owner requests empiric therapy rather than definitive diagnostic testing. Metronidazole is only approximately 70% effective in eliminating *Giardia* from dogs, however; so if a positive diagnosis is made, fenbendazole or febantel represents a better choice. Potential side effects of metronidazole include anorexia, vomiting, and neurologic problems (ataxia, vestibular problems, seizures). In my experience these side effects are not common. They are more likely to occur when the anti-*Giardia* dose is used (12 to 15 mg/lb orally every 12 hours for 5 to 7 days). *The total dose per day should not exceed 30 mg/lb.* A lower dose (5 to 10 mg/lb every 12 hours) is used in treatment of intestinal bacterial overgrowth and IBD. Side effects are infrequent at this dose. In the past if a 5- to 7-day course of metronidazole failed to eliminate *Giardia,* a longer follow-up course (10 to 14 days) was often used. With the availability of fenbendazole and febantel, it is recommended that one of these drugs be used instead in this situation. Metronidazole is suspected of being teratogenic and should therefore not be administered to pregnant patients. Fenbendazole is recommended in this situation.

Fenbendazole has also been shown to be effective in eliminating *Giardia*. The same dose that is used to treat roundworms, hookworms, whipworms, and the tapeworm *Taenia pisiformis* (22 mg/lb orally once daily for 3 to 5 consecutive days) is used to treat *Giardia*. Fenbendazole has a proven record for being very safe and is thought not to have any teratogenic effects. Therefore fenbendazole would be the drug of choice for treatment of *Giardia* in pregnant animals. Fenbendazole is now the preferred treatment for *Giardia* in cats (Drontal Plus is approved for use only in dogs).

Drontal Plus is now recognized as an excellent drug for treatment of *Giardia,* as well as nematodes and tapeworms. This product includes febantel in addition to praziquantel and pyrantel pamoate. Febantel is the drug component that treats *Giardia.* Febantel is metabolized into fenbendazole and oxyfenbendazole after oral administration. Drontal Plus is administered once daily for 3 to 5 consecutive days in dogs for treatment of *Giardia.*

Oral furazolidone has proven to be an effective drug for treating *Giardia* in cats at a dose of 2 mg/lb orally twice daily for 5 to 10 days. Furazolidone causes vomiting and/or diarrhea in some cats. It should not be used in pregnant queens.

In addition to use of pharmacotherapy to eradicate *Giardia,* it is important to consider environmental control to minimize chances of reinfection, especially in kennel or cattery situations. Cysts that are present in a cool, wet environment can remain infective for a period. Cages and runs should be thoroughly cleaned of all solid fecal material. Steam cleaning and treatment with a quaternary ammonium compound are both very effective measures for killing cysts. Allowing time for thorough drying is important to desiccate any remaining cysts. Finally, patients should be bathed before they are returned to the kennel area to wash out any cysts that may be present in the hair coat. In kennel or cattery environments where *Giardia* is recognized as a significant problem an additional step that can be undertaken is to use a quaternary ammonium compound topically. The hair in the perineal and perianal regions can be washed with a quaternary ammonium compound once the shampoo has been rinsed out. These compounds do not seem to cause any significant skin irritation as long as they are left on for no more than 3 to 5 minutes and then thoroughly rinsed out and allowed to dry. These compounds can inactivate *Giardia* cysts within 1 minute at room temperature. In addition, a second 5-day course of treatment for *Giardia* is administered to ensure that each animal is parasite free before being returned to the kennel or cattery. Any newcomers are treated with fenbendazole or Drontal Plus (dogs) and a topical quaternary ammonium rinse as previously described before being placed in the environment.

In home environment situations bathing the patient at the conclusion of drug therapy may also be helpful. Patients may be reinfected with cysts that are in the hair coat or the environment. Bathing will help remove cysts that could be licked from the hair coat by the patient and help reduce the chances of reinfection.

Zoonotic Potential. Zoonotic potential definitely exists with *Giardia.* Children may be especially at risk due to their proclivity for playing in grass and soil areas where cysts may be present. They also are more likely to put their fingers or hands in their mouths, and this can occur anytime after they have had direct contact with an animal's hair coat, including in the perineal area. This is why it is so important for veterinarians to perform quality laboratory tests to investigate companion animals for parasitic infections, including *Giardia,* on a routine basis whenever there are children in contact with family pets. When both animals and humans living in the same environment become infected, a common source of infection rather than direct transmission must also be considered.

The question whether patients that are asymptomatic carriers of *Giardia* should be treated is often asked. *Giardia* cysts have been found in many patients with well-formed feces. *Giardia* is clearly not pathogenic in some patients, whereas in others it causes significant enteritis. Because the public health considerations must still be considered, it is strongly recommended that all patients with fecal samples that contain *Giardia* be treated and then retested to ensure that the infection has been cleared.

Vaccination

In 1999 a new vaccine was released for control of *Giardia.* The vaccine is a killed product containing chemically inactivated trophozoites. Efficacy studies showed that vaccinated dogs were less severely affected clinically and shed cysts for a shorter time following challenge with infective cysts, compared with nonvaccinated dogs. In addition, chronic giardiasis resolved after dogs were vaccinated with this product. In these studies clinical signs of infection were less severe by 21 to 35 days after vaccination, and cysts were no longer detected in the feces by 21 to 70 days. This is not expected to be a "core" vaccine (i.e., recommended for annual vaccination of all dogs and cats), but there definitely is a place for it in our armamentarium. The vaccine has been approved for use in both dogs and cats.

The following are important points regarding *Giardia* vaccine:

- Both cellular and humoral immunity are important for the following purposes:
  - Preventing *Giardia* infections.
  - Elimination of the parasite.
- Specific immunity to *Giardia* is slow to develop in natural infections.
- Some animals with persistent *Giardia* infections do not develop a sufficient antibody response.
- Anti-*Giardia* IgA and IgG coat the trophozoites in the small intestine, thus preventing adhesion of the parasite to the intestinal mucosa.
- Anti-*Giardia* IgG and IgM are cytotoxic to the trophozoites, with or without the presence of complement.
- Response to vaccine:
  - It was shown in the studies that the *Giardia* vaccine produced a strong IgG response, whereas saline-treated puppies had a weak or absent response.
  - There was technical difficulty in determining specific IgA in the study puppies, but a specific response was clearly shown in cats.
  - It may be possible for the vaccine to be used to immunostimulate patients with chronic *Giardia* infections, thus enabling the patients to clear the infection. Further work still needs to be done to confirm this. Of course, it is necessary that a correct diagnosis be made before stating/confirming that a patient has a "chronic infection."

Which Animals Should Be Considered Candidates for Vaccination?

Pets considered at higher risk of exposure to *Giardia* (and therefore candidates for vaccination) include dogs that frequently visit parks or play areas frequented by other dogs, dogs and cats living in multipet households, dogs living in endemic areas, hunting dogs, dogs and cats that travel to pet shows, farm dogs, dogs that board at training kennels, dogs and cats that board frequently at boarding facilities, and animals that have chronic giardiasis with poor response to therapy.

∎ INFLAMMATORY BOWEL DISEASE

Historical Perspectives

IBD is now well recognized as one of the most common causes of chronic vomiting and diarrhea in cats and dogs. Our knowledge about the various manifestations of this syndrome has expanded greatly over the last 20 years. Before the mid-1980s there was very little information in the veterinary literature about inflammatory bowel disorders. Early reports included an overview of clinical observations of malabsorption in the cat (1969) and a single case report on a cat with what was described at that time as ulcerative colitis (1972). Textbooks on small animal medicine published in the 1970s included only short and vague discussions about malassimilation syndromes (primarily lymphangiectasia, lymphosarcoma, and exocrine pancreatic insufficiency), and most of this information pertained only to dogs. Several of the earliest reports on IBD in dogs, centering on histiocytic ulcerative colitis in boxers, appeared in human journals in 1967 and 1970. Our recognition that IBD is a truly common disorder in cats and dogs did not really occur until the 1980s.

In humans a type of IBD known as ulcerative colitis was described as early as 1859 in England. It was not until 1932, however, that small intestinal inflammatory disease, specifically ileitis, was defined as a separate entity. It is now apparent in humans that the prevalence of inflammatory bowel disorders has increased dramatically over the past several decades, such that thousands of Americans and hundreds of thousands of patients worldwide are affected. Currently in the human field there are entire textbooks devoted to IBD, some encyclopedic in extent and containing tremendous diversification of viewpoints by their many authors.

To what factors do we owe our rather dramatic increase in awareness of the clinical manifestations of this syndrome in cats and dogs over the past 20 years? Is IBD a relatively new disease, or rather have we as clinicians simply become more skilled at recognizing it? I believe that the latter is much more likely. Our recognition that IBD commonly occurs directly parallels our increased use of endoscopy to investigate more thoroughly patients with such clinical signs as vomiting, diarrhea, weight loss, and change in appetite. In the not too distant past, the diagnostic work-up of a patient with chronic vomiting and/or diarrhea was commonly limited to such tests as fecal examination for parasites, fecal cultures, hematologic studies, and survey and contrast radiography, or in some cases simply fecal tests and a series of empiric pharmaceutical maneuvers. Now, however, an understanding of the absolute importance of histologic evaluation of GI tissues in patients whose symptoms are not readily explained by routine tests and dietary trials is thankfully well entrenched in our thinking. Indeed, IBD is a diagnosis that can be made only by biopsy specimen analysis. I suspect that in the past many patients with what was described as "nonspecific enteritis" may actually have had some type of IBD. Without specific treatment, many patients with chronic vomiting and/or diarrhea with subsequent wasting disease were euthanized or died prematurely as a result of "unknown causes."

My personal experience parallels that of other veterinary gastroenterologists working in the early 1980s. Beginning in 1980 as pediatric-sized endoscopes became more readily available and as we gained the necessary skills to routinely guide an endoscope through the pylorus and into the duodenum of cats and dogs, we rapidly became more capable of obtaining GI tissue samples both more *safely* (endoscopy is less invasive than exploratory surgery, with procurement of full-thickness biopsy specimens) and more *readily* (owners are much more likely to allow endoscopy than they are to approve a laparotomy). Once it became apparent that significant inflammatory bowel changes were present in a number of patients with GI symptoms (especially vomiting and/or diarrhea), it followed that procurement of gastric and intestinal biopsy samples should be strongly recommended in any patient with chronic (lasting as little as 4 weeks) unexplained signs. Indeed, the more we looked, the more we found.

On a personal note, I have had the good fortune to have worked at two large high-caseload institutions (Angell Memorial Animal Hospital in Boston and the VCA West Los Angeles Animal Hospital) in urban areas where a majority of animal owners tend to demonstrate a strong desire to provide the best medical care that they can for their pets. Many of our owners have embraced the idea of reaching a definitive diagnosis as early as possible. With the availability of endoscopy, we have been able to recommend and perform GI biopsies much earlier on the "chronicity curve" of disease. Our patients and their owners have no doubt benefited greatly from this approach. As a result of these experiences, I have had the opportunity to study the various clinical manifestations of IBD in quite a large number of cats and dogs. The information that follows represents a compilation of my experiences as a clinician along with observations of other specialists in gastroenterology who have also managed a significant number of cases.

We are in the midst of an exciting era of research in the field of the various inflammatory bowel disorders. It must be realized, however, that despite our ever-increasing knowledge in this area in both the human and the veterinary fields, we are still at the frontier. We have much to learn!

Terminology and Pathogenesis

The term *inflammatory bowel disease* describes a group of chronic intestinal disorders that are characterized by a diffuse infiltration within the lamina propria by various populations of inflammatory cells, including lymphocytes, plasma cells, eosinophils, neutrophils, and macrophages. The most commonly identified idiopathic inflammatory bowel disorders in cats are lymphocytic-plasmacytic enteritis, benign lymphocytic enteritis (an apparently distinct disorder from intestinal lymphosarcoma), and lymphocytic-plasmacytic colitis. Two different classifications of eosinophilic IBD have been identified in cats: eosinophilic enteritis and hypereosinophilic syndrome.

Eosinophilic enteritis is characterized by diffuse or focal infiltration of inflammatory cells that are almost entirely eosinophils into one or more layers of the alimentary tract. The stomach, small intestine, and colon may all be involved in some cases (eosinophilic gastroenterocolitis). Eosinophilic enteritis in cats is similar in clinical manifestations and response to treatment (very favorable) to the same condition in dogs.

Hypereosinophilic syndrome is a *severe* type of IBD in cats that involves massive infiltration of eosinophils in the alimentary tract and other parts of the body. Dramatic bowel thickening often results.

The eosinophilic disorders are not seen very commonly in cats. Of the two, hypereosinophilic syndrome is less common and more life threatening. Occasionally, mixed populations of inflammatory cells (e.g., lymphocytic-plasmacytic-eosinophilic, lymphocytic-eosinophilic) are identified. Inflammatory disease may be localized to the small intestine (enteritis), specific areas of the small intestine (e.g., duodenitis, ileitis), or colon (colitis). Although some cats have generalized intestinal involvement (enterocolitis), many cats with IBD have only small intestinal disease.

In dogs the most common types of IBD are lymphocytic-plasmacytic enteritis and lymphocytic-plasmacytic colitis. Pure lymphocytic enteritis is rarely identified in dogs. Eosinophilic enteritis is occasionally seen, but definitely not as commonly as was once speculated.

It is essential that the clinician understand that identifying an increase in inflammatory cells on intestinal biopsy specimen analysis does *not* automatically warrant a diagnosis of IBD. Inflammatory cells may be present in increased numbers simply as a normal response to a variety of inciting factors. Potential underlying causes include hyperthyroidism (thyrotoxicosis may generate an inflammatory response); various infectious agents, including bacteria, viruses, and parasites (including *Giardia*); food antigens; presence of a foreign body; and GI neoplasia, which may be associated with a blanket of inflammatory cells surrounding neoplastic cells (e.g., this may occur with lymphosarcoma).

It is my impression that tissue samples that are characterized by moderate to severe inflammation represent true idiopathic disease in a majority of cases. Specimens that reveal only mild inflammation, however, could be consistent with either mild idiopathic IBD or any number of underlying disorders. It is the clinician's responsibility to investigate thoroughly (see section on diagnosis) for underlying causes, whenever possible, before settling on a final diagnosis of idiopathic IBD. By taking this approach, we will most certainly better serve both our patients (by definitively diagnosing and specifically treating any underlying disorders) and our combined efforts in more accurately defining the diverse group of inflammatory bowel disorders. *The term IBD is used here to describe a chronic disorder in which no specific cause can be determined.*

The definitive cause of IBD, despite years of major research in humans and some recent work in animals, remains unknown. It is likely that a cytopathic immunologic response results in the bowel from chronic antigenic challenge. It appears that immune activation in IBD is largely confined to the GI tract, so the search for the "antigenic trigger" has focused on the intestinal lumen. Although the specific inciting factor or factors for these host hypersensitivity responses are still un-

clear, the most commonly speculated causes include defective mucosal immune responses, changes in mucosal permeability, dietary influences, and intestinal microorganisms.

Recently research in human medicine has focused on a possible autoimmune response in the pathogenesis of IBD. It has been proposed that there may be a specific immune response against an antigen expressed on the patient's own cells, particularly on intestinal epithelial cells. In this theory the patient mounts an appropriate immune response against some luminal antigen (e.g., dietary or microbial). However, because of similarities between proteins on the epithelial cells and the luminal antigens, the patient's immune system also attacks the epithelial cells. The immune response may be directed specifically at the epithelial cell. A defect in immunoregulation may be involved in this process (i.e., in individuals with IBD there may be a failure to suppress the inflammatory response). Thus, as a result of failure of normal suppressor mechanisms, there may be a prolonged and vigorous response to some normal luminal antigens.

Although theories abound, there is still no defined cause for IBD. Active research in both the human and the animal fields for pathogenic mechanisms continues.

Patient Profile

Although IBD most commonly occurs in middle-age to older cats and dogs, it has occasionally been diagnosed in patients as young as 4 months. The predominant clinical sign in young cats with IBD tends to be diarrhea, whereas in young dogs I have found vomiting to be the more predominant sign. Attempts to perform intestinal biopsies on young patients are made only after meticulous effort is taken to rule out intestinal parasites (including *Giardia* and *Cryptosporidium*), infectious agents (including viruses and bacteria, including *Campylobacter, Salmonella,* and *Shigella*), adverse food reactions, and metabolic derangements. No breed or sex predilections have been identified in animals with IBD.

History and Clinical Signs

One of the most common clinical signs observed in patients with idiopathic small intestinal IBD is vomiting. Vomiting is a common presenting complaint seen in clinical practice, and clinicians should give careful attention to patterns observed by the owner. In inflammatory bowel disorders, vomiting is most often recognized as an intermittent occurrence for weeks, months, or years. Often as the disorder progresses, there is an increased frequency of vomiting and other clinical signs, which leads the owner to seek veterinary attention. Alternatively, an occasional patient with even moderate to severe inflammatory changes on biopsy specimen analysis may be presented with clinical signs limited to an acute onset of vomiting and lethargy, with no past history of GI signs.

Vomiting episodes are usually associated with retching, are nonprojectile, and may produce clear fluid, bile, or foam. Vomiting of food, either fresh or partially digested, is sometimes observed. In patients with concurrent gastric hypomotility that is either idiopathic or secondary to chronic gastritis or IBD, vomiting of undigested food may occur many hours after eating. Blood is rarely present. Hematemesis may indicate concurrent gastric involvement (e.g., erosions, foreign body, gastritis, neoplasia) or superficial erosive changes in the proximal small intestine.

Vomiting in IBD can occur at variable times after eating. Many patients with mild IBD go about their daily routine showing no untoward effects from any of the vomiting episodes. The vomiting and associated nonspecific signs may be *cyclical* in nature. Clinical signs may be evident on one or several days and then spontaneously disappear, indicating that untreated IBD runs a course often characterized by exacerbations and remissions. Successes therefore should not automatically be attributed to the symptomatic treatment that is often given in these cases (nothing by mouth, bland diets, antiemetics). It is owing to this cyclic nature that some patients with IBD are not presented until signs are more frequent or severe. If a pattern of intermittent vomiting in a cat causes owner concern, a work-up to determine its cause should be undertaken, even if it is not a long-standing clinical sign. Without question, IBD is one of the leading differentials of chronic vomiting in cats and dogs.

In my experience the second most common sign observed in feline IBD is diarrhea. It may be the most common sign in dogs. Diarrhea may be the sole clinical sign or may occur in conjunction with intermittent vomiting. Diarrhea may be acute or chronic, but most cases are evaluated because of chronic diarrhea that is responsive or only temporarily responsive to diet changes or nonspecific symptomatic treatment. The first step in diagnosis of a disorder characterized by diarrhea is to decide whether the process is principally affecting small or large intestine or both. This helps determine the direction of further work-up and is done by combining information from history, physical examination, and stool characteristics (frequency, volume, consistency, odor, color, composition).

Small bowel diarrhea is most often characterized by large quantities of soft-formed, bulky, or watery stool. Steatorrhea may be evident, and more chronic cases are often accompanied by weight loss and listlessness. In contrast, diarrhea of large bowel origin most often has a loose, stringy consistency due to increased mucus content, and intermittent streaks of fresh blood may be present. Owners are often not aware of the presence of blood. Other signs include increased frequency of attempts to defecate (cat owners may misinterpret this as attempts to urinate), defecating in abnormal places, and hiding (cats). Cats with large intestinal inflammation sometimes begin defecating outside the litter box. Dogs sometimes demonstrate a sense of urgency to defecate.

If the disease is limited to the large intestine, most patients remain active and alert, have a normal appetite, and do not lose weight. Some patients have both small and large intestinal disease, with similar histologic changes, yet only small intestine or large intestine signs *predominate*. *If biopsy specimens are to be obtained in chronic diarrhea cases, obtaining tissue samples from both small and large intestine is strongly recommended.* Treatment for only small or large intestinal disease is not likely to result in complete resolution of signs if generalized involvement is present.

In some cats with chronic IBD, diarrhea does not occur until some stressful episode (e.g., change in environment, queening) causes an exacerbation of clinical signs. In these cases of acute diarrhea, initial testing is naturally directed toward ruling out dietary indiscretions, parasites, foreign bodies, and infectious agents (e.g., *Campylobacter*). Often no definitive diagnosis can be made, and feeding trials and empirical treatment fail to effect lasting resolution of the diarrhea. Further work-up involving intestinal biopsy in these cases may reveal chronic moderate to severe inflammatory bowel changes. A review of the history again may surprisingly not show any past occurrence of vomiting or diarrhea. Diarrhea, once apparent, usually does not resolve until specific treatment for IBD is instituted in these cases.

In addition to vomiting and diarrhea, other clinical signs that may be observed in IBD include changes in attitude or activity, altered appetite, and weight loss. Many patients tend to be more depressed during periods of increased vomiting. As with the sign of vomiting, these activity-level changes are often cyclic. In some cats with chronic diarrhea, listless behavior is the predominant attitude. An owner may describe decreased tendencies to play, decreased interest in surroundings, and more frequent hiding or sitting near heating units for long periods of time.

Appetite changes in cats with IBD vary from decreased to complete anorexia to ravenousness. Inappetence seems to occur more commonly in cats that have vomiting as the primary clinical sign and usually occurs during exacerbations of clinical signs. In some cats, anorexia is the primary clinical sign and vomiting or diarrhea is not observed until later or not at all. The three leading differential diagnoses for a cat with a ravenous appetite, diarrhea, and weight loss are IBD, hyperthyroidism, and exocrine pancreatic insufficiency (an uncommon disorder in cats). I have also seen cats with chronic low-grade lymphocytic lymphoma of the small intestine exhibit identical clinical signs (Box 7-2). Dogs with IBD tend to have a normal to decreased appetite, depending on the degree of disease that is present. One notable exception is that Chinese shar-peis with IBD frequently have an increased to ravenous appetite (see further information about shar-peis later in this chapter).

The clinical course of IBD in many dogs and cats, at least fairly early in the course, is characterized by unpredictable exacerbations and remissions. This makes accurate assessment of disease burden difficult. It is important that an early assessment be made for patients that demonstrate GI symptoms so that the best course of therapy can be instituted early rather than later, when more intensive therapy might be needed.

Diagnosis

The differential diagnosis for IBD is listed in Box 7-3. A definitive diagnosis of IBD can only be made based on intestinal biopsy specimen analysis. Other tests are run to evaluate the overall health status of the patient and to rule out other disorders. Recommended baseline tests include a complete blood count, complete biochemical profile, urinalysis, and fecal examinations for parasites and in cats a serum thyroxine (T_4) test and tests for feline leukemia virus antigen and feline immunodeficiency virus antibody.

Baseline test results frequently are normal or negative, but abnormalities that may be identified include mild nonregenerative anemia (anemia of chronic inflammatory disease); leukocytosis (20,000 to 50,000 cells/μl) without a left shift (suggests active chronic inflammatory disease); eosinophilia (mild to dramatic increase) in some cats and dogs with eosinophilic enteritis and in all cats with hypereosinophilic syndrome; and hypoproteinemia (increased loss of protein through a damaged intestinal lining) *or* mild hyperproteinemia (due to increased globulin fraction in idiopathic

BOX 7-2	**Differential Diagnosis of Disorders Causing Chronic Diarrhea, Weight Loss, and Ravenous Appetite in Cats**

Hyperthyroidism
Inflammatory bowel disease
Intestinal lymphoma
Exocrine pancreatic insufficiency

BOX 7-3	**Differential Diagnosis of Disorders Resembling Inflammatory Bowel Disease in Dogs and Cats**

Chronic giardiasis
Hyperthyroidism (cats)
Dietary sensitivity (e.g., food allergy or intolerance)
Bacterial overgrowth
Clostridium perfringens enterotoxicosis
Lymphangiectasia (dogs)
Lymphoma
Pythiosis
Functional bowel disorder (e.g., irritable bowel syndrome)
Histoplasmosis
Exocrine pancreatic insufficiency
Feline infectious peritonitis (gastrointestinal involvement)
Adenocarcinoma
Stagnant loop (secondary intestinal obstruction) (e.g., adenocarcinoma, mesenteric adhesions)

IBD or feline infectious peritonitis with intestinal involvement).

Hypoproteinemia (total protein less than 6.0 g/dl, with albumin and globulin fractions proportionately decreased) occurs much less commonly in cats with IBD than in dogs and usually indicates moderate to severe intestinal involvement when it is identified in a cat with IBD. A work-up should be expedited to determine the cause. The most common cause of hypoproteinemia in cats with a total protein level less than 5.0 g/dl in my case series is intestinal lymphoma. The most common cause of PLE in dogs is lymphocytic-plasmacytic enteritis.

Fecal α_1-protease inhibitor (Fα_1-PI) is an assay that will help detect evidence of excessive intestinal protein loss in dogs before hypoproteinemia develops. α_1-PI is a plasma glycoprotein. It is not present in the intestinal lumen above trace background concentrations unless there is abnormal transmucosal loss of plasma, lymph, or intracellular fluid as a result of GI disease. Fα_1-PI can reach abnormal concentrations before there is enough protein loss from the intestine to cause panhypoproteinemia. α_1-PI is excreted in the stool with minimal loss of its immunoreactivity, because it is largely resistant to degradation in the intestinal lumen by virtue of its inhibitory activity.

This assay is useful in dogs with chronic diarrhea that have normal or slightly decreased serum protein levels, as a screening tool for evidence of the presence of a potentially severe PLE disorder. The assay is available at the GI laboratory at Texas A&M University.* Contact the laboratory for special fecal sample submission tubes. Samples are submitted frozen. The level of Fα_1-PI in healthy dogs has been determined to be no more than 5.7 μg/g. Values as high as 53.2 μg/g have been observed in dogs with PLE sufficiently severe to cause panhypoproteinemia. Values in the range of 6.0 to 15.0 μg/g have been observed in dogs with PLE not sufficiently severe to cause panhypoproteinemia.

Hyperthyroidism should always be ruled out in any cat older than 5 years of age that has manifest unexplained GI signs. Hyperthyroidism is occasionally diagnosed in cats younger than 5 years of age, so this possibility should always be considered.

Testing for hyperthyroidism may include running a free T_4 by equilibrium dialysis or a thyroid hormone (T_3) suppression test in cats with clinical signs suggestive of hyperthyroidism but that have a baseline T_4 level in the high normal range. Interestingly, thyrotoxicosis can cause inflammatory changes in the intestinal tract, and this may explain why some cats with hyperthyroidism have vomiting or diarrhea. These changes often resolve after treatment for hyperthyroidism is instituted. Failure of vomiting or diarrhea to resolve, however, within 4 to 6 weeks of institution of treatment for hyperthyroidism suggests the possibility of ongoing inflammatory disease or some other disorder that likely requires primary therapy.

I have observed cats with moderate to severe lymphocytic-plasmacytic enteritis or lymphocytic enteritis that were also hyperthyroid. Intestinal biopsy specimens were obtained from these patients after treatment for hyperthyroidism effectively decreased serum thyroid hormone concentrations into the normal range but had little effect in resolving ongoing GI symptoms (generally primarily vomiting and/or diarrhea, although in several cats the predominant sign was inappetence). It has been my impression that cats with such significant degrees of inflammation have both hyperthyroidism and idiopathic IBD rather than a single problem.

It is also recommended that all dogs and cats exhibiting chronic signs of GI disease have the serum cobalamin concentration measured. Several studies have demonstrated that some patients with GI disease have a significant deficiency of tissue-level cobalamin. This is particularly important in any case in which there has already been a suboptimal response to previous therapy, because supplementation with cobalamin may be helpful to such patients. Clinical signs of cobalamin deficiency include chronic wasting or failure to thrive, lethargy, and diarrhea. Subnormal cobalamin levels may result from intestinal mucosal disease, reduced intrinsic factor availability, or bacterial competition. Cobalamin therapy in patients with subnormal levels may be an important key to improved weight gain and a decrease in signs such as vomiting and diarrhea. Dose recommendations are described in the treatment section for IBD.

Patients with chronic diarrhea should also be thoroughly evaluated for intestinal parasites, including *Giardia* and *Cryptosporidium,* and *Clostridium perfringens* enterotoxicosis (CPE). A panel of fecal tests is run, including zinc sulfate centrifugal

---

*GI Laboratory at Texas A&M University, College of Veterinary Medicine, TAMU 4474, College Station, TX 77843-4474; Telephone: (979) 862-2861; www.cvm.tamu.edu/gilab.

flotation, *Giardia* antigen test, *C. perfringens* enterotoxin assay, and *Cryptosporidium* indirect fluorescent antibody test. Dogs and cats with IBD may have multiple GI disorders concurrently, and it is important that each problem be identified so that the most comprehensive treatment regimen can be instituted. Dogs should also be tested for intestinal bacterial overgrowth (described later in this chapter).

Survey abdominal radiographs and barium contrast study results are often unremarkable. Because cost containment is so often an important factor in clinical practice, barium series are often not performed unless clinical signs or abdominal palpation findings (e.g., obstruction) indicate that this procedure should be done. In many cases, money is best spent on baseline tests and intestinal biopsies. Abnormal findings that may be identified on a barium series include diffuse mucosal irregularities or spicular small intestinal mucosal changes and thickened bowel segments. Positive findings do not provide a definitive diagnosis; rather, they confirm the need for direct examination and biopsy of the affected areas. Radiographs can also suggest false-positive findings.

Intestinal biopsies can be performed either under endoscopic control or by exploratory laparotomy. Among the many advantages of endoscopy are that it is relatively quick and noninvasive. Multiple biopsy samples can be obtained, and the stomach, proximal small intestine (and frequently the proximal jejunum in cats), and colon can be thoroughly evaluated. In many cats, ileum samples can be obtained blindly, with the endoscope tip situated in the ascending colon or at the junction of the transverse and ascending colon. In most dogs larger than 8 to 10 lb, a pediatric-sized endoscope can be advanced into the ileum. A total of 8 to 10 small bowel biopsy specimens are usually obtained at endoscopy, depending on the gross appearance of the mucosa. Biopsies of proximal small intestine, as well as stomach, should *always* be done in patients with chronic vomiting that are undergoing endoscopy. It is not uncommon for cats and dogs with inflammatory changes involving only the small intestine to be presented with signs limited to chronic intermittent vomiting. If only gastric biopsy samples are obtained, the diagnosis may be missed.

The gross appearance of the mucosa in IBD can range from normal (primarily cream to slightly pink in color) to mildly erythemic to varying degrees of mucosal irregularity (Figure 7-1). Mucosal irregularity may appear as fissures or resemble a cobblestone texture in more advanced cases (Figure 7-2). Focal erosions may also be observed. The mucosa may be friable and may bleed from direct contact with the endoscope tip as it is advanced. Endoscopic biopsy techniques useful in the small intestine have been described in detail elsewhere. Biopsy samples vary in size. They are often small when the intestinal mucosa is

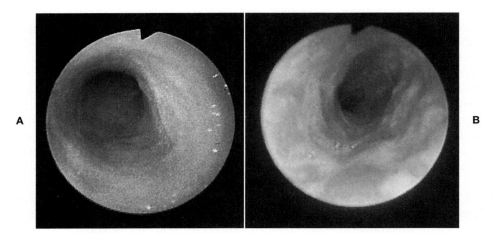

FIGURE 7-1 *A,* Endoscopic photograph of normal duodenal mucosa in a dog. Normal small intestinal mucosa is primarily cream to slightly pink in cats and pinkish white to light red in dogs. The mucosa often appears slightly irregular or velvety as a result of its makeup of digitate villi. *B,* Mild mucosal irregularity, increased graininess, and patchy erosive mucosal changes in a dog with moderate lymphocytic-plasmacytic enteritis. There was a history of chronic intermittent vomiting that had recently become more frequent.

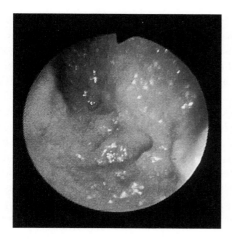

FIGURE 7-2 Severe mucosal irregularity (note sizable troughs) in a 9-month-old cat with a ravenous appetite, voluminous loose stools, and weight loss. Endoscopy was done after there was no response to empirical treatment for exocrine pancreatic insufficiency and occult gastrointestinal parasitism. The histologic diagnosis was severe lymphocytic-plasmacytic enteritis.

normal. When the intestinal mucosa is compromised by some disorder, sample size is invariably larger. Occasionally a long linear strip (2 to 3 cm) of tissue is lifted off when marked inflammatory disease causes altered mucosal and submucosal integrity. A greater than normal amount of hemorrhage may occur at the site after mucosal samples are obtained. This is rarely of any concern. The risk of gastric or intestinal perforation by endoscopic biopsy forceps is extremely low and would only be expected to occur if tissue samples are obtained from the depths of ulcerated areas.

The abdomen should be carefully palpated before endoscopy when the patient is under general anesthesia to examine for abnormalities that may have been missed during palpation when it was awake. A disadvantage of endoscopy is that extraluminal lesions cannot be evaluated. This is not a significant problem, however, if the decision to perform endoscopy rather than exploratory laparotomy is based on careful patient evaluation, including baseline testing and abdominal palpation. In addition, ultrasound can be used to examine for intestinal masses and to evaluate wall thickness.

If it appears that an intestinal mass is present, greater consideration is given to doing an exploratory laparotomy. If exploratory laparotomy is

performed, a total of three full-thickness biopsy samples are obtained (one each from the duodenum, jejunum, and ileum). *At laparotomy, a majority of patients with IBD have grossly normal bowel. If clinical signs warrant abdominal exploratory, intestinal biopsy specimens must be obtained regardless of the gross appearance of the intestines.* A lymph node biopsy should also be done if there is any lymphadenopathy. Biopsy samples of other tissues (e.g., liver, pancreas, kidney) are obtained if indicated based on abnormal laboratory test results or abnormal gross appearance.

The reason for obtaining multiple biopsy samples from the small bowel is that intestinal diseases may have varying degrees of severity in different parts of the intestinal tract. There may also be segmental lesions with some normal areas still present. It is even possible to find patchy normal zones of intestine in a patient with a life-threatening intestinal disease. Therefore there is no guarantee that representative tissue samples will be obtained from a patient that in fact does have intestinal lesions, especially when there are no grossly evident lesions to guide the clinician to a site that is more likely to yield significant information. By obtaining multiple samples and using techniques best suited for procuring high-quality samples, diagnostic yield will be enhanced.

Interpretation of Pathologic Findings

In inflammatory bowel disorders, increased numbers of inflammatory cells are present in the lamina propria. Infiltrations of either single-cell or mixed-cell type may be involved. Often one to two cell types predominate (e.g., lymphocytic-plasmacytic enteritis, lymphocytic enteritis). Neutrophils are not commonly identified in IBD but, when present, probably indicate an inflammatory response to a microbial component of the disorder. Histologic changes are usually reported as mild, moderate, moderate to severe, or severe, and the percentages of various inflammatory cells are noted. Other abnormalities that may be observed include mucosal atrophy, villous atrophy without cryptal hyperplasia, villous fusion, epithelial erosion, and fibrosis.

In general, "mild" IBD refers to increased inflammatory cells without architectural disruption, glandular necrosis, or fibrosis in the lamina propria. "Moderate" IBD refers to increased numbers of inflammatory cells with attendant separation and distortion of glands or crypts. There may also be mild villous blunting. "Severe" IBD is manifest by architectural distortion of the mucosa, marked villous blunting, marked separation of glands or crypts, necrosis, and fibrosis. Studies are ongoing to further define the criteria for various degrees of IBD.

Severe cases of lymphocytic-plasmacytic enteritis or lymphocytic enteritis can be difficult to differentiate histologically from lymphoma, especially in cats, when endoscopic-sized biopsy samples are evaluated. There are serious implications as to what type of therapy to prescribe in such cases. Changes that tend to suggest lymphoma include absolute uniformity of the lymphocyte population, mitotic cells, pleomorphism, and attendant ablation of villous arches. Areas of necrosis may be present. Overlying mixed inflammatory cell infiltrates may make it difficult to differentiate benign from malignant disease. If a diagnosis is unclear from evaluation of endoscopic biopsy samples, it may be necessary to repeat the procedure to obtain more samples (generally 2 to 4 weeks later) or to obtain full-thickness intestinal samples at laparotomy. Use of immunohistochemical staining techniques may also be helpful. Histologic differentiation of IBD and lymphoma is summarized in Table 7-1.

A major, and probably underappreciated, problem related to interpretation of pathologic findings by clinicians is the lack of uniformity with which pathologists assess intestinal biopsy specimens. Variability in the histologic assessment of the general group of inflammatory bowel disorders has raised many questions about the significance of certain findings. Part of the basis for the confusion is that little information is available regarding normal cellularity of the lamina propria or normal villus length in dogs and cats of different breeds and ages, that eat different diets, that live under different conditions, and so on. This then makes it difficult to *clearly* define and describe various degrees of normal and abnormal intestinal histologic findings. One pathologist's interpretation may be quite different from that of another. The difficulty becomes somewhat greater when inadequate endoscopic samples (too small or damaged) are submitted or when a pathologist is inexperienced or disinterested in evaluating other than full-thickness intestinal samples. It is therefore recommended that clinicians select their pathologists carefully and that consistent efforts be made to obtain the best-quality tissue samples. There are veterinary pathologists who specialize in GI tissue pathology, just as there are specialists in dermatologic pathology. Most pathologists are eager to discuss cases with clinicians, and indeed this opportunity to compare observations is an invaluable means of making the best use of the available information for determining a patient's treatment and prognosis. In some situations it may be best to obtain a second or third opinion before deciding on a final diagnosis.

In recent years investigators have begun some very important work centered on developing specific criteria for histologic grading of various inflammatory bowel disorders in small animals. In one study it was shown that there can be

TABLE 7-1   Features of Lymphocytic-Plasmacytic Enteritis/Colitis and Intestinal Lymphosarcoma

	Lymphocytic-Plasmacytic Enteritis/Colitis	Intestinal Lymphosarcoma
Gross features		
Thickened bowel wall	±	±
Involvement of other organs	−	±
Histologic features		
Cell population	Heterogeneous	Homogeneous
Lamina propria infiltration	+	±
Submucosal infiltration	±	±
Muscularis infiltration	−	±
Serosal infiltration	−	±
Involvement of other organs	−	±

From Roth L: Pathologic atlas of selected gastrointestinal disorders. In August JR, ed: *Consultations in feline internal medicine,* Philadelphia, 1991, WB Saunders.
±, May be present; −, absent; +, present.

substantial interobserver variation among pathologists when evaluating the same intestinal histologic sections. Biopsy specimen interpretation can be notoriously subjective from one pathologist to the next. Most clinicians are well aware of the importance of obtaining intestinal biopsy specimens from patients with signs that may be consistent with intestinal disease. As we go forward we need to focus more on two important areas, namely, we need more consistency among pathologists regarding how different pathologists interpret the same tissue specimens, and there is a need for some correlation between the pathologist's description of the tissue and the clinical state of the patient.

We need to know whether or not a clinically significant disorder exists in a particular tissue, because in some instances a pathologist may interpret a sample as being abnormal, suggesting the presence of intestinal disease, and yet the patient may be known to have no signs that correlate with these findings.

Variation in the interpretation of intestinal biopsy specimens among pathologists has also been described in human medicine, in which there are also sometimes blatant differences in diagnostic criteria. It is certainly acknowledged that histologic evaluation of the digestive tract is difficult. Continued collaboration between clinicians and pathologists is essential if we hope to develop a more accurate and predictable set of criteria for consistent interpretation of intestinal biopsy samples.

Treatment

It is important that the clinician formulate a treatment protocol based on a correlation of clinical course, laboratory and gross findings, and histologic findings rather than relying on histologic changes alone. Although treatment principles for cats and dogs with IBD are similar, drug selection and dosage regimens vary between these two species in some situations. For the sake of clarity, treatment recommendations for cats and dogs are discussed separately.

Cats

Dietary Therapy

Because dietary allergens may play a role in the cause of IBD, specific dietary therapy may be beneficial. Dietary therapy is instituted at the outset for all cats with IBD, and in cats with mild IBD, dietary therapy alone may be sufficient for resolu-

tion of clinical signs. In one study, which evaluated 55 cats with various GI symptoms, of which vomiting and diarrhea were the most common signs, 16 cats (29%) were classified as food sensitive based on response to feeding of a novel protein source (either chicken or lamb in this particular study). Resolution of GI signs occurred fairly quickly in these cats, and then signs recurred once the original diet was reintroduced. All of the cats with food sensitivity had inflammation, identified on endoscopic biopsy specimens, in at least one region of their intestinal tract. Gastric mucosal biopsy specimens were abnormal in 66% of the food-sensitive cats, and duodenal samples were abnormal in 50%. This study provides further confirmation of the importance of dietary therapy in cats with inflammatory GI disorders. Clearly, long-term control of IBD with minimal drug administration may be aided by specific dietary management. However, some cats will be only temporarily responsive or only minimally responsive to careful dietary manipulations. Therefore some cats with mild disease will require some form of pharmacologic therapy in addition to dietary manipulation. Most cats with moderate to severe IBD will require pharmacologic therapy, and this is started in conjunction with dietary therapy as soon as a diagnosis is made.

There is no single diet that can be universally recommended for management of IBD in cats. The diet must be chosen based on the dietary history, and then an assessment has to be made as to how well the affected patient embraces the recommended diet. Adjustments may need to be made over time. We now have the advantage of having a wide variety of very palatable commercial diets available, and using commercial diets, compared with home-prepared diets, reduces concern about dietary imbalances significantly. Using commercial diets is also much more convenient for owners.

In general the first step is to select a diet with a novel protein source, that is, something the animal has not been fed before (e.g., duck, venison, lamb, rabbit, whitefish, turkey). The effects of this diet should be assessed over a 3- to 4-week period for therapeutic response and palatability. If there is not a satisfactory response to the first diet *and* the cat's condition remains very stable, then an alternate diet can be tried, or, alternatively, drug therapy can be instituted at this point as well. Most owners are anxious for prompt resolution of their pet's clinical signs, and so I usually try to make a determination as to whether ongoing strict dietary trials will be practical or not.

Many of the commercially available therapeutic diets have been enriched with omega-3 fatty acids. Altering the dietary ratio of omega-6 to omega-3 polyunsaturated fatty acids may affect the inflammatory response of IBD. Omega-3 fatty acids competitively inhibit formation of prostaglandins and leukotrienes derived from arachidonic acid, resulting in decreased concentrations of proinflammatory fatty acid metabolites. It remains unclear, however, if dietary supplementation with fatty acids is truly beneficial.

Hydrolyzed protein diets have become available for dietary therapy. The theory is that because these diets contain no intact proteins, only peptides of sizes ranging from 6,000 to 15,000 daltons, which are proposed to be nonantigenic, no adverse reaction to the diet will occur. It is still possible, however, for an antigenic response to one of the epitomes of the peptides to occur. Further investigation is needed; however, these diets certainly do represent an attractive option for feeding to some patients with dietary sensitivities or true food allergy.

Recent studies conducted in dogs and cats have shown that cell mediated immunity declines with age. Dietary supplementation with vitamin E appears to enhance this function. Other potential benefits of vitamin E include reduction of oxidative damage and correction of a deficiency of vitamin E that may naturally occur in animals with severe GI disease. Therefore it may be beneficial to provide vitamin E supplementation for dogs and cats with moderate to severe IBD. At this time it is still unclear what dose of vitamin E is best for antioxidant effects in the GI tract. A dose of 100 IU per 10 lb per day is suggested.

For cats with concurrent large bowel disease and symptoms, fiber supplementation may be helpful. Beneficial effects of fiber supplementation include improved fecal character, improved colonic motility, binding of potential colonic irritants, and production of beneficial short-chain fatty acids that positively influence large intestinal structure and function.

Once the disease has been in remission for 6 or more months, adjustments in the type of foods offered can be attempted, based on owner and patient preferences. New ingredients should be added one at a time, and the owner should observe for any adverse effects. If any adverse effects occur, the offending ingredients are removed. Usually several palatable and effective diets can be identified that will be well tolerated over time.

Pharmacologic Therapy for Cats With IBD

Corticosteroids are the cornerstone of pharmacologic therapy for idiopathic inflammatory bowel disorders. Mild to moderate cases often respond to prednisone or prednisolone at a starting dose of 0.5 to 1 mg/lb divided twice daily for 2 to 4 weeks, followed by a gradual decline in 50% increments at 2-week intervals. Cats with inflammatory changes graded as mild usually respond quite well to the lower dose, and alternate-day or every-third-day treatment can often be achieved by 2 to 3 months. In many but not all cats with mild disease, treatment can be discontinued altogether by 3 to 6 months.

If biopsy specimen analysis reveals disease that is moderate to severe, a dose of 1 to 2 mg/lb divided twice daily is used for the first 4 weeks or until clinical signs resolve. Some clinicians feel that better bioavailability will be achieved in cats with use of prednisolone rather than prednisone. Therefore for more severe cases it may be best to prescribe prednisolone specifically. This dose of corticosteroid is generally very well tolerated in cats. In these cases a dose of 0.5 to 1 mg/lb/day may be necessary long-term (months to years) to maintain clinical remission. Use of combination drug therapy (e.g., prednisolone and metronidazole, or prednisolone and azathioprine) may also be required at the outset to control clinical signs and prevent progression of the disease. Cats with hypoproteinemia and histologic changes graded as severe often respond quite well when an aggressive therapeutic course is undertaken. Dexamethasone (0.15 to 0.25 mg/lb orally every 24 hours) may be useful in cats that are poorly responsive to increased doses of prednisolone.

It has been my experience that young cats (less than 5 years of age) with IBD often do not need to be treated as long as do many middle-age to older cats. This may be due in part to the fact that by the time older cats are diagnosed, the disease is often long-standing and often of a moderate to severe degree. Earlier diagnosis of these older cats in conjunction with appropriate therapy will likely provide a better opportunity for lower daily or alternate-day dosage levels to be successful in maintaining control. I have found that many older cats with moderately severe to severe IBD require prednisone or prednisolone at 1 mg/lb/day for life for adequate control of all symptoms related to IBD. Combination drug therapy may also be required (see subsequent information). Many clinicians who treat empirically for suspected IBD often use inadequate dosages of corticosteroids (initial dose either not high enough or tapered too early). *The importance of evaluating biopsy samples, including periodic follow-up biopsy specimens in some cases, to best tailor a treatment program cannot be overemphasized.*

Methylprednisolone acetate (Depo-Medrol) can be used as sole treatment for cats with mild to moderate IBD or as adjunctive therapy when oral prednisolone and/or metronidazole are used as the primary treatment and flare-ups of clinical signs occur. Consistent control of clinical signs in cats with moderate to severe IBD is more difficult to maintain when methylprednisolone acetate is used alone, however. It is recommended that sole use of methylprednisolone acetate be reserved for situations in which the owner is unable to consistently administer tablet or liquid preparations orally. Initially 20 mg is given subcutaneously or intramuscularly and is repeated at 2-week intervals for two to three doses. Injections are then given every 4 to 6 weeks or as needed for control.

Budesonide is a glucocorticoid that represents a new alternative for management of IBD in dogs and cats, especially in severe cases that have proven to be refractory to prednisolone, metronidazole, azathioprine, and dietary management; or that are intolerant of the corticosteroids discussed previously. Budesonide is a new and recently approved corticosteroid for use in humans. It is one of a group of novel corticosteroids that have been in development for use in humans in an attempt to make available alternative preparations that will help limit toxicity associated with corticosteroid use. Others include fluticasone propionate, tixocortol pivalate, and beclomethasone dipropionate.

Budesonide undergoes high first pass metabolism in the liver, and 90% is converted into metabolites with low corticosteroid activity. It has minimal systemic availability. The potential for typical corticosteroid side effects is significantly reduced as a result of decreased bioavailability and the resulting limited systemic exposure, which makes this a particularly attractive drug for use in humans and animals that are poorly tolerant of other corticosteroids. Budesonide also has a high receptor-binding affinity in the mucosa. It has been referred to as a "locally acting" corticosteroid.

Therapeutic results with budesonide have been promising in humans with Crohn's disease, collagenous colitis and lymphocytic colitis, ulcerative colitis, either when administered as a retention enema or in oral form, and primary biliary cirrhosis. Budesonide has been used by some veterinary clinicians in recent years to treat IBD in dogs and cats. Dosage recommendations vary. In humans, a range of 6 to 9 mg per day has been used during initial therapy. The following general recommendations have been made for dogs and cats. In general, budesonide is administered to cats and small dogs at 1 mg once per day. It has been used at higher doses (3 mg per small dog or cat per day), but the lower dose is frequently effective. Large dogs receive 3 mg twice daily initially, and the dosage is later tapered to 3 mg once daily, and then to alternate day administration for longer term use.

Budesonide can be used in combination with other drugs. Since cats tolerate corticosteroids very well, there is little indication to use budesonide as a primary therapy for IBD. However, this may be a very attractive option for use in diabetic cats that also have IBD.

Potential adverse effects include PU/PD, when budesonide is used at the high end of the dose range, and GI ulceration. These reactions have been observed in some human patients. These problems would be more likely to occur in dogs than in cats. It appears to be very safe when used at the levels listed above.

When combination therapy is indicated, metronidazole is usually the first choice to be used in conjunction with prednisolone. It can also be used as sole treatment in some cases (e.g., in the unusual event that a cat cannot tolerate corticosteroids, or if their use is contraindicated). Metronidazole's mechanism of action includes an antiprotozoal effect, inhibition of cell-mediated immune responses, and anaerobic antibacterial activity. A dosage of 5 to 10 mg/lb twice daily is used for IBD. Ideally at least several months of metronidazole therapy is given once it is started. In some cats with severe disease, long-term consecutive use (months to years) or 1- to 2-month cycles of treatment may be required.

Side effects of metronidazole at this low dose are uncommon in cats. Adverse reactions that have been observed include primarily GI (inappetence, nausea, and occasionally vomiting and/or diarrhea) and neurologic (ataxia, seizures, disorientation) problems. In my experience, neurologic side effects are very rare when the dose range recommended here is used, for whatever duration (weeks to months to years). I have observed two cats that were treated with prednisone and metronidazole (5 mg/lb twice a day in one, and 7 mg/lb twice a day in the other) for IBD that developed rear limb ataxia within 3 to 4 days of the start of therapy. In both cases the metronidazole was discontinued within 24 hours and the ataxia completely resolved within 2 to 4 days. Metronidazole was not reinstituted in either cat.

The most troublesome problem that the owners of my patients have encountered with metronidazole is excessive salivation after pill administration in cats. Metronidazole is known to have a sharp, unpleasant metallic taste. Most cats are given half to one quarter of a 250-mg tablet per dose, and the taste of broken sections is apparently quite bitter. Salivation does not occur when the medication is administered directly to the back of the mouth and quickly swallowed. If, however, the pill is retained in the oral cavity for even the shortest time, the battle is most likely lost! Recompounding metronidazole into a tasty suspension form often makes the task of administering metronidazole much easier.

Metronidazole has shown evidence of carcinogenic activity in studies involving chronic oral administration in mice and rats. There are reports of humans with Crohn's disease who have been treated with high doses of metronidazole for prolonged periods of time and in whom breast or oral cancer subsequently developed. A cause-and-effect relationship has *not* been established. To date I am aware of no cases of GI or mammary cancer that have occurred in dogs or cats in conjunction with metronidazole use. I consider it to be a safe drug for prolonged use (months to years) in patients with chronic disorders for which long-term therapy is required.

If remission cannot be maintained with use of corticosteroids and metronidazole, azathioprine (Imuran) should be added to the treatment regimen. There is no need to reduce the prednisolone dose in cats when azathioprine is used in conjunction. It may not be necessary to continue metronidazole after completion of the first 4 weeks of azathioprine therapy. This decision is best made on an individual case basis. Azathioprine is a potent immunosuppressive drug. It is metabolized to 6-mercaptopurine, its active metabolite, which functions to interfere with antigenic triggering of lymphocytes. Replication of rapidly dividing cells,

including immunoblasts, is inhibited, and there is interference with cellular function. Azathioprine is usually used in cats only when the previously discussed therapeutic measures fail to control the disease. The most important side effect of azathioprine in cats is bone marrow suppression.

I use a maximum starting dose of azathioprine in cats of 0.15 to 0.23 mg/lb once every other day. At this low dose, side effects are very uncommon in my experience, but I have seen one cat develop significant pancytopenia within 4 weeks of the start of therapy. The cat gradually recovered after immediate cessation of azathioprine. One blood transfusion was required. Alternatively, if clinical signs of IBD do not resolve on the initial azathioprine dose, the dose can gradually be increased if there is no evidence of bone marrow suppression. Because of lag effect, beneficial therapeutic results from azathioprine are often not apparent until 3 to 4 weeks after treatment is started. Azathioprine is generally used for 3 to 9 months or longer in cats. A majority of cats with IBD do not require azathioprine treatment.

A complete blood count and platelet count should be run to monitor for anemia, leukopenia, and thrombocytopenia before the start of therapy with azathioprine and at 3- to 4-week intervals for the first 2 months, and then once every 2 months. Significant side effects are most often identified during the first 3 to 6 weeks of treatment. There is usually no physical evidence of early azathioprine toxicity in cats. Mild leukopenia (e.g., 3000 to 4000 cells/μl) is usually the first abnormality that is identified. Azathioprine is currently available only as 50-mg tablets. Because it is too difficult to break azathioprine into a consistent fragment size for cats, it should always be recompounded into an oral suspension form for administration to cats. A major advantage of administering azathioprine in this manner is that any required increase in dosage can be done very accurately. If azathioprine is well tolerated and there has been inadequate clinical improvement, the dosage can be increased from 0.15 mg/lb to 0.2 mg/lb to 0.25 mg/lb every 48 hours.

Another immunosuppressive drug that is used in some cats with severe IBD is chlorambucil (Leukeran). Some clinicians use chlorambucil as an alternative to azathioprine (they are not used in conjunction). Chlorambucil is an alkylating agent. Alkylating agents alter DNA synthesis and inhibit rapidly proliferating cells. Chlorambucil is administered initially at 0.05 to 0.1 mg/lb/day in conjunction with prednisolone at 1 mg/lb/day. The small pill size of chlorambucil (2 mg) allows for easy dosing. Most cats receive one-half tablet (1 mg) per day. Various dosage schedules for cats have been published. An alternate schedule is 0.07 to 0.15 mg/lb every 72 hours. Toxicities are uncommon in cats but may include anorexia, vomiting, and diarrhea, but these problems generally resolve rapidly when chlorambucil is reduced from daily to every-other-day administration. Bone marrow suppression is possible but uncommon and is mild and rapidly reversible when it does occur. Once the desired clinical response is achieved, chlorambucil is gradually tapered over several months while prednisolone is continued as the primary maintenance drug.

Colostrum is currently recognized as an emerging therapy for various inflammatory disorders in human medicine. Some patients with infectious diarrhea caused by *Cryptosporidium parvum* have also benefited from bovine colostrum immunoglobulin concentrate. Animal studies have shown promise, and so colostrum also represents a potential alternative therapy for various disease conditions in animal patients. Colostrum is particularly rich in immunoglobulins, antimicrobial peptides (e.g., lactoferrin and lactoperoxidase), and other bioactive molecules, including growth factors. Recent studies have suggested that the peptide growth factors in colostrum might provide novel treatment options for a variety of GI conditions, as well as other disorders. The growth factors in colostrum include insulinlike growth factor I and II (IGF-1 and IGF-2), epithelial growth factor (EGF), transforming growth factors A and B (TGFs A and B), growth hormone (GH), fibroblast growth factor (FGF), and platelet derived growth factor (PDGF). Bovine colostrum is an excellent source of growth factors and immunoglobulins, and it will most likely be the main source for therapeutic supplies of colostrum, since it is readily available in large supplies, as opposed to human colostrum. The growth factors in bovine colostrum reportedly boost cell and tissue growth by stimulating DNA and RNA formation, and also assist in repairing and replacing cell structures. Other beneficial effects include increases in T cell numbers. Antiaging effects are currently under investigation in humans.

Proposed mechanisms of action for colostrum in IBD include inhibition or prevention of reproduction of pathogenic invaders and protection against toxins through the action of immunoglob-

ulins, lactoferrin, and other immune factors, and stimulation of repair of intestinal membranes at the cellular level through actions of epithelial growth factors. There may also be an enhanced effect of assimilation of nutrients.

Currently colostrum can be considered as an alternative therapeutic option for animals with IBD that are poorly responsive to conventional medications and dietary trials. Colostrum has been effective in improving the stool consistency of some animals with chronic diarrhea caused by IBD. Results in human trials have been promising, and use of colostral-derived preparations may become more prevalent in the next several years. Studies are needed to help determine the most effective dose. Various preparations are currently available in health food stores.

Cats with *hypereosinophilic syndrome* should be treated aggressively as soon as a diagnosis is established. Prednisolone (1.5 to 2 mg/lb divided twice a day for 2 to 4 weeks, then reduced to a maintenance dose of 1 to 1.5 mg/lb/day), metronidazole, and azathioprine should be used in conjunction. Contrary to early reports that characterize this severe eosinophilic enteritis syndrome as very poorly responsive to treatment, *early* aggressive therapy can help achieve a state of remission in some patients that can last for months to several years or more. Cats with *eosinophilic enteritis,* which is a much milder disease than hypereosinophilic syndrome, generally respond well to corticosteroids alone (follow guidelines for treatment of mild to moderate IBD).

Antibacterial therapy can be quite beneficial in some situations, most notably for treatment of patients that are suspected of having a bacterial cause or component of IBD and CPE. Indications for use of antibiotics include histologic changes that include presence of neutrophils or evidence of crypt abscesses or poor initial response to antiinflammatory therapy. Intestinal bacterial problems occur more commonly in dogs than in cats. CPE can cause intermittent or chronic diarrhea (see Chapter 8). Definitive diagnosis requires identification of *C. perfringens* enterotoxin in fresh feces (assay available at commercial laboratories). Amoxicillin, metronidazole, and tylosin appear to be the most effective antibiotics for treatment of CPE. Occasionally only tylosin is effective ($^1/_{16}$ tsp Tylan Soluble powder administered in capsule form twice a day for cats). Cats generally will not eat food to which tylosin powder has been added. Antibiotics used most commonly for bacteria-related intestinal problems in cats include amoxicillin, metronidazole, enrofloxacin, and trimethoprim-sulfa.

Usually a 2- to 4-week course of antibacterial therapy is adequate (adjunctive treatment in cases in which the inflammatory disease is considered most significant). In cats with IBD that experience intermittent flare-ups of diarrhea, the most commonly successful therapeutic maneuvers are use of antibiotics for 2 to 3 weeks at a time or use of more aggressive antiinflammatory measures. Because metronidazole has both antibacterial and antiinflammatory activity, it is an excellent choice for use in cats in which symptoms are not well controlled by corticosteroids alone. Metronidazole is often used in these situations for several months or more at a time.

Some cats with concurrent IBD and colitis may show minimal or no clinical signs of colitis. Initiation of treatment specific for colitis (sulfasalazine [Azulfidine] at 5 to 7 mg/lb two times daily for 7 to 10 days at a time and increased dietary fiber) may result in dramatic improvement in cats with enterocolitis. It is interesting to note, however, that cats with colitis generally demonstrate a much better response to corticosteroids than do dogs. Therefore sulfasalazine is used much less commonly in cats that in dogs.

As described earlier, significant tissue-level cobalamin deficiency is present in some patients with GI disease. This is usually secondary to reduced cobalamin absorptive capacity. Therapy involves administering injectable cobalamin at the following schedule for cats: 250 µg subcutaneously once a week for 6 weeks, then every 2 weeks for the next six doses, then once monthly. Most generic cobalamin preparations contain 1 mg/ml (1000 µg/ml). It is important to note that multivitamin and B-complex injectable formulations contain significantly lower concentration of cobalamin and they also cause pain when injected. Therefore it is recommended that these preparations not be used for cobalamin supplementation. Unless the intestinal disease is totally resolved, long-term and perhaps lifelong supplementation with cobalamin may be necessary. The frequency of injections on a long-term basis is determined by regular measurement of serum cobalamin concentration.

Poor responses to treatment of cats with IBD usually result from the following:

1. Inadequate initial or long-term maintenance corticosteroid dosage

2. Failure to use ancillary medications (metronidazole, azathioprine, chlorambucil) in cases in which disease is moderate to severe

3. Failure to recognize and treat a concurrent condition (e.g., gastric hypomotility disorder that may either be secondary to IBD or idiopathic in nature, hyperthyroidism, parasitism [e.g., *Giardia, Cryptosporidium*], CPE)

4. Poor owner compliance

5. Treatment for only small intestinal inflammatory disease when colitis is present as well (colitis that might respond better to sulfasalazine than to corticosteroids or metronidazole)

6. Failure to recognize and treat low body cobalamin levels (measure serum cobalamin)

7. Failure to identify an effective diet

Management of Dogs With IBD

Specific treatment recommendations for dogs with IBD are as follows. Corticosteroids are the initial treatment of choice for lymphocytic-plasmacytic and eosinophilic enteritis. Mild to moderate cases (as determined by clinical signs, *normal* protein levels, and degree of inflammatory cell infiltrate on biopsy specimens) often respond to prednisone at a dose of 0.25 to 0.75 mg/lb divided twice daily for 2 to 4 weeks, followed by a gradual decrease in 50% increments at 2-week intervals. Alternate-day or every-third-day treatment can often be reached by 2 to 3 months. Occasionally treatment can be discontinued altogether by 3 to 6 months.

Moderate to severe cases and any case in which the total protein is less than 5.5 g/dl should be treated more aggressively using an initial prednisone dose of 1 mg/lb/day for 2 to 4 weeks before an attempt is made to decrease the dose. Dogs in this category often require long-term therapy (months to years) on an every-other-day or every-third-day basis to maintain remission. Use of combination drug therapy (prednisone and metronidazole) in these cases at the outset is recommended to improve chances of controlling clinical signs more quickly and to prevent progression of the disease.

If significantly bothersome side effects are caused by prednisone (e.g., severe polyuria/polydipsia, panting, lethargy), either oral dexamethasone or budesonide can be used instead. Budesonide is a new oral corticosteroid that was described earlier in the section on management of IBD in cats. Its use should be considered in any case where conventional corticosteroids may be problematic, for example, where side effects are very significant or in diabetic animals or those with Cushing's disease that also require management for IBD. In general, budesonide is administered to small dogs at 1 mg once per day. It has been used at higher doses (3 mg per small dog per day), but the lower dose is frequently effective. Large dogs receive 3 mg twice daily initially, and the dosage is later tapered to 3 mg once daily, and then to alternate day administration for longer term use. In some dogs, dexamethasone is much better tolerated than prednisone and side effects are minimal or nonexistent. If prednisone side effects are judged to be severe, it is generally discontinued for 12 to 36 hours to allow for adequate metabolism and clearance. Prednisone may then be reintroduced at 25% to 50% of the previous dose, or, alternatively, dexamethasone can be instituted at a conservative level (0.005 to 0.01 mg/lb/day orally). Some dog breeds are very sensitive to steroids and are poorly tolerant of prednisone doses over 0.5 to 0.75 mg/lb/day. Arctic breeds and rottweilers are often in this category.

As was discussed in the section on treatment of cats with IBD, metronidazole has both antibacterial and antiinflammatory effects. It is very useful in treatment of IBD in dogs, as well as in cats. Metronidazole is administered at 5 to 10 mg/lb two times daily. A major advantage of using combination therapy is that the corticosteroid dose can usually be decreased from the high initial dose in a timely manner, thus decreasing the likelihood of significant corticosteroid-related side effects. Also, I have successfully managed on a long-term basis canine patients with mild to moderate lymphocytic-plasmacytic enteritis that were intolerant to corticosteroids on metronidazole alone.

When prednisone and metronidazole are used in combination, the dosage level of each drug is generally gradually decreased as the patient's condition improves and laboratory parameters (especially protein levels and white blood cell count) return to normal. Corticosteroids are decreased gradually for several months before any reduction is made on the metronidazole dose. If there has been an excellent response, it is possible that metronidazole can be discontinued after several months. Alternatively, if chronic therapy is required, metronidazole can often be administered on a once-daily basis and eventually on an every-

other-day basis. If it is not possible to discontinue medication altogether owing to recurrence of symptoms when no medication is given, control can be maintained with prednisone and/or metronidazole given on an alternate-day basis. If both drugs are used, I often recommend giving prednisone on one day and metronidazole on the alternate day. Occasionally in dogs with moderate to severe IBD or in a case in which both IBD and chronic bacterial overgrowth are present, it is necessary to continue metronidazole on a long-term (months to years) basis (5 to 7 mg/lb twice daily). I have observed no instances of significant complications when this protocol has been used.

Dogs with marked hypoproteinemia (total protein less than 4.5 g/dl) caused by severe lymphocytic-plasmacytic enteritis often respond well when an aggressive therapeutic course is undertaken (prednisone, metronidazole, and azathioprine used in combination). This aggressive approach has led to control of clinical signs and return to a total protein level of greater than 6.0 g/dl (by 2 to 4 months) in a number of cases. One exception to this approach in my experience is that patients with hypoproteinemia resulting from eosinophilic enteritis often respond well to corticosteroids alone.

Combination drug therapy is used early in severe cases or if a side effect to one drug requires that it be used at a lower dose. If corticosteroids are poorly tolerated (e.g., excessive polyuria/polydipsia, listlessness, panting, inappetence associated with steroid hepatopathy) or if corticosteroids and metronidazole are unable to achieve remission, azathioprine should be added to the regimen. Azathioprine is started *early* in the course for cases of lymphocytic-plasmacytic enteritis that cause a protein-losing enteropathy and result in a total protein level less than 4.5 g/dl.

The *canine* dose of azathioprine is 1 mg/lb/day (note significant difference in dose between cats [0.15 mg/lb once every other day] and dogs). If azathioprine is used at the outset, the prednisone dose is decreased by 50% from 1 mg/lb/day after 3 to 4 weeks or based on clinical improvement (i.e., remission of signs and increase in protein levels) and degree of tolerance of this dose of prednisone. Subsequent decreases in the prednisone dose can usually be made at monthly intervals until an alternate-day schedule is reached. If azathioprine is started in any type of IBD case because of significant corticosteroid side effects, the prednisone is initially decreased by 50% to

75% but is not stopped completely unless absolutely necessary because loss of remission might result.

Azathioprine is generally used for 3 to 9 months in dogs. Once adequate control is achieved, the daily dose is decreased by 50%, and subsequently alternate-day therapy is used. Side effects are uncommon in dogs but may include anorexia, jaundice (hepatic damage), poor hair growth, and bone marrow suppression. In addition, it is suspected that azathioprine has the potential to induce pancreatitis (this is an uncommon occurrence, however, in my experience). A complete blood count should be run to monitor for evidence of anemia or leukopenia at 3-week intervals for the first 2 months and then once every several months. Routine monitoring also includes periodic (once every 4 to 6 weeks initially) evaluation of hepatic enzyme levels (increases may be due to corticosteroids and occasionally azathioprine) and protein levels.

Colostrum, which is currently recognized as a potential new adjunctive therapy for IBD patients that do not respond fully to more conventional therapies, was described in the section on management of IBD in cats. There may be indications for use of colostrum in dogs as well. Therapeutic trials in dogs are needed to determine whether or not this is a useful option to consider.

IBD that is initially graded as moderate to severe can usually be managed quite successfully and can be maintained in remission but not often cured. Sometimes follow-up biopsy specimen analyses in severe cases reveal only slight to moderate histologic resolution of inflammatory infiltrates despite excellent clinical control even on lower drug doses. Alternatively, dramatic histologic resolution has been noted in other cases. Treatment decisions (e.g., can treatment be discontinued completely?) ideally are based on a thorough review of clinical response to date (control of clinical signs, levels of medication required, and resolution of hypoproteinemia if it was initially present) and follow-up endoscopic biopsy specimen information.

As a general clinical rule of thumb, an attempt can be made to discontinue therapy after 2 to 3 months of successful control on twice-weekly medication. If signs recur, medication is resumed on a daily basis for 7 to 14 days before a gradual reduction program is started. In some dogs with severe lymphocytic-plasmacytic enteropathy and marked hypoproteinemia, therapy can be successfully discontinued as early as 6 months to 1 year. In others, lifelong treatment is required.

Cobalamin deficiency and associated clinical signs were described in the section on IBD in cats. For dogs that are thought to be deficient in cobalamin, supplementation is as follows: dogs up to 10 lb, 250 μg per injection; 10 to 30 lb, 500 μg per injection; and over 30 lb, 1000 μg per injection. As with cats, injections are administered once weekly for 6 weeks, then every 2 weeks for six doses, and then once monthly. The incidence of low tissue cobalamin levels in dogs with chronic intestinal disease is not known, but it is recommended that dogs with a history of chronic GI disease be investigated for this possibility by running serum cobalamin assays.

Dietary Therapy

In some patients with mild lymphocytic-plasmacytic enteritis or eosinophilic enteritis, dietary modification may lead to partial or complete resolution of clinical signs and even improvement in histologic lesions. In others, dietary therapy may be an important adjunct to pharmacotherapy in the control of clinical signs related to chronic IBD. It is also possible that dietary management used on a long-term basis will effectively help maintain control once drug therapy is discontinued. Potential benefits of dietary therapy include reduction of hypersensitivity reactions to dietary antigens, alteration of bowel motility, and effects on composition of the bowel flora and mucosal morphology and function.

Dietary therapy for IBD may involve use of a strict elimination diet or a balanced commercial diet that contains minimal additives. In most cases, diets that are highly digestible and have low residue work best for small intestinal disease. If a decision is made to manage a patient initially with dietary therapy alone, the dietary trial should be conducted for a minimum of 3 to 4 weeks. Some patients require 6 weeks or more before clinical improvement occurs. If biopsy results reveal moderate to severe IBD and/or if there is any degree of patient compromise, pharmacotherapy should be included in the treatment regimen along with dietary management. In my experience, patients with this degree of disease rarely respond to dietary manipulation alone.

Diets that often work well include those that supply a single source of protein to which the patient has not previously been exposed (i.e., "novel" proteins). These may include lamb, rabbit, venison, duck, whitefish, or low-fat cottage cheese. A single digestible carbohydrate such as boiled rice should be added to home-prepared diets. Many of the premium commercial diets now include optimum levels of omega-6 and omega-3 fatty acids. These agents may be useful in reducing inflammation in the intestine. Dividing feedings into two to three meals per day will help maximize dietary assimilation.

Unusual Complications in Patients With Inflammatory Bowel Disease

Several complications associated with IBD or its treatment have been reported. These include the potential for IBD to progress to lymphoma, hemorrhagic diathesis secondary to intestinal malabsorption of fat and the fat-soluble vitamin K, and toxoplasmosis in cats on immunosuppressive therapy for treatment of IBD.

Lymphoma. It has been recognized in cats, dogs, and humans that IBD can progress to lymphoma. In one report, three of nine cats with lymphocytic-plasmacytic gastroenteritis confirmed by full-thickness biopsy, diagnosed during a 1-year period, subsequently developed GI lymphoma 9 to 18 months after the initial diagnosis. Clinical signs initially resolved in all cats in response to management with hypoallergenic diets but later recurred in the three cats with lymphoma.

To date the progression has been found overall to be an *uncommon* occurrence. No one type of IBD is recognized as more likely than others to progress to lymphoma. It has occurred in cats with an original diagnosis of lymphocytic enteritis, lymphocytic-plasmacytic enteritis, or lymphocytic-plasmacytic-eosinophilic enteritis.

In my four feline cases in which progression occurred, initially there was excellent control of the inflammatory bowel disorder with conventional treatment. All four cats required chronic medication to control clinical signs, and at a range of 1 to 3 years, clinical remission was lost. Follow-up histologic evaluation is recommended in patients with IBD if previous treatment is no longer successful in controlling clinical signs in order to detect and treat lymphoma as early as possible.

Hemorrhagic Diathesis. One report described two cats with hemorrhagic diathesis that was thought to be related to a chronic malabsorp-

tion of fat and the fat-soluble vitamin K. Both cats experienced a sudden onset of bleeding. In one there was an acute intraabdominal bleeding episode, whereas in the other there was spontaneous and extensive subcutaneous hemorrhage. Both cats had marked lymphocytic-plasmacytic enteritis with villous atrophy.

Spontaneous bleeding is an infrequent but well-documented complication of intestinal malabsorption in humans. The acquired hemorrhagic diathesis is characterized as a hypoprothrombinemic disorder secondary to malabsorption of vitamin K. The fact that this occurs infrequently in patients with malabsorption is probably attributable to absorption of bacterially derived vitamin K_2 from the ileum and colon.

Treatment involves subcutaneous injections of vitamin K (oral administration should be avoided because the active absorption of vitamin K from the duodenum is unpredictable in patients with malabsorption). Its use is also indicated before surgery when abnormal clotting is detected. Chronic maintenance therapy (oral vitamin K) may also be required. Dietary fat requirements of patients with malabsorption should be met by short- or medium-chain saturated fatty acids, because absorption of vitamin K is reduced by progressively longer chain fatty acids and greater degrees of unsaturation.

Toxoplasmosis. Intensive immunosuppressive therapy for IBD can potentiate reactivation of latent infections. Toxoplasmosis was reported in two cats that were initially diagnosed with and treated for IBD. *Toxoplasma gondii* was found on follow-up biopsy (full thickness) of the intestine in one cat 9 weeks after endoscopic biopsy specimens had revealed severe lymphocytic-plasmacytic gastroenteritis. Treatment had included prednisone, metronidazole, and azathioprine. Both cats had serologic evidence of active toxoplasmosis. In cats treated with azathioprine, it is hypothesized that active toxoplasmosis was attributable to reactivation of a prior infection, resulting from the immunosuppressive effects of prednisolone and azathioprine. Both cats had no signs of illness other than GI tract disease (diarrhea, weight loss). Recent coincidental infection was considered highly unlikely because both cats were kept strictly indoors and were fed controlled diets.

Experience from these two cases indicates that toxoplasmosis should be considered in cats with IBD if signs of illness (i.e., GI type of signs) occur during treatment with immunosuppressive drugs.

Recurrent signs of IBD may actually *not* be due to failure of the current treatment regimen. Diagnosis of toxoplasmosis is based on serologic documentation of active toxoplasmosis (IgM titers should be done because they may permit earlier diagnosis than is possible with IgG titers) and response to an anti-*Toxoplasma* drug (clindamycin is recommended). Treatment for IBD is continued as needed.

SMALL INTESTINAL BACTERIAL OVERGROWTH

Small intestinal bacterial overgrowth (SIBO) is a syndrome in which there are excessive numbers of bacteria (more than 10^5 organisms per milliliter of intestinal contents) in the duodenum and jejunum in a fasting state. This overproliferation of microflora can result in malabsorption and diarrhea. SIBO is well recognized in dogs and humans, but there are no reports of SIBO in cats.

The normal small intestinal microflora consists of a small but stable population of aerobic and facultative anaerobic bacteria. Population size is influenced by factors such as the host's immune system, bacterial interactions, dietary composition, and the action of normal mechanisms that help to limit bacterial overgrowth (secretion of gastric acid, the dynamic process of intestinal motility and continuous aborad flow of ingesta, and antibacterial factors in pancreatic juice). Causes of overgrowth of bacteria may include anatomic factors such as obstruction (e.g., partial stricture, presence of a mass), segmental hypomotility, conditions associated with decreased secretion of gastric acid, intestinal mucosal disease, immunodeficiency states, and concurrent exocrine pancreatic insufficiency, or it may result from some unidentifiable cause. A state of immunodeficiency may be one of the reasons that SIBO might be more commonly diagnosed in German shepherds and shar-peis than in other breeds. These breeds appear to have a higher incidence of IgA deficiency. The most common problems in dogs with IgA deficiency are recurrent infections and atopic dermatitis. The infections associated with IgA deficiency are generally not severe or life threatening, and treatment is symptomatic.

Although any species of bacteria may be found, *Escherichia coli,* enterococci, and lactobacilli are more common in dogs. Obligate anaerobic species are rarely found in the proximal small intestine of the dog, whereas in cats there may be up to 10^5 to 10^8 bacteria per milliliter of fluid, commonly including obligate anaerobic bacteria such as *Bacteroides, Eubacterium,* and *Fusobacterium.* In cats *Pasteurella* spp. are the most common bacteria isolated.

The pathophysiology of SIBO is very complex and is related to both the effects of proliferation of bacteria in the intestinal lumen and direct damage to enterocytes. Potential mechanisms include direct injurious effects on brush border enzymes and carrier proteins, secretion of enterotoxins, deconjugation of bile acids, hydroxylation of fatty acids, and competition for nutrients.

The most common clinical signs of SIBO are diarrhea and weight loss. Vomiting, flatulence, and anorexia may also occur. Diarrhea is usually of small bowel type of consistency and may be watery to soft formed and malodorous. Stools may also be lighter in color than normal, but this is a nonspecific sign. Blood and mucus are usually not present (if they are, a large bowel disorder of any type should be considered). Other clinical signs that might be present occur as a result of a primary disorder (e.g., ravenous appetite associated with exocrine pancreatic insufficiency, decreased appetite, frequent vomiting, and lethargy associated with obstruction).

Diagnosis

Establishing a *definitive* diagnosis of SIBO is difficult in a private-practice setting. Ideally, *quantitative* duodenal fluid cultures should be done to determine if SIBO is present. This is difficult to do properly and is also expensive. Aliquots of duodenal fluid need to be obtained either at laparotomy or by using a sterilized endoscope to obtain samples from the small intestine. A positive response to antibiotics (e.g., amoxicillin, metronidazole, tetracycline, tylosin) for 2 to 4 weeks can be used as a presumptive diagnosis of SIBO.

The best screening tests for use in private practice involve serum analysis of fasting cobalamin (vitamin B_{12}) and folate levels, although these tests are not regarded as very sensitive, because many affected dogs do not have abnormal test results. Abnormalities that suggest SIBO include elevated folate levels (due to increased production by abnormal microflora) and decreased cobalamin levels (due to utilization by microflora). It is not common for this combination of results to be found. In many patients only one of the two tests is abnormal. In patients with SIBO that is not present in conjunction with exocrine pancreatic insufficiency, elevated folate level is found in approximately 50% of the cases, and decreased cobalamin level alone in about 25% of cases. These tests should be considered in any patient that has chronic diarrhea, including those with exocrine pancreatic insufficiency (these dogs commonly have SIBO). Cobalamin levels that are below the control range may also be consistent with disease affecting the distal small intestine (cobalamin is absorbed only in the last 25% of the distal small intestine). Folate levels *below* the control range may indicate infiltrative disease affecting the proximal small intestine (folate is absorbed in the proximal small intestine only).

A new test for SIBO is serum unconjugated cholic acid (SUCA). Many of the species of bacteria that increase in number in SIBO have the capacity to unconjugate bile acids. Unlike the conjugated bile acids that are normally present in the small intestinal lumen, bile acids that are unconjugated diffuse across the intestinal mucosa into the blood. In dogs, SUCA values greater than 72 nm/L are suggestive of bacterial overgrowth or disturbance of the normal flora of the upper small intestine. The SUCA test is currently available at the Texas A&M University GI Lab.

The sample should be shipped overnight on ice, ideally on the same day on which the sample is obtained. Dogs should be fasted for 12 hours before sampling. When testing for SIBO, it is recommended that serum for cobalamin, folate, and SUCA assays should be run concurrently. Trypsin-like immunoreactivity (TLI) assay should be done as well if pancreatic exocrine insufficiency has not already been ruled out.

It is not uncommon for a dog with IBD to have SIBO as well. Intestinal biopsy specimens from patients with SIBO are normal or may show minimal morphologic mucosal changes. Minor changes may include mild atrophy of villi and a slight increase in inflammatory cells. If intestinal biopsy samples in a dog or cat with chronic diarrhea are normal or exhibit only mild changes, the presence of SIBO should definitely be considered.

Treatment

Treatment of SIBO involves use of selected antibiotics, and treatment time may vary from several weeks to many months. Some patients require intermittent treatment. Sometimes once-daily antibiotic administration is adequate in patients that require long-term therapy. Any identifiable causes should be removed (e.g., surgical removal of blind or stagnant loops of bowel). Antibiotics that have broad-spectrum effect that includes anaerobic bacteria are selected (amoxicillin, metronidazole, tetracycline, and tylosin are good choices). If there is a rapid response to therapy, an attempt to discontinue antibiotic administration can be made after 2 to 3 weeks.

If long-term antibiotic administration seems to be necessary, my preference is usually to use either metronidazole or tylosin powder. The recommended dose of tylosin is 5 to 10 mg/lb orally every 12 hours mixed with food. Tylosin powder has a bitter taste, and some dogs will accept it better if it is mixed in the food initially in very small amounts.

It is emphasized that concurrent problems may be present with SIBO, and even if the bacterial overgrowth is adequately treated, an underlying disorder not yet diagnosed and managed may itself cause persistence of clinical signs.

CHRONIC ENTEROPATHY IN SHAR-PEIS

Shar-peis with chronic diarrhea frequently have PLE due to moderate to severe IBD, and some also likely have intestinal bacterial overgrowth as well. Typical signs in shar-peis often include persistent diarrhea weeks to months in duration, weight loss, and an increased to ravenous appetite. There is almost always evidence of small bowel diarrhea, but in some dogs large intestinal signs such as hematochezia, mucoid feces, and dyschezia are evident as well. I have seen shar-peis that concurrently have vomiting that is due to gastric hypomotility, and occasionally reflux esophagitis is diagnosed as well, based on endoscopic findings of esophageal lesions. Energy level often remains normal or nearly normal until the disease is severe.

The prognosis for successful clinical control of symptoms is excellent as long as a definitive diagnosis is made before the disease becomes too severe. Clinicians are reminded that although a great majority of shar-peis with chronic diarrhea have IBD and some also likely have SIBO, an occasional case of intestinal lymphoma, histoplasmosis, or other disorder may still be found in this breed. Clinical signs and baseline laboratory parameters may be similar in all of these disorders. Therefore it is always best to make every effort to establish a definitive diagnosis rather than simply assuming that the most common problem is indeed present and subsequently administering empiric therapy. This issue should be thoroughly discussed with owners who may initially be reluctant to support the diagnostic testing that is necessary to make a diagnosis.

The most consistent laboratory parameters are panhypoproteinemia (usually ranging from 2.8 to 5.0 g/dl), indicating significant small intestinal involvement, and low cobalamin (vitamin B_{12}) levels, which are very commonly found in shar-peis, and which could be consistent with SIBO. Folate levels are usually either normal or mildly elevated (increased folate is also consistent with SIBO). There may be leukocytosis (often 20,000 to 40,000 cells/μl) with mature neutrophilia (inflammatory leukogram) and mild anemia (most consistent with anemia of chronic disease, rarely blood loss). Eosinophilia is occasionally present. Although the triad of signs of chronic diarrhea, weight loss, and ravenous appetite is strongly suggestive of exocrine pancreatic insufficiency, I have found this disease to be quite uncommon in shar-peis (based on TLI assay results).

In addition to a complete blood count, serum biochemical profile, fecal examinations for parasites (including *Giardia* and *Cryptosporidium*), fecal cytologic examination, fecal analysis for *C. perfringens* enterotoxin, TLI assay for exocrine pancreatic insufficiency, and cobalamin, folate, and SUCA assays for intestinal bacterial overgrowth, shar-peis with chronic diarrhea should undergo upper and lower GI endoscopy to obtain biopsy specimens from the stomach, duodenum, jejunum (if it can be reached), ileum, and colon. Even if there are no clinical signs consistent with large bowel disease, colonoscopy is still done because it is important that biopsy samples be obtained from the ileum. Usually there is diffuse involvement of the small intestine. However, histologic lesions will occasionally be found only in the lower small intestine (this highlights the importance of doing both upper and lower GI endoscopy). Other findings may include esophagitis (grossly evident at endoscopy), gastric hypomotility, and colitis.

Treatment

Treatment of shar-peis usually includes management of IBD and SIBO (prednisone, metronidazole, and amoxicillin or tylosin, which is administered for 1 month if there is laboratory evidence of SIBO). In severe cases of IBD it may be necessary to use azathioprine (see guidelines described earlier in this chapter). It may be useful to administer tylosin powder if the diarrhea is poorly responsive to initial therapy (reasons for poor response may include persistent bacterial overgrowth or CPE that did not respond to metronidazole and/or amoxicillin).

Esophagitis is managed with a restricted-fat diet, H_2-receptor antagonist therapy (e.g., famotidine once daily 30 minutes before food), and metoclopramide. Treatment for gastric hypomotility includes a restricted-fat diet provided in divided feedings two to three times daily and a promotility drug (metoclopramide or cisapride). Colitis is managed with metronidazole, and in some cases sulfasalazine is used as well. Anemia often resolves as the inflammatory disease comes under control. Dietary therapy guidelines previously described for IBD are followed.

Most shar-peis can be managed on a long-term basis, once remission has been achieved, with maintenance doses of prednisone (every 2 to 3 days) and metronidazole (once daily to every other day). In some cases, medication can be discontinued altogether after 6 to 24 months. Hematologic parameters and overall clinical condition should be consistently back to normal before all medication is stopped. Dogs with gastric motility disease (hypomotility) may require lifelong promotility therapy. If there are periodic flare-ups of large intestinal signs, sulfasalazine is used as needed, generally for 7 to 21 days at a time (dose and frequency of administration depend on severity of clinical signs).

▌ GERMAN SHEPHERD DOG ENTEROPATHY

German shepherd dogs appear to be predisposed to an increased incidence of GI diseases such as IBD and SIBO. Practitioners who see German shepherds with any frequency no doubt recognize that these dogs have an increased incidence of diarrhea and sometimes weight loss and other symptoms. It is not known for sure why German shepherds are predisposed to IBD and SIBO, but there are several theories, and perhaps there are at least several factors involved concurrently. Possible factors include the following:

- Genetic susceptibility, as a result of major histocompatibility complex class II antigens
- A breakdown in immunologic tolerance to endogenous bacterial components
- Mucosal permeability and brush border enzyme defects, which may allow increased antigen exposure to the mucosal immune system
- Underlying selective IgA deficiency—German shepherd dogs with small intestinal disease have been shown to have a relative deficiency of IgA secretion from the small intestinal mucosa
- IBD in German shepherd dogs is accompanied by marked disturbances in inflammatory cell populations and the cytokine profile

It is possible that IBD and SIBO in German shepherds are part of a single disease syndrome. It is also possible, given that SIBO is more common in young animals and IBD is more common in older dogs, that SIBO can predispose to IBD. There is currently no substantiation of this hypothesis, but studies are ongoing.

Clinical signs in German shepherds are variable. The most common signs of SIBO are diarrhea and weight loss or failure to thrive. Signs of IBD are more variable and in addition to diarrhea and weight loss may include vomiting, flatulence, decreased appetite, and other signs. German shepherd dogs with GI signs should be investigated in the same manner as has been described for intestinal disease earlier in this chapter. Problems other than SIBO and/or IBD may be present, so a thorough diagnostic work-up should be recommended. In addition to a baseline of a complete blood count, biochemical profile, and urinalysis, other tests should include fecal tests for nematode parasites, *Giardia, Cryptosporidium,* and *Clostridium perfringens* enterotoxin, TLI assay if exocrine pancreatic insufficiency has not already been ruled out, determination of serum cobalamin and folate levels, and SUCA or other currently recommended indirect test for SIBO, and upper and lower GI endoscopy for procurement of intestinal biopsy specimens. Alternatively, if there are minimal signs and the dog's condition remains good overall, a trial with antibiotics (see treatment section) for 4 to 6 weeks may be attempted. A positive response would be suggestive of SIBO. It will then need to be deter-

mined if antibiotics should be continued on a long-term or intermittent basis.

Treatment

If it is thought that the problem is limited to SIBO and/or IBD, it is generally recommended that antibiotics alone be used initially, unless there is a moderate or of course severe degree of IBD present, in which case immunosuppressive therapy is also indicated. Antibiotics may include oxytetracycline, metronidazole, or tylosin. Initially a course of 4 to 6 weeks is prescribed, and then if there has been a good response, the medication can be discontinued. The dog is then observed for relapse, and if this occurs, the antibiotic therapy should be reinstituted. Again, it is important that other causes of diarrhea be ruled out, if they have not been already, and an effort to look for evidence of CPE must be made. CPE sometimes responds to metronidazole and more consistently, especially in chronic cases, to tylosin. Fiber supplementation is also very beneficial in management of CPE. For SIBO and IBD, a highly digestible low-residue diet is generally preferred, so dietary trials may be necessary, along with a thorough diagnostic effort, to determine which type of diet is most indicated. If there is an excellent response to antibiotics and the diarrhea recurs when they are discontinued, antibiotics can be used either continuously on a low-dose basis (I prefer to use tylosin in this situation as a first choice and metronidazole as a second choice), or pulse therapy may be used, in which case antibiotics are administered once daily two to three times a week. In some dogs this is sufficient to maintain control.

If IBD is present and not responsive to antibiotics and dietary management, immunosuppressive drugs are used following the guidelines described earlier in this chapter. In general I rarely find it necessary to use a prednisone dose greater than 0.5 mg/lb per day in German shepherd dogs.

LYMPHOCYTIC-PLASMACYTIC ENTERITIS OF BASENJIS

Lymphocytic-plasmacytic enteritis of basenjis is an immunoproliferative process involving primarily the small intestine. This is a potentially severe form of IBD that is thought to result from a genetic disorder of immune regulation. There is an intense infiltration of lymphocytes and plasma cells in the intestinal mucosa. Other changes often include gastric rugal hypertrophy, lymphocytic gastritis and/or gastric mucosal atrophy, blunting and widening of intestinal villi, and mild dilation of lacteals.

The disorder is often progressive in nature. Clinical signs may tend to be intermittent for a period of time before they worsen and become more persistent. GI signs may be exacerbated by episodes of "stress," such as traveling, boarding, or other medical disorders. Clinical signs usually include small intestinal diarrhea, which may become intractable, vomiting, and/or inappetence. Weight loss can become significant as the disease progresses. Ulcerative dermatitis of the pinnae occasionally occurs in conjunction with this disease. Most affected basenjis demonstrate clinical signs by 3 to 4 years of age.

Basenji enteropathy is commonly associated with hypoalbuminemia and hyperglobulinemia, especially in advanced cases. Neutrophilic leukocytosis and mild nonregenerative anemia are commonly present as well. Early in the disease course, basenji enteropathy may mimic other forms of IBD (e.g., mild symptoms, no significant laboratory abnormalities).

As the disease becomes more advanced, signs and laboratory parameters are characteristic; however, clinicians should be aware that other forms of intestinal disease, such as lymphoma, lymphangiectasia, or histoplasmosis, may be present, and the symptoms of any of these diseases can mimic basenji enteropathy. Therefore it is always best to confirm the diagnosis by doing intestinal biopsies before instituting aggressive immunosuppressive therapy.

Treatment of basenji enteropathy is based on control of the inflammatory bowel component (see guidelines for treatment of IBD in dogs described earlier in this chapter), management of intestinal bacterial overgrowth if it is present, and feeding a controlled or hypoallergenic diet. Because the disease is often progressive, basenjis with this disorder should be carefully monitored. Over time, treatment may need to include combination immunosuppressive drugs and use of long-term antibiotics (e.g., metronidazole, tylosin). If there is evidence of gastric hypomotility, a promotility drug (metoclopramide or cisapride) is also used. Most basenjis die within 2 to 3 years of diag-

nosis, although some affected dogs can be maintained for a period of years with careful monitoring and ongoing therapy. Affected dogs should not be bred.

LYMPHANGIECTASIA

Intestinal lymphangiectasia is a chronic protein-losing enteropathy of dogs that results in malabsorption. It is characterized by obstruction and dysfunction of the intestinal lymphatic network. Lymphatic obstruction leads to stasis of chyle within dilated lacteals and lymphatics of the bowel wall and mesentery. Lymphatic hypertension results, and overdistended lacteals release intestinal lymph into the intestinal lumen either by extravasation or by rupture, resulting in loss of protein, lymphocytes, and chylomicrons. Although proteins may be digested and resorbed to some extent, loss in patients with a significant degree of lymphatic obstruction eventually exceeds the normal recovery mechanism, and hypoproteinemia results.

At the time of presentation, dogs with lymphangiectasia frequently have marked hypoproteinemia. Prominent clinical consequences include body cavity effusions (ascites, hydrothorax) and dependent pitting edema of the subcutis and limbs. In addition to hypoproteinemia, leakage of fat (chylomicrons) from the lacteals may cause inflammation and granuloma formation in the intestinal wall, which may further exacerbate lymphatic obstruction.

Potential causes of lymphatic obstruction include congenital malformation of the lymphatic system; infiltration or obstruction due to an inflammatory, fibrosing, or neoplastic process; obstruction of lymph flow through the thoracic duct; and pericarditis or congestive heart failure. Generalized inflammatory disease of the intestinal lymphatic network is probably the most common factor in pathogenesis of the disease. The cause of this inflammation is undetermined in most cases. Most dogs with lymphangiectasia also have mild to moderate lymphocytic-plasmacytic infiltration in the lamina propria. The fact that patients with lymphangiectasia often respond better when corticosteroids are included in the treatment regimen adds credence to the theory that an inflammatory process is involved in the pathogenesis of the disease.

Lymphangiectasia is not commonly encountered in clinical practice. Of the diseases that cause protein-losing enteropathy, IBD (especially severe lymphocytic-plasmacytic enteritis) is by far the most common. Although some dogs with lymphangiectasia respond well to treatment, this disease is not as consistently responsive to therapy as is IBD. Breed predilections for intestinal lymphangiectasia are not documented, but there seems to be an increased incidence in Yorkshire terriers, soft-coated wheaten terriers, lundehunds, and rottweilers. Lymphangiectasia should be a leading consideration if hypoproteinemia is detected in any of these breeds.

Clinical Signs

The most common clinical manifestations of lymphangiectasia are diarrhea and weight loss. It is important to note, however, that some dogs do not have diarrhea until the disease process is advanced, or there may be no incidence of diarrhea at all. Initial presentation may be directly related to signs associated with significant hypoalbuminemia and the effects of reduced colloidal osmotic pressure, including peripheral edema, ascites, and increased respiratory rate and/or distress secondary to hydrothorax. The onset of clinical signs may be acute (less than 21 days in 10 of 17 dogs in one reported case series) or chronic (greater than 21 days in 7 of 17 dogs).

When present, diarrhea is usually watery to semisolid in consistency. It may be persistent or intermittent. Vomiting may be observed in dogs with lymphangiectasia (11 of 17 dogs in one case series). Progressive weight loss is common.

Diagnosis

A definitive diagnosis of lymphangiectasia is made only on intestinal biopsy specimen analysis. The index of suspicion is heightened when the following test results are identified:

- Panhypoproteinemia (often between 2.5 and 5.0 g/dl total protein at the time of diagnosis, with albumin frequently in the range of 0.8 to 1.6 g/dl)
- Absolute lymphopenia (found in approximately 70% of cases and due to loss of lymphocytes into the gut lumen)
- Hypocholesterolemia
- Hypocalcemia

Lymphopenia is also a common hematologic finding in "stressed" patients however, and this factor should not be overlooked when the hemogram

is reviewed (a "stress" leukogram also includes neutrophilia and eosinopenia).

Lymphangiectasia must be differentiated from other protein-losing enteropathies and from nonintestinal causes of hypoproteinemia (primarily liver and kidney disease). If hypoproteinemia occurs in association with kidney and liver disease, it is usually primarily due to a decrease in the albumin fraction (impaired synthesis in liver disease and increased loss through the glomeruli in protein-losing glomerulonephropathy). Liver function testing (e.g., serum bile acids assay) and urine protein determinations (e.g., urine protein-creatinine ratio) are very useful in evaluating for presence of liver and kidney disease.

Intestinal biopsy specimens can be obtained at either endoscopy or surgery. Endoscopy offers a safer approach to obtaining small bowel biopsy samples in protein-losing enteropathy cases in which there is concern that full-thickness biopsy sites may heal slowly. This is an especially important consideration in patients with a total protein level less than 3.5 g/dl. Lymphangiectasia has a characteristic histologic appearance. The severity of lesions is usually graded as mild, moderate, or severe. Lymphangitis may be present as well. Concurrent inflammatory cell infiltrates are usually found on histologic examination.

In some cases pronounced gross changes can be seen at endoscopy (white "cottony" appearance or multifocal white granular foci of the mucosa, occasional presence of pooled mucoid lymph fluid in the intestinal lumen). Occasionally a diagnosis of lymphangiectasia is missed if only the descending duodenum is examined and sampled during biopsy. In dogs with hypoproteinemia associated with chronic diarrhea, it is best to examine *both* upper (duodenum, and jejunum if it can be reached) and lower small intestine (the ileum can be entered after traversing the colon) to obtain samples from as many areas as possible. This approach maximizes the likelihood that representative biopsy samples will be obtained.

Gross lesions that may be observed at laparotomy include a prominent weblike network of dilated milky-white lymphatic channels; small yellow-white granulomas (lipogranulomas) adjacent to lymphatics; patchy, foamy white deposits on the serosa; and diffuse intestinal thickening. As is the case any time full-thickness intestinal biopsy samples are obtained from a hypoproteinemic patient, serosal patch grafting and nonabsorbable suture material should be used to minimize chances of dehiscence and peritonitis.

I have found that it is very difficult to diagnose lymphangiectasia in rottweilers endoscopically. This is primarily because lesions in this breed are frequently most prominent in the jejunum, an area of the small intestine that is difficult to reach in large-breed dogs with an endoscope. Typical clinical signs in rottweilers include weight loss, chronic intermittent diarrhea, decreased appetite, and occasionally peripheral edema. There is usually significant hypoproteinemia (often ranging from 2.8 to 4.0 g/dl). The lymphocyte count is frequently but not always low. Biopsy specimens from duodenum and ileum often reveal only mild lymphocytic-plasmacytic enteritis in rottweilers with lymphangiectasia. This mild degree of inflammatory infiltrate is not enough to explain the degree of hypoproteinemia and clinical signs that are often present, and this finding certainly should raise suspicions that a more significant process is involved.

If a disorder that is consistent with the clinical presentation is diagnosed at endoscopy (e.g., moderate to severe IBD), treatment for that disorder should be instituted. If there is suspicion that a disease other than what was diagnosed at endoscopy is present, ideally exploratory surgery should be done next to evaluate the serosa and mesentery for gross evidence of lymphangiectasia and to obtain full-thickness intestinal biopsy samples. If the dog is judged to be a poor surgical candidate, treatment for lymphangiectasia and IBD should be instituted. The prognosis for reasonable control in rottweilers is guarded to fair. The prognosis is better if the dog eats enough of the prescribed diet to effect weight gain.

Treatment

The cornerstone of treatment for lymphangiectasia is dietary management. Corticosteroids are used to reduce the intestinal inflammation that is often present. As is true any time there is a chronic enteropathy, an effort is made to investigate as thoroughly as possible for other disorders that may be present at the same time. For example, I have treated dogs with lymphangiectasia that concurrently had CPE and intestinal parasites. Bacterial overgrowth should always be considered as well. Response to treatment is best when all disorders are adequately treated.

The ideal diet for lymphangiectasia should contain minimal fat (long-chain triglycerides) and provide an ample quantity of high-quality protein.

Absorption of long-chain triglycerides from the diet stimulates an increase in intestinal lymph flow, thus promoting further engorgement of intestinal lacteals and subsequent loss of more protein. Fat restriction helps decrease lymphatic hypertension by decreasing lymph flow and aids in controlling diarrhea, presumably by reducing steatorrhea.

Initially a home-prepared diet that includes nonfat or low-fat cottage cheese as the primary protein source and carbohydrate sources such as boiled rice, potatoes, and pasta is fed (one part cottage cheese and three parts carbohydrate source). White turkey and potatoes is a formulation that also works well for some dogs. Yogurt can also be used as a source of protein. Diets should be supplemented with a fat-soluble vitamin.

One of the greatest difficulties encountered in managing dogs with lymphangiectasia is that some tend to be inappetent, even when corticosteroids are included in the treatment regimen. Owners should be encouraged to try a variety of low-fat foods until they find something that the dog will eat. Sometimes breakfast cereals are readily ingested. Persistent coaxing may be required. Once a dog with lymphangiectasia begins to eat well, there is often noticeable clinical improvement and the prognosis gradually begins to improve. For example, removal of ascitic fluid from a significantly distended abdomen may promote a return to a normal appetite. An appetite stimulant such as cyproheptadine is sometimes effective. Frequent divided feedings should be provided initially.

As improvement in overall condition occurs (increase in weight, resolution of diarrhea if it was present, increase in serum protein levels), commercial foods can be added gradually on a trial basis. Some clinicians elect to feed commercial diets at the outset of therapy. Special commercial diets such as Innovative Veterinary Diets (IVD) Select Care Canine Sensitive formula, IVD Vegetarian Diet, Iams Low Residue (Iams Food Co), and Prescription Diet i/d and/or w/d (Hill's Pet Products) can be tried. One significant disadvantage of feeding low-fat calorie-restricted diets such as Prescription Diet r/d in dogs with lymphangiectasia is that when this type of food is used as the primary diet, it is difficult to meet the patient's total energy requirements. Palatability can also be a problem. Some dogs do best when fed a combination of home-prepared and commercial foods. Long-term dietary management is required in most cases.

Most dogs with lymphangiectasia benefit from corticosteroid therapy. Prednisone is administered at 1 to 1.5 mg/lb daily for 2 to 4 weeks and then gradually decreased to a maintenance level of 0.1 to 0.2 mg/lb every other day. If there is an excellent response to dietary management and corticosteroids, the corticosteroids can often be discontinued after 3 to 6 months' total treatment time.

If there is poor weight gain despite adequate food intake, it is sometimes beneficial to supplement the diet with medium-chain triglycerides (MCT Oil). Medium-chain triglycerides are hydrolyzed more rapidly and efficiently than long-chain triglycerides and are absorbed directly into the portal system, thus bypassing the diseased lymphatics. The primary purpose of supplementing the diet with medium-chain triglycerides is to supply extra calories. MCT Oil contains 8 kcal/ml. The recommended dose is 0.5 to 1 ml/lb mixed in food. Because most dogs (and humans!) do not like the taste of MCT Oil, gradual introduction and thorough mixing in the food are recommended. I do not routinely recommend using MCT Oil with dogs other than those that I feel will significantly benefit from its use.

▌PYTHIOSIS

Pythiosis is a severe and often fatal cause of chronic GI or cutaneous disease in dogs living mostly in tropical or subtropical climates. In the United States most cases are seen in the Gulf Coast region, but it has been seen as far north as southern Indiana, Missouri, Kentucky, and North Carolina. There are also rare cases in cats that involve mostly invasive subcutaneous lesions. Pythiosis is caused by the aquatic oomycete *Pythium insidiosum*. The infective stage of *P. insidiosum* is thought to be the zoospore, which is released into warm water environments. Infection is caused either through encystment in the skin or through ingestion. GI pythiosis causes severe segmental transmural thickening of the GI tract with variable mucosal ulceration and mesenteric lymphadenopathy.

There are other fungal agents of the class Zygomycetes that can cause severe intestinal and skin disease. It is difficult to differentiate some of the agents, however, and so the general term *zygomycosis* is often used. Dogs with zygomycosis oftentimes are undifferentiated from those cases with pythiosis. These infections were formerly misnamed *phycomycosis* (outdated name that should no longer be used).

Historically, definitive diagnosis of pythiosis and zygomycosis has been difficult because of the challenges inherent in obtaining a culture-based confirmation of these organisms. Therefore a presumptive diagnosis has often been made (i.e., "suspected pythiosis") based on histopathologic findings. Newer tests are now available that are making specific diagnosis somewhat easier.

Clinical signs include chronic intractable diarrhea and vomiting, loss of appetite, depression, and chronic weight loss. The diarrhea may become bloody due to intestinal necrosis and ulceration. Extensive granulomatous reaction may cause palpable enteromesenteric masses to develop. There may eventually be spread to other abdominal viscera.

Baseline laboratory tests may reveal mild to moderate nonregenerative anemia, neutrophilic leukocytosis, and panhypoproteinemia. Survey abdominal radiography may reveal a mass effect, and barium contrast radiography may identify an area of obstruction. Abdominal ultrasonography can identify intestinal thickening and lymphadenopathy. Rectal scraping cytologic analysis may reveal organisms as may a fecal culture. Historically diagnosis has been dependent on histologic identification of characteristic hyphae in biopsy samples of stomach, intestine, or abdominal lymph nodes. Diagnostic tissue samples are best obtained surgically, because endoscopic biopsy techniques do not reliably harvest adequate tissue in all cases for diagnosis of pythiosis. Extensive tissue reaction may be evident at laparotomy, and this should not be mistaken for neoplasia. It is best to obtain tissues and await a histologic diagnosis rather than making assumptions based on visual inspection alone.

The clinical faculty at Louisiana State University has extensive experience in diagnosis and management of pythiosis and zygomycosis, and some promising new tests have recently been developed in their laboratory. These include polymerase chain reaction (PCR)-based assays and serologic analysis. There is now a PCR test available for identification of *P. insidiosum*. This assay can be applied to DNA extracted either from cultured isolates or from appropriately preserved infected tissue samples. The test will reliably differentiate *P. insidiosum* from other *Pythium* species. A new highly specific and sensitive mycelial antigen-based ELISA assay for the detection of anti–*P. insidiosum* antibodies is also now available for use on samples from both dogs and cats. This test provides an excellent means for making an early, noninvasive diagnosis and also provides an excellent means for monitoring response to therapy. This is especially important with regard to the GI form of the disease because, unlike skin lesions, the lesions cannot be visually monitored by the owner.

Treatment

The treatment of choice for pythiosis is aggressive surgical removal of lesions. Complete resection provides the best chance for long-term cure. For intestinal lesions the goal is to resect infected tissues with 4- to 6-cm margins. Postoperative medical management is also necessary, because there is always a chance for local recurrence. Medical management using itraconazole either with or without terbinafine is recommended for a period of 2 to 4 months after surgery. Drug cost is a significant concern for some owners. If medical management cannot be afforded, then ELISA serologic analysis is recommended at several-month intervals for up to a year after surgery to monitor for evidence of recurrence.

Medical management alone is often unrewarding, but this is the only choice in patients that have diffuse nonresectable disease. The internal medicine service at Louisiana State University has reported that in recent years about 15% of their cases of pythiosis in dogs have responded to either itraconazole at 5 mg/lb every 24 hours for 3 to 6 months or amphotericin B lipid complex (Abelcet) 1 to 1.5 mg/lb administered intravenously over several hours every other day to a cumulative dose of 11 to 12.5 mg/lb. The drugs can also be used in combination, or, alternatively, itraconazole and terbinafine (2.5 to 5 mg/lb per 24 hours) can be used in combination. Combination has been shown to achieve a better response overall, although the prognosis still remains very guarded.

SHORT BOWEL SYNDROME

Short bowel syndrome refers to the clinical consequences of massive small bowel resection, with or without some additional loss of large intestine. Short bowel syndrome frequently results when 75% or more of the small intestine is resected. Reasons for massive bowel resection include intussusception, intestinal infarction secondary to strangulation or vascular thrombosis, loss of blood supply due to injury, and intestinal neoplasia. Clinical manifestations of short bowel syndrome persist when the remaining intestine is unable to undergo adequate compensatory changes. SIBO may also become a significant complicating factor, especially if the ileocolic valve is removed.

Affected patients usually have unrelenting small bowel diarrhea and progressive weight loss in the face of a ravenous appetite. It should be noted, however, that not all patients that lose a large amount of small intestine have signs of short bowel syndrome. It is not always the amount of bowel loss that determines whether or not a patient will be affected. The response to bowel loss is often unpredictable. Clinically, sometimes a patient will do surprisingly well when it was anticipated that the prognosis would be poor, and in other cases a patient will do unexpectedly poorly. Several important factors are involved in determining clinical course. These include the following:

1. Status of the ileocolic valve (symptoms are consistently worse if the valve is lost)
2. The extent and site of bowel resection
3. The functional capacity of the remaining bowel and other digestive organs
4. The degree of adaptation that subsequently occurs in the remaining small and large intestine

The ileocolic valve is important for preventing SIBO, and it may also play an important role in slowing small intestinal transit time.

Maldigestion and malabsorption are prominent features of short bowel syndrome. Factors causing malabsorption include decreased absorptive surface area; reduced transit time, which results in inadequate intestinal mucosa–nutrient contact time; decreased bile salt reabsorption, especially if the ileum is lost, resulting in decreased fat absorption; and decreased fatty acid absorption, which results in impairment of colonic water absorption.

Maldigestion results from decreased nutrient contact time with digestive enzymes; deficiency of cholecystokinin and secretin in patients with significant resection of duodenum and jejunum, which subsequently causes decreased release of pancreatic and biliary exocrine secretions; and loss of important mucosal brush border digestive enzymes, which follows massive bowel resection. Gastric acid hypersecretion may also occur after massive small bowel resection, for unknown reasons. Consequences of acid hypersecretion may include inactivation of pancreatic lipase and increased osmolarity in the small intestinal lumen.

The degree of adaptation that occurs in the small intestine is an important factor in determining whether or not a patient will be able to recover sufficiently to maintain adequate fluid balance and body weight. Over time following massive bowel resection, compensatory changes that increase the absorptive surface of the remaining intestine occur. The fact that it takes time for compensation to occur is an important clinical point, because it is important that a decision resulting in too early euthanasia of a patient not be made too hastily. These include increased bowel diameter, lengthening of villi, and crypt enlargement to maximize the number of mucosal cells per unit length of gut. One of the most important factors in promoting adaptation is the presence of intraluminal nutrients (long-chain triglycerides or long-chain free fatty acids have been shown to have the greatest trophic effect, but any nutrient may promote a stimulatory effect). Pancreaticobiliary secretions, GI and other hormones, and prostaglandin E_2 also play a role in stimulating bowel adaptation. Corticosteroids probably do not have any significant effect on promoting bowel adaptation.

Clinical Signs

In patients that have undergone extensive resection, persistent diarrhea that is often watery in nature is the predominant early sign. Dehydration and electrolyte deficiencies can readily occur. Postoperative treatment is directed at preventing these factors from becoming significant. Malabsorption predominates during the ensuing weeks, and major weight loss and nutritional deficiencies develop. Later, as intestinal adaptation begins to occur, body weight frequently stabilizes, although at levels that are mildly to moderately below preresection levels. Diarrhea and steatorrhea persist in most patients. In some patients, especially those that have lost the ileocolic valve, steatorrhea and malabsorption continue to be severe and the prognosis for stabilization becomes very poor.

Treatment

The primary goal of medical therapy for patients with short bowel syndrome involves providing adequate nutritional support and controlling diarrhea through use of antidiarrheal agents. Gastric acid hypersecretion can be an important causative factor of diarrhea and should be controlled with H_2-receptor antagonists (e.g., famotidine). Intestinal bacterial overgrowth is managed with antibiotics (metronidazole and amoxicillin or enrofloxacin are often used initially; metronidazole and/or tylosin are often used if long-term antibiotics are required). It is sometimes useful to provide pancreatic enzyme replacement therapy (e.g., Pancrezyme). If diarrhea is persistently watery, an antidiarrheal agent such as loperamide is used. The dose for dogs is 0.05 to 0.1 mg/lb orally two to three times daily. Loperamide can be used in cats at 0.025 to 0.04 mg/lb every 12 hours. In some patients, it may be necessary to use loperamide on a long-term basis.

If the treatments listed above are not considered reasonably effective, several other maneuvers can be tried. Research work published in Japan in 1992 suggested that ursodeoxycholate (UDCA) is beneficial in some dogs with short bowel syndrome. The study involved resection of 75% of the small intestine in healthy beagle dogs followed by separation of the dogs into one of three treatment groups:

1. 300 mg UDCA plus 0.375 µg of vitamin D_3 every other day
2. 0.375 µg vitamin D_3 every other day
3. Control group, no drug therapy

Dogs medicated with UDCA experienced significant improvements in body weight, fecal characteristics, and overall nutritional status. The beneficial effect of UDCA may be in prolongation of intestinal transit time. Other investigators have also found that UDCA has an inhibitory effect on GI smooth muscle.

Finally, use of a hydrophilic laxative may help decrease fluidity of the existing bowel content and increase fecal bulk. Among the compounds that may be tried are methylcellulose (Citrucel), psyllium (Metamucil, Siblin), Karaya gum, and calcium polycarbophil (Fiberall, Fiber Con). Calcium polycarbophil reportedly absorbs 60 to 100 times its weight in water.

The ideal form of nutritional support during the early postoperative period is total parenteral nutrition (TPN) (see Chapter 12). TPN is routinely used in humans with short bowel syndrome to maintain caloric intake, electrolyte balance, and acid-base balance for as long as 1 to 2 months of the initial phase of therapy. This is not feasible in most veterinary patients.

Partial parenteral nutrition can also be used to help provide adequate early nutritional support.

ProcalAmine (McGaw, Inc) is a protein-sparing product that is very convenient for use in clinical practice because no mixing or additives are required. It is a combination of 3% amino acids, 3% glycerol, and electrolytes. If infused at maintenance rates (30 ml/lb/day), this product provides approximately 20% of a patient's caloric needs and 0.6 to 0.9 g/lb/day of protein. ProcalAmine contains inadequate sodium (35 mEq/L) and chloride (41 mEq/L) for total maintenance requirements. Addition of 65 ml of 7.2% hypertonic saline to a liter of ProcalAmine increases electrolyte levels sufficiently (sodium, 115 mEq/L). ProcalAmine does contain adequate potassium (24 mEq/L). A peripheral vein can be used. ProcalAmine is hypertonic, and the catheter site should be watched carefully for any evidence of phlebitis. Catheters are not left in place any longer than 60 to 72 hours.

Limited oral intake is instituted as soon as possible after surgery to begin stimulation of intestinal adaptation. Elemental or polymeric diets are often fed in the initial phase. Long-term feeding involves diets that are low in fat and highly digestible. Small amounts should be fed frequently (three to four meals per day). Vitamin B$_{12}$ (cobalamin) as well as fat-soluble vitamins should be supplemented indefinitely.

If intestinal adaptation occurs, a stable body weight and a reasonable stool consistency can be maintained on a long-term basis. Some patients, however, never stabilize despite all treatment efforts and careful dietary manipulation, and their prognosis becomes poor. *The prognosis seems to be better in patients that are aggressively managed in the early stages.* Because it can be very difficult to predict accurately how well a patient with short bowel syndrome will respond to therapy, every effort should be made to maintain treatment for a reasonable period of time before euthanasia is recommended.

Careful consideration about how much bowel will be resected should be given at the time of surgery. Prevention of situations that may end with development of short bowel syndrome begins with avoiding unnecessarily extensive resection of small intestine, considering conservative resection of ischemic bowel with the option of follow-up surgery if necessary, and making every effort to leave the duodenum and ileocolic valve intact. Early diagnosis and timely surgical intervention in situations that might end up requiring intestinal resection are extremely important in mini-mizing the amount of intestine that will need to be removed.

NEOPLASIA OF THE SMALL INTESTINE

Neoplasia of the small intestine is discussed in detail in Chapter 11. A summary is provided here.

Tumors of the small intestine occur uncommonly. GI neoplasms account for approximately 2% of all canine and feline neoplasms. Intestinal neoplasms of dogs and cats are usually malignant. Although neoplasia is uncommon overall, in cats intestinal lymphoma is now diagnosed with increased frequency. This is important to recognize because cats with intestinal lymphoma, especially the type now referred to as chronic low-grade lymphocytic lymphoma, often respond well to chemotherapy if the diagnosis is made relatively early in the disease course. The most common malignant neoplasms of the intestinal tract are lymphoma and adenocarcinoma. Other tumors affecting the intestinal tract include mast cell tumor, fibrosarcoma, leiomyoma, leiomyosarcoma, undifferentiated sarcoma, carcinoids, plasmacytoma, and neurolemmoma.

Most dogs with intestinal neoplasia are middle-age or older (7 years or more). A majority of dogs with lymphoma and adenocarcinoma are males. There is no apparent sex predilection in cats with intestinal neoplasia. Siamese cats appear to be at greater risk for developing adenocarcinoma of the intestine.

The most common clinical signs of intestinal neoplasia are weight loss, vomiting, diarrhea, and lethargy. Inappetence is often apparent as the disease advances. Other signs may include melena, hematemesis, anemia, fever, icterus, and abdominal effusion. Although clinical signs in most patients are slowly progressive, dogs with intestinal adenocarcinoma are occasionally presented because of acute signs that may mimic intestinal obstruction (e.g., acute frequent vomiting, anorexia, lethargy).

Physical examination may reveal pallor, cachexia, thickened intestinal loops, an isolated intestinal mass, intraabdominal lymphadenopathy, dilated intestinal loops, organomegaly (liver, spleen), abdominal effusion, and peripheral edema (most often due to hypoproteinemia associated with diffuse intestinal lymphoma).

Hematologic and biochemical parameters are often normal, although anemia (anemia of chronic disease or anemia consistent with blood loss) and hypoproteinemia may be present. Hypoproteinemia may be due to either blood loss into the intestine or diffuse infiltrative intestinal disease. Neutrophilic leukocytosis and elevated hepatic enzymes may also be present.

Useful procedures in evaluating patients for evidence of intestinal neoplasia include survey radiography, ultrasonography, and endoscopy. Pulmonary metastases are rarely detected on thoracic radiography in patients with small intestinal neoplasia. Survey abdominal radiographs may reveal a soft tissue opacity consistent with a mass or lymphadenopathy, or signs of intestinal obstruction. Contrast radiography can be helpful for delineating regions of significant mucosal irregularity, luminal narrowing, and intramural thickening. Narrowing of the lumen is commonly seen with carcinoma, which has a tendency to be annular (Figure 7-3). Annular indicates that there is 360-degree constriction. Intramural disease usually produces radiographic signs of thickening, rigidity of the wall, and narrowing of the lumen.

Abdominal ultrasonography is useful for defining abdominal mass lesions (e.g., confirming presence of a mass effect, delineating intestinal versus lymph node involvement, examining for hepatic involvement).

A definitive diagnosis of intestinal neoplasia can be made only on histologic examination of biopsy material. Biopsy specimens are most commonly obtained via either endoscopy or exploratory laparotomy. Percutaneous fine-needle aspiration under either ultrasound or laparoscopic guidance can be used in selected cases in which the involved area can be isolated and stabilized for needle insertion. Endoscopy is particularly useful for examining and procuring biopsy samples from the duodenum and terminal ileum. Intestinal lymphoma (either diffuse or focal) can be reliably diagnosed in a majority (approximately 90%) of dogs and cats when proper biopsy instrumentation and technique are used. Mass lesions can be very reliably diagnosed (samples should be obtained as deeply as possible). Laparotomy offers the advantage of thorough exploration of the abdomen with biopsy and possibly complete excision of involved areas.

Intestinal lymphoma in cats and dogs will be discussed here, and the reader is referred to Chapter 11 for a more detailed discussion of neoplasia of the small intestine. Intestinal lymphoma is discussed here as well because clinically it can appear very similar to IBD in cats.

Lymphoma

In cats chronic low-grade lymphocytic lymphoma can be very similar to IBD in the way it manifests itself clinically. It can only be differentiated based on biopsy specimen analysis. Because cats with chronic low-grade lymphocytic lymphoma often have a reasonably good prognosis when indicated treatment is administered, it is incumbent on veterinarians to make the correct diagnosis early in the disease course, rather than later, when it may be more difficult to successfully manage the patient.

The GI tract is a common site of extranodal lymphoma in dogs and cats. In cats intestinal lymphoma is caused by feline leukemia virus, although as few as 12% to 30% have been reported to be viremic. However, more recent studies using PCR methods suggest that the incidence of feline leukemia virus in lymphoma may be as high as 63%. The cause in dogs is unknown. GI lymphoma reportedly arises from B lymphocytes of the gut-associated lymphoid tissue (GALT) in most cases in dogs and cats.

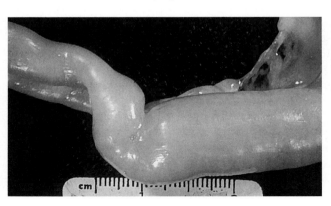

FIGURE 7-3 Adenocarcinoma involving the ileum of a cat. Note annular constriction and dilation of the segment proximal to the tumor site. (Courtesy Dr. David C. Twedt, Colorado State University, Ft. Collins, Colo.)

Morphologically there are two forms of GI lymphoma: diffuse (multifocal) lymphoma and nodular (solitary) lymphoma. In *diffuse* lymphoma there is a diffuse proliferation of the lamina propria and submucosa with neoplastic lymphocytes. The mesenteric lymph nodes are usually affected. There is occasionally deep ulceration of the intestinal mucosa, and malabsorption is common as the disease becomes advanced. The diffuse form occurs commonly in both dogs and cats. In the *nodular* form a single expanding tumor mass is present that causes progressive luminal obstruction. The most common site is the ileocecocolic region. The mesenteric lymph nodes may or may not be involved.

More recently three grades of GI lymphoma have been described in cats. These are referred to as well differentiated (low grade or lymphocytic), poorly differentiated (high grade, lymphoblastic, or immunoblastic), and intermediate (or mixed). Rare forms, such as large granular lymphocytic lymphoma, also exist.

Intestinal lymphoma in dogs and cats is discussed separately because there are both clinicopathologic and epizootologic differences between the two species. In my experience, cats with intestinal lymphoma respond much better to chemotherapy than do dogs. As a result, I strongly recommend to cat owners that chemotherapy be attempted unless there is significant debilitation at the time of diagnosis. Unfortunately, intestinal lymphoma in dogs is often advanced at the time of diagnosis and malabsorption and panhypoproteinemia are commonly present. Response to chemotherapy is not often very favorable in dogs with advanced disease.

Feline Lymphoma

The most common clinical sign in my series of feline intestinal lymphoma cases is chronic diarrhea. Occasionally, vomiting is the sole or predominant sign (in many of these cats, gastric biopsy results are unremarkable or reveal only mild inflammation), whereas in others vomiting and diarrhea occur with similar frequency. Occasionally the lymphoma involves stomach and/or colon, as well as small intestine. Other signs may include decreased appetite and weight loss (especially as the disease becomes more advanced) and lethargy. Interestingly, some cats have an increased appetite early in the course. Clinical signs may actually be very similar in cats with hyperthyroidism, IBD, and lymphoma. Therefore it is strongly recommended that middle-age to older cats with chronic (more than 1 to 2 months) GI signs be thoroughly evaluated (complete blood count, biochemical profile, urinalysis, feline leukemia and feline immunodeficiency virus testing, T_4 analysis, and endoscopy to obtain GI biopsy samples if hyperthyroidism is not present) to establish a definitive diagnosis.

Most cats with intestinal lymphoma are older, with an age range of 6 to 18 years. There does not seem to be a breed or sex predilection. Most cats are domestic short hair cats.

Cats with intestinal lymphoma can survive (and thrive!) for many months to years if the diagnosis is established and chemotherapy is administered early enough. *Cats with IBD and lymphoma can demonstrate similar clinical signs. Careful consideration must be given before corticosteroids are used empirically to treat cats with chronic diarrhea.* Without question, IBD occurs much more commonly than intestinal lymphoma. Without a histologic diagnosis, however, it is not possible to differentiate a cat with IBD from one with lymphoma. Therefore in middle-age to older cats the best recommendation for owners who wish to do everything possible for their cat is to make a definitive diagnosis before instituting long-term corticosteroid therapy empirically.

Laboratory test results in cats with intestinal lymphoma are variable. Frequently, test results are unremarkable unless there is chronic disease. Abnormalities may include anemia, neutrophilic leukocytosis, lymphocytosis, and hypoproteinemia. Unlike dogs, cats rarely have hypoproteinemia with chronic small intestinal disease. When hypoproteinemia does occur in cats, it is indicative of severe disease, especially when the total protein level is less than 5.5 g/dl. The most common cause of panhypoproteinemia with a total protein of less than 5.0 g/dl in cats is intestinal lymphoma (the primary disorder to rule out is IBD).

Radiographic changes are nonspecific. Abnormalities may include evidence of an abdominal mass or GI obstructive pattern. Contrast studies are not frequently done. Careful abdominal palpation, endoscopy, ultrasonography, and aspiration cytologic analysis of any palpable masses are the most valuable diagnostic aids. Abdominal palpation may be unremarkable or may detect thickened intestines or a mass effect (intestinal mass or lymphadenopathy). Lymphadenopathy is sometimes mild and not readily apparent on palpation. It may occur in conjunction with both IBD and lymphoma. Fine-needle aspiration of a mass may yield sufficient material to make a definitive diagnosis.

Endoscopy is a very safe and reliable means of diagnosing diffuse intestinal lymphoma in cats. Small intestinal masses are not often accessible to endoscopic evaluation, however; if present, exploratory surgery is recommended. As previously stated, aspiration cytologic analysis of a mass may provide a diagnosis, but surgery is still recommended for detailed evaluation and resection of an intestinal mass, where feasible, if there is concern that the mass may cause significant luminal obstruction. Mass resection also provides effective tumor debulking before chemotherapy. Full-thickness intestinal biopsies and mass resection should be done with careful surgical technique, because dehiscence of the suture line may occur. Nonabsorbable suture should be used.

If endoscopy is done, as much of the small intestine as possible is examined. In many cats the tip of the endoscope can be extended to the jejunum. Proper instrumentation and biopsy technique are essential for making a definitive diagnosis of lymphoma on endoscopic biopsy specimen analysis. Gross appearance varies from normal to variable degrees of mucosal irregularity. Erosions or ulcerative changes are occasionally present. As was discussed in the section on IBD, it is sometimes difficult for a pathologist to differentiate diffuse intestinal lymphoma from IBD. This is especially true when severe lymphocytic enteritis is present. Immunoperoxidase studies to assess the clonality of the lymphoid population are often helpful in confirming whether or not lymphoma is present. Pathologists can request that these special stains be done at an academic institution if they are not available at their own laboratory. T-cell and B-cell stains often show presence of virtually 100% of *either* T lymphocytes or B lymphocytes in lymphoma cases, with a virtually negative stain for the other lymphocyte type. An alternative approach is to proceed to obtaining full-thickness intestinal biopsy samples if it is not clear from evaluation of endoscopic samples what disease process is present.

Lymphocytic-plasmacytic gastroenteritis may constitute a prelymphomatous disorder (see discussion earlier in this chapter in the section on feline IBD). In my experience, however, eventual transition from benign to malignant disease is rare.

There are few detailed reports in the literature of treatment response among cats with GI lymphoma. One recent report described diagnosis and management of 67 cats with GI lymphoma. In this series the histologic grade was determined to be lymphocytic in 75% of cases (50 cats) and lymphoblastic in 25% of cases (17 cats). Several therapeutic protocols have been described. Two of these are discussed here. Multiagent chemotherapy is recommended for all affected cats. Survival times in excess of 12 to 18 months are not unusual. In some cats the response is somewhat shorter (3 to 6 months). The prognosis for longer survival time is much better if the diagnosis is made before clinical signs become chronic and debilitation results. The protocol that I have used most often is described in Table 7-2. This protocol uses cyclophosphamide, vincristine (Oncovin), and prednisolone (COP). It can be easily managed in any practice setting. An alternate protocol that was used in the series of 67 cats used mostly prednisolone and chlorambucil. (See guidelines that follow.)

COP Protocol. Vincristine is administered intravenously at a dose of 0.75 mg/m^2 once weekly for 4 consecutive weeks and then once every 3 weeks. The initial doses are often decreased by approximately 25% for cats that are inappetent or debilitated. If well tolerated, the dose can then be

TABLE 7-2	COP Protocol for Treatment of Lymphoma												
						Week							
	1	2	3	4	5	6	7	8	9	10	11	12	13-52
Cyclophosphamide	1			1			1			1			1
Vincristine (Oncovin)	1	1	1	1			1			1			1
Prednisolone		Daily											

Modified from Cotter SM: Treatment of lymphoma and leukemia with cyclophosphamide, vincristine, and prednisone. II. Treatment of cats, *J Am Anim Hosp Assoc* 19:159, 1983.
Outline of the COP protocol *with current dose recommendations:* cyclophosphamide 225 mg/m² PO (round off to nearest 25 mg on the low side of that dose), vincristine 0.75 mg/m² IV (see text), prednisolone 1 mg/lb PO continued as long as the cat remains in continuous remission, every 3 weeks for 1 year. For patients 1-5 kg: m² = 0.5 × wt in kg + 0.05.

gradually increased. Care is taken to ensure that none of the vincristine is given extravascularly. The average volume that is administered is quite low (0.1 to 0.15 ml for many cats, using a vincristine concentration of 1 mg/ml). Cyclophosphamide is given orally at a single dose of 225 mg/m^2 every 3 weeks (50-mg tablets are used, with dose adjusted to the nearest 25 mg on the low side of the calculated dose). Prednisolone is given orally at 1 mg/lb/day. Although cyclophosphamide and vincristine can be given on the same day, I often prefer to have the owner administer the cyclophosphamide 2 to 3 days after the vincristine. This allows a little recovery time between treatments.

A complete blood count is done several times during the first month and then every 3 weeks to be sure that adequate granulocytes are present before treatment. At least 3000 granulocytes/μl must be present before cyclophosphamide is given. If the granulocyte count drops to less than 1000/ μl 5 to 7 days after cyclophosphamide, the dose for subsequent treatments is reduced by 25%. The highest nontoxic dose is most likely to result in the greatest tumor cell kill.

The COP protocol is generally well tolerated, although side effects may occur and dosage or interval adjustments may be necessary. Side effects of COP in cats may include anorexia, vomiting, lethargy, and severe tissue irritation if any vincristine is given extravascularly. Also, the hair coat may become thinner, but complete hair loss does not occur. Cats do tend to lose whiskers. Cats should be carefully observed for sepsis, especially during the induction phase. Prophylactic antibiotics are not indicated, but any infections that occur should be treated aggressively.

Advantages of this protocol include hospital visits at only 3-week intervals after the first 4 weeks, lower cost to the owner, and a treatment interval that allows recovery of normal cells between treatments. I would like to emphasize that with careful monitoring and use of a dosage schedule that is tailored to each individual cat, few problems are encountered. It is my general practice to *encourage* owners of most cats with GI lymphoma to pursue treatment that includes chemotherapy.

Nutritional and metabolic support is also important. If inappetence is a problem, cyproheptadine can be administered as an appetite stimulant (1 to 2 mg orally every 12 to 24 hours) on an as needed basis (long-term if necessary). If there is concurrent renal disease with azotemia or if dehydration is a problem, owners are taught how to administer subcutaneous fluids at home (e.g., lactated Ringer's solution, 100 to 150 ml every 24 hours to 48 hours, based on the individual cat's needs). Injections of B-complex vitamins are sometimes helpful as well.

Rarely, chemotherapy can be discontinued after 1 year. This is done only if follow-up endoscopic intestinal biopsy samples indicate that there is no remaining lymphoma. Most cats remain on treatment for the rest of their lives. If chemotherapy is poorly tolerated and reduced dosages and increased intervals between treatment times are unsuccessful in adequately decreasing side effects, chemotherapy should be suspended. Prednisolone should be continued, however, because it may help maintain remission for a period of time. L-Asparaginase can also be used if cyclophosphamide and vincristine are poorly tolerated. Doxorubicin (Adriamycin) can also be used in cats.

Prednisone and Chlorambucil for Lymphocytic Lymphoma. Lymphocytic lymphoma may also be treated with prednisone (or prednisolone) at 10 mg/day orally and chlorambucil (Leukeran) at a dosage of 15 mg/m^2 orally once per day for 4 days, repeated every 3 weeks.

Many cats go into remission for a number of months. Cyclophosphamide can be used for "rescue" (225 mg/m^2 every 21 days). Adverse reactions on this protocol are rare but may include vomiting, diarrhea, anorexia, and leukopenia.

Monitoring includes running a complete blood count on days 10 and 21 of the first 3-week cycle. If there is no neutropenia (less than 3,000/μl), the same dosage of chlorambucil is continued. Subsequently a complete blood count is obtained on the tenth day on every second or third cycle thereafter.

Canine Lymphoma

GI lymphomas occur less commonly in dogs than in cats. The GI tract may be involved as either a primary or a secondary site. GI lymphoma appears to be somewhat more common in males than in females.

Clinical signs commonly include vomiting, diarrhea, decreased appetite, weight loss, and lethargy. Signs are usually slowly progressive and poorly responsive to symptomatic therapy. Hematologic findings include anemia and panhypoproteinemia, especially in dogs with diffuse intestinal lymphoma. Lymphoma must be considered in any dog with hypoproteinemia that occurs in conjunction with GI signs (IBD, lymphangiectasia, and histoplasmosis are the main disorders to rule out).

Endoscopy has been very reliable for diagnosing diffuse intestinal lymphoma in dogs in my experience. As opposed to cats, dogs rarely have the nearly pure lymphocytic form of IBD; therefore there are not many cases in which a pathologist will have difficulty in differentiating IBD from lymphoma. However, it is essential that biopsy samples be obtained as deeply in the intestinal mucosa as possible. Proper instrumentation and technique are very important. To maximize my efforts to obtain adequate amounts of tissue for diagnosis, I routinely perform upper and lower GI endoscopy in dogs with hypoproteinemia caused by intestinal disease. After complete colonoscopy, a pediatric endoscope can be advanced through the ileocolic sphincter and into the ileum of most dogs as small as 8 to 10 lb. I have had several dogs in which lymphoma was identified only on biopsy samples of the ileum. If only upper endoscopy had been done on these dogs, the diagnosis would have been missed.

Eight to 10 or more biopsy samples are obtained from each general intestinal region examined. In some patients more samples are obtained, especially if it seems difficult to get adequate-size samples. Every effort is made to provide the pathologist with diagnostic-quality samples. The importance of making the effort to obtain biopsy specimens as deeply as possible cannot be overemphasized. Lymphocytic-plasmacytic inflammation commonly occurs in conjunction with intestinal lymphoma. Specifically, in one report, marked to severe lymphocytic-plasmacytic infiltration was present adjacent to or occasionally distant from the neoplastic foci in 8 of 15 dogs (53%) with primary lymphoma. The junctional region between neoplastic and nonneoplastic tissue was not sharply demarcated, and often an inflamed mucosa overlaid a submucosal lymphomatous focus.

Exploratory surgery should be considered for dogs with GI signs and concurrent hypoproteinemia in which there is a poor response to treatment of IBD that was diagnosed via endoscopy. It may be that the poor treatment response is due to lymphoma that has not yet been identified.

Treatment involves multiple-agent chemotherapy. Unfortunately, prolonged remission (more than 3 to 4 months) is uncommon in dogs. Occasionally, prolonged remission (8 to 12 months) can be achieved. Clinical experience indicates that dogs with diffuse intestinal lymphoma have a worse prognosis than those with localized disease. Further information can be found in Chapter 11.

REFERENCES

Barr SC, Bowman DD: Giardiasis in dogs and cats, *Compend Contin Educ Pract Vet* 16:603, 1994.

Cotter SM: Treatment of lymphoma and leukemia with cylophosphamide, vincristine, and prednisone. II. Treatment of cats, *J Am Anim Hosp Assoc* 19:159, 1983.

Couto CG: Gastrointestinal neoplasia in dogs and cats. In Bonagura JB, Kirk RW, eds: *Current veterinary therapy XI*, Philadelphia, 1992, WB Saunders.

Couto CG, Rutgers C, Sherding RG: Gastrointestinal lymphoma in 20 dogs: a retrospective study, *J Vet Intern Med* 3:73, 1989.

Dow SW et al.: Central nervous system toxicosis associated with metronidazole treatment of dogs: five cases (1984-1987), *J Am Vet Med Assoc* 195:365, 1989.

Gardner SA: Use of colostrum in patients with IBD. Personal communication, 2001.

Garvey M: Management of short bowel syndrome. Personal communication, 1999.

German AJ, Hall EJ, Day MJ: Immune cell populations within the duodenal mucosa of dogs with enteropathies, *J Vet Intern Med* 15:14, 2001.

Greenberg PD, Cello JP: Treatment of severe diarrhea caused by *Cryptosporidium parvum* with oral bovine immunoglobulin concentrate in patients with AIDS, *J Acquir Immune Defic Syndr Hum Retrovirol* 13:348, 1996.

Grooters AM: Phycomycosis revisited: new developments in canine pythiosis. Proceedings of the twentieth annual forum of the American College of Veterinary Internal Medicine, 2002.

Grooters AM et al.: Development and evaluation of an enzyme-linked immunosorbent assay for the serodiagnosis of pythiosis in dogs, *J Vet Intern Med* 16:142, 2002.

Inamura-Mikio, Yamauchi-Hidemi: Effects of massive bowel resection on metabolism of bile acids and vitamin D_3 and gastrin release in dogs, *Tohoku J Exp Med* 168:515, 1992.

Jergens AE: Clinical staging for severity of inflammatory bowel disease. Proceedings of the nineteenth annual forum of the American College of Veterinary Internal Medicine, 2001.

Jergens AE et al.: Cytologic examination of exfoliative specimens obtained during endoscopy for diagnosis of gastrointestinal tract disease in dogs and cats, *J Am Vet Med Assoc* 213:1755, 1998.

Krecic MR: Feline IBD: diagnostic challenges, treatment, and monitoring. Proceedings of the forum of the American College of Veterinary Internal Medicine, 2002.

Kull PA et al.: Clinical, clinicopathologic, radiographic, and ultrasonographic characteristics of intestinal lymphangiectasia in dogs: 17 cases (1996-1998), *J Am Vet Med Assoc* 219:197, 2001.

Littman MP et al.: Familial protein-losing enteropathy and protein-losing nephropathy in soft-coated wheaten terriers: 222 cases (1983-1997), *J Vet Intern Med* 14:68, 2000.

Payne JT, Jones BD: Short bowel syndrome. In Bojrab MJ, ed: *Disease mechanisms in small animal surgery,* Philadelphia, 1993, Lea & Febiger.

Playford RJ, Macdonald CE, Johnson WS: Colostrum and milk-derived peptide growth factors for the treatment of gastrointestinal disorders, *Am J Clin Nutr* 72:5, 2000.

Rhodes KH: Feline immunomodulators. In Bonagura JB, Kirk RW, eds: *Current veterinary therapy XII,* Philadelphia, 1995, WB Saunders.

Sherding RG: Intestinal lymphangiectasia. In Kirk RW, ed: *Current veterinary therapy IX,* Philadelphia, 1986, WB Saunders.

Sherding RG: Intestinal histoplasmosis. In Bonagura JB, Kirk RW, eds: *Current veterinary therapy IX,* Philadelphia, 1992, WB Saunders.

Sherding RG, Johnson SE: Diseases of the intestines. In Birchard SJ, Sherding RG, eds: *Manual of Small Animal Practice,* ed 2, Philadelphia, 2000, WB Saunders.

Stenson WF, MacDermott RP: Inflammatory bowel disease. In Yamada T, ed: *Textbook of gastroenterology,* vol 2, Philadelphia, 1991, JB Lippincott.

Strombeck DR, Guilford WG: Maldigestion, malabsorption, bacterial overgrowth, and proteinlosing enteropathy. In Strombeck DR, Guilford WG, eds: *Small animal gastroenterology,* Davis, Calif, 1990, Stonegate.

Tams TR: Feline inflammatory bowel disease, *Vet Clin North Am* 23:569, 1993.

Tams TR: Endoscopic examination of the small intestine. In Tams TR, ed: *Small animal endoscopy,* ed 2, St. Louis, 1999, Mosby.

Twedt DC: *Clostridium perfringens*–associated enterotoxicosis in dogs. In Bonagura JB, Kirk RW, eds: *Current veterinary therapy XI,* Philadelphia, 1992, WB Saunders.

Washabau R: Management of short bowel syndrome. Personal communication, 1999.

Willard MD: Disorders of the intestinal tract. In Nelson RW, Couto CG, eds: *Essentials of small animal internal medicine,* ed 2, St. Louis, 1998, Mosby.

Willard MD et al.: Intestinal Crypt lesions associated with protein-losing enteropathy in the dog, *J Vet Intern Med* 14:298, 2000.

Willard MW et al.: Interobserver variation among histopathologic evaluations of intestinal tissues from dogs and cats, *J Am Vet Med Assoc* 220:1177, 2002.

Zajac AM: Giardiasis, *Compend Contin Educ Pract Vet* 14:604, 1992.

DISEASES OF THE LARGE INTESTINE

Robert G. Sherding

The large intestine comprises the cecum, colon, rectum, and anal canal. In the carnivores such as the dog and cat, the colon is relatively small and the cecum is only a vestigial component. In the ventrodorsal plane, the colon has the shape of a question mark and is anatomically subdivided into a short proximal ascending colon with ileocolic and cecocolic junctions or sphincters, a middle transverse colon, and a long descending colon that is continuous with the rectum and anal canal.

The two principal functions of the colon are (1) the absorption of electrolytes and water from the luminal content and (2) the temporary storage and periodic elimination of the resulting feces. Absorption is mostly a function of the proximal colon, whereas storage is mostly a function of the rectum and distal colon. The principal function of the anus is to maintain fecal continence between defecations.

Colonic mucosal cells actively absorb sodium and chloride; water follows passively. Within the colonic mucosa, tubular glands called the *crypts of Lieberkühn* contain numerous mucus–secreting goblet cells. The circular and longitudinal muscle layers of the colon are responsible for the normal motility and "tone" of the colon, under the influence of intrinsic and extrinsic innervation and gastrointestinal (GI) hormones. Retrograde peristaltic contractions (cats only) and phasic segmentation contractions (both dogs and cats) mix and delay passage of the bowel contents, thereby promoting optimal absorption, whereas peristaltic contractions (mass movements) propel the bowel contents downstream, eventually resulting in defecation. Defecation is a well-controlled act involving the colon, rectum, and anus under nervous system control.

In general, most diseases of the colon are manifested as either diarrhea or constipation, and thus colonic diseases are categorized as such for the purposes of discussion in this chapter. Perforation and volvulus of the colon are rare causes of an acute abdominal distress presentation. Diseases in or near the anus generally cause dyschezia, often accompanied by constipation and sometimes fecal incontinence.

DISEASES OF THE COLON WITH DIARRHEA AS THE PRINCIPAL SIGN

Diarrhea is the most common sign associated with colonic disease in the dog and cat. Inflammatory diseases (colitis), which may be dietary, traumatic, parasitic, infectious, immune, or idiopathic, are the most important causes of large bowel diarrhea.

251

Other causes include neoplastic (lymphoma, adenocarcinoma), obstructive (intussusception, volvulus), and functional (irritable bowel syndrome) disorders. The principal causes and categories of large bowel diarrhea are summarized in Box 8-1.

Clinical Signs of Large Bowel Diarrhea

The first step in the recognition and diagnosis of large bowel diarrhea is the anatomic localization of the disease process to the colon based on the evaluation of the patient's defecation pattern and fecal characteristics (frequency, volume, consistency, color, odor, and composition). Large bowel diarrhea is characterized by frequent urges to defecate (usually greater than three times normal frequency), with each defecation producing small quantities of feces that often contain excessive mucus and sometimes fresh red blood. Urgency, resulting from irritability or inflammation of the distal colon, causes frequent premature expulsions of small quantities of feces that would otherwise be insufficient to trigger the defecation reflex. In addition, lapses in house training ("accidents")

may be caused by urgency and inability to control urges to defecate. The owner may also notice straining (tenesmus) as the patient remains in a squatting posture for an extended period of time after defecation or makes repeated attempts to defecate within a period of a few minutes. These attempts may produce little or no feces, or sometimes a small amount of feces composed almost entirely of mucus, exudate, and blood.

Because many colonic diseases are associated with mucosal injury, inflammation, or ulceration, abnormal fecal constituents are frequently found in large bowel diarrhea. These include (1) fresh red blood (hematochezia), which originates from sites of erosion or ulceration; (2) mucus, which originates from the abundant goblet cells in the colon that respond to mucosal injury by an outpouring of mucus; and (3) exudate (leukocytes), which originates from sites of inflammation. Blood may coat the feces, streaks of blood may be mixed within the feces, or drops of blood may be passed at the end of defecation. Excessive mucus may give the feces a glistening or jellylike appearance. Exudates are detected by the positive identification of fecal leukocytes on conventional cytology stains. These abnormal constituents—red blood, mucus,

---

BOX 8-1 Causes of Large Bowel Diarrhea

Dietary factors
  Abrasive colitis (ingestion of foreign material—e.g., bones, hair)
  Dietary hypersensitivity (food allergy?)
  Fiber-responsive diarrhea
Helminths
  Whipworms *(Trichuris vulpis)*
  Hookworms *(Ancylostoma caninum)*
  Strongyloides tumefaciens
Protozoa
  Entamoeba histolytica
  Balantidium coli
  Trichomonas sp.
  Giardia sp. (?)
Viruses
  FIP coronavirus (pyogranulomatous colitis)
  Retroviruses (FeLV; FIV)
Bacteria
  Salmonella sp.
  Campylobacter jejuni
  Clostridium perfringens, Clostridium difficile (?)
  Yersinia enterocolitica, Yersinia pseudotuberculosis
  Bacillus piliformis (Tyzzer's disease)

Mycobacteria
  Enteropathogenic *Escherichia coli* (?)
Fungi
  Histoplasma capsulatum
  Others (pythiosis, *Candida albicans, Aspergillus* sp.)
Algae (*Prototheca* sp.)
Idiopathic inflammatory bowel disease
  Lymphocytic-plasmacytic colitis
  Eosinophilic colitis
  Suppurative (neutrophilic) colitis
  Granulomatous colitis
  Histiocytic (PAS+) ulcerative colitis of boxer dogs
Drug-induced colonic ulceration
  Steroidal and nonsteroidal antiinflammatory drugs
Pancreatitis-associated colitis
Ischemia
  Trauma, infarction, volvulus, strangulation
Intussusception
  Cecocolonic, ileocolonic
Neoplasia
  Benign (adenomatous polyp)
  Malignant (adenocarcinoma, lymphoma, others)
Motility dysfunction—irritable bowel syndrome

FIP, Feline infectious peritonitis; *FeLV,* feline leukemia virus; *FIV,* feline immunodeficiency virus; *PAS,* periodic acid–Schiff.

and leukocytes—are localizing signs indicative of colonic disease.

Because the principal function of the colon is absorption of water and electrolytes rather than digestion and absorption of nutrients, nutrient malabsorption and steatorrhea are absent in large bowel diarrhea. Thus dramatic weight loss and wasting are unlikely if the patient is eating, and the daily fecal output (volume or weight of feces) is usually only minimally increased. This contrasts with the substantial increase in fecal output of dogs with small intestinal disease. The characteristics of small bowel diarrhea are discussed in Chapter 1. Diffuse diseases of the GI tract may produce concurrent small and large bowel signs and sometimes gastric signs as well. It has been estimated that vomiting is an associated sign in about 30% of patients with colitis.

Diagnostic Approach for Large Bowel Diarrhea

Diarrhea as a clinical sign is relatively nonspecific; however, once it is localized to a disorder of the large bowel, a logical diagnostic approach can be followed. Specific treatment or intervention is usually necessary, and this generally requires either a specific diagnosis or at least a histopathologic characterization. Initial evaluations should be aimed at diagnosis of dietary, parasitic, and infectious causes of diarrhea. This should include multiple fecal examinations for whipworm ova and protozoa, therapeutic deworming trials (fenbendazole, 22 mg/lb orally daily for 3 days), fecal examinations for *Clostridium perfringens* spores and toxin, and a 4-week dietary trial using a highly digestible commercial or homemade GI diet alone and with fiber added (psyllium). If diarrhea persists and the cause is not apparent, the next phase of diagnostic evaluations should include a complete blood count (CBC), serum chemistry profile, urinalysis, additional fecal examinations for infectious agents (cytologic examination, toxin assay, cultures), and abdominal imaging (radiography and ultrasonography). Finally, complete colonoscopic examination and biopsy are performed. The various diagnostic procedures for animals with large bowel diarrhea are summarized in Table 8-1.

Physical Examination

A complete physical examination may reveal important clues about the severity, nature, and cause of diarrhea, although in many patients the findings

are nonspecific. An effort should be made to identify underlying extraintestinal diseases that may be a cause or consequence of diarrhea. The colon and rectum should be thoroughly examined by palpation, and if abnormalities are identified, additional diagnostic studies, such as colonoscopy, radiography, or ultrasonography, are usually indicated. For example, abdominal palpation of the colon (and small intestines as well) may reveal masses, thickenings, intussusception, distention, fecal impaction, pain, or associated changes in abdominal lymph nodes and other abdominal organs. Digital palpation of the rectum may reveal foreign objects, intramural or extramural masses, strictures, or abnormalities of mucosal texture. In addition, the fecal material obtained on the palpation glove can be inspected for abrasive particles (such as bone chips), blood, or mucus. Fecal material also can be examined microscopically for parasites and inflammatory cells and submitted for culture if indicated.

Consideration of Dietary, Parasitic, and Infectious Causes

Before hospitalizing a patient with large bowel diarrhea for an in-depth diagnostic work-up, the possibilities of dietary, parasitic, or infectious causes should initially be considered. Ingestion of abrasive materials such as bones or chew toys can injure the rectocolonic mucosa, producing abrasive colitis and signs of diarrhea and hematochezia that typically last 2 to 3 days. The diagnosis can usually be made from a thorough dietary history and inspection of the feces for abrasive particles.

Acute nonspecific large bowel diarrhea often resolves with restriction of food intake for 24 to 48 hours followed by gradual resumption of feeding using a bland digestible diet. Chronic nonspecific diet-responsive diarrhea can be resolved in many cases by strict feeding of a balanced, highly digestible diet using one of the commercially available "GI diets," such as Low Residue Formula (Iams), Select Care Sensitive (IVD), Prescription i/d (Hill's), EN (Purina), or Low Fat (Waltham), or using a comparable homemade diet following published recipes. In dogs if diarrhea persists after a 4-week feeding trial, then add fermentable soluble fiber in the form of psyllium (Metamucil, 1 to 3 tbsp/day) or oat bran (1 to 3 tbsp/day) to determine if the patient has fiber-responsive large bowel diarrhea.

In dogs, whipworms are the most common cause of colitis in many practice areas and should be ruled out by fecal flotation or, if occult infection is

TABLE 8-1	Diagnosis of Large Bowel Diarrhea
Procedures	**Diagnostic Findings**
Dietary history	Ingestion of bones or other foreign materials, which may cause abrasive colitis
	Dietary hypersensitivity as a potential cause of inflammatory bowel disease
Abdominal palpation	Intestinal masses, thickenings, distention, pain, or associated lymphadenopathy
Rectal palpation	Foreign objects, masses, strictures, or abnormalities of mucosal texture
Fecal examinations	
Gross inspection	Blood, mucus, ingested foreign material
Flotation	*Trichuris* ova
Saline smear	Protozoan trophozoites
Cytologic examination	Inflammatory cells, *Histoplasma* organisms, clostridial endospores, *Campylobacter* organisms
Bacteriologic examination	*Campylobacter, Salmonella,* etc.
Enterotoxin assays	*Clostridium perfringens* enterotoxin
Hemogram	Anemia, eosinophilia, neutrophilia, neutropenia
Serum biochemistry studies	Hyperkalemia/hyponatremia of whipworm (pseudo-Addison's syndrome)
	Hypoproteinemia (enteric protein loss)
	Underlying renal failure or pancreatitis
	Other metabolic and systemic alterations that could cause or result from colonic disease
Serologic examination	*Histoplasma* titer (in endemic areas)
Barium enema radiography	Intussusceptions, neoplasms, polyps, strictures, and inflammatory lesions (colonoscopy is generally preferred over barium enema)
Abdominal ultrasonography	Intestinal and abdominal masses, intussusception, mesenteric lymphadenopathy, pancreatitis
Colonoscopy	Visual examination and biopsy for definitive or histopathologic diagnosis in most neoplastic or inflammatory diseases of the colon
Therapeutic trials	Response to fenbendazole suggests occult whipworm infection
	Response to dietary trials with novel protein diets suggests dietary hypersensitivity as a cause of lymphocytic-plasmacytic colitis
	Response to dietary fiber supplementation indicates fiber-responsive enteropathy

suspected, by a therapeutic trial of an effective anthelmintic such as fenbendazole (Panacur). Hookworms can also cause colitis. Although less common, protozoan causes of colitis (e.g., *Trichomonas*) can be detected rapidly by examination of saline fecal smears for the presence of motile trophozoites. In warm, humid regions endemic for *Strongyloides tumefaciens* in cats (e.g., parts of the southern United States), sedimentation or Baermann techniques can be used to identify larvae in the feces.

Campylobacter, Salmonella, and *C. perfringens* are becoming recognized as important bacterial causes of enterocolitis. *Campylobacter* and *Salmonella* can be diagnosed by specialized fecal cultures. Such cultures are particularly indicated when examination of fecal cytologic preparations reveals the presence of numerous fecal leukocytes or when there is an outbreak of diarrhea in groups of animals. *C. perfringens* enterotoxigenic diarrhea is suggested by the presence of large numbers of endospores

(more than five spores per high-power oil immersion field) with a "safety pin" or "tennis racket" configuration in fecal cytologic preparations stained with Diff-Quik; however, fecal assays for *C. perfringens* enterotoxin are probably a more reliable means of diagnosing clostridial diarrhea (see section on *C. perfringens*).

Histoplasmosis is an important cause of chronic colitis in areas endemic for this mycotic infection. The diagnosis is usually based on either positive serologic study (immunodiffusion or complement fixation) or identification of the organisms in exfoliative cytology specimens from rectocolonic mucosa. Sabouraud's medium can be used to culture feces for *Histoplasma* and other fungi or for *Prototheca,* a rare cause of colitis, but culture growth is slow (up to 2 weeks) and the isolation rate is low.

Hematology and Serum Biochemistry

In addition to fecal examinations, the initial database for undiagnosed chronic large bowel diarrhea should include a complete hemogram (CBC) and serum biochemistry profile. Significant CBC findings may include (1) anemia, which could result from enteric blood loss or depressed erythropoiesis due to chronic disease; (2) eosinophilia, which could suggest parasitism, eosinophilic enterocolitis, or sometimes other inflammatory or neoplastic intestinal diseases; (3) regenerative neutrophilia, which could suggest bowel inflammation (particularly involving the deeper layers), necrosis, or neoplasia; and (4) degenerative or toxic neutropenia, which could suggest overwhelming sepsis or endotoxemia, such as occurs with bowel ischemia, necrosis, or perforation.

A serum biochemistry profile and urinalysis should be considered to identify metabolic or extraintestinal disorders that could cause or result from diarrhea. For example, underlying systemic diseases that can cause diarrhea may be detected, such as renal failure (increased levels of blood urea nitrogen and creatinine), pancreatitis (increased amylase and lipase levels), liver disease (e.g., abnormal serum liver enzymes levels), or hypoadrenocorticism (hyperkalemia and hyponatremia). In addition, serum chemistry findings can be used to evaluate potential complications of large bowel diarrhea, such as dehydration, electrolyte abnormalities, and hypoproteinemia. Because of the high incidence of hyperthyroidism in cats older than 5 years of age and because this disorder is occasionally manifested as unexplained diarrhea, cats in this age-group with diarrhea should have a screening serum thyroxine (T_4) level measured.

Colonoscopy and Biopsy

Most cases of chronic large bowel diarrhea in which extraintestinal, dietary, parasitic, and infectious causes have been excluded require colonoscopic examination and mucosal biopsy for definitive diagnosis or accurate characterization of the disease. Colonoscopy allows direct visualization of the lumen of the colon, sampling of luminal content, and directed forceps biopsy of the mucosa. Suitable rigid colonoscopes are relatively inexpensive and easy to use. Because colonic diseases are often diffuse, examination of the descending colon with a rigid instrument is sufficient for diagnosis in many patients. However, when lesions are located predominantly in the ascending or transverse colon, areas that are inaccessible with a rigid colonoscope, a flexible fiberoptic colonoscope must be used. The normal colonic mucosa through a colonoscope appears pale pink and reflects light

uniformly. The mucosa should be nonfriable, thin enough that the submucosal vessels are visible, and free of ulcers, thickened folds, masses, or strictures. Cultures, exfoliative cytology specimens, and biopsy specimens of the colonic mucosa are easily obtained through the instrument.

There are occasions when colonoscopy cannot be used to evaluate adequately or to perform deep enough biopsies of lesions in the proximal colon, especially when deep inflammatory or neoplastic lesions involve the region of the ileocecocolic junction. Under these circumstances, examination and biopsy by laparotomy are required for accurate diagnosis.

Radiography and Ultrasonography

Plain abdominal radiography is indicated for detection of foreign material in the colon, intestinal masses, intussusception, or an abnormal gas-fluid pattern that would suggest obstruction or volvulus. Barium enema contrast radiography is useful in selected cases of large bowel diarrhea for detection of ileocolonic intussusceptions, cecal inversions, neoplasms, polyps, strictures, colonic displacement, colonic shortening, and chronic inflammatory lesions. Some of these lesions can also be detected in the latter phases of an upper GI barium contrast radiographic series; however, the lower bowel is generally evaluated better by a barium enema study. (See Chapter 2 for a more detailed discussion of contrast radiography.) However, it must be emphasized that if flexible fiberoptic colonoscopy is available, it is generally preferred over barium radiography for evaluation of the proximal colon because it is easier to perform and yields more definitive diagnostic information.

Abdominal ultrasonography can be a useful diagnostic aid in selected cases of unexplained diarrhea for noninvasively defining intestinal and other abdominal or perirectal masses, for diagnosis of intussusceptions, and for evaluating the mesenteric lymph nodes, pancreas, liver, and prostate (see Chapter 2).

Therapeutic Trials

Therapeutic trials can sometimes support a tentative diagnosis when accompanied by other supportive clinical evidence. For example, occult whipworm infection is often diagnosed circumstantially by rapid resolution of signs in response to fenbendazole therapy. In some patients, nonspecific diet-responsive large bowel diarrhea is resolved by feeding a highly digestible diet or a diet supplemented with fiber as described previously in this section. Similarly, the response to trial-and-error test diets plays an important role in establishing dietary hypersensitivity as a cause of lymphocytic-plasmacytic colitis.

Abrasive Colitis

Ingested bone particles, pieces of chew toys, or other indigestible abrasive foreign materials (stones, hair, plants, wood, cloth, carpeting, foil, plastic), when incorporated into the fecal mass, may cause abrasive colitis because of a traumatizing sandpaper-like effect on the rectocolonic mucosa during transit. Abrasive injury is usually transient and self-limiting after 2 to 3 days, although repeated episodes in patients that have frequent dietary indiscretions may mimic other causes of chronic intermittent colitis. Dietary history and examination of the feces for abrasive particles are usually sufficient to establish the diagnosis. Management is based on eliminating the source of ingested abrasive material.

Diet-Responsive and Fiber-Responsive Large Bowel Diarrhea

These conditions are characterized by chronic nonspecific large bowel diarrhea. The diagnosis is based on a complete absence of abnormal findings on diagnostic evaluations, minimal abnormalities on colonoscopy, and complete response to dietary manipulation. A 4-week feeding trial of a new diet is usually adequate to determine response. Some of these patients respond simply to feeding of a balanced, highly digestible diet (i.e., moderate to restricted fat level with digestible protein and carbohydrate) using one of the commercially available "GI diets," such as Low Residue Formula (Iams), Select Care Sensitive (IVD), Prescription i/d (Hill's), EN (Purina), or Low Fat (Waltham), or using a comparable homemade diet. One example of a homemade diet combines turkey, rice, and safflower oil. Other acceptable recipes for homemade "GI diets" are published elsewhere. The advantage of a highly digestible diet would be less undigested "residue" presented to the colon from the small intestines. This helps to prevent unabsorbed fat from reaching the colon, where it can be metabolized to hydroxy fatty acids that produce diarrhea.

In dogs the diagnosis of fiber-responsive large bowel diarrhea is based on an absence of abnormal diagnostic findings, minimal abnormalities on colonoscopy, and responsiveness to supplementation of a digestible diet with fermentable soluble fiber in the form of psyllium (Metamucil, 1 to 3 tbsp/day) or oat bran (1 to 3 tbsp/day). Some of these patients may actually have so-called irritable bowel syndrome (see later section). Fermentable soluble fiber is fermented by colonic bacteria to short-chain fatty acids (SCFAs) that provide an energy source for colonic epithelium, protect against mucosal injury, and acidify bowel contents, which may reduce proliferation and sporulation of enteropathogenic bacteria such as *C. perfringens*. Fiber also has other beneficial effects on fecal water content, fecal bulk, and colonic myoelectrical function.

Novel protein diets are used in diagnostic trials and treatment for chronic colitis related to dietary hypersensitivity. This is discussed in the section on lymphocytic-plasmacytic colitis.

Parasitic Colitis
Whipworm Colitis

Whipworm *(Trichuris vulpis)* infection is a common cause of acute, chronic, or intermittent signs of large bowel diarrhea in dogs in many practice areas. The adult nematode has a predilection for the proximal colon and cecum, where its distinctive thread like head end or "whip" firmly embeds deep within the mucosa to feed on blood and tissue fluids, thereby resulting in colitis and typhlitis.

Whipworms infect dogs of all ages. Although there may be minimal clinical signs in light infestations, trichuriasis frequently causes mucoid large bowel type of diarrhea with urgency and sometimes hematochezia. Because of these signs, whipworm infection is often mistaken for other, more serious forms of colitis or colonic neoplasia. In addition, a condition of pseudohypoadrenocorticism characterized by hyperkalemia and hyponatremia in the presence of normal adrenal function has been associated with severe whipworm diarrhea in several dogs. The feline whipworms, *Trichuris campanula* and *Trichuris serrata*, are considered to be very rare and usually are not associated with clinical signs.

Whipworm infections occur by ingestion of infective ova, and the life cycle is direct. The prepatent period is approximately 3 months. Because ova may survive and remain infectious in the environment for 4 to 5 years, contaminated ground is probably the major reservoir of infection.

Definitive diagnosis of whipworm infection necessitates identification of the characteristic brown, bipolar-operculated, football-shaped ova by routine fecal flotation. Repeated fecal examinations may be necessary to identify ova because of the unusually long prepatent period and also because it is not uncommon for active infection to be characterized by prolonged periods when ova are not shed in the feces. It is estimated that up to 50% of dogs presenting with whipworm diarrhea have ova-negative or so-called occult infections. Alternative means of diagnosis are directly by colonoscopic observation of adult whipworms in the bowel lumen or indirectly by observing resolution of signs in response to a therapeutic trial of an effective anthelmintic.

Whipworms are treated with fenbendazole (22 mg/lb orally for 3 consecutive days). Treatment should be routinely repeated at 3 weeks and 3 months because whipworms are difficult to eradicate. In refractory cases, a 5-day course of fenbendazole is recommended. Febantel is an alternative treatment for whipworms. Regular use of milbemycin (Interceptor, Sentinel) for heartworm prevention also helps to control whipworm infections. Because whipworm ova survive so well in the environment, frequent reinfection is a common problem. Therefore feces should be collected and disposed of properly whenever possible. In dogs with frequent access to ground that has been heavily contaminated with whipworm ova, a common situation in many public parks and backyards, reinfection is so frequent that retreatment every 2 to 3 months may be necessary. It is virtually impossible to eradicate the parasite from infected ground; however, concrete runs can be disinfected with dilute sodium hypochlorite solution or by flaming.

Rarely trichuriasis has been associated with severe transmural granulomatous typhlitis, which may be palpable as a tender right midabdominal mass. This lesion may be refractory to anthelmintics and require typhlectomy.

Hookworm Colitis

Although the common canine hookworm, *Ancylostoma caninum,* is primarily a small intestinal parasite, it occasionally parasitizes the colon in large numbers. Hookworms embed their mouthparts in the mucosa to suck blood, leaving bleeding punctiform ulcers as they "graze." When they involve the colon, they produce a bloody mucoid diarrhea characteristic of colitis.

Young dogs are most often affected, and the diagnosis is usually readily established by identification of the characteristic hookworm ova by routine fecal flotation. Eosinophilia is a common ancillary finding on CBC.

There are many anthelmintics that are effective for eradicating hookworms, including the standard recommended dosages (4.5 mg/lb for patients under 5 lb; 2.25 mg/lb for patients over 5 lb) of pyrantel pamoate (Nemex), fenbendazole, or febantel. Most heartworm preventatives also control hookworms.

Strongyloides Colitis

S. tumefaciens is a tiny nematode parasite of cats in warm, humid tropical regions such as the Gulf region of the United States. The adult parasites burrow within the mucosa of the large intestine. Infection is usually asymptomatic, but in some cats the parasite causes peculiar tumorlike, white, 2- to 3-mm nodular proliferations in the colonic mucosa and submucosa that are associated with signs of chronic diarrhea and debilitation.

Ova that contain first-stage *Strongyloides* larvae can be identified in feces by flotation techniques, and free larvae may be identified by direct microscopic examination of feces or by a Baermann technique. In addition, the diagnosis can be established by colonoscopic observation and biopsy of the mucosal nodules, which are filled with adult worms.

Strongyloidiasis can be treated with a 5-day course of fenbendazole (23 mg/lb/day orally).

Protozoan Colitis

Pentatrichomonas hominis, Entamoeba histolytica, and *Balantidium coli* are large bowel protozoal parasites that are occasionally associated with colitis and large bowel diarrhea in animals. In addition, *Giardia,* which is primarily a small bowel parasite (see Chapter 6), has been associated with bloody-mucoid large bowel diarrhea on very rare occasions. All of these protozoa are responsive to treatment with metronidazole (Flagyl).

Trichomoniasis

Trichomonas spp. are motile, pear-shaped, flagellated protozoa that inhabit the colon and cecum of dogs and cats and have been found in both normal and diarrheic feces. The pathogenicity of these protozoa in dogs has not been conclusively established, but massive numbers of trichomonads are sometimes found in diarrheic feces of puppies and are especially associated with unsanitary overcrowded kennel conditions and coinfection with other parasites. *Tritrichomonas foetus* has recently been identified as a frequent cause of chronic large intestinal diarrhea in young cats, especially cats confined in crowded cattery conditions. The diarrhea may wax and wane, may be malodorous, and may contain blood or mucus. The diagnosis of trichomoniasis is based on identification in saline fecal smears or in fecal culture (Modified Diamond's Media or InPouch TF kit) of motile, pear-shaped, flagellated trophozoites with characteristic wavelike motion of an undulating membrane and a constant erratic turning and rolling motion. Feces for detecting trichomonads should be taken directly from the rectum or examined within minutes of defecation, while trophozoites are still motile. Trichomonads lack a cyst stage. Fecal polymerase chain reaction (PCR) testing has also been used in cats. *Trichomonas* are extremely difficult to eradicate in cats. Numerous antibiotic agents have been evaluated without success. Treatment can reduce the number of organisms and improve clinical signs, but it usually does not eliminate the infection. The patient should also be evaluated and treated for concurrent infection with other parasites and enteropathogens. Proper sanitation measures should be instituted to control infection in animals housed in groups.

Amebic Colitis

E. histolytica, primarily a human pathogen, may rarely cause amebic colitis in dogs and cats. Amebic invasion of the colonic mucosa and submucosa results in ulceration and signs of bloody-mucoid large bowel diarrhea with tenesmus. Diarrhea is usually severe and may simulate other forms of chronic colitis or is manifested as an acute dysentery. Both forms of *Entamoeba,* the trophozoite and cyst, are infectious for animals. Infection is most likely acquired from ingestion of food or water contaminated with human feces, such as drinking from polluted water sources (free-roaming animals) or toilets (house pets). The diagnosis is based on identification of ameboid trophozoites with pseudopodial movement in saline smears of fresh diarrheic feces, amebiccysts in zinc sulfate flotation of formed feces, or trophozoites in colon biopsy specimens. Amebic colitis responds to metronidazole (12 to 15 mg/lb orally two times a day for 5 to 10 days) or furazolidone (1 mg/lb orally three times a day for 7 days).

Balantidiasis

B. coli, a ciliated protozoan that primarily infects swine, is a rare cause of chronic ulcerative colitis in dogs. Rural dogs in contact with swine feces are most at risk for the disease. Humans can also be infected. Dogs with balantidiasis are usually coinfected with whipworms, and thus it has been suggested that whipworm-induced damage to the colonic mucosa may be a predisposing factor. The diagnosis is based on identification of extremely large (40-80 × 25-45 μm), oval, brown, rapidly swimming ciliated trophozoites with prominent macronuclei in saline smears of fresh feces or on identification of protozoal cysts in zinc sulfate or sedimentation preparations of feces. As with *Entamoeba* and *Giardia,* the trophozoite stage of *Balantidium* can be seen in diarrheic feces, whereas cysts are more likely to be found in formed feces. Balantidiasis is treated with metronidazole (10 to 15 mg/lb orally twice a day for 5 to 10 days).

Viral Colitis

The colon may be significantly involved in generalized viral infections of the intestinal tract. Lesions of acute colitis are especially common in parvoviral infections of both the dog and the cat. In addition, the colon may be involved in some of the multisystemic viral diseases. For example, in dogs the epitheliotropic attack of canine distemper virus may involve the colon, whereas cats infected with feline leukemia virus (FeLV), feline immunodeficiency virus (FIV), or feline infectious peritonitis (FIP) virus sometimes have diarrhea associated with enterocolitis that varies from necrotizing to ulcerative to pyogranulomatous. (See Chapter 6 for further discussion of viral infections of the GI tract.)

Bacterial Colitis

Invasive enteropathogenic bacteria primarily invade the colon and distal small bowel, where the mucosal damage they cause leads to inflammation, exudation, mucus secretion, and bleeding. Thus typical signs of large bowel diarrhea and hematochezia are characteristic of these infections. Bacterial enterotoxins may also play a role in the pathogenesis of diarrhea. Although the clinical importance of the various enteropathogenic bacteria in animals has not yet been fully defined, *Salmonella* sp., *Campylobacter jejuni, Yersinia* sp., *Bacillus piliformis,* and *Clostridium* sp. may be associated with colitis and large bowel diarrhea in dogs and cats.

Salmonellosis

Manifestations of *Salmonella* infection may be categorized into three syndromes: (1) the subclinical carrier state, (2) enterocolitis, and (3) enterocolitis with bacteremia. Clinical salmonellosis is relatively uncommon compared with the prevalence of the subclinical carrier state. When it does occur, *Salmonella* enterocolitis is characterized by acute watery or mucoid diarrhea (containing blood in severe cases), vomiting, tenesmus, fever, anorexia, lethargy, abdominal pain, and dehydration. Most patients recover within 3 to 4 weeks, although shedding of organisms often persists for up to 6 weeks, sometimes longer. *Salmonella* also appears to cause chronic or intermittent diarrhea in some patients. Rarely, acute enterocolitis may develop into a potentially fatal bacteremia or endotoxemia with signs of endotoxic shock and even disseminated intravascular coagulation (DIC).

The diagnosis of salmonellosis should be suspected in patients that develop acute diarrhea and have identifiable risk factors, such as known or probable exposure, young age, immune deficiency, debilitating illness, or housing in overcrowded or unsanitary conditions. A severe acute febrile illness with hemorrhagic diarrhea in cats has been linked to a highly fatal *Salmonella* outbreak in songbirds and transmission to cats via ingestion of dead birds. In addition, nosocomial outbreaks with high morbidity and mortality have been recorded in hospitalized patients, with the greatest risk occurring in those patients with severe illness, those undergoing major surgery, those hospitalized for 5 or more days, and those receiving glucocorticosteroids, anticancer chemotherapy, or oral antibiotics (such as ampicillin) that upset the normal flora. Routine diagnostics are usually noncontributory, except that in severe cases with bacteremia and endotoxemia a degenerative neutropenia may be found. Confirmation of the diagnosis depends on isolation of *Salmonella* sp. from properly cultured fecal specimens or from blood cultures in bacteremic animals.

The use of antibiotics in the treatment of salmonellosis is controversial. *Salmonella* invasion that is confined locally to the mucosa produces enterocolitis that is both self-limiting and not likely to be affected by antibiotics. In fact, antibacterial therapy, especially oral nonabsorbable antibiotics that alter the flora, may actually prolong shedding of organisms and encourage development of a prolonged convalescent carrier state. However, antibiotics are indicated whenever *Salmonella* invasion becomes severe or complicated by bacteremia and endotoxemia, as indicated by signs such as shock, dehydration, high fever or hypothermia, and extreme depression, or by laboratory findings such as azotemia, electrolyte imbalances, neutropenia, hypoglycemia, hypoproteinemia, or coagulopathy. Peracute onset and severe hematochezia also may be indications of impending systemic invasion and should prompt antibiotic therapy. The choice of an antibiotic may be based on culture and sensitivity, although most isolates are susceptible to enrofloxacin (Baytril, 2.5 mg/lb two times a day) or trimethoprim-sulfadiazine (7 mg/lb two times a day). Fluoroquinolones such as enrofloxacin can be effective for treating both active disease and the carrier state. In addition to antibiotics, fluid and electrolyte replacement and identification and correction of underlying predisposing conditions are important aspects of therapy. Antibiotics should be continued for 7 to 10 days, and feces should be recultured 1 and 4 weeks after treatment. The prognosis for most patients with salmonellosis is good, although the mortality rate can be high in outbreaks in extremely susceptible populations (e.g., hospital patients, neonates). Proper hygiene in handling infected patients is necessary to prevent feco-oral or fomite transmission of infection to other animals or to humans.

Campylobacteriosis

C. jejuni are fastidious, microaerophilic, gram-negative, motile, slender, curved bacteria that have emerged as important pathogens of animals and humans worldwide. In dogs and cats the full spectrum of clinical manifestations remains to be defined because it is known that the number of clinically normal animals that shed *Campylobacter* in their feces is comparable to the incidence of shedding by diarrheic animals. Isolation rates vary widely, from less than 1% in confined pet populations to 50% or more in some animal pounds and shelters. Thus conditions of close confinement or poor sanitation apparently provide the greatest opportunity for exposure.

Because it is difficult to produce enteritis with *Campylobacter* experimentally in dogs and cats and because many of the animals that harbor these organisms are asymptomatic, it has been debated whether *Campylobacter* by itself even causes diarrhea in the dog and cat unless superimposed on other enteropathogenic infections, such as viruses, other bacteria, *Giardia*, or helminths. Nevertheless, clinical signs that have been associated with *Campylobacter* infection in dogs and cats have been attributed to superficial erosive enterocolitis or enterotoxin-mediated secretory diarrhea and are characterized by a 5- to 15-day course of watery-mucoid diarrhea that occasionally contains blood and may be accompanied by vomiting or tenesmus. Fever is usually mild or absent. In some patients the diarrhea appears to be chronic or intermittent.

A presumptive diagnosis of campylobacteriosis can be made by identification of slender, curved, gram-negative rods that have a characteristic W shape in stained fecal smears. The presence of fecal leukocytes may also be noted. In fresh saline smears, an experienced examiner may be able to tentatively identify *Campylobacter* with darkfield or phase-contrast microscopy as highly motile, darting, spiral or S-shaped bacteria; however, they should not be confused with spirochetes and other motile bacteria that are part of the normal flora. Definitive diagnosis requires isolation of *Campylobacter* from fresh feces with special selective media. Because *Campylobacter* are microaerophilic and difficult to isolate, fecal specimens should be obtained directly from the rectum and cultured or placed in transport media immediately after collection.

The antibiotic of choice for treating campylobacteriosis is erythromycin (5 to 7 mg/lb orally three times a day for 7 days); however, resistant strains have occasionally been isolated. Anorexia and vomiting are frequent side effects of erythromycin. Other effective oral antibiotics include neomycin (Biosol, 5 to 10 mg/lb orally three times a day), enrofloxacin (2.5 mg/lb orally two times a day), chloramphenicol, furazolidone, and doxycycline. Although fatalities in dogs and cats have been reported, the prognosis is considered good, and antibiotics are rapidly effective for eliminating fecal shedding of the organisms. Fecal cultures should be repeated 1 and 4 weeks after treatment. Because contact with feces from infected animals is a potential source of infection for humans as well as other animals, owners of infected pets should be advised to take standard precautions, such as proper disposal of potentially infectious feces, hand washing after handling infected animals, and separating infected animals from infants and small children until posttreatment cultures confirm that infection has been eliminated.

Yersiniosis

Yersinia enterocolitica, a motile, gram-negative rod, is recognized as a cause of acute and chronic enterocolitis in humans and has been isolated from small numbers of dogs and cats, mostly in Japan and Scandinavia. The majority of positive fecal isolations from dogs and cats have been from clinically healthy animals. On rare occasions in young dogs, *Y. enterocolitica* has been associated with enterocolitis characterized by bloody-mucoid large bowel diarrhea, tenesmus, and an absence of fever or systemic signs. An association with clinical disease in cats has not been established.

Y. enterocolitica grows best at colder temperatures, and special isolation methods are needed to culture the organism from feces. It also may be cultured from infected tissues or blood if the patient is bacteremic. Treatment for 7 to 10 days with trimethoprim-sulfadiazine (7 mg/lb two times a day), tetracycline, chloramphenicol, or an aminoglycoside is usually effective; however, antibiotic sensitivity testing is recommended. *Yersinia* infection of pets may be a public health concern.

In cats *Yersinia pseudotuberculosis* infection is a disseminated pyogranulomatous disease that is acquired from ingestion of infected rodent and avian prey and that primarily involves the GI tract, abdominal lymph nodes, and liver. Consequently the clinical signs are vomiting, diarrhea, weight loss, depression, fever, and icterus. Feline pseudotuberculosis is usually progressive and fatal, although clinically healthy carriers of the organism also have been found. Treatment consists of a prolonged course of an antibiotic such as trimethoprim-sulfadiazine, tetracycline, or chloramphenicol, but the prognosis is guarded.

Bacillus Piliformis

Tyzzer's disease, caused by a pleomorphic, gram-negative, spore-forming, obligate intracellular bacillus called *B. piliformis*, is a rare but fatal disease characterized by hemorrhagic-necrotizing enterocolitis and hepatic necrosis. The principal reservoirs of infection are rodents. Puppies and kittens are most often affected, and the disease may complicate parasitism and viral infections such as parvovirus, FeLV, and canine distemper virus. The progression of Tyzzer's disease is rapid; most patients die within 48 hours after the initial onset of signs of anorexia, depression, and diarrhea. Successful therapy has not been reported.

Definitive diagnosis of Tyzzer's disease is difficult because *B. piliformis* cannot be cultured on artificial media. Instead, mouse inoculation or embryonated egg culture techniques must be used to isolate the organisms. Most cases have been diagnosed at necropsy by the histologic identification of typical-appearing bundles of intracellular filamentous bacilli at the margins of necrotic foci within liver and intestinal lesions with special stains such as methenamine silver, Giemsa, or periodic acid–Schiff (PAS).

Clostridial Diarrhea

Enterotoxigenic *C. perfringens* is an important cause of acute and chronic large bowel diarrhea in dogs and cats. In addition, *Clostridium difficile,* the primary cause of antibiotic-associated pseudomembranous colitis in humans, is also found in dogs and cats and may occasionally be associated with diarrhea.

Diarrhea Associated With *Clostridium Perfringens*

C. perfringens is a large anaerobic gram-positive bacillus that normally exists in the intestinal tract of most dogs and cats. Enterotoxin-producing strains of *C. perfringens* can be associated with nonspecific episodes of diarrhea, acute hemorrhagic diarrhea, chronic or recurrent diarrhea, and outbreaks of diarrhea in animal groups. These bacteria normally reside in the bowel in the vegetative form, but they can release their toxin during sporulation endogenously within the bowel or exogenously in contaminated food. The *cpe* gene that regulates production of *C. perfringens* enterotoxin (CPE) is up-regulated by factors that activate sporulation; thus the presence of clostridial endospores in feces or food has been suggested as an indirect marker for the presence of CPE. Whether derived endogenously or ingested, CPE causes diarrhea by binding to intestinal epithelium and causing increased permeability, hypersecretion, and cell damage (cytotoxicity). Endogenous sporulation and the production of CPE can be associated with alteration of the intraluminal environment caused by sudden changes in diet, antibiotic administration, alkaline conditions, immunosuppression, inflammatory bowel disease (IBD), or concurrent intestinal infections.

Clinical Signs

Enterotoxigenic *C. perfringens* infection is associated with large bowel diarrhea that varies from watery to soft and may contain mucus or blood. Increased frequency is common, and tenesmus may be seen. In dogs enterotoxigenic *C. perfringens* has also been associated with a syndrome of acute hemorrhagic gastroenteritis (HGE) accompanied by severe hemoconcentration. Infection can also cause diarrhea in groups of animals confined together and nosocomial outbreaks in hospitalized patients. Clostridial diarrhea is usually self-limiting after a few days, but in some patients diarrhea can persist chronically for weeks to months. Some patients have recurrent episodes of diarrhea.

Diagnosis

Routine hematologic and serum chemistry evaluations are usually normal in patients with clostridial diarrhea. Colonoscopy is not routinely necessary in these cases, but endoscopic findings are usually nonspecific (diffuse hyperemia, increased friability, fresh bleeding, and increased mucus). Biopsy results range from minimal abnormalities to catarrhal, lymphocytic-plasmacytic, or suppurative colitis.

A definitive diagnostic test for *C. perfringens*–induced diarrhea is lacking. Further work is needed to determine the role of CPE in canine and feline diarrhea and to define the optimal diagnostic parameters for clostridial diarrhea. Fecal spore counts in stained fecal smears are commonly used for routine cage-side screening; however, studies have not shown a correlation between spore counts and positive assays for CPE or a correlation between either of these diagnostic procedures and the presence or absence of diarrhea. In humans, fecal assays for CPE are considered more accurate than spore counts; however, the commercially available CPE assays used in humans need to be validated for dogs and cats. In principle, CPE assays should be valid across species.

The identification of more than five clostridial endospores per oil immersion field (identified by their "safety-pin" appearance with Diff-Quik or Wright's staining, see Chapter 6) is considered by many to be presumptive evidence for a diagnosis of enterotoxigenic diarrhea caused by *C. perfringens*. Clostridial spores are generally larger than other bacilli found in feces. Malachite green can be used as a special stain for endospores. Fecal leukocytes also may be present. Unfortunately, the appearance or absence of clostridial spores in the feces does not correlate well with CPE assays or signs; thus it might be advisable to take into account spore counts, CPE assays, and clinical information before making a diagnosis of clostridial diarrhea.

Commercial fecal assays for *C. perfringens* enterotoxin are available in kit form as either an enzyme-linked immunosorbent assay (ELISA) or reverse passive latex agglutination (RPLA Kit).★ The ELISA assay is recommended as easier to use and interpret than the RPLA assay, and possibly more sensitive. It is recommended that fresh feces be used whenever possible and transported without delay to the laboratory in prechilled diluent at 4° C (but freezing should be avoided). Assays for CPE are generally considered to be more specific than fecal spore counts.

Cultures are not helpful because *C. perfringens* are normally found in the feces of most normal dogs and cats, and cultures do not reliably distinguish toxigenic and nontoxigenic strains. Assays using molecular probes and polymerase chain reaction are currently being evaluated as improved diagnostic procedures for enterotoxigenic *C. perfringens*.

Treatment

Diarrhea caused by enterotoxigenic *C. perfringens* can be effectively treated with ampicillin (10 mg/lb orally every 8 hours), amoxicillin-clavulanate (6 to 12.5 mg/lb orally every 12 hours), tylosin (10 to 20 mg/lb orally every 12 hours), or clindamycin (2.5 to 5 mg/lb orally every 12 hours) for 5 to 7 days. Metronidazole (5 to 10 mg/lb orally every 12 hours) can also be effective but seems to work less consistently. Clostridial diarrhea is usually self-limiting or responsive to antibiotics in 2 to 3 days; however, chronic or recurrent clostridial diarrhea may require long-term antibiotics (e.g., tylosin once daily or every other day) and a fiber-supplemented diet to prevent relapses. Commercial fiber-containing diets or regular diets supplemented with psyllium (Metamucil; dogs: 1 to 2 tbsp/day) may help to reduce bacterial proliferation and sporulation because fiber is fermented to SCFAs that acidify bowel contents. Alkaline rather than acid conditions are most favorable for *C. perfringens*. In addition, SCFAs nourish colonic epithelium and protect against injury.

Diarrhea Associated With *Clostridium Difficile*

A severe form of pseudomembranous colitis in humans is caused by colonic overgrowth of cytotoxin-producing *C. difficile,* usually subsequent to suppression of the normal flora by antimicrobials or anticancer agents. Toxigenic *C. difficile* and

its toxin have been isolated from normal dogs and cats and from a few patients with mild diarrhea; however, this organism does not appear to be significant as an enteropathogen in dogs and cats. *C. difficile* can be cultured using selective medium; however, infection can be established more rapidly by fecal PCR assay for the toxin gene or by latex agglutination assay of feces for toxin.

Mycotic Colitis
Histoplasma Colitis

Histoplasma capsulatum, a dimorphic soilborne fungus endemic to regions bordering the Mississippi River and its tributaries, primarily causes pulmonary and macrophage-monocyte system infection and occasionally intestinal tract infection. Widespread dissemination to virtually any tissue or organ system also can occur. The intestinal form of histoplasmosis occurs most often in young dogs and cats and is characterized by extensive transmural granulomatous inflammation of the bowel with mucosal ulceration and involvement of associated lymph nodes. The macrophages in these lesions contain *Histoplasma* organisms.

Intestinal histoplasmosis may be manifested as either small or large bowel diarrhea, or a combination of both when the disease is diffuse. Small bowel involvement is characterized by malabsorption syndrome and sometimes protein-losing enteropathy (see Chapter 7). When the colon is affected, severe bloody-mucoid large bowel diarrhea and tenesmus are seen. The disease is usually chronic, and associated signs may include fever, pallor, inappetence, lethargy, and progressive weight loss. Abdominal palpation may reveal diffuse thickening of the colon or small intestines, focal tumorlike (granulomatous) thickenings in the intestinal tract or mesentery, mesenteric lymphadenopathy, or abdominal effusions. When the rectum is involved, mucosal proliferations may be detected by digital palpation. Physical examination may also detect other extraintestinal sites of dissemination (e.g., liver, spleen, or eyes).

Histoplasmosis should be suspected in young patients in endemic areas with chronic intractable diarrhea. The results of diagnostics are variable but may reveal nonregenerative anemia, regenerative neutrophilia, monocytosis, and hypoproteinemia. Contrast radiography may demonstrate an irregular mucosal pattern indicative of a diffuse infiltrative lesion. Ultrasonography may reveal diffuse or focal thickening of the colon with associated lym-

---

★Oxoid, Unipath, Ogdensberg, NY.

phadenopathy. Colonoscopy usually reveals severe granulomatous ulcerative colitis. Definitive diagnosis depends on identification of *Histoplasma* organisms in cytologic preparations (rectal mucosal smears, colonic biopsy impressions, aspirates of lymph nodes or abdominal masses), colonoscopic biopsy specimens, or cultures of feces or affected tissues on Sabouraud's medium. In addition, serologic tests (immunodiffusion, complement fixation) that detect anti-*Histoplasma* antibodies can be used to establish a presumptive diagnosis; however, reliability of these tests is questionable because false-negative results are frequent.

Histoplasma colitis is progressive without treatment. Oral itraconazole (2.5 mg/lb orally every 12 hours) is the treatment of choice for histoplasmosis. Ketoconazole (5 mg/lb every 12 hours with food) can also be used as a more economical alternative, but it has less consistent efficacy and greater risk of side effects. Treatment with either of these antifungal drugs is continued for at least 2 to 3 months beyond remission, usually for a total of 4 to 6 months, while monitoring for hepatotoxicity. For symptomatic relief of colonic inflammation and tenesmus, 5-aminosalicylates (5-ASA) (e.g., sulfasalazine, olsalazine, mesalamine) can be administered as described later under treatment of idiopathic IBD.

Other Mycoses

Other than histoplasmosis, mycotic infections of the colon are rare; however, opportunistic fungi sometimes invade devitalized tissue (such as mucosa traumatized by passage of a foreign body) or infect young patients already compromised by predisposing factors such as immunodeficiency, malnutrition, preexisting debilitating illnesses (such as parasitism or parvovirus), or prolonged therapy with antimicrobials or corticosteroids. Opportunistic fungi can infect any portion of the intestinal tract of the dog and cat, and they include *Candida albicans, Aspergillus* sp., *Pythium* sp., and various fungi of the Zygomycetes class.

Both *Aspergillus* and *Candida* cause chronic diarrhea with mucosal ulceration and necrotizing lesions that extend into the deeper layers of the bowel wall. Pseudomembrane formation and vascular invasion by hyphae have been seen in cats with aspergillosis.

The term *pythiosis* is often used to designate GI infections caused by *Pythium* sp. and Zygomycetes. Pythiosis is most prevalent in the Gulf region of the United States, especially in young large-breed dogs, and it is characterized by extensive necrotizing transmural granulomatous inflammation of the bowel. The lesions may result in tumorlike thickening of the affected segment of the GI tract. The stomach, small intestines, and mesentery are most often affected; however, the colon is occasionally involved and may result in chronic bloody-mucoid large bowel diarrhea.

The antemortem diagnosis of any of these intestinal mycoses is difficult, usually requiring histologic identification of the fungi in colonic biopsy specimens. The branching hyphae of *Aspergillus* sp. or the sparsely septate hyphae of *Pythium* sp. and Zygomycetes are best demonstrated in tissue specimens by Gridley's or methenamine silver stains. *Candida* may form yeastlike cells or septate mycelia (pseudohyphae), which can be seen with fungal stains or Gram stain (gram-positive). Feces or biopsy specimens can be cultured on Sabouraud's medium for fungi, but this is slow and often unrewarding.

Most cases of intestinal aspergillosis and candidiasis have been diagnosed at necropsy; thus information on which to base treatment is limited. Treatment with oral itraconazole is suggested. Successful treatment of pythiosis is rare; thus the prognosis must be considered poor. When feasible, surgical excision of the severely involved segments of bowel with follow-up therapy using oral itraconazole or intravenous (IV) lipid-complexed amphotericin B is suggested.

Prothecal Colitis

Prototheca sp. are ubiquitous unicellular algae that may rarely colonize the lamina propria and submucosa of the intestinal tract of dogs and cause severe necrotizing or ulcerating enterocolitis. These algae appear to have a predilection for initially invading the colon, resulting in signs of chronic large bowel diarrhea with hematochezia. Typically the prothecal organisms then disseminate widely throughout the body and most frequently involve other visceral organs, the eyes, and the central nervous system (CNS). Only a cutaneous form has been described in cats.

Colonoscopy reveals thickened, corrugated mucosal folds, and the mucosa may be friable or ulcerated. *Prototheca* organisms can be identified in feces, cytologic preparations (Wright's or Gram stain), and biopsy specimens (Gomori's or PAS stain) as clusters of endosporulated ovoid structures (5 to 16 μm in length). *Prototheca* can also be cultured on Sabouraud's cycloheximide-free dextrose medium. Successful treatment of systemic prototthecosis in animals is rare. A combination of IV lipid-complexed amphotericin B with either itraconazole, ketoconazole, or tetracycline is suggested.

Chronic Idiopathic Colitis (Inflammatory Bowel Disease)

The terms *chronic idiopathic colitis* and *inflammatory bowel disease (IBD)* are generally used interchangeably to refer to a diverse group of chronic disorders characterized by diffuse infiltration of the colonic mucosa and sometimes submucosa with inflammatory cells. The types of colitis are classified histopathologically on the basis of the predominant infiltrating cells as lymphocytic-plasmacytic colitis, eosinophilic colitis, neutrophilic colitis, granulomatous colitis, and histiocytic ulcerative colitis. Thus definitive diagnosis depends on colonoscopic biopsy in conjunction with establishing the idiopathic nature of the condition. Sometimes there is a mixture of inflammatory cells in the lesion that makes classification difficult. The most common form of IBD in dogs and cats is lymphocytic-plasmacytic colitis. In some animals with IBD, infiltrative lesions may also involve the small intestines and/or stomach. It is unclear whether these are variants of the same disease process or not. Chronic idiopathic inflammatory diseases of the stomach and small bowel are discussed in Chapter 5 and 7, respectively.

The etiology of colitis (IBD) in dogs and cats is not determined in most cases, but genetic, dietary, bacterial, immunologic, and mucosal permeability factors have been implicated. The pathogenesis may involve altered mucosal permeability and a hypersensitivity response to antigens derived from food, intestinal bacteria, or the intestine itself. This may result either from a primary disorder of the intestinal immune system or its regulation or from immune events that occur secondary to mucosal injury and permeability. It has been suggested that chronic inflammation of the bowel becomes self-perpetuating when loss of mucosal integrity allows bacterial or dietary proteins to enter the lamina propria, where they act as antigens (or cross-react with self-antigens) that incite ongoing immune-mediated recruitment of inflammatory cells.

Most animals with IBD involving predominantly the colon have chronic or recurrent large bowel diarrhea; thus IBD must be differentiated from parasitic and infectious causes of colitis. Even though the cause of IBD is unknown, dietary manipulation and medical treatment are often effective in controlling the disease.

Lymphocytic-Plasmacytic Colitis

The most common form of IBD in both dogs and cats is characterized by diffuse infiltration of the lamina propria by lymphocytes and plasma cells in association with mucosal damage and abnormalities of mucosal epithelium and permeability. Idiopathic lymphocytic-plasmacytic IBD is generally considered to be the most common finding in dogs and cats evaluated for chronic vomiting and diarrhea. The stomach, small intestines, and colon may be involved separately or together. This discussion will focus on lymphocytic-plasmacytic colitis; the reader is referred to other chapters in this book for further information regarding IBD of the stomach and small intestine.

Etiology

The etiology of lymphocytic-plasmacytic IBD is unknown, but genetic, dietary, bacterial, immunologic, and mucosal permeability factors have been suggested to play a role. The disease involves either a primary disorder of the intestinal immune system or its regulation, or immune responses that occur secondary to mucosal injury and permeability. Chronic inflammation of the bowel may become self-perpetuating when loss of mucosal integrity and increased permeability allow bacterial or dietary proteins to enter the lamina propria, where they incite further immune reaction and inflammation.

In some cases this lesion can be associated with dietary hypersensitivity, enteric pathogens, or lymphoma. Some patients with lesions of lymphocytic-plasmacytic enterocolitis respond to protein elimination diets or antibiotics such as metronidazole or tylosin; however, in most patients lymphocytic-plasmacytic colitis is idiopathic.

Clinical Signs

The most frequent presenting clinical signs of lymphocytic-plasmacytic IBD are vomiting, diarrhea, and weight loss. The signs vary with the regions of the GI tract that are involved and the severity of mucosal infiltration and damage. The typical historical pattern is one of GI problems that wax and wane over periods ranging from a few weeks to several years. Animals of all ages are susceptible. Chronic intermittent vomiting is the most frequent sign of lymphocytic-plasmacytic

IBD in cats. Colitis usually causes large bowel diarrhea characterized by increased frequency of defecation, urgency, tenesmus, increased fecal mucus, and hematochezia. Fecal consistency varies. Intermittent hematochezia without diarrhea may be the only sign of IBD. A change in defecation habits or loss of litter training without diarrhea can also occur. Physical examination is usually unremarkable, except for cachexia in severe cases. Intestinal loops can occasionally be palpably thickened and firm when the small intestine is involved. The literature reports some patients with concurrent food allergic dermatopathy, but this has been extremely rare in my experience.

Diagnosis

Precise criteria for the diagnosis of idiopathic lymphocytic-plasmacytic colitis have not yet been established. In general the clinical criteria for diagnosis are (1) chronic signs of colonic disease, (2) characteristic mucosal lesions of IBD in colonoscopic biopsy specimens, (3) failure to respond to dietary trials, and (4) exclusion of known causes of chronic inflammation of the intestinal tract based on thorough diagnostic evaluation. This last criterion emphasizes that IBD is a diagnosis of exclusion and not a catch-all label to be used as a substitute for diagnostic evaluation. Because lymphocytic-plasmacytic inflammation is a nonspecific lesion, only a thorough diagnostic work-up can establish that it is truly idiopathic and not merely an inflammatory response to an undiagnosed condition. A well-planned diagnostic approach could include routine fecal examinations (for parasites, *C. perfringens* spores, *Campylobacter*, and fecal leukocytes), a therapeutic trial of fenbendazole for occult whipworm infection, elimination dietary trials, routine screening for extraintestinal disease (CBC, serum chemistry profile, urinalysis, retrovirus tests in cats, and baseline serum T_4 level in cats over 5 years of age), abdominal imaging (radiography, ultrasonography), and colonoscopy with biopsy under anesthesia.

Laboratory Evaluations

Routine hematologic and serum biochemical parameters are normal in most patients with lymphocytic-plasmacytic colitis; however, some are found to have mild nonspecific laboratory abnormalities such as mild anemia, stress leukogram (mature neutrophilia, lymphopenia), stress hyperglycemia, mild hypoproteinemia (hypoalbuminemia, hypoglobulinemia, or both), and hypokalemia. Unexplained thrombocytopenia has been observed occasionally. Eosinophilia is occasionally found in cats. Cats with IBD often have mild-to-moderate elevations of serum liver enzymes (especially alanine aminotransferase), which in some cases is due to associated cholangiohepatitis and/or pancreatitis. Hypoproteinemia related to protein-losing enteropathy sometimes is noted in dogs with small intestinal involvement but is rare in cats.

Radiography and Ultrasonography

In most cases radiographic and ultrasonographic findings are unremarkable and do not aid in diagnosis. Some patients have a nonspecific finding of fluid- and gas-distended bowel loops on plain abdominal radiography. Barium-contrast radiography occasionally demonstrates diffuse mucosal irregularity, and ultrasonography may reveal intestinal thickening, but these are nonspecific findings that merely suggest an infiltrative lesion. In selected cases contrast radiography and ultrasonography can be helpful nonetheless, because they may discover an unexpected diagnosis other than IBD, for example, pancreatitis, hepatobiliary disease, or intestinal tumors, polyps, granulomas, or malformations (e.g., diverticulum, short colon).

Endoscopic Examination

In patients with GI disease, the spectrum of clinical signs usually suggests the most appropriate region of the GI tract for endoscopic examination. In IBD, however, signs do not always correlate with the region of greatest cellular infiltration, especially in cats. It is not uncommon to find significant involvement of the colon in cats that present for vomiting. Conversely, cats with hematochezia or other colonic signs may have unexpected gastroduodenal lesions. Therefore it may be advisable in many cases to obtain biopsy specimens from the stomach, duodenum, jejunum (if possible), colon, and ileum (if the ileocolic sphincter can be navigated during colonoscopy).

Endoscopically the mucosa in colitis may appear to be normal or it may have any of the following abnormalities: erythema, petechiae, increased mucus, increased friability, increased surface granularity, decreased visibility of the submucosal vessels, thickened or increased folds, erosions/ulcers, or decreased distensibility. The mucosal lesions may be apparent only microscopically; thus a normal endoscopic appearance does not rule out IBD, and multiple biopsy specimens should be taken even if there are no endoscopically visible abnormalities.

Mucosal Histopathologic Examination

The histopathologic lesion of lymphocytic-plasmacytic IBD is characterized by diffuse infiltration of the lamina propria with mature lymphocytes and plasma cells in association with mucosal damage. In some cases the inflammation is mostly lymphocytic; in others the infiltrate also contains a mixture of other types of inflammatory cells (neutrophils, eosinophils, macrophages). The cellular infiltrate is usually confined to the mucosa but occasionally may extend to the submucosa. Additional findings indicative of mucosal damage include architectural distortion, fibrosis, and epithelial abnormalities (hyperplasia, degeneration, necrosis, erosion, ulceration, glandular dilation, loss of globlet cells). Pathologists may differ in their interpretation of endoscopic biopsy specimens and in their definition of how many lymphocytes and plasma cells within the lamina propria are too many. Infiltrates assessed to be minimal or mild by an inexperienced pathologist may not be truly abnormal. For definitive diagnosis of lymphocytic-plasmacytic colitis there must be abnormal infiltration of lymphocytes and plasma cells, as well as evidence of mucosal damage. Various grading systems have been proposed, but these have not correlated well with clinical disease activity. A severe infiltration of lymphocytes that extends beyond the mucosa into the submucosa and muscularis should raise the suspicion of early lymphoma mimicking IBD, and further diagnostics should be recommended.

Evaluation for Dietary Hypersensitivity

Dietary hypersensitivity or food allergy is an immunologically mediated adverse reaction to a protein component in food. A well-controlled dietary trial using a protein elimination diet is the basis for diagnosis of dietary hypersensitivity as a cause of IBD. The diet is changed to a well-defined, additive-free, highly digestible diet that contains a single source of protein not found in the patient's normal diet. Intake of all other foods or sources of antigen must be completely eliminated throughout the feeding trial, including table scraps, treats, and flavored medications such as vitamin supplements. The goal is to feed a single protein source to which the patient is not yet sensitized. Although many commercial hypoallergenic diets are available (see the section on treatment), home-prepared single-protein diets are preferred for diagnostic testing purposes. Examples of novel protein sources not likely found in the patient's regular diet might include turkey, duck, lamb, rabbit, venison, fish, or soybean (tofu). Once dietary hypersensitivity is confirmed with a home-prepared diet, commercial hypoallergenic diets can

be substituted for more convenience for long-term management.

A cooperative and patient owner is required for a successful elimination diet trial. A minimum of 3 to 4 weeks should be allowed for initial response to an elimination diet. If no improvement has occurred during this time, then dietary hypersensitivity is unlikely and medical therapy should be instituted. If some improvement has been observed, then the trial should continue, because it may require 6 to 10 weeks before improvement is complete.

If there is a substantial improvement with the elimination diet, then the patient can be rechallenged with its original diet. Recurrence of clinical signs confirms dietary intolerance or hypersensitivity. In addition, once remission is restored with the controlled diet, the patient can then be challenged sequentially with individual dietary components to identify the specific offenders. To do this, individual components of the original diet are added one at a time to the controlled diet while the patient is in remission. With each challenge the patient is monitored for recurrence of signs for 7 to 10 days. If signs recur, then that substance is implicated as an offender.

After several weeks of remission of the controlled diet, some patients can be returned to their original diet and remain asymptomatic; but in most cases specially formulated or hypoallergenic diets may need to be continued indefinitely to prevent relapse. If there is no response to dietary management within 4 to 6 weeks, the patient can be returned to its original diet and medical therapy instituted.

Treatment

Well-controlled therapeutic trials for chronic colitis in animals are lacking; thus treatment is largely empirical and based on clinical experience. Because dietary hypersensitivity, parasites (see previous section), and bacterial enteropathogens (see previous section) may cause lymphocytic-plasmacytic colitis, it is appropriate to first consider evaluation and treatment for these possibilities. In most cases of lymphocytic-plasmacytic colitis an underlying cause cannot be identified and the most effective treatment is an antiinflammatory regimen of either a corticosteroid or mesalamine (5-aminosalicylate derivative) combined with dietary modification (e.g., novel protein diet or fiber-enriched diet). If diet and antiinflammatory drugs fail to control the disease, metronidazole is added for its antibacterial and immunomodulatory properties. Metronidazole can also be used as a single drug to induce or maintain remission in less severe cases. For the most refractory cases a cytotoxic immunosuppressive agent such as azathioprine is added to the corticosteroid regimen.

Dietary Therapy

Various strategies for dietary modification have been used for treatment of chronic colitis, including novel protein diets, fiber-enriched diets, and diets with adjusted omega-6 and omega-3 fatty acid levels. In some patients with IBD, dietary modification produces a complete or partial resolution of the signs and sometimes regression of the lesions. Potential explanations for a beneficial response to dietary modification include the effects of the diet on bowel motility, composition of the microflora, mucosal structure and function, and exposure to foodborne antigens or additives.

The treatment of IBD associated with dietary hypersensitivity is based on the controlled feeding of a well-defined, additive-free, highly digestible diet that contains a single source of protein not found in the patient's normal diet (i.e., a novel protein to which the patient is not yet sensitized). Home-prepared diets (turkey, duck, lamb, rabbit, venison, whitefish, or tofu) are most suitable for diagnostic testing purposes (see previous section on diagnosis); however, if the home-prepared diet suggests diet-responsive disease, then a commercial "hypoallergenic" novel protein diet can be substituted and is more convenient and balanced for long-term feeding. Many commercial diets that contain novel protein sources are now marketed for dietary hypersensitivity. A relapse rate of approximately 15% to 20% is to be expected when switching from a home-prepared to a commercial hypoallergenic diet. For long-term feeding of a home-prepared diet, recipes for balanced diets containing novel protein sources can be found in standard veterinary therapy and nutrition textbooks, or various reliable websites under supervision of Diplomates of the American College of Veterinary Nutrition.

In cases in which hypoallergenic novel protein diets have not been effective, other dietary adjustments may be beneficial as an adjunct to medical therapy for IBD. This includes fiber supplementation (psyllium, bran, canned pumpkin) of the regular diet or switching to a commercial diet enriched with fermentable fiber (e.g., beet pulp) marketed for improving colonic function and ameliorating diarrhea in patients with colitis. Fiber has many beneficial effects on colonic function and helps to keep enteropathogens in check. Colonic bacteria metabolize fermentable fiber to SCFAs that nourish colonic epithelium and protect against mucosal injury. Adjustment of the levels of omega-6 and omega-3 fatty acids in the diet has been proposed to manage bowel inflammation through decreasing inflammatory mediators, although evidence for this is lacking.

Corticosteroids

Oral prednisolone is the most consistently effective medical therapy (dogs: 0.5 to 1 mg/lb/day; cats: 1 to 2 mg/lb/day or 5 mg total dose every 12 hours) for inducing remission of idiopathic lymphocytic-plasmacytic colitis. Clinical improvement using this dosage should be noted within 1 to 2 weeks. After 2 weeks of remission, the dosage is tapered in 2- to 4-week increments to the lowest effective alternate-day dosage. In cats that are too difficult to medicate orally, periodic injections of methylprednisolone acetate (20 mg intramuscularly or subcutaneously every 2 to 4 weeks) may be substituted for oral treatment, or dermal preparations formulated by a compounding pharmacist may be applied topically. Corticosteroid therapy may be discontinued on a trial basis after 6 to 12 weeks of remission; however, continuous alternate-day therapy is often required to prevent relapse. In refractory cases metronidazole or mesalamine (see following sections) should be added to the prednisolone regimen. If this fails to control the disease, then the combination of azathioprine (see later section) and prednisolone may be more effective in achieving remission of the disease.

5-Aminosalicylic Acid

Derivatives of 5-ASA, also known as mesalamine, exert an antiinflammatory effect in colitis through local inhibition of mucosal leukotrienes and prostaglandins. Many gastroenterologists regard these as the initial drugs of choice for treatment of colitis, particularly in dogs. Orally administered 5-ASA derivatives are designed to be minimally absorbed during passage through the small intestine so that they reach the colon. These drugs should be used cautiously in cats because some salicylate absorption occurs and cats metabolize salicylates very slowly.

In sulfasalazine (Azulfidine), 5-ASA is combined with sulfapyridine by an azo bond that prevents significant absorption of the drug so that 75% of it reaches the colon, where colonic bacteria split the bond and release the 5-ASA for its local effect in the colon. Sulfasalazine dosages of 10 to 20 mg/lb (maximum of 1 g per dose) every 8 hours are used in dogs; 5 to 10 mg/lb every 12 hours or 250 mg total dose every 24 hours have been effective and relatively well tolerated in cats. The most common adverse side effect of sulfasalazine is keratoconjunctivitis sicca, which can be irreversible. For this reason it is recommended that a baseline Schirmer's tear test be performed at the start of therapy and then monitored subsequently at monthly intervals if treatment is long-term. Less common side effects include allergic dermatitis, nausea and vomiting, and cholestatic jaundice. Rarely cats may develop anemia.

Newer formulations of 5-ASA include olsalazine (Dipentum) and polymer-coated mesalamine tablets (Asacol) and capsules (Pentasa). The advantages of these newer formulations over sulfasalazine are that a greater percentage of the drug (80% to 90%) reaches the colon and these formulations do not contain sulfapyridine so they have fewer side effects. Unfortunately, these products are much more expensive than sulfasalazine and they are not available in convenient dosage sizes for most patients. Safe and effective dosages remain to be determined. Sulfasalazine, olsalazine, or mesalamine can also be combined with corticosteroids or metronidazole to treat refractory colitis.

Metronidazole and Other Antibiotics

Low-dose metronidazole therapy (Flagyl, 5 to 7 mg/lb every 12 hours) is often beneficial either alone or in combination with prednisolone to treat IBD. The beneficial effects of metronidazole in any patient with diarrhea might be attributable to an antibacterial effect on enteropathogens (e.g., enterotoxigenic *C. perfringens*), an antiprotozoal effect (e.g., *Giardia*), a reduction of bacterial-derived antigens that could be involved in the immunopathogenesis of IBD, or the immunomodulating effect of the drug on cell-mediated immunity and neutrophil chemotaxis. Metronidazole tablets have an unpleasant taste and provoke salivation in most cats and sometimes vomiting. For ease of administration and accurate dosing, a liquid suspension can be formulated on request by many pharmacists or the tablets can be split and placed in gel capsules. Dosages of metronidazole exceeding 25 mg/lb/day for prolonged periods (weeks) occasionally cause signs of reversible CNS toxicity (ataxia, weakness, seizures). Other antibiotics that might be helpful to control intestinal microflora include tylosin or doxycycline (2.5 mg/lb every 12 hours).

Azathioprine

In IBD patients refractory to prednisone alone or in combination with metronidazole or mesalamine, the combination of azathioprine (Imuran) with prednisolone may be a more effective immunosuppressive regimen for producing remission of the disease. In addition to treating refractory IBD, the addition of azathioprine may enable use of a lower dose of corticosteroid to control the disease and thereby minimize steroidal side effects. Azathioprine is usually given as an alternate-day treatment (alternating with every-other-day prednisolone) at a dosage of 0.5 to 1 mg/lb orally in dogs and 0.15 to 0.25 mg/lb orally in cats. Azathioprine should be prepared as an oral suspension to facilitate accurate and safe dosing for cats. Because of its myelosuppressive toxicity (leukopenia), the CBC should be monitored periodically, every 2 to 3 weeks for the first 2 months.

Future Possibilities for Immune Modulation in Colitis

Cyclosporine is a potent immunosuppressive drug (inhibits interleukin-2 and T-cell recruitment) and has shown promise in treating human IBD. New types of antiinflammatory drugs used to treat airway inflammation in asthmatics might find use in treating chronic GI inflammation as well. Zileuton (Zyflo) inhibits the formation of leukotrienes by inhibiting 5-lipoxygenase. Zafirlukast (Accolate) and montelukast (Singulair) are leukotriene receptor antagonists that reduce inflammatory cell influx. The effects of these so-called leukotriene blockers are comparable to steroids without steroidal side effects.

Eosinophilic Colitis

Eosinophilic colitis is an uncommon form of IBD that may occur alone or as part of a generalized syndrome of eosinophilic gastroenterocolitis. The lesion is characterized by segmental or diffuse infiltration of one or more layers of the colon with mature eosinophils, often accompanied by peripheral eosinophilia but not in all cases. Allergy and parasitism have been proposed as causes, but in most patients evidence for these is lacking and the disease must be considered idiopathic.

The colon may also be involved in the feline hypereosinophilic syndrome, in which there is widespread infiltration of eosinophils throughout the GI tract and in numerous extraintestinal tissues (see Chapter 7). Associated findings in cats with hypereosinophilic syndrome can include palpation of thickened intestinal loops, hepatosplenomegaly, lymphadenopathy, pulmonary infiltration, and bone marrow infiltration.

Transmural eosinophilic granulomas in the colon occasionally produce focal tumorlike thickenings or masses that can bleed and cause partial intestinal obstruction. Surgical excision is usually advisable.

Diagnosis

The clinical signs of eosinophilic colitis are typical of acute or chronic large bowel diarrhea. Hematochezia is common due to bleeding from mucosal ulceration. If the stomach and small intestine also are involved, vomiting and small bowel diarrhea also may be seen. The history may indicate dramatic responsiveness to prior corticosteroid therapy. The diagnosis is based on peripheral eosinophilia (although not present in all cases), lesions of eosinophilic inflammation in colonoscopic mucosal biopsy specimens, and the exclusion of underlying parasitism. The endoscopic appearance of the colon is similar to that described for lymphocytic-plasmacytic colitis, except mucosal ulceration is found more often in eosinophilic colitis.

Treatment

It is especially important to rule out occult whipworm or hookworm infection as a cause of eosinophilic colitis in dogs with a therapeutic trial of fenbendazole (22 mg/lb orally daily for 3 days). A larvacidal dose of ivermectin (100 mg/lb subcutaneously once) has been suggested to empirically treat for migrating larvae of *Toxocara canis* as a potential cause; however, the usual precautions for ivermectin should be taken, including avoidance of use in collies and related breeds.

Because eosinophilic gastroenteritis may potentially be due to food allergy, a feeding trial using an elimination or hypoallergenic diet (as described for lymphocytic-plasmacytic colitis) may be considered initially; however, dietary therapy alone has seldom been effective for eosinophilic colitis in my experience.

Most dogs and cats with idiopathic eosinophilic colitis respond rapidly to oral prednisolone at an initial dosage of 0.5 to 1 mg/lb/day for dogs and 1 to 2 mg/lb/day for cats. Once remission has been maintained for 2 weeks, this dosage is gradually tapered over an additional 2 to 4 weeks to the lowest effective maintenance dose. In some patients the treatment can eventually be discontinued, whereas in others alternate-day maintenance therapy is required. In some patients it may be necessary to add azathioprine to the corticosteroid

regimen as described for lymphocytic-plasmacytic colitis to facilitate reduction of corticosteroid dosage and side effects or to provide more effective control of the disease.

Obstructing transmural eosinophilic granulomas involving a localized area of bowel should be surgically excised and treated with follow-up corticosteroid therapy. The prognosis for this atypical form of the disease is less favorable than for diffuse eosinophilic enterocolitis.

Neutrophilic (Suppurative) Colitis

Some patients with signs of acute or chronic colitis have been found by colonoscopic biopsy to have an infiltrate of predominantly neutrophils without evidence of an infectious cause. Associated findings in some cases may include mucosal ulceration, necrosis, or crypt abscesses. These lesions should prompt an evaluation for the presence of bacterial enteropathogens. Too few patients with neutrophilic colitis have been characterized to draw conclusions; however, antibiotics (e.g., metronidazole and enrofloxacin or regimens consisting of sulfasalazine, mesalamine, or antiinflammatory-immunosuppressive drugs as discussed for lymphocytic-plasmacytic colitis (see Table 8-2) appear to be effective for controlling the disease.

Regional Granulomatous Colitis

Regional granulomatous colitis is a rare form of IBD characterized by transmural granulomatous inflammation that usually involves the ileum and colon and results in a stenosing, masslike thickening of a region of the bowel wall. In some dogs the granulomatous lesion also contains numerous eosinophils (eosinophilic granuloma). Regional granulomatous enterocolitis of animals is idiopathic and has been compared with human regional enteritis known as Crohn's disease; however, despite the resemblance, it is not known if these are related.

The principal clinical sign of regional granulomatous enteritis is chronic large bowel diarrhea containing mucus and fresh blood, sometimes accompanied by tenesmus and abdominal pain. Additional signs may include weight loss, anorexia, and depression. The diseased segment of bowel may be palpable as a firm mass in the midabdomen. The adjacent intestinal loops and mesentery also may be thickened, and regional lymph nodes may be enlarged. Rectal masses may be

TABLE 8-2	Drugs Used for Treatment of Idiopathic Colitis		
Drug	**Product (Manufacturer)**	**Preparations**	**Dosage (D, dog; C, cat)**
ANTIINFLAMMATORIES/IMMUNOSUPPRESSIVES			
Sulfasalazine*	Azulfidine (Kabi Pharmacia)	Tab: 500 mg	D: 5-20 mg/lb PO q8h C: 5-10 mg/lb PO q12-24h
Olsalazine	Dipentum (Kabi Pharmacia)	Cap: 250 mg	D: 5-10 mg/lb PO q12h
Mesalamine	Asacol (Procter & Gamble)	Cap: 400 mg	D: 5-10 mg/lb PO q12h
	Pentasa (Shire)	Cap: 250 mg	
Prednisone†	Various	Tab: 5, 10, 20, 50 mg	D: 0.5-1 mg/lb PO q24h C: 1-2 mg/lb PO q24h
Methylprednisolone acetate	Depo-Medrol (Upjohn)	Inj: 40 mg/ml	C: 20 mg IM q2-4wk
Azathioprine‡	Imuran (Prometheus)	Tab: 50 mg	D: 0.5-1 mg/lb PO q24-48h C: 0.15-0.25 mg/lb PO q48h
ANTIINFLAMMATORY RETENTION ENEMAS§			
5-Aminosalicylic acid	Rowasa (Solvay)	Enema: 4 g/60 ml	Needs to be determined
Hydrocortisone	Cortenema (Reid-Rowell)	Enema: 100 mg/60 ml	20-60 ml rectally q24h
ANTIBIOTICS			
Metronidazole	Flagyl (Searle)	Tab: 250 mg, 500 mg	5-7 mg/lb PO q8-12h
Tylosin‖	Tylan Soluble (Elanco)	Powder	D: 10-20 mg/lb PO q12h
OPIOID MOTILITY MODIFIERS			
Loperamide	Imodium (McNeil)	Cap: 2 mg; liq: 0.2 mg/ml	D: 0.05-0.1 mg/lb PO q8-12h C: 0.05 mg/lb PO q12h
FIBER SUPPLEMENT			
Psyllium	Metamucil (Procter & Gamble)	Powder	D: 1-3 tbsp/day (in food) C: 1-3 tsp/day (in food)

Tab, tablets; *PO*, orally; *cap*, capsules; *inj*, injectable.

*Sulfasalazine dosage may need to be increased to 25 mg/lb q8h to achieve effect in some dogs; may cause sicca in dogs and salicylate toxicosis in cats.

†In some cats with severe colitis, prednisone dosage may need to be increased to 2.3 mg/lb/day, divided bid. In dogs, if steroidal side effects become a problem, decrease the dosage and combine with azathioprine or metronidazole or both.

‡Azathioprine may cause myelotoxicity, so monitor CBC; tablet can be crushed and compounded into a favorite liquid for accurate dosing of cats.

§Retention enemas for topical therapy of the distal colon may relieve signs of tenesmus and urgency in some patients with proctitis.

‖Tylosin powder is bitter tasting and thus best tolerated when mixed with food. It should be mixed in capsules for administration to cats.

identified by digital rectal palpation when this area is involved.

Diagnosis

Regional granulomatous colitis must be differentiated from intestinal neoplasia and from infectious causes of pyogranulomatous bowel lesions, such as histoplasmosis, pythiosis, and mycobacteriosis. In cats FIP coronavirus can occasionally cause pyogranulomatous colitis manifesting as a large tumorlike mass. Barium contrast radiography or ultrasonography of the ileum and colon may delineate a thickened or stenosed segment of bowel. A routine CBC may reveal eosinophilia, neutrophilia, or monocytosis. Panhypoproteinemia due to chronic intestinal bleeding and protein loss may be found in some patients.

Definitive diagnosis of granulomatous colitis depends on biopsy by colonoscopy or laparotomy. Colonoscopic findings include thickened and corrugated folds, proliferative mucosal masses, ulceration, loss of distensibility, and partial obstruction. The key histopathologic feature is transmural granulomatous inflammation. Fibrosis and aggregates of epithelioid cells, giant cells, and eosinophils are often found deep in the lesion. Deep ulceration is common. Whenever granulomatous lesions are found in the bowel, infectious causes should be ruled out with special stains that identify fungi and acid-fast organisms. In cats polymerase chain reaction assay for detection of coronavirus in biopsy specimens should be considered.

Treatment

Medical treatment of regional granulomatous colitis is based on the use of antiinflammatory and immunosuppressive agents such as olsalazine or sulfasalazine, prednisone, azathioprine, and metronidazole, as described for treatment of lymphocytic-plasmacytic colitis (see Table 8-2). If the degree of thickening and cicatrization of the affected segment of bowel is producing severe stenosis and obliteration of the lumen, surgical excision of the lesion may be necessary. Surgery should be followed by long-term medical therapy for 6 to 8 weeks or longer to prevent recurrence of the lesion at the surgical site. The prognosis is guarded.

Histiocytic Ulcerative Colitis

Histiocytic ulcerative colitis is a chronic idiopathic IBD of young boxer dogs characterized by infiltration of the lamina propria and submucosa of the colon by distinctive histiocytes engorged with deposits that stain positive with PAS stain. A mixture of other types of inflammatory cells also is found in the lesion, and there is usually severe mucosal ulceration. Affected boxers generally develop a severe unresponsive bloody-mucoid large bowel diarrhea before 2 years of age. Colonoscopy reveals diffuse severe mucosal inflammation with corrugation, ulceration, bleeding, and thickened folds. Weight loss and moderate hypoproteinemia may occur in dogs with long-standing disease. The diagnosis is based on the known breed predisposition and the presence of numerous PAS-positive histiocytes in a colonoscopic biopsy specimen.

The disease is treated with olsalazine or sulfasalazine, prednisone, azathioprine, and metronidazole in single-agent or combination regimens as described for lymphocytic-plasmacytic colitis (see Table 8-2); however, lifetime therapy is needed and the prognosis for effective control of the disease is poor. In general these dogs seem to have less diarrhea on a highly digestible diet than on a high-fiber diet.

There have been isolated case reports of histiocytic colitis in a cat and a French bulldog, but it is not known if these represent the same disease as occurs in boxers.

Colitis Associated With Pancreatitis

Necrotizing hemorrhagic colitis occurs occasionally in dogs with acute pancreatitis. It is presumed that because the transverse colon lies adjacent to the inflamed pancreas, it can sometimes become secondarily involved in the local inflammatory and vascular-compromising processes in that region of the abdominal cavity.

The diagnosis is based on colonoscopic demonstration of lesions of colitis in the transverse colon in a patient that has laboratory, radiographic, and ultrasonographic evidence of pancreatitis. Olsalazine, sulfasalazine, or metronidazole can be added to the treatment regimen for pancreatitis, but corticosteroids should be avoided in acute pancreatitis.

Cecocolonic Intussusception (Cecal Inversion)

Cecocolonic intussusception results in invagination of the cecum into the lumen of the colon, where the mucosa of the inverted cecum then becomes congested, inflamed, hemorrhagic, and ulcerated. Whipworm infection has been suggested as a predisposing cause. With partial ileocolonic obstruction, chronic or intermittent bloody-mucoid diarrhea is usually the presenting sign; thus cecal inversion can often mimic colitis or colonic neoplasia. When cecal inversion causes complete ileocolic obstruction, the signs are acute depression, anorexia, vomiting, and dehydration.

The inverted cecum can sometimes be palpated as a firm, painful, right cranial abdominal mass, but usually the diagnosis is made by identification of the inverted cecum during colonoscopic examination of the proximal colon by ultrasonography or by demonstration of an intraluminal filling defect at the ileocolic junction on a barium contrast radiographic study. Surgical excision of the cecum is the treatment of choice.

Short Colon

Short colon, a malformation resulting from developmental errors in rotation and elongation of the embryonic gut, has been reported in both cats and dogs. The animals were diagnosed with colitis, and the malformation was apparently an incidental finding, although there had been a lifelong history of soft feces. Barium contrast radiography and colonoscopy revealed an abnormally short colon with absence of the ascending and transverse colons and location of the ileocolic junction and cecum in the left hemiabdomen at the proximal end of the descending colon. A digestible low-residue diet alleviated the soft feces.

Colonic Neoplasia

Colonic polyps and tumors usually cause hematochezia, dyschezia, and tenesmus, sometimes with mucoid diarrhea; thus they are easily confused with inflammatory diseases of the colon. Benign tumors, which include adenomatous polyps, adenomas, and leiomyomas, occur most commonly in the rectum and terminal colon of dogs. The most common malignant neoplasms of the colon are adenocarcinoma and lymphosarcoma. Carcinoid tumors, leiomyosarcoma, fibrosarcoma, hemangiosarcoma, and anaplastic sarcoma occur rarely. Metastasis to regional lymph nodes is common with all malignancies of the colon.

Adenocarcinomas are locally invasive and slow growing, and they occur primarily in older patients. There are three forms of adenocarcinoma: (1) the infiltrative type, which produces a thickened stenotic region of the colon that eventually obstructs the lumen; (2) the ulcerative type, which produces a deep indurated mucosal ulcer with raised edges; and (3) the proliferative type, which produces a lobulated mucosal mass.

Colonic lymphosarcomas usually cause a diffuse infiltration and thickening of the colon with mucosal ulceration and corrugation. Most colonic lymphomas occur in the descending colon and rectum of dogs younger than 4 years of age and at the ileocolic junction in cats older than 8 years of age.

Colonic neoplasia should be considered in any dog or cat with rectal bleeding or unresponsive large bowel diarrhea and hematochezia and therefore must be differentiated from colitis. Stenosing or polypoid rectal masses can usually be detected by digital rectal palpation. Most adenomatous polyps can be exposed at the anus by everting the rectal mucosa with gentle traction. Polyps usually appear dark red and lobulated, they are extremely friable, and they bleed easily. More proximal lesions, including most malignant colonic tumors, are identified by colonoscopy, ultrasonography, or barium contrast radiography. Biopsy is needed for definitive diagnosis. Colonoscopic biopsies can reveal the neoplastic cells in many cases, but in some patients the tissue obtained by the biopsy forceps is not adequate or deep enough for confirmation of the diagnosis. Surgical biopsy is then needed.

Surgical resection is the treatment of choice for benign tumors such as polyps and, when feasible, for adenocarcinomas. Excised tissue should always be submitted for thorough histopathologic examination. Unfortunately, most malignant tumors of the colon are too advanced for successful resection by the time they are recognized clinically. Some benign polypoid lesions recur months following excision as malignant (adenocarcinoma). Colonic lymphosarcoma may be treated with anticancer chemotherapy.

Colonic neoplasia is discussed in more detail in Chapter 11.

Irritable Bowel Syndrome

Irritable bowel syndrome (IBS) is characterized by noninflammatory, mucoid large bowel diarrhea associated with episodic disturbances of colonic myoelectrical function. Humans with an irritable colon seem to be hyperreactive to psychological and emotional stress and anxiety. Neurogenic pathways are presumably involved in the pathogenesis of the diarrhea and colonic dysfunction in IBS.

The clinical signs in humans with IBS are alternating patterns of diarrhea, constipation, and abdominal cramping. Evidence for the existence of IBS in animals is mostly circumstantial; thus it is a controversial topic in veterinary medicine. Nonetheless, it seems that a comparable syndrome exists at least in dogs with the most frequent clinical sign being intermittent mucoid diarrhea. Hematochezia is uncommon in IBS and should stimulate a search for other diagnoses. Large-breed dogs, especially those under stress as working dogs (e.g., police dogs, seeing eye dogs), and temperamental or excitable dogs may be predisposed to IBS.

The diagnosis of irritable bowel syndrome should be suspected primarily in dogs with chronic intermittent large bowel diarrhea when a thorough diagnostic evaluation, including colonoscopy, fails to identify a definitive cause. As a diagnosis of exclusion, IBS can be established only by normal colonoscopic biopsy and diligent exclusion of the other known causes of colonic disease such as dietary, parasitic, infectious, and idiopathic colitis (IBD). At colonoscopy the colon may appear to be hypermotile or spastic. The mucosa appears normal except for an erythematous response to insufflation and increased intraluminal mucus.

Treatment of IBS is based on dietary adjustment, motility-modifying drugs, and drugs that relieve anxiety or stress, such as various sedatives and psychotropic drugs. The initial approach should be to manage IBS with dietary modification alone. Supplement dietary fiber in the form of psyllium (Metamucil, 1 to 3 tbsp/day in the food), unprocessed wheat bran (1 to 5 tbsp/day), or a commercial high-fiber diet. Fiber-enriched diets can have a normalizing effect on colonic myoelectrical activity, thereby improving functional diarrhea in some dogs. If dietary fiber supplementation is unsuccessful, episodes of diarrhea can usually be controlled with a brief period of fasting and an opioid antidiarrheal drug such as loperamide (Imodium; dogs: 0.05 to 0.1 mg/lb orally every 8 to 12 hours; cats: 0.05 to 0.15 mg/lb orally every 24 hours). Once an episode has abated, loperamide can be discontinued and remission maintained by dietary and stress management. Stress management may require consultation from an animal behavior expert. Sedative and psychotropic drugs are used to produce anxiety relief and light sedation during stressful times. Standard dosages of benzodiazepines, acepromazine, chlorpromazine, or phenobarbital may be helpful in excessively nervous or excitable patients. Amitriptylin (Elavil, 0.5 to 1 mg/lb orally every 12 hours) has been highly effective in treating some dogs with IBS. The concept of "neurogenic inflammation" associated with stress may lead to new strategies for management of IBS in the future.

COLONIC DISORDERS THAT CAUSE ACUTE ABDOMEN

Perforation of the Colon

Perforation of the colon allows leakage of fecal material containing massive numbers of anaerobic and gram-negative bacteria into the abdominal cavity. This produces rapidly progressive bacterial peritonitis, sepsis, and endotoxemia. Death occurs in a matter of hours from septic shock. Colonic perforation may be caused by penetrating trauma (e.g., gunshot wounds), erosive tumors, complications of colonic surgery or biopsy procedures, and high doses of corticosteroids following neurosurgical procedures. Rectal perforation leads to retroperitoneal leakage of fecal material and may be caused by displaced bone fragments of a fractured pelvis or by iatrogenic puncture from a thermometer, enema infusor, or biopsy instrument.

The clinical signs of colonic perforation are the result of septic peritonitis and include acute abdominal pain, severe depression, fever (hypothermia occurs terminally), vomiting, hemorrhagic diarrhea, and rapidly progressive signs of shock. A CBC usually reveals a neutropenia with a degenerative left shift and circulating toxic neutrophils. Serum electrolyte imbalances and prerenal azotemia are likely. Survey abdominal radiographs may indicate free air within the abdominal cavity or retroperitoneal space, loss of abdominal contrast due to peritoneal effusion, and gas-distended bowel loops due to ileus. Acute septic peritonitis (indicating probable bowel perforation) is confirmed by cytologic findings (toxic neutrophils and intracellular and extracellular bacteria), abdominocentesis, or peritoneal lavage.

Rapid recognition of colonic perforation as a life-threatening intraabdominal crisis in need of immediate surgical intervention is required. On the basis of signs of acute abdominal distress and radiographic or laboratory indication of perforation, the patient is treated for shock and emergency laparotomy is performed. Parenteral antibiotics are initiated immediately to cover anaerobic and gram-negative enteric bacteria; for example, penicillin, ampicillin, or clindamycin combined with enrofloxacin, an aminoglycoside, or a cephalosporin. The colon is surgically repaired, the abdomen is copiously lavaged, and the septic peritonitis is treated vigorously postoperatively. The prognosis for survival from colonic perforation is guarded to poor.

Volvulus of the Colon

Torsion or volvulus of the colon results in complete distal bowel obstruction, rapidly progressive ischemic necrosis of the bowel, eventual septic peritonitis, and finally death from septic shock; thus early recognition and immediate surgical intervention are necessary. This is a rare condition in dogs and cats. When it occurs, the signs are those of acute abdominal distress with pain, vomiting, raspberry jam–like hemorrhagic diarrhea, and acute collapse. Radiographs generally reveal a gas-distended lower bowel, which, taken together with the clinical signs, is indication to proceed with emergency laparotomy. Measures to treat hypovolemic and septic shock also should be initiated immediately.

CONSTIPATION AND DYSCHEZIA

Constipation is a clinical sign characterized by absent, infrequent, or difficult defecation associated with retention of feces within the colon and rectum. When feces are retained in the colon for a prolonged period of time, the mucosa continues to absorb water from the fecal mass, which gradually results in impacted feces that become progressively harder and drier. Obstipation is a condition of intractable constipation in which the colon and rectum become so impacted with excessively hard feces that defecation cannot occur. Megacolon is a term that refers to a disorder (not a sign) in which the colon becomes extremely dilated and hypomotile, usually irreversibly so, and it is an important cause of chronic constipation/obstipation in cats.

Dyschezia, a clinical sign often associated with constipation, is defined as difficult or painful evacuation of feces from the rectum and is usually associated with lesions in or near the anal region. Tenesmus is a clinical sign characterized by ineffective or painful straining to defecate; thus it usually accompanies dyschezia.

Etiology

Underlying causes or predisposing factors for constipation are listed in Table 8-3 and include

(1) ingested foreign material, (2) environmental factors, (3) painful anorectal or orthopedic conditions, (4) anorectal or colonic obstruction, (5) neuromuscular diseases, (6) fluid and electrolyte disturbances, and (7) drug-related effects.

Ingested foreign material such as indigestible fibrous material (especially hair in cats from their grooming behavior) or abrasives (especially bones in dogs) may become incorporated into the fecal mass and result in the formation of hard fecal impactions that are difficult or painful to evacuate from the colon.

Environmental factors that are not conducive to defecation or that vary from the daily routine to which the patient is accustomed may cause the patient to inhibit the urge to defecate, leading to constipation. This occurs, for example, when a patient is placed in strange surroundings such as a kennel or veterinary hospital or when the patient's daily outdoor exercise routine is changed. Indoor cats will often suppress the urge to defecate when their litter box is too dirty or there is territorial competition with other cats in the household.

Painful defecation caused by anorectal diseases (e.g., anal sacculitis or perianal fistulae; see section on anorectal disease) or by orthopedic disorders that limit positioning for defecation (e.g., disorders of pelvis, spine, or hips) can result in voluntary inhibition of defecation and lead to constipation.

Rectocolonic obstructions that mechanically impede passage of feces may occur from intraluminal causes, such as foreign bodies, perineal hernia, or stenosing neoplastic or inflammatory lesions (i.e., strictures), and from extraluminal causes, such as prostatic enlargement, paraprostatic cysts, compressive pelvic fractures, perianal tumors, or pseudocoprostasis (feces matted to the hair of the perianal area).

Neuromuscular disorders may lead to constipation by interfering with colonic innervation, colonic smooth muscle function, or simply the ability of the patient to assume the normal defecation stance—for example, disease or injury of the lumbosacral spinal cord (e.g., canine intervertebral disk disease), spinal deformity (as occurs in Manx cats), endocrine disease (hypothyroidism), or dysautonomia, a progressively fatal autonomic polyneuropathy of young cats. When innervation of the anus is also impaired, fecal incontinence may be an associated clinical sign. The pathogenesis of idiopathic megacolon appears to involve smooth muscle dysfunction. Studies have demonstrated decreased

TABLE 8-3	**Classification and Causes of Constipation**
Classification	**Cause**
Dietary	Ingested foreign material mixed with feces (hair, bones, cloth, garbage, cat litter, rocks, plant material, etc.)
	Inadequate water intake
Environmental/psychologic	Dirty litter box
	Prolonged inactivity
	Confinement (hospitalization, boarding)
	Change in habitat or daily routine
Painful defecation	Anorectal disorders
	Anal sac impaction, infection, or abscess
	Anorectal stricture, tumor, or foreign body
	Myiasis
	Perianal fistulae
	Perianal bite wound cellulitis or abscess
	Pseudocoprostasis
	Orthopedic disorders
	Spinal disease or injury
	Injuries of the pelvis, hip joints, or pelvic limbs
Rectocolonic obstruction	Extramural
	Prostatic hypertrophy, prostatitis, abscess, or tumor
	Paraprostatic cyst
	Pelvic fracture (malunion)
	Pelvic collapse due to nutritional bone disease
	Perianal tumor
	Pseudocoprostasis
	Intramural or intraluminal
	Rectocolonic stricture, tumor, foreign body, or fecolith
	Rectal diverticulum or perineal hernia
Neuromuscular dysfunction	Lumbosacral spinal cord disease (injury, deformity, degeneration, neoplasia)
	Bilateral pelvic nerve injury
	Dysautonomia (Key-Gaskell syndrome)
	Hypothyroidism
	Idiopathic megacolon
Fluid and electrolyte abnormalities	Dehydration (e.g., chronic renal failure)
	Hypokalemia
	Hypercalcemia (hyperparathyroidism)
Drug-induced	Anticholinergics
	Adrenergic blockers
	Calcium channel blockers
	Phenothiazines and benzodiazepines
	Opiates and opioids
	Diuretics
	Antihistamines
	Aluminum hydroxide antacids
	Sucralfate
	Kaolin-pectin
	Barium sulfate
	Iron
	Laxatives (chronic overuse)

active contraction (in vitro) of smooth muscle from cats with megacolon in response to neurotransmitters (acetylcholine, substance P, cholecystokinin), membrane depolarization (potassium), and electrical stimulation. Innervation of the colon, however, appears to be normal in these cats.

Fluid and electrolyte disorders may predispose to constipation, particularly dehydration, which can cause the feces to become excessively dry and hard, and hypokalemia or hypercalcemia, either of which can affect colonic smooth muscle function. A combination of these may explain the frequent constipation seen in chronic renal failure, especially in cats.

Drug-induced constipation may occur as a side effect of motility-modifying drugs (anticholinergics, opiates, opioids), antihistamines, barium sulfate, aluminum hydroxide, and diuretics.

Clinical Signs

Constipated patients are usually presented for failure to defecate over a period of days. The owner may notice tenesmus or frequent attempts to defecate with little or no passage of feces. Other signs may include anorexia, lethargy, vomiting, dehydration, and hunched-up appearance caused by abdominal discomfort. Dyschezia usually indicates anorectal disease (see section on anorectal disease). The patient first may cry out as it attempts to defecate, usually with straining (tenesmus) during the attempt, then it ceases the effort, walks around anxiously, and repeatedly tries again. Mucosal irritation caused by impacted feces may provoke a secretion of fluid and mucus that bypasses the retained fecal mass and is expelled paradoxically as diarrhea during attempts to defecate. Constipation tends to be a recurrent problem in some patients.

Megacolon mostly occurs in middle-age cats (mean age of 5.8 years in one case survey). The same study found a predilection in male cats (70%) over females (30%). The most frequently affected breeds were domestic short hair (46% of cases), domestic long hair (15%), and Siamese (12%). Megacolon in most cats is idiopathic; however, irreversible colonic dilation can also be caused by persistent mechanical obstruction (e.g., pelvic canal stenosis caused by malunion, anorectal stricture, anorectal neoplasia) or neuromuscular dysfunction caused by lumbosacral spinal cord disease.

Diagnosis

Constipation is generally established as a problem from the history and confirmed by rectal and abdominal palpation of a colon distended with hard feces. The goal of diagnosis is to identify predisposing factors (see Table 8-3). The owner should be carefully questioned to identify any of the potential dietary, environmental, behavioral, psychologic, or medication-related factors or predispositions listed in Table 8-3 that might be involved.

Physical examination may also reveal the cause or predisposition for constipation. Digital anorectal examination should be performed to detect painful or obstructive lesions of the anorectal area and pelvic canal (sedation may be required). The rear limbs, coxofemoral joints, pelvis, and lumbosacral spine should be evaluated for orthopedic problems that could cause either painful defecation or difficulty for the patient to maneuver into the defecation stance. In addition, a neurologic examination with emphasis on candal spinal cord function should be performed to identify neurologic causes of constipation. In cats with constipation due to dysautonomia (Key-Gaskell syndrome), additional manifestations of progressive autonomic failure that may be seen include urinary/fecal incontinence, megaesophagus, bradycardia, mydriasis, decreased lacrimation, and prolapse of the nictitating membranes.

A routine serum biochemistry profile, urinalysis, and CBC should be evaluated in patients with recurrent constipation or signs indicating the potential for underlying systemic conditions (e.g., chronic renal failure) that could cause dehydration and electrolyte disturbances. These laboratory evaluations are also helpful in patients that are severely constipated or obstipated, especially those that are vomiting or markedly depressed, to detect the metabolic consequences of prolonged fecal retention (e.g., fluid and electrolyte imbalances, endotoxemia, azotemia) and to guide supportive treatment. Thyroid function should be evaluated in dogs with recurrent constipation and other signs compatible with hypothyroidism.

Abdominal radiography can be used in the constipated patient to identify the following: (1) extent of colonic impaction with densely packed feces; (2) extreme dilation of the colon that would indicate megacolon; (3) radiopaque foreign material (e.g., bone chips) in the retained feces that would indicate a dietary cause of constipation; (4) pelvic, coxofemoral, or spinal lesions that may be predisposing causes of constipation; and (5) enlargement of the prostate that may be an underlying cause of constipation.

Additional specialized diagnostic studies may be indicated in selected patients. When intraluminal obstructive lesions are suspected, barium enema contrast radiography (see Chapter 2) or colonoscopy (see Chapter 3) may be used after the retained feces have been evacuated to evaluate the lumen of the colon. Myelographic and electrodiagnostic evaluations of the lumbosacral spinal cord and spinal nerves should be considered in patients with evidence of impaired anorectal innervation. When prostatic disease or paraprostatic cysts are suspected to be the cause of constipation, further evaluations might include caudal abdominal ultrasound examination, contrast cystourethrography, and cytology/culture studies of the prostate. Computed tomography (CT) and magnetic resonance imaging (MRI) scans can be useful for imaging pelvic canal structures and the lumbosacral spine.

Treatment

Mild constipation resolves spontaneously or is treated on an outpatient basis by dietary adjustment and oral or suppository laxatives. Severe constipation is treated initially by evacuation of impacted feces from the colon by means of enemas and/or manual extraction along with correction of complicating dehydration and electrolyte imbalances. Follow-up therapy is aimed at eliminating or controlling any of the underlying causes of constipation that are identified from Table 8-3 and at preventing recurrences by means of dietary adjustments and laxative therapy (Table 8-4). Surgical correction is required for obstructing neoplasms and strictures and many anorectal disorders. Finally, long-term management of megacolon or

TABLE 8-4	Treatments for Constipation*†	
Treatment	**Product (Manufacturer)**	**Dosage**
ORAL CATHARTICS		
Bulk-Forming Laxatives		
Coarse bran	All-Bran (Kellogg's) and others	1-5 tbsp daily with food
Canned pumpkin	Pie filling (Libby's)	1-5 tbsp daily with food
Psyllium	Metamucil (Procter & Gamble); Fiberall (CIBA)	1-3 tbsp daily with food
Lubricant Laxatives		
White petrolatum	Laxatone (Evsco)	1-5 ml daily PO
Emollient Laxatives		
Docusate sodium	Colace (Shire)	Dog: 50-200 mg daily PO Cat: 50 mg daily PO
Docusate calcium	Surfak (Geneva)	Dog: 100-240 mg daily PO Cat: 50-100 mg daily PO
Saline Laxatives		
Magnesium hydroxide	Phillips' Milk of Magnesia (Glenbrook)	Dog: 2-8 tablets daily PO
Osmotic Laxatives		
Lactose	Milk	Add to diet to effect
Lactulose	Duphalac (Reid Rowell); Cephulac (Merrell Dow)	0.25-0.5 ml/lb PO, q8-12h
Polyethylene glycol and electrolytes‡	Colyte (Schwarz); Golytely (Braintree)	12-20 ml/lb PO repeated in 2-4h (for bowel prep)
Stimulant Laxatives		
Bisacodyl	Dulcolax (Boehringer Ingelheim)	Dog: 5-20 mg daily PO Cat: 5 mg daily PO

Continued

TABLE 8-4	Treatments for Constipation*†—Cont'd	
Treatment	**Product (Manufacturer)**	**Dosage**
Promotility Laxatives		
Cisapride	Available from compounding pharmacies	Dog: 0.25-0.5 mg/lb q8-12h, PO Cat: 0.5 mg/lb q8h or 0.7 mg/lb q12h, PO
Ranitidine	Zantac (GlaxoSmithKline)	Dog: 1 mg/lb q8-12h, PO Cat: 1.5 mg/lb q12h, PO
Nizatidine	Axid (Lilly)	1-2 mg/lb q12-24h, PO
ENEMAS AND SUPPOSITORIES		
Enemas		
Warm tap water	—	2.5-5 ml/lb
Isotonic saline solution	—	2.5-5 ml/lb
Docusate sodium	Colace (Shire)	5-30 ml
Mineral oil	Various	5-30 ml or 0.5-1 ml/lb
Lubricant jelly	Various	5-30 ml
Lactulose	Duphalac; cephulac	5-30 ml
Sodium phosphate§	Fleet	0.5-1 ml/lb or 1 enema unit
Bisacodyl	Fleet	0.5-1 ml/lb or 1 enema unit
Rectal Suppositories		
Glycerin	Various	1-3 pediatric suppositories
Docusate sodium	Colace (Shire)	1-3 pediatric suppositories
Bisacodyl	Dulcolax (Boehringer Ingelheim)	1-3 pediatric suppositories

*Ancillary treatment measures:
1. Regular grooming to prevent ingestion of loose hair (especially cats).
2. Prevent ingestion of abrasive foreign materials.
3. Provide fresh drinking water.
4. Provide clean litter for cats.
5. Encourage regular exercise.
†For severe recurrent or refractory cases: total or subtotal colectomy.
‡Used mainly to prepare the colon for radiography or endoscopy.
§Should not be used in cats or small dogs.

recurrent obstipation that is unresponsive to medical therapy in the cat may involve colectomy surgery.

Initial Relief of Constipation

Simple constipation with mild to moderate impaction of feces and without accompanying systemic signs (depression, vomiting, dehydration) can often be managed on an outpatient basis using dietary adjustment, measures to increase water intake, and oral laxatives. Oral laxatives can be prescribed as discussed later in this chapter and the animal reevaluated in 48 hours. To promote initial evacuation of the distal colon when impaction is not severe, one to three pediatric suppositories consisting of docusate sodium, bisacodyl, or glycerin also can be used or a therapeutic enema can be administered.

In severe constipation/obstipation, fluid and electrolyte balance should initially be restored par-

enterally. The colon is then evacuated manually under general anesthesia with a combination of colonic irrigation with warm isotonic saline as an enema solution to soften the impacted feces and extraction of retained fecal masses by gentle transabdominal manipulation to milk the feces into the distal rectum for digital extraction or removal with sponge or whelping forceps. To avoid excessive bowel trauma in patients with extensive fecal impaction, it may be advisable to evacuate the colon manually in stages over a period of 2 to 3 days.

Enema Solutions

Enema solutions can be used to soften hard, impacted feces and promote evacuation. The enema solutions should be warmed prior to instillation, and the calculated dose administered slowly so as not to induce vomiting. The following are commonly used enema solutions:

1. Warm isotonic saline or tap water (2.5 to 5 ml/lb body weight), with or without the addition of a mild soap to stimulate defecation by an irritant effect (soap must not contain hexachlorophene because of its neurotoxicity if absorbed).
2. Docusate as an emollient (5 to 10 ml in cats and small dogs; 10 to 20 ml in medium-sized dogs; 20 to 30 ml in large dogs).
3. Mineral oil as a lubricant (5 to 10 ml in cats and small dogs; 10 to 20 ml in medium-sized dogs; 20 to 30 ml in large dogs).
4. Sodium phosphate solution (Fleet Children's Enema), which has softening, bulk-producing, and irritant effects (use only in medium-sized or large dogs with normal renal function; not safe for use in cats or small dogs).

Mineral oil and docusate should not be mixed because docusate promotes mucosal absorption of mineral oil, and mineral oil coats the feces, reducing the emollient effect of docusate. Sodium phosphate enemas must never be used in cats and small dogs because they can cause dangerous hypernatremia, hyperosmolality, hyperphosphatemia, and hypocalcemia.

Measures to Prevent Recurrence of Constipation

Following evacuation of retained feces from the colon, measures are instituted to prevent and control recurrences of constipation. If underlying causes or predisposing factors (see Table 8-3) can be identified, they should be eliminated or corrected if at all possible. For example, ingestion of potential abrasive materials such as bones should be prevented. In cats, if hair ingestion is a potential contributing factor, the owner should be instructed to adopt a routine of regular grooming to remove loose hair from the cat's hair coat before it can be ingested. A daily routine of exercise and frequent opportunities to defecate should be provided for dogs, and clean litter should be provided at all times for cats, to encourage regular defecation. Water intake should be encouraged by providing access to fresh water at all times. The use of any medications that promote constipation should be adjusted or discontinued. Predisposing prostatic, endocrine (e.g., thyroid), spinal, or orthopedic disorders should be treated. Whenever possible, painful or obstructing anorectal lesions (see section on anorectal diseases) should be corrected, even surgically if necessary.

Oral Laxatives

Oral laxative medications and dietary supplements can be prescribed as needed for control of constipation (see Table 8-4). Laxatives act through interrelated effects on both intestinal mucosal fluid transport and colonic motility and are classified by their properties and mechanisms of actions as (1) bulk-forming, (2) lubricant, (3) emollient, (4) osmotic, and (5) stimulant. The use of an oral laxative often needs to be individualized by adjusting the dose until the desired frequency of defecation and fecal consistency are obtained.

High-Fiber Bulk-Forming Laxatives. These should be added to the food to promote soft feces and normal colonic motility as the initial approach for prevention and control of constipation. Bulk-forming agents consist of indigestible polysaccharides and cellulose that exhibit hydrophilic properties within the bowel. Insoluble fiber is derived principally from wheat bran or psyllium seed coat. Beneficial effects include increased fecal water content, increased fecal weight and frequency, softer fecal consistency, decreased intestinal transit time, and reduction of the intracolonic pressure required for normal defecation. Adequate water intake and patient hydration are required for these beneficial actions and to prevent impaction of fiber in the colon. For long-term control of constipation, a commercially prepared high-fiber diet can be fed, or the regular diet can be supplemented with unprocessed wheat bran, oat bran, or pumpkin (1 to 5 tbsp per meal) or commercial sources of psyllium (Metamucil or Fiberall, 1 to 5 tsp per meal). Dietary adjustments alone are not usually sufficient to control constipation in cats with megacolon.

Lubricant Laxatives. Mineral oil and flavored white petrolatum products can be used to soften and lubricate the feces to facilitate evacuation. These should be administered between meals so that they do not interfere with the absorption of fat-soluble vitamins. Mineral oil should be used only in enema form. Oral administration should be avoided because of the risk of aspiration lipid pneumonia.

Emollient Laxatives. Docusate sodium available in enema and oral forms (Colace), and docusate calcium (Surfak) are mild laxatives that promote water penetration into the feces, thereby softening the feces. Although relatively inert, docusate may increase intestinal loss of fluid; thus its use should be avoided in the presence of dehydration. For the reasons mentioned previously (see section on enema solutions), docusate and mineral oil should not be mixed.

Osmotic Laxatives. These consist of poorly absorbed disaccharides (such as lactose or lactulose), ions (such as magnesium hydroxide, magnesium citrate), or inert osmotic agents (polyethylene glycol) that osmotically retain water in the bowel lumen to produce soft or fluid feces. A mild osmotic laxative effect can be produced in some patients by the addition of milk (lactose) to the diet in a quantity that exceeds the digestive capacity of small intestinal lactase. The nonabsorbable disaccharide lactulose (Duphalac, Cephulac, 0.25 to 0.5 ml/lb orally three times a day) is an excellent choice as a safe and effective all-purpose laxative for short- or long-term use in both dogs and cats. Unabsorbed dissacharides such as lactulose are fermented by colonic bacteria to lactic acid and other organic anions, thereby producing an osmotic catharsis and acidification of the colon. The dosage of lactulose needs to be adjusted to effect. If the dosage is too high, abdominal discomfort, flatulence, and diarrhea may occur. These side effects resolve with lowering the dosage.

Magnesium hydroxide is available as an over-the-counter drug (Phillips' Milk of Magnesia). Magnesium is contraindicated in renal failure. Magnesium citrate and polyethylene glycol–electrolyte solutions (Colyte, GoLYTELY) are available commercially for preparation of the colon for endoscopy, but the large oral doses required are too impractical for therapeutic use.

Stimulant Laxatives. These increase propulsive motility of the bowel by a variety of mechanisms. They are generally contraindicated in the presence of an obstructive lesion and are less appropriate for long-term use than other categories of laxatives. A useful stimulant laxative for the dog and cat is bisacodyl (Dulcolax, daily dose of 5 mg for cats and small dogs, 10 mg for medium-sized dogs, and 15 to 20 mg for large dogs), which works by stimulating colonic smooth muscle and the myenteric plexus. Although beneficial on a short-term basis in conjunction with measures to soften the feces, long-term use of bisacodyl may damage the myenteric plexus. Castor oil, another stimulant laxative, is hydrolyzed in the intestines to ricinoleic acid, which stimulates colonic motility and secretion. Castor oil is not very useful for outpatient treatment because of poor patient acceptance, but it can be used effectively in hospitalized patients to prepare the bowel for radiographic or endoscopic procedures.

Promotility Therapy. Cisapride (Propulsid) is a benzamide derivative that promotes GI motility by stimulating colonic smooth muscle, increasing the physiologic release of acetylcholine from postganglionic nerve endings of the myenteric plexus, and acting as a $5-HT_4$-serotonergic agonist. These actions lead to improved propulsive motor activity of the esophagus, the stomach, and the small and large intestines. Cisapride is a highly effective laxative for both cats (0.5 mg/lb every 8 hours or 0.7 mg/lb every 12 hours orally) and dogs (0.25 to 0.5 mg/lb every 8 to 12 hours orally) (see Table 8-4). It can be administered alone or combined with stool-softening measures such as a fiber-augmented diet or lactulose. Cisapride is the most effective medical therapy for megacolon in cats. The colon in cats with megacolon may even resume normal diameter radiographically under treatment with cisapride. Unfortunately, megacolon commonly becomes refractory to cisapride after several months of therapy, necessitating increasing the dosage to 1 mg/lb every 8 hours or higher. Eventually after several months to years, many cats with megacolon become completely refractory to cisapride and require colectomy.

Cisapride is contraindicated in the presence of GI obstruction or perforation. It is ineffective if used with anticholinergics. Side effects are uncommon, but nausea, vomiting, diarrhea, flatulence, and abdominal discomfort are occasionally reported. Cisapride appears very safe for long-term use in animals; however, it is no longer approved for use in humans in the United States because of its association with serious arrhythmias. This side effect has not been a problem in animals. Cisapride can be obtained in the United States from compounding pharmacies for animal use.

Ranitidine (Zantac) and nizatidine (Axid) are H_2-receptor antagonists that also stimulate GI and colonic motility at standard dosages (see Table 8-4). They increase acetylcholine by inhibiting synaptic acetylcholinesterase. These are not as potent as cisapride as promotility agents; however, they may be useful when a mild laxative effect is needed.

Colectomy

For megacolon and severe recurrent constipation/obstipation that is unresponsive to medical management, especially in cats, subtotal colectomy is the most effective method of treatment. This procedure involves the removal of 95% or more of the colon. In cats with obstipation from pelvic fracture malunion, pelvic osteotomy or reconstructive surgery can allow return of normal colonic function if obstipation has been a problem for less than 6 months; otherwise, subtotal colectomy is recommended. After subtotal colectomy, diarrhea and frequent defecation are common; however, bowel function gradually improves during the 2 to 4 weeks following surgery in most cats. In dogs, diarrhea, frequent defecation, hematochezia, and tenesmus often persist after colon removal.

ANORECTAL DISEASES

The presenting signs of anorectal disease may include any of the following: dyschezia, hematochezia, constipation, anal discomfort (licking, scooting), ribbonlike feces, fecal incontinence, anal discharge, foul perianal odor, matting of perianal hair, and perianal dermatitis. Physical examination establishes the diagnosis of anorectal disease in most cases. In many of these disorders, surgery is required for effective treatment.

Anorectal Prolapse

Anorectal prolapse is usually a consequence of an underlying disorder that produces persistent straining; thus it is associated with (1) intestinal diseases that cause diarrhea and tenesmus, (2) anorectal diseases that cause dyschezia, (3) lower urinary tract and prostatic diseases that cause stranguria, and (4) dystocia. Partial prolapse involves only the rectal mucosa and appears as a red, swollen, donut-shaped ring of prolapsed mucosa. Complete prolapse involves all layers of the rectal wall and appears as an edematous cylindric-shaped mass. The prolapsed tissue may be viable (pink or red and moist) or necrotic (blackened and dry). A thermometer or finger should be inserted in the space between the prolapsed tissue and the anal sphincter to probe for a cul-de-sac. If there is none and resistance is not met, the prolapsed tissue is an intussusception of ileum or colon rather than an anorectal prolapse.

Management of anorectal prolapse involves both repair of the prolapse and treatment of the underlying cause. Minor prolapses in which the tissue is viable are treated by reduction and medical therapy to reduce tenesmus and prevent reprolapse, such as an anticholinergic-antispasmodic drug, hydrocortisone retention enema, mesalamine enema, or mild sedation. See Table 8-2 for dosages. A temporary (2 to 3 days) anal purse-string suture may be required in patients with persistent straining that produces recurrence of the prolapse. Amputation is performed when the prolapsed tissue is nonviable. For recurrent prolapse, a prophylactic colopexy should be considered. Successful management requires identification and treatment of the underlying cause; thus the anus, rectum, intestines, and urogenital tract should be evaluated by palpation, urinalysis, fecal examinations, proctoscopy, and radiographic studies as deemed appropriate.

Perineal Hernia

Perineal hernia occurs when weakness of the pelvic diaphragm muscles fails to support the rectal wall, resulting in persistent rectal distention and impaired defecation. The pathogenesis of the weakened pelvic diaphragm is poorly understood. Older male dogs are almost exclusively affected, although perineal hernia has also been reported in cats. The hernia usually contains outpouched rectum and can be either unilateral or bilateral; unilateral hernias are predominantly right-sided. The rectal defects associated with perineal hernia have been classified as (1) sacculation, when unilateral loss of support allows expansion of the rectal wall to one side; (2) dilation, when bilateral loss of support allows generalized distention of the rectum; (3) deviation or flexure, when the rectum curves or bends to one side within the hernia sac; and (4) diverticulum, when there is an outpouching of mucosa through a defect in the rectal wall. The hernia sac may also contain retroperitoneal fat, prostate gland, or rarely abdominal organs such as the urinary bladder.

The clinical signs of perineal hernia include constipation, obstipation, dyschezia, and tenesmus. Stranguria may occur with herniation of the urinary bladder and associated urethral obstruction. The diagnosis is based on palpation of a reducible swelling ventrolateral to the anus and rectal palpation of the weakened pelvic diaphragm and rectal dilation.

Initial treatment is aimed at evacuating retained feces from the rectum as described in the section on constipation and dyschezia. Urethral catheterization or cystocentesis also may be necessary initially to relieve urinary obstruction. In some dogs with perineal hernia, normal defecations can be maintained by laxative therapy and stool-softening diets (see Table 8-4); however, perineal herniorrhaphy surgery combined with castration provides the best, longer-lasting results in most cases. Even with surgery, the recurrence rate is fairly high.

Anorectal Foreign Bodies and Fecoliths

Ingested foreign bodies such as bones, toys, sticks, or sewing needles can sometimes pass unobtrusively through the GI tract and become lodged transversely within the rectum or at the anal sphincter. In addition, foreign objects are occasionally inserted into the anus of an animal by a malicious or deranged person. Older cats are sometimes presented for inability to pass a firm lump of feces (fecolith) that lodges in the anal canal between the internal and the external sphincter. Whenever a foreign body or fecolith is lodged in the anal canal or rectum, defecation becomes painful or impossible and signs of dyschezia, tenesmus, and secondary fecal impaction occur.

Most anorectal foreign bodies and fecoliths can be detected and removed by rectal palpation, although sedation or anesthesia is often necessary. In some cases a proctoscope may facilitate foreign body extraction. There are two potentially serious complications of anorectal foreign bodies: rectal laceration, resulting in retroperitoneal cellulitis, and anorectal stricture.

Anorectal Stricture (Stenosis)

Strictures of the anus or rectum may result from the trauma caused by passage of sharp foreign bodies (especially bones), from postsurgical scarring after anorectal surgery, and from the chronic inflammation of anal sac disease, perianal fistulae, or proctitis. Anorectal strictures cause dyschezia, tenesmus, hematochezia, and secondary constipation. The stricture can usually be identified by digital rectal palpation, proctoscopy, or barium enema contrast radiography. Surgical correction is usually required.

Anal Spasm

Some authors report a rare form of severe dyschezia, in which the anal sphincter appears to contract in spasm when the patient attempts to defecate; the patient may cry out in pain, move about frantically before stopping to make another attempt to defecate, turn and stare at its hindquarters, and appear extremely anxious. A cycle seems to occur of painful defecation, leading to defensive contraction of the anal sphincter, leading to more pain. Digital palpation of the rectum is vigorously resented, and the anal sphincter muscle feels hypertrophied and tightly contracted in spasm. Even visually the external sphincter muscle appears hypertrophied. Most affected dogs have been German shepherds of temperamental disposition. To attribute dyschezia to anal spasm, it is important to rule out structural causes of dyschezia (such as anal sac disease and perianal fistulae) and to exclude anal stricture (stenosis) by thorough rectal examination under anesthesia. Conservative treatment involving anal sac evacuation, topical analgesics, antispasmodic-sedative drugs, and stool softeners has not been very successful; thus resection of one or both anal branches of the pudendal nerve has been required for palliation in most dogs. Fecal incontinence is often a postoperative problem.

Congenital Defects of the Anus and Rectum
Imperforate Anus and Rectal Agenesis

Imperforate anus and rectal agenesis are uncommon congenital malformations of cloacal development that result in an absence of a patent anal opening for defecation. Consequently, within days or weeks of birth the affected puppy or kitten shows signs of abdominal distention and discomfort, tenesmus, restlessness, vomiting, and loss of appetite. The diagnosis is established by absence of an anal opening. The variations in the malformation range from an imperforate anal membrane covering the anal opening (atresia ani) to varying degrees of rectal agenesis (rectal atresia), in which the rectum ends in a blind pouch at some distance cranial to the anus. The terminal end of the rectum can be delineated radiographically by the intraluminal air when a lateral radiograph is exposed with the patient's hind end slightly elevated. In some patients, imperforate anus is associated with genitourinary defects such as rectovaginal fistula.

The treatment for atresia ani is surgical opening and removal of the retained anal membrane, usually producing favorable results. For rectal atresia, surgical correction is more difficult and requires combined abdominal surgery and rectal pull-through; thus the prognosis is guarded.

Rectovaginal Fistula

Rectovaginal fistula is a rare congenital malformation of females characterized by passage of fecal material from the vaginal opening. In many cases there also is an imperforate anus. Persistent fecal incontinence through the vagina leads to perivulvar dermatitis. Colonic distention usually occurs once the puppy or kitten begins eating solid food. The defect can be surgically corrected, but the prognosis is guarded. Other related anorectal anomalies that are very rare include rectovestibular fistula, anovaginal cleft, and rectourethral fistula.

Anal Sac Disease

Disorders of the anal sacs are the most common problem of the anal area in small animals, especially in dogs. Anal sac disease has been classified into impaction, inflammation (sacculitis), infection, abscess, and rupture. These probably represent a continuum such that impacted anal sacs tend to become inflamed and infected, which may then lead to abscessation and finally to rupture or fistulation. All breeds of dogs can be affected. Anal sac disease is uncommon in cats and usually involves only impaction.

The specific cause of anal sac disease is poorly understood. It is believed to be associated with conditions that promote inadequate emptying of the sacs, which should normally occur during defecation when feces of normal consistency are forced through a normally functioning anal sphincter. It is therefore the abnormal retention of anal sac secretions that leads to the impaction-inflammation-infection cycle.

The most frequent clinical signs of anal sac disease are related to anal discomfort and include scooting the hind end on the floor, tenesmus, and licking and biting the anal area, perineum, or base of the tail. Chewing and licking may result in areas of self-inflicted (pyotraumatic) dermatitis. In addition, tail chasing, malodorous perianal drainage, and change in temperament may be noted.

The diagnosis of anal sac disease is based on historical signs and examination of the anal sacs. The anal sacs are best examined by palpation with a gloved index finger inserted in the rectum and a thumb compressed against the skin ventrolateral to the anus. Impaction is usually bilateral and indicated by sacs that are distended, mildly painful on palpation, and not readily expressed. The impacted contents are usually thick and pasty and dark brown or grayish brown. Anal sacculitis is associated with moderate to severe pain on palpation, and the sacs contain a thinner-than-normal, yellowish or blood-tinged purulent fluid.

Anal sac abscess is usually unilateral and characterized by marked distention of the sac with pus, cellulitis of surrounding tissues, erythema of the overlying skin, and fever. Abscessed anal sacs may rupture through the adjacent skin, producing a draining fistulous tract.

Treatment of anal sac impaction and anal sacculitis by manual evacuation of the sac contents to reestablish drainage may be all that is required in many patients. Follow-up examination and expression of the anal sacs again in 1 to 2 weeks are advisable. A high-fiber diet may help to prevent recurrences. For recurrence of impaction or sacculitis, irrigation with povidone-iodine solution with a lacrimal needle and instillation of an antibiotic (e.g., an otic or ophthalmic antibiotic ointment) into the sac may be helpful, along with follow-up expression of the sacs every 3 to 4 days. Culture and sensitivity testing of the sac contents also should be considered for patients with troublesome recurrences. Anal sac abscesses are drained, irrigated with povidone-iodine solution, and treated with systemic antibiotics. Recurrent anal sacculitis or abscess is treated by surgical excision of the sacs. Chemical cautery and cryosurgery also have been used as alternatives to surgical excision for ablation of the sacs.

Perianal Fistulae

Perianal fistulae is a chronic progressive disease characterized by deep ulcerating fistulous tracts and suppuration in the perianal tissues. The disease occurs primarily in the German shepherd, although it has been reported sporadically in Irish setters, Labrador retrievers, and various other breeds. The proposed pathogenesis involves infection and abscessation of the various glandular elements in and around the anus as promoted by the moist contaminated environment of the area and a broad-based, low-slung tail conformation.

Dogs with perianal fistulae usually have signs of anal discomfort (licking the anal area, scooting, dyschezia, tenesmus) along with any of the following: hematochezia, constipation, fecal incontinence, or foul-smelling purulent perianal discharge. Examination of the perianal area establishes the diagnosis. The fistulas usually first appear as small draining puncture holes in the perianal skin with inflammation and hyperpigmentation of the surrounding skin. These small tracts then enlarge and coalesce to form large, interconnecting fistulas and areas of ulceration and granulation tissue. The fistulous tracts may extend deep into the perirectal tissues, and the anal sacs may also be infected or ruptured. Histopathologically, there is hidradenitis, chronic necrotizing pyogranulomatous inflammation of skin and hair follicles, cellulitis, necrosis, and fibrosis.

Surgery is the traditional method of treatment for perianal fistulae. Numerous surgical techniques have been advocated, including varying degrees of excision and debridement of diseased tissue, chemical cautery and electrocautery, and cryosurgery. It is advisable to tailor the aggressiveness of the technique to the extensiveness of the lesions and to preserve as much normal tissue and anal function as possible. Postoperative complications such as fecal incontinence, anal stenosis, and recurrence of the lesions can lead to an unacceptable outcome. Recent studies have shown that medical therapy using cyclosporine (Sandimmune, 0.8 mg to 1.4 mg/lb orally every 12 hours) produces a high rate of healing within 16 weeks, although the recurrence rate is 40%, necessitating additional treatment or surgery. In general, early diagnosis and medical or surgical intervention allows a less radical excision than is required in advanced disease, which in turn means less risk of postoperative complications and a better prognosis.

Pseudocoprostasis

Pseudocoprostasis is a condition of obstruction of the anal opening when the surrounding hair becomes densely matted with feces. It occurs most often in long-haired breeds of dogs and cats, especially during bouts of diarrhea. The anal obstruction leads to anal irritation, inability to pass feces, and constipation. The patient is usually restless and attempts to bite or lick at the anal region. The owner may complain of an unexplained foul odor from the patient. In addition, the matted hair often results in an underlying dermatitis and in warm weather attracts flies that may produce a maggot infestation (myiasis) of the anal area. Examination of the anal region is sufficient for diagnosis. For treatment the hair mats are clipped away and the underlying irritated skin is cleansed and treated topically. Once the obstructing hair mats are removed, defecation should occur normally; however, if the patient has severe colonic impaction of feces, measures to evacuate the colon, as discussed in the Constipation and Dyschezia section may be required.

Perianal Dermatitis

Anal irritation, a common consequence of anal sac disease and other anorectal disorders, often causes licking and biting at the anal area, which may lead to perianal dermatitis. Any pruritic skin condition, most notably fleas, also may cause local dermatitis in this area. Finally, the mucocutaneous junction where the perianal skin and anal mucosa join may be severely inflamed and ulcerated similarly to other mucocutaneous junctions of the body in any of the systemic mucocutaneous dermatologic disorders such as pemphigus vulgaris, bullous pemphigoid, systemic lupus, candidiasis, and cutaneous drug eruption. Eosinophilic granuloma complex of cats also may involve the perianal region. Perianal dermatitis itself can often be treated topically, but the key is to recognize that it is usually secondary to some other anorectal or dermatologic disorder that must be identified and treated.

Anal and Perianal Tumors

The most common tumor of the anal region is the perianal (circumanal) gland adenoma of dogs. These androgen-dependent tumors occur most often in older intact male dogs, and they usually appear as small, firm, well-circumscribed nodules in the skin surrounding the anus. Perianal gland adenomas may be incidental findings unassociated with clinical signs or they may cause anal irritation with scooting and licking at the anal area. In addition, they sometimes ulcerate and periodically bleed. The treatment of choice is excisional or cryosurgical removal and adjunctive castration because of their hormone dependency. Castration alone can produce regression of these tumors; however, excisional biopsy at the time of castration is the only way to rule out malignancy. Estrogens also are inhibitory for perianal gland adenomas; however, they cannot be recommended for prolonged use because of their myelotoxic effects. Other benign tumors of the anal area are rare but include lipoma and leiomyoma.

The two most important anal malignancies are the perianal (circumanal) gland adenocarcinoma and the apocrine gland (anal sac, anal gland) adenocarcinoma. Perianal gland adenocarcinomas occur most often in older male dogs and may resemble an ulcerated perianal gland adenoma, except they are locally invasive and may cause diffuse thickening of surrounding tissues. They eventually metastasize to regional lymph nodes (sublumbar) and beyond. Their appearance can also be confused with a perianal fistula lesion or a ruptured anal sac. Apocrine gland adenocarcinomas arise in the anal sac and most often affect older spayed female dogs. They are unique in that they can be an ectopic source of parathyroid hormone–like protein; thus even very small apocrine adenocarcinoma nodules often produce a hypercalcemia of malignancy syndrome with polyuria and polydipsia. Other malignant tumors of the anal region include squamous cell carcinoma, melanoma, and mast cell neoplasia.

For potentially malignant lesions of the perianal area, excisional biopsy is the diagnostic procedure of choice. Thoracic and abdominal radiography and abdominal ultrasonography of the sublumbar region are indicated to evaluate for metastasis. Early excision of malignant tumors of the anal region can be effective, but once extensive local invasion or regional lymph node metastasis has occurred, the prognosis for a cure is poor. Repeated partial excisions, radiation therapy, cryosurgery, and chemotherapy have been used for palliative therapy of inoperative malignancies of the anal region.

REFERENCES

Dennis JS, Kruger JM, Mullaney TP: Lymphocytic/plasmacytic colitis in cats: 14 cases (1985-1990), *J Am Vet Med Assoc* 202:313, 1993.

Dibartola SP et al.: Regional enteritis in two dogs, *J Am Vet Med Assoc* 181:904, 1982.

Gookin JL et al.: Diarrhea associated with trichomoniasis in cats, *J Am Vet Med Assoc* 215:1450, 1999.

Guilford WG: Idiopathic inflammatory bowel diseases. In Guilford WG et al., eds: *Strombeck's small animal gastroenterology* ed. 3, Philadelphia, 1996, WB Saunders.

Guilford WG et al.: Food sensitivity in cats with chronic idiopathic gastrointestinal problems, *J Vet Intern Med* 15:7, 2001.

Hall EJ: Dietary sensitivity. In Bonagura JD, ed: *Kirk's current veterinary therapy* XIII, Philadelphia, 2000, WB Saunders.

Hall EJ et al.: Histiocytic ulcerative colitis in boxer dogs in the UK, *J Small Anim Pract* 35:509, 1994.

Hasler AH, Washabau RJ: Cisapride stimulates contraction of idiopathic megacolonic smooth muscle in cats, *J Vet Intern Med* 11:313, 1997.

Jergens AE: Inflammatory bowel disease: current perspectives, *Vet Clin North Am* 22(2):501, 1999.

Jergens AE et al.: Idiopathic inflammatory bowel disease in dogs and cats: 84 cases (1987-1990), *J Am Vet Med Assoc* 201:1603, 1992.

Johnson SE: Canine eosinophilic gastroenteritis, *Semin Vet Med Surg* 7:145, 1992.

Leib MS: Chronic colitis in dogs. In Bonagura JD, ed: *Kirk's current veterinary therapy* XIII, Philadelphia, 2000, WB Saunders.

Leib MS et al.: Plasmacytic lymphocytic colitis in the dog, *Semin Vet Med Surg* 4:241, 1989.

Marks SL, Fascetti AJ: Nutritional management of diarrheal diseases. In: Bonagura JD, ed: *Kirk's current veterinary therapy* XIII, Philadelphia, 2000, WB Saunders.

Marks SL et al.: Evaluation of methods to diagnose *Clostridium perfringens*–associated diarrhea in dogs, *J Am Vet Med Assoc* 214:357, 1999.

Mathews KA, Sukhiani HR: Randomized controlled trial of cyclosporine for treatment of perianal fistulas in dogs, *J Am Vet Med Assoc* 211:1249, 1997.

Nelson RW, Dimperio ME, Long GG: Lymphocytic-plasmacytic colitis in the cat, *J Am Vet Med Assoc* 184:1133, 1984.

Nelson RW, Stookey LJ, Kazacos E: Nutritional management of idiopathic chronic colitis in the dog, *J Vet Intern Med* 2:133, 1988.

Roth L et al.: A grading system for lymphocytic plasmacytic colitis in dogs, *J Vet Diagn Invest* 2:257, 1990.

Sherding RG: Diseases of the intestines. In Sherding RG, ed: *The cat: diseases and clinical management* New York, 1994, Churchill Livingstone.

Simpson JW, Maskell IE, Markwell PJ: Use of a restricted antigen diet in the management of idiopathic canine colitis, *J Small Anim Pract* 35:233, 1994.

Washabau RJ, Holt D: Feline constipation and idiopathic megacolon. In Bonagura JD, ed: *Kirk's current veterinary therapy* XIII, Philadelphia, 2000, WB Saunders.

Washabau RJ, Sammarco J: Effect of cisapride on feline colonic smooth muscle function, *Am J Vet Res* 57:541, 1996.

Washabau RJ, Stalis IH: Alterations in colonic smooth muscle function in cats affected with idiopathic megacolon, *Am J Vet Res* 57:580, 1996.

DISEASES OF THE LIVER AND HEPATOBILIARY SYSTEM

Keith P. Richter

Hepatic disease is often treatable and has a predictable prognosis when a definitive diagnosis is made. The many complex functions of the liver are reflected in a multitude of pathophysiologic derangements that occur with hepatic disease. An understanding of these derangements is necessary for accurate interpretation of laboratory tests, making clinical decisions regarding further diagnostic tests, and determining management of the patient. A brief discussion of some of the important pathophysiologic abnormalities is included at the beginning of this chapter. Recent advances in noninvasive imaging of the liver and biopsy methods have made hepatic biopsy a routine and essential tool in the management of patients with hepatic disease. This can lead to a definitive diagnosis, which allows the clinician to make appropriate decisions regarding management.

PATHOPHYSIOLOGIC DERANGEMENTS OCCURRING WITH HEPATIC DISEASE

Bile Pigment Metabolism

Bilirubin Metabolism

Hepatobiliary excretion of bilirubin requires adequate uptake, conjugation, and secretion by the hepatocyte. Hepatic failure leads to hyperbilirubinemia and icterus. Bilirubin is formed primarily from breakdown products of red blood cells, from other hemoproteins, and other enzymes such as the cytochromes. Red blood cells have a finite life span (usually 120 days in the dog, 90 days in the cat), after which they are removed from the circulation by the body's reticuloendothelial system (especially in the spleen and liver). In the Kupffer's cells of the liver, senescent red blood cells are degraded to free hemoglobin. Similarly, circulating hemoglobin bound to several carrier proteins is phagocytized by Kupffer's cells. The enzyme heme oxygenase catabolizes hemoglobin to biliverdin, which is then converted to bilirubin by the enzyme biliverdin reductase. This lipid-soluble free bilirubin crosses the cell membrane and is released into the circulation, where it is bound to albumin. This circulating complex (termed unconjugated or indirect bilirubin) is eventually actively taken up by hepatocytes. Bilirubin is then bound to intracellular carrier proteins and undergoes conjugation, primarily with glucuronide. Conjugated bilirubin (also called direct bilirubin) is secreted into the bile canaliculus and transported to the gallbladder for storage.

There must be considerable hepatocellular disease or increase in the bilirubin load (hemolysis) to result in hyperbilirubinemia, because the liver's reserve capacity for bilirubin processing is up to 30 times the normal bilirubin load. Therefore the serum bilirubin concentration is an insensitive indicator of hepatocellular function, only increasing with severe hepatocellular disease. In general, total bilirubin concentrations above 2 to 3 mg/dl are detectable clinically as jaundice, whereas concentrations above 0.6 to 0.8 mg/dl result in abnormal bilirubinuria and spun serum or plasma to be visibly icteric.

Because unconjugated bilirubin circulates in plasma bound to albumin, it does not undergo glomerular filtration and does not appear in the urine (unless there is coexisting glomerular disease). Conjugated bilirubin, however, is freely filtered and appears in the urine and is readily detected with urine dipsticks. The dog has a very low renal threshold for conjugated bilirubin excretion; thus urine concentration of bilirubin increases far more readily than plasma concentration. It is normal to find a small amount of bilirubin in the urine of dogs, especially in a concentrated sample. Therefore there must be a considerable increase in the bilirubin load to increase plasma concentrations. Slight elevations in plasma bilirubin are significant, suggesting hepatobiliary disease. In the cat the renal threshold is much higher, so the finding of any degree of bilirubinuria is always abnormal. Renal tubular cells of the dog also possess a limited ability to convert hemoglobin into unconjugated bilirubin, which then appears in the urine. This can thus account for some of the bilirubinuria that occurs with hemolytic disease.

Hyperbilirubinemia is categorized into prehepatic, intrahepatic, and posthepatic causes. Prehepatic hyperbilirubinemia occurs when production exceeds the liver's capacity for metabolism and secretion. Causes of this include immune-mediated hemolytic anemia, heavy metal toxicity (lead, copper), and methylene blue toxicity. There will be evidence on the hemogram of increased production of bilirubin, with the most notable change being a decreased hematocrit.

Intrahepatic causes of hyperbilirubinemia occur when there is abnormal hepatic uptake, conjugation, or secretion of bilirubin. In most hepatocellular diseases there is usually coexisting impairment of bilirubin uptake, conjugation, and secretion. Therefore there is usually a mixture of conjugated and unconjugated hyperbilirubinemia. The increase in conjugated bilirubin results from impaired bilirubin secretion from damaged hepatocytes or from impairment of bile flow through bile canaliculi due to hepatocyte swelling, inflammation, or fibrosis. The increase in unconjugated bilirubin results from coexisting impairment of hepatic uptake and conjugation or from deconjugation of conjugated bilirubin by lysosomal enzymes released from injured hepatocytes or by inflammatory cells invading the liver. Therefore there can be an increase in primarily unconjugated bilirubin, conjugated bilirubin, or a mixture of both depending on the nature of the intrahepatic lesion.

Intrahepatic or extrahepatic biliary obstruction causes posthepatic hyperbilirubinemia. When this occurs, conjugated bilirubin is regurgitated into the systemic circulation, so that there is primarily a conjugated hyperbilirubinemia. However, there can also be concurrent unconjugated hyperbilirubinemia with posthepatic causes. This can result from deconjugation of bilirubin by damaged hepatocyte lysosomal and inflammatory cell enzymes (bile is hepatotoxic and cholestasis results in secondary hepatocellular damage and inflammation) or because conjugated bilirubin once absorbed into the systemic circulation recirculates and competes with unconjugated bilirubin for uptake by hepatocytes. The causes of extrahepatic biliary obstruction are listed in Box 9-1.

The relative increases of conjugated or unconjugated bilirubin are variable with all three general categories of hyperbilirubinemia and therefore do not aid the clinician in localizing the nature of the lesion. Ultrasonography, laparoscopy, and laparotomy localize the cause of hyperbilirubinemia.

> ### BOX 9-1 | Causes of Extrahepatic Bile Duct Obstruction in the Dog and Cat (in Order of Frequency)
>
> Pancreatitis
> Pancreatic neoplasia
> Other neoplasms arising near the common bile duct
> Bile duct carcinoma
> Inspissated bile plugs
> Abscess or granuloma in area of common bile duct
> Cholelithiasis
> Choledocholithiasis
> Cholecystitis
> Duodenal foreign body
> Parasite migration

Delta-Bilirubin. Delta-bilirubin is a novel form of bilirubin first noticed when the sum of conjugated and unconjugated bilirubin was less than the total bilirubin concentration when measured by high-performance liquid chromatography. The difference has been attributed to conjugated bilirubin covalently bound to albumin, subsequently called delta-bilirubin. This form of bilirubin is mainly seen with cholestatic hepatic diseases. The life span of delta-bilirubin is dependent on the half-life of albumin (approximately 14 days). Because of the strong covalent bond to albumin, delta-bilirubin does not appear in the urine or have significant hepatocellular uptake. Thus, because of these features and the long half-life of albumin, delta-bilirubin remains elevated even after cholestasis is completely resolved. There is marked variability in the amount of delta-bilirubin among dogs. This explains the persistent elevation in total bilirubin concentration (and clinical icterus) following surgical correction of biliary obstruction in some patients. The finding of increased total bilirubin concentration without concurrent hyperbilirubinuria suggests the presence of delta-bilirubin (excluding artifact). In these patients resolution of bilirubinuria may be the best marker of resolution of cholestasis.

Bile Acid Metabolism and Pathophysiology

Bile is composed of bile acids (salts), bile pigments (primarily bilirubin), cholesterol, phospholipids (primarily lecithin), and hepatic enzymes (such as alkaline phosphatase). Of these, bile acids are the most abundant and are the major solute in bile, constituting three fourths of the total solids. They are synthesized in the liver as a result of cholesterol metabolism and secreted into the bile. Feeding is a normal stimulus for bile acid secretion. They enter the intestine and undergo an efficient enterohepatic circulation following passive and active absorption from the ileum. Both unaltered bile acids and those deconjugated and dehydroxylated by intestinal bacteria are reabsorbed and enter the enterohepatic circulation. They are efficiently removed by the liver, reconjugated if necessary, and resecreted in bile. Hepatocellular uptake is a highly efficient process with large excess capacity, operating far from saturation under physiologic conditions. During a typical meal the total bile acid pool is recycled two to three times through this enterohepatic pathway. Only small amounts of bile acids are lost in the feces. Normally the liver synthesizes enough bile acids to compensate for fecal losses, which are minimal with respect to the total bile acid pool. Although bile acid formation depends on hepatic synthesis, the liver reserve capacity for this is never exceeded because of the small amounts needed for physiologic purposes.

Fecal loss of bile acids represents the major pathway for cholesterol excretion from the body. In addition to their role in lipid absorption, bile acids also stimulate pancreatic enzyme release and activity.

Factors important in governing bile acid metabolism include hepatic function, the portal blood supply, the small intestine, intestinal bacteria, and dietary factors. *The pathophysiologic effects of bile acids are hepatotoxicity, gastric hyperacidity, and diarrhea.*

Abnormal hepatic function, biliary excretion, or portal circulation can interrupt the normal enterohepatic circulation and lead to an increase in serum bile acid concentration. This occurs with many hepatobiliary diseases. When the liver parenchyma is diseased, the inability of normal uptake, conjugation, and secretion results in decreased extraction of bile acids from the portal circulation and leads to increased systemic concentrations. With intrahepatic or posthepatic cholestasis, bile acids diffuse from bile into the systemic circulation in a manner similar to that of bilirubin. With portosystemic shunting (either congenital or acquired), the enterohepatic circulation is directly interrupted and bile acids fail to be extracted by the bypassed liver. In this setting, hepatic synthesis of bile acids continues in order to maintain a normal bile acid pool. This can result in tremendous increases in systemic concentrations, especially following feeding. As will be discussed in the section on laboratory evaluation of hepatic disease, *serum bile acid concentrations represent a sensitive indicator of hepatic function.*

Protein Metabolism
Albumin Metabolism
Albumin is an important protein synthesized by the liver that is important in many homeostatic functions, such as maintenance of plasma colloid oncotic pressure and as a plasma transport carrier for many electrolytes, hormones, pigments, and drugs. Albumin represents approximately 25% of all the proteins synthesized by the liver. Because albumin has a relatively high priority for synthesis, the synthesis of other proteins will decrease before that of albumin with hepatocellular disease or with protein-calorie malnutrition.

Albumin concentration decreases with severe hepatic disease because of decreased synthesis and because ammonia (when elevated with hepatic disease) inhibits albumin release from hepatocytes. In addition, the abnormal insulin and glucagon concentrations that occur with hepatic disease also result in inhibition of albumin release from hepatocytes. Also, when ascites is present, there is an increased volume of distribution of albumin.

Clotting Factors
The liver is responsible for synthesizing many of the clotting factors, including factors I, II, V, VII, IX, and X. The liver also synthesizes activators and inhibitors of the fibrinolytic system (such as antiplasmins). In addition, the liver is involved in the synthesis, catabolism, and clearance of both procoagulants and anticoagulants (such as antithrombin III, fibrin degradation products, and plasminogen activators). With hepatic disease, derangements of these processes can lead to a variety of hemostatic abnormalities. Causes of coagulopathies associated with hepatic disease are listed in Box 9-2.

Although spontaneous bleeding in patients with hepatic disease is unusual, excessive bleeding following surgical trauma or liver biopsy may occur. In clinical cases of hepatic disease, there may be multiple abnormal hemostatic tests. Prothrombin time, partial thromboplastin time, and activated clotting time can be prolonged with hepatic failure because of lack of synthesis of clotting factors. This usually occurs with massive

BOX 9-2	Causes of Coagulopathies With Hepatic Disease

Decreased synthesis of clotting factors
Disseminated intravascular coagulation (DIC)
Decreased antithrombin III synthesis
Excessive fibrinolysis (decreased antiplasmin synthesis, decreased clearance of plasminogen activator)
Circulating anticoagulants normally removed by the liver remain elevated, such as fibrin degradation products (FDPs)
Decreased vitamin K availability
Increased tissue thromboplastin with massive hepatic destruction
Abnormal platelet function

acute hepatic necrosis and with cirrhosis. In a published study, dogs with chronic hepatitis that died within 1 week of presentation had significantly prolonged prothrombin and partial thromboplastin time compared with dogs that survived.

Decreased absorption of fat-soluble vitamin K leads to prolongation of clotting times. This cofactor is necessary for the hepatic synthesis and activation of factors II, VII, IX, and X. Chronic biliary obstruction can cause vitamin K malabsorption. However, intestinal bacteria synthesize vitamin K, making a deficiency of this vitamin a less common cause of bleeding during hepatic disease (unless the use of long-term intestinal antibiotics decreases bacterial vitamin K synthesis). If clotting times are prolonged, administration of parenteral vitamin K_1 followed by normalization of clotting times within 24 hours confirms vitamin K deficiency as a contributor to the coagulopathy. Recently reported studies in dogs and cats using the PIVKA test (proteins induced by vitamin K antagonism/absence) suggest that this test is the most sensitive in detecting coagulopathies in patients with hepatic disease. In these studies the PIVKA test was more than twice as sensitive in detecting coagulopathies in dogs and more than three times as sensitive in detecting coagulopathies in cats compared with routine coagulation tests (prothrombin time, activated partial thromboplastin time). Vitamin K administration may be helpful in certain situations. In one report, Vitamin K administration improved PIVKA times in 10 of 23 dogs with hepatic disease and normalized PIVKA times in 12 of 48 cats. It has been my experience that bleeding following hepatic biopsy does not correlate with coagulation findings, including the PIVKA test. Patients with coagulopathies are no more likely to bleed than patients without coagulopathies. In most cases of significant bleeding following hepatic biopsy, there are technical problems. In my experience, the rapidity of bleeding and/or necropsy examination suggest that a large vessel has been damaged rather than hemorrhage being due to persistent oozing from needle biopsy sites. The exception to this is that patients with disseminated intravascular coagulation (DIC) often have significant hemorrhage regardless of biopsy technique used. Controlled studies in veterinary patients will be necessary to make final conclusions regarding postbiopsy hemorrhage in the patient with a coagulopathy.

DIC is the most common coagulopathy occurring with hepatic disease in my experience and the one most likely to result in hemorrhage following hepatic biopsy. Thrombosis and hemorrhage are both potential sequellae of DIC. DIC can result from decreased hepatic synthesis of antithrombin III, decreased clearance of activated clotting factors, and increased release of tissue thromboplastin associated with massive hepatic destruction. These mechanisms may be further complicated by events leading to excess fibrinolysis. The latter situation can occur from excessive activity of the fibrinolytic enzyme plasmin (occurring because of increased plasminogen activator and decreased antiplasmin concentrations). The net result of excessive fibrinolysis is the formation of fibrin degradation products (FDPs), which have potent anticoagulant effects and are not cleared efficiently by a diseased liver. Laboratory test results suggesting the presence of DIC include prolongation of prothrombin, partial thromboplastin, and thrombin times, thrombocytopenia, elevated FDPs, hypofibrinogenemia, and schistocytosis.

Abnormal platelet function can also occur with hepatic disease. These defects may be evaluated by platelet aggregation studies, but these studies are not routinely performed in clinical patients because of the lack of equipment availability. Platelet function defects may explain bleeding tendencies in patients with normal coagulation tests. Platelet function can be estimated by evaluating toenail or lip bleeding time.

Spontaneous hemorrhage is unusual with hepatic disease with the exception of gastrointestinal (GI) hemorrhage. The latter can result from increased gastrin concentration (due to decreased hepatic clearance of gastrin and increased gastrin release stimulated by elevated bile acid concentrations), which causes an increase in gastric acid production. In addition, DIC can lead to abnormal GI mucosal microcirculation due to microthrombi formation, thus decreasing the ability of the mucosa to withstand injury. One of the consequences of GI hemorrhage is exacerbation of hepatic encephalopathy because blood is a substrate for ammonia production in the large intestine. In addition, GI hemorrhage can result in partial depletion of clotting factors, and, when reduced further by hepatic biopsy, massive or prolonged bleeding can result.

When evaluating patients with hepatic disease for hemostatic abnormalities, the clinician must be aware of the relative insensitivity of clotting times. *These times are prolonged only when coagulation factors are reduced to 30% of normal.* In addition, multiple defects may be present, some of which are not detected by routine coagulation tests, such as abnormal platelet function and excessive fibrinolysis. Sudden demand for clotting factors, as would occur following hepatic biopsy or laparotomy, may precipitate massive or prolonged hemorrhage in a patient with normal coagulation test results. Because the exact nature of the defect is often unknown or multifactorial, treatment with fresh whole blood collected in a plastic blood collection bag (to preserve platelet activity and prevent activation of factor XII) is usually indicated to treat these patients. If possible, efforts such as this should be taken before hepatic biopsy to correct a known coagulopathy.

Ammonia Metabolism

Ammonia has long been considered one of the most important encephalopathic toxins in patients with hepatic disease. The most important source of ammonia is the large intestine, where intraluminal bacteria convert proteins and other nitrogen-containing compounds to ammonia. Once the ammonia is absorbed into the portal circulation, the liver normally extracts most of it, converting it to urea via the urea cycle. Hepatic failure results in increased blood ammonia and decreased blood urea nitrogen (BUN) concentrations.

Gram-negative enteric bacteria are quantitatively the most important organisms for converting nitrogenous substrates to ammonia, although certain anaerobes are also capable of synthesizing ammonia. Dietary proteins are the most important substrate for ammonia production, but other substrates such as urea (which freely diffuses from the systemic circulation into the colon), sloughed intestinal epithelial cells, and GI hemorrhage are also quantitatively important. Therefore reduction of these substrates and of large intestinal bacterial numbers will have a beneficial effect on ammonia absorption. Treatment measures used to decrease ammonia absorption are discussed in the section on management of hepatic disease.

Portal blood in the dog normally contains approximately 350 μg/dl of ammonia (and about double this in the cat because of the higher dietary protein content of this species). The liver is normally able to extract approximately 85% of this, resulting in a systemic venous ammonia concentration of approximately 50 μg/dl (± 30 μg/dl). Because the liver has a large capacity for ammonia removal, there must be considerable hepatic dysfunction or abnormal portal circulation to raise systemic plasma concentrations. The normal liver can tolerate up to twice the normal ammonia load. This degree of tolerance can be a sensitive indicator of hepatic function and is used clinically when performing the ammonia tolerance test.

Hepatic Encephalopathy

Hepatic encephalopathy is defined as a clinical syndrome characterized by abnormal mental status occurring in patients with severe hepatic insufficiency. This can result from primary hepatocellular disease or from portosystemic shunting of blood away from the liver. Clinical signs in patients with this condition include a wide variety of behavioral changes, ranging from only mild depression and anorexia to coma. Many signs are nonspecific and can be seen with a wide variety of unrelated disorders. These include depression, anorexia, vomiting, diarrhea, polydipsia, and polyuria. Neurologic signs are also common. These signs are variable and often cannot be localized to a specific anatomic lesion. When this occurs, or when the nature of the neurologic abnormalities vary with time, hepatic encephalopathy should be considered as a cause. The most common neurologic manifestation is decreased mentation and responsiveness. Often patients will appear confused, have compulsive pacing and wandering, and appear transiently blind. Some patients will have abnormal patterns of urination

and defecation and appear no longer housebroken. Signs can progress to include seizures, severe dementia, and coma. The severity of these signs often wax and wane, sometimes in response to feeding, but do not always correlate with the severity of the hepatic lesion.

Etiology of Hepatic Encephalopathy

Several factors have been implicated in contributing to hepatic encephalopathy. Most of these factors relate to an accumulation of neurotoxic substances that have not been metabolized properly by the liver, including ammonia, benzodiazepine-like substances, amino acids, mercaptans, and fatty acids. Other causes include changes in the blood-brain barrier, abnormal neurotransmitter balance, abnormal cerebral metabolism, and metabolic abnormalities.

There is experimental and clinical evidence that hepatic encephalopathy is multifactorial. The concentrations of ammonia, mercaptans, and free fatty acids necessary to produce coma individually are much higher than when more than one or all are elevated. Both mercaptans and free fatty acids will increase ammonia concentration. Likewise hyperammonemia will contribute to amino acid imbalances. *In addition to the synergistic effects of encephalopathic toxins, metabolic derangements augment these effects. These changes include azotemia, hypoxia, electrolyte imbalances, hypoglycemia, tranquilization, alkalosis, and hypovolemia. Patients with these derangements are more likely to develop encephalopathy, and correction of these derangements will significantly improve the encephalopathic state.* For example, the hypokalemia that frequently accompanies hepatic failure is one of the most common metabolic derangements that contribute to depression and anorexia. With potassium supplementation there is often dramatic clinical improvement in appetite and attitude. Factors that can precipitate metabolic changes that lead to encephalopathy include increased dietary protein intake, GI hemorrhage, diuretic administration, sedative administration, uremia, infection, constipation, large intestinal bacterial overgrowth, and methionine administration.

The importance of synergistic effects and multiple interactions of encephalopathic factors help explain the different clinical presentations and severity of encephalopathy with varying blood concentrations of encephalopathic toxins. It also explains the occurrence of encephalopathy in the absence of a striking abnormality in any single factor, including ammonia concentration. The therapeutic manipulations of all these factors represent the cornerstone of symptomatic management of hepatic encephalopathy. These will be discussed in the section on management of hepatic disease.

Ascites and Portal Hypertension

Ascites (the accumulation of free fluid in the peritoneal cavity) is a common sign of hepatic disease and occurs as a result of chronic portal hypertension, hypoalbuminemia, and increased renal salt and water retention. The development of ascites occurs when there is an alteration of Starling's forces, including increased venous or lymphatic hydrostatic pressure, decreased capillary oncotic pressure, increased vascular permeability, and increased intraperitoneal oncotic pressure.

Portal hypertension is one of the most important factors leading to the development of ascites in patients with hepatic disease. Portal hypertension can be caused by increased total portal blood flow; increased resistance to portal, intrahepatic, or posthepatic blood flow; or a combination of these changes. The most common cause of portal hypertension is cirrhosis, resulting in increased resistance in sinusoidal vessels caused by swelling of hepatocytes or fibrosis around sinusoids causing postsinusoidal outflow block. The combination of increased portal pressure and blood flow causes an increase in hepatic lymph formation. When this is excessive, ascites results. Another common effect of chronic portal hypertension is the development of acquired portosystemic shunts. Unlike congenital portosystemic shunts, acquired shunts are usually multiple, extremely tortuous, and variable in their location.

It was formerly thought that portal hypertension and hypoalbuminemia initiate ascites formation. This results in decreased effective circulating plasma volume. The compensatory response to this is renal conservation of fluid and electrolytes, mediated by changes in renal blood flow, glomerular filtration rate, and activation of the renin-angiotensin-aldosterone axis. This retention of salt and water perpetuates the problem by leading to increased splanchnic lymph and portal blood flow.

However, more recent evidence contradicts this theory and suggests that the renal mechanisms leading to retention of water and electrolytes are the primary initiating events in the formation of ascites with hepatic disease. In this setting there is

renal salt and water retention before the development of ascites, thus expanding the circulating plasma volume and contributing to the development of portal hypertension. Eventually portal hypertension leads to the development of ascites, with hypoalbuminemia continuing to perpetuate it. Factors that may initiate renal salt and water retention include increased sensitivity to aldosterone and failure to release or respond to natriuretic hormone in response to an expanded circulating plasma volume. The latter situation results in the inability to excrete a salt and water load in response to volume expansion. In addition, the normal negative feedback system that governs the renin-angiotensin-aldosterone system does not shut off and reduce aldosterone secretion in the presence of portal hypertension and ascites. This is because the high concentrations of aldosterone do not return effective circulating plasma volume to normal in the presence of ascites, despite the retention of sodium. Because of these mechanisms, therapeutic interventions for managing ascites include salt restriction and inhibition of the renin-angiotensin-aldosterone axis with drugs such as spironolactone, enalapril, and benazepril. This will be discussed in the section on management of hepatic diseases.

The presence of ascites acts to increase albumin's volume of distribution, which lowers blood albumin concentration. This lowers plasma oncotic pressure and exacerbates the formation of ascitic fluid. The presence of portal hypertension is necessary for the development of ascites and leakage of albumin into the abdominal cavity. In this setting, ascites is present when plasma albumin concentrations are higher than when ascites can be attributed to hypoalbuminemia alone. With normal portal pressure, plasma albumin concentration must be below approximately 1.5 g/dl to result in ascites, as occurs with GI or renal protein loss. When this occurs, subcutaneous edema often predominates over ascites.

Other Metabolic Abnormalities
Carbohydrate Metabolism

The liver plays a central role in carbohydrate metabolism. It is the primary organ for glucose storage (converting glucose by glycogenic enzymes) and also provides glucose during fasting (through glycogenolysis). When there are inadequate stores of glycogen, as might occur with hepatic disease, the glucose need is supplied through catabolism of muscle proteins to amino acids and conversion to glucose via gluconeogenic pathways. This causes muscle wasting and increases the nitrogen load and aggravates hyperammonemia. Because of the importance of gluconeogenesis in the liver for maintaining blood glucose concentrations, complete hepatectomy rapidly results in death from hypoglycemia.

Hepatic failure can result in either preprandial hypoglycemia or postprandial hyperglycemia. Loss of approximately 70% of the hepatic mass may cause fasting hypoglycemia because of inadequate glycogen storage and gluconeogenesis. Additional causes of hypoglycemia include congenital deficiency of glycogen-metabolizing enzymes (as occurs with glycogen storage diseases), tumor hypoglycemia, and portosystemic shunts (associated with decreased hepatic mass and lack of tropic portal blood to the liver). In patients with hypoglycemia associated with hepatic disease, it is usually easy to get the blood glucose concentration into the normal range with intravenous glucose supplementation, in contrast to patients with insulin-producing tumors in which it can be very difficult to get the blood glucose concentration into the normal range despite aggressive intravenous glucose administration.

Causes of postprandial hyperglycemia with hepatic disease include deficient hepatic enzymes to handle the carbohydrate load, leading to inadequate glycogenesis, and increased plasma concentration of glucocorticoids (because of decreased hepatic clearance).

Fibrinogen

Fibrinogen is a protein that is synthesized by the liver. Synthesis of fibrinogen is diminished only in the late stages of severe hepatic failure. Other factors are usually more important in determining fibrinogen concentration than the rate of hepatic synthesis. Factors that will more commonly lead to decreased fibrinogen concentration include increased fibrinogen consumption, as occurs with DIC or primary fibrinolysis. Factors that result in increased fibrinogen concentration include inflammatory diseases (involving or not involving the liver) and major surgery. In this setting there is increased synthesis and release by the hepatocyte.

Drug and Hormone Metabolism

The microsomal enzyme system of the liver is important for drug and hormone metabolism. Hepatic failure can result in abnormally delayed drug metabolism and clearance. In addition, drugs that are highly protein bound can have increased biologic effects when there is hypoalbuminemia associated with hepatic disease. In this setting there is less albumin to bind to the drug and therefore more unbound (active) drug to exert its effects. Therefore drugs that undergo hepatic clearance or that are highly protein bound should be administered with caution in patients with hepatic failure.

Many hormones are metabolized by the liver and can be abnormally elevated with hepatic disease. The more important hormones to have prolonged clearance are the steroid hormones, including cortisol, estrogens, androgens, and progesterones. As with many drugs, the degree of protein binding and therefore the concentration of unbound, active hormone can be altered with hypoalbuminemic states. Other hormones that undergo altered metabolism in patients with hepatic disease include insulin, glucagon, thyroxine, pituitary hormones, gastrin, and aldosterone. Many of these alterations were discussed in reference to their specific physiologic effects.

Reticuloendothelial System Function

The reticuloendothelial system (RES) removes toxic or foreign substances, cellular debris, bacteria, drugs, and endotoxins from the blood. The hepatic RES is more important than that in the rest of the body for appropriate processing of these materials. Primary hepatocellular disease or portosystemic shunting (either congenital or acquired) can cause failure of the hepatic RES. With hepatic disease other tissues with RES activity can only partially compensate for the diminished hepatic RES function. Deficiencies of specific roles of the hepatic RES function can lead to characteristic changes that other RES tissues cannot compensate for. The liver is directly responsible for clearing absorbed GI products, because they pass through the liver before gaining access to the systemic circulation. These products include intestinal bacteria, endotoxins, and GI mucosal antigens. The effects of decreased clearance of GI products can be the systemic access of bacteria or their toxins, resulting in potential sepsis and/or endotoxemia. In addition, there can be positive bacterial growth from hepatic biopsy specimens even when the underlying cause of hepatic disease is not bacterial in origin. In my experience it is not unusual to culture *Escherichia coli* or other enteric bacteria from hepatic biopsy specimens obtained from patients with various hepatic diseases.

One of the consequences of abnormal exposure of GI antigens to the systemic circulation is the development of hyperglobulinemia. These immunoglobulins are produced by nonhepatic tissues in response to the systemic antigen load. Another potential source of hyperglobulinemia occurring with hepatic disease is the release of antigens from injured hepatocytes. Many of the intracellular structures of the hepatocyte, especially the nucleus and mitochondria, are recognized as foreign and elicit an immune response characterized by an influx of lymphocytes and plasma cells. The effects of this cellular infiltration include the potential for further hepatocyte damage and thus perpetuate a vicious cycle (this will be discussed further in the section on chronic active hepatitis). In addition, the plasma cells will manufacture gamma globulins, which lead to a hyperglobulinemia.

Loss of Compartmentalization Function

The maintenance of the integrity of the hepatocyte membrane is an important function. Any insult that damages the cell membrane can lead to loss of intracellular contents, including organelles, enzymes, and antigens. In addition to loss of intracellular contents, hepatocyte function may be compromised.

Loss of intracellular enzymes (with the exception of certain proteases) does not lead to abnormal function or clinical signs but can be a useful laboratory test for diagnostic purposes. Those enzymes that leak into plasma following increased hepatocellular membrane permeability include alanine aminotransferase (ALT, formerly glutamic-pyruvic transaminase [GPT]), aspartate aminotransferase (AST, formerly glutamic-oxaloacetic transaminase [GOT]), arginase, sorbitol dehydrogenase (SDH), lactic dehydrogenase (LDH), and ornithine carbamoyltransferase (OCT). Enzyme activities that increase with biliary obstruction include alkaline phosphatase (ALP), gamma glutamyl transpeptidase (GGT), and 5'-nucleotidase.

DIAGNOSTIC EVALUATION OF HEPATIC DISEASE

Historical Findings

Historical findings in patients with hepatic disease are often vague and nonspecific. In patients with toxic hepatopathies, there may be a history of exposure to known hepatotoxins, including corticosteroids, anticonvulsants, thiacetarsemide, mebendazole, acetaminophen, or certain chemicals. Clinical signs associated with hepatic disease are listed in Box 9-3. The most common signs in cats with hepatic disease are nonspecific, including lethargy and inappetence. In some patients manifesting neurologic signs, signs may be precipitated by eating (especially high-protein meals), thus suggesting hepatic encephalopathy as the cause. This historical finding is often absent, however, even in severe cases of hepatic failure, including terminal hepatic cirrhosis and portosystemic shunts. The presence of signs and laboratory abnormalities suggestive of hepatic disease in certain breeds may suggest diseases for which these breeds are predisposed, such as copper-storage disease in the Bedlington terrier, West Highland white terrier, and possibly Doberman pinscher.

Physical Examination Findings

Physical examination findings in patients with hepatic disease are often variable and nonspecific. The findings most suggestive of hepatic disease include icterus, ascites, and abnormal hepatic size. However, these signs may be seen in other diseases unrelated to the liver.

BOX 9-3	Clinical Signs Associated With Hepatic Disease	
Depression Lethargy	Acholic feces Dark or orange urine	Behavior changes Dementia
Anorexia	Jaundice	Other neurologic disturbances
Vomiting Diarrhea	Petechiae Bleeding tendencies	Polyuria Polydipsia
Weight loss	Melena	Ascites

Icterus

Prehepatic causes of increased bilirubin concentration, such as immune-mediated hemolytic anemia, can result in icterus (jaundice). The presence of icterus in a patient *without* anemia is diagnostic of hepatic or posthepatic biliary disease. The clinical manifestation of icterus usually occurs when serum total bilirubin concentration reaches 2 to 3 mg/dl, although this varies with the individual. Mucous membranes and skin appear yellow at lower serum bilirubin concentration if most is present in the conjugated state. The sclerae, soft palate, area under the tongue, and penis are usually the most sensitive areas to look for icterus. The magnitude of elevation in bilirubin concentration does not always correlate with the intensity of icterus observed on physical examination. Likewise, it can take several days for icterus to resolve following return of serum bilirubin to normal. This is especially true following resolution of biliary obstruction due to the presence and persistence of delta-bilirubin (see earlier section on pathophysiologic derangements occurring with hepatic disease).

Ascites

Portal hypertension, hypoalbuminemia, and renal retention of salt and water cause ascites in patients with hepatic disease. It is important to consider other causes of ascites in the differential diagnosis, including right-sided heart failure, pericardial disease, hypoalbuminemia resulting from nonhepatic causes, abdominal neoplasia, heartworm disease, pancreatitis, increased lymphatic or vascular permeability, and certain infectious diseases (such as feline infectious peritonitis and abdominal abscesses). The presence of ascites can be confirmed with radiography, ultrasonography, or abdominal paracentesis. Subsequent fluid analysis is helpful to rule out many of the disorders mentioned above.

Abnormal Hepatic Size

Hepatomegaly may be detected on physical examination, but normal or small hepatic size cannot be palpated. Causes of increased hepatic size include neoplasia, passive congestion (secondary to right-sided heart failure), increased corticosteroid concentration (exogenous or endogenous), lipid accumulation (diabetes mellitus, feline hepatic lipidosis, other metabolic abnormalities), diffuse inflammation, glycogen storage diseases, hepatic abscess, hepatic or biliary cyst, or liver lobe torsion. Puppies and kittens normally have a larger liver relative to their body size than adults. Causes of decreased hepatic size include portosystemic shunts (congenital or acquired), cirrhosis, or hepatic necrosis. Apparent decreased hepatic size may also be normal in some patients.

Laboratory Evaluation of Hepatic Disease

Laboratory tests are often essential to identify that hepatic disease exists, to assess its severity, and to monitor progression. An understanding of the pathophysiology of hepatic disease is necessary to interpret laboratory test results and to make clinical decisions regarding further diagnostic efforts and patient management. No laboratory test identifies a specific problem, helps determine specific therapeutic management, or predicts outcome. This is because different diseases produce similar alterations in hepatic function or in laboratory test results. Biochemical tests usually determine the liver's excretory or functional ability or measure the integrity of the hepatocyte by virtue of leakage of intracellular enzyme systems. Once biochemical tests identify that hepatic disease exists, the diagnosis must be pursued with a morphologic diagnosis obtained by biopsy specimen analysis. Results of laboratory tests in various disease states are summarized in Table 9-1.

Tests of Hepatic Function

Many biochemical tests are available to evaluate the liver's anabolic and/or catabolic functions and hepatic circulation. These include measurement of serum bile acid concentrations, plasma ammonia concentration, bile pigment (bilirubin) concentration, and the ability to excrete organic dyes. Hepatic function can be markedly abnormal despite maintenance of the hepatocellular membrane (and therefore normal serum activities of hepatic enzymes). Examples include portosystemic shunts, terminal cirrhosis, and metastatic hepatic neoplasia. Likewise, the liver can continue normal anabolic or catabolic function despite severe hepatocyte leakage of intracellular enzymes because of its marked reserve capacity. For example, this situation can occur with certain cases of hepatocellular necrosis, primary hepatic neoplasia, or trauma.

Serum Bile Acids

See the earlier section on pathophysiologic derangements occurring with hepatic disease for a detailed discussion of normal bile acid metabolism and changes occurring with hepatic disease. Briefly,

TABLE 9-1 Serum Hepatic Enzyme Activities and Chemistry Values in Various Disease States

	SALT	SAST	ALP	GGT	Total Bilirubin	BUN	Glucose	Albumin	Bile Acids
Chronic active hepatitis	++-+++	++-+++	+-+++	+-+++	N-+++	Dec-N	Dec-N	Dec-N	+-+++
Steroid hepatopathy	N-++	N-++	++-+++	+-+++	N	N	N-+	N	N-+
Feline cholangiohepatitis	+-+++	+-++	N-++	N-++	N-+++	N	N	N	N-+++
Feline hepatic lipidosis	+-+++	+-+++	+-+++	+-++	+-+++	N	N	N	N-+++
Primary hepatic neoplasia	+-+++	+-+++	+-+++	+-+++	N-+++	N	Dec-N	N	N-+++
Metastatic neoplasia	N-++	N-++	N-++	N-+	N-++	N	Dec-N	N	+-+++
Portosystemic shunt	N-+	N-+	N-+	N-+	N	Dec-N	Dec-N	Dec-N	+-+++
Cirrhosis	N-++	N-++	N-++	N-++	N-+++	Dec-N	Dec-N	Dec-N	++-+++
Hepatic necrosis	++-+++	++-+++	+-+++	+-+++	N-++	N	N	N	N-+++
Bile duct obstruction	+-+++	+-++	+++	+++	++-+++	N	N	N	+-+++

SALT, Serum alanine aminotransferase; *SAST*, serum aspartate aminotransferase; *ALP*, serum alkaline phosphatase; *GGT*, gamma glutamyl transpeptidase; *BUN*, blood urea nitrogen; + *mild increase;* ++, *moderate increase;* +++, *severe increase;* Dec, *decrease;* N, *normal.*

bile acids are synthesized in the liver as a result of cholesterol metabolism and secreted into bile. Feeding is a normal stimulus for bile acid secretion. Bile acids enter the intestine and undergo an efficient enterohepatic circulation following active absorption from the ileum. Once absorbed, they are removed from the portal circulation by the liver and reexcreted into bile. During a typical meal, the total bile acid pool is recycled two to three times through this enterohepatic pathway. Only small amounts of bile acids are lost in the feces. Normally the liver synthesizes enough bile acids to compensate for fecal losses, which are minimal with respect to the total bile acid pool. Although bile acid formation depends on hepatic synthesis, the liver reserve capacity for this is never exceeded because of the small amounts needed for physiologic purposes. Thus measurement of bile acid concentration is a reliable test even in end-stage liver disease.

Abnormal hepatic function, biliary excretion, or portal circulation can interrupt the normal enterohepatic circulation and thus lead to an increase in serum bile acid concentration. This occurs with many hepatobiliary diseases. When the liver parenchyma is diseased, the abnormal uptake, conjugation, and secretion of bile acids result in decreased extraction from the portal circulation and lead to increased systemic concentrations. With intrahepatic or posthepatic cholestasis, bile acids diffuse from bile into the systemic circulation in a manner similar to that of bilirubin. With portosystemic shunting (either congenital or acquired), the enterohepatic circulation is directly interrupted and bile acids fail to be extracted by the bypassed liver. In this setting, hepatic synthesis of bile acids continues in order to maintain a normal bile acid pool. This can result in tremendous increases in systemic concentrations, especially following feeding.

Both solid-phase radioimmunoassay (RIA) and direct enzymatic spectrophotometric methods of bile acid determinations have been validated for the dog and cat. These methods have made serum bile acid determinations a routine part of evaluating hepatic function. In my laboratory, normal fasting concentrations are approximately 2.5 μmol/L in the dog, and 1.5 μmol/L in the cat. Two-hour postprandial concentrations rise to approximately 8.5 μmol/L in the dog and cat. Serum is stable for measurement for several days at room temperature. Several artifacts can affect bile acid measurement. Moderate to marked lipemia artifactually increases the serum bile acid measurement determined by the enzymatic method but artifactually decreases the measurement when determined by the RIA method. Moderate to marked hemolysis artifactually decreases the serum bile acid value determined by the enzymatic method but probably does not affect the measurement determined by the RIA method. Bilirubin has little effect on the measurement of bile acid concentration unless the serum bilirubin concentration is greater than 5 mg/dl, in which case there may be a small (less than 20%) decrease in measurement at low bile acid concentrations. If there is hyperbilirubinemia due to hepatic disease, measurement of serum bile acids is not indicated.

Bile acid measurements have certain advantages over other tests of hepatic function. They do not require the administration of exogenous compounds (such as sulfobromophthalein [BSP] and indocyanine green [ICG] dyes and oral ammonium chloride) or meticulous sample handling (as is required for plasma ammonia determination).

The indications for measuring serum bile acid concentrations include the identification of occult hepatic disease when enzyme determinations are normal (as can occur with portosystemic shunts, cirrhosis, and metastatic hepatic neoplasia), evaluation for the possibility of a portosystemic shunt in patients with suggestive symptomatology, monitoring of hepatobiliary function to assess progression of hepatic disease, and identification of abnormal hepatic function in patients in which enzyme activity elevations may be due to extrahepatic causes.

To maximize the diagnostic information from total serum bile acid measurement, both a 12-hour fasting and a 2-hour postprandial sample should be obtained. In general it is recommended that a normal-size meal be fed. However, minimum amounts of food that should be consumed have been established. Patients weighing 10 lb or less should be fed a minimum of 2 tsp, and those over 10 lb, 2 tbsp. Foods that are high in protein and fat should be fed because they most consistently challenge the bile acid enterohepatic circulation at the 2-hour postprandial level.

If inappetence is a problem, it may be necessary to force-feed the patient. For cats, special steps to avoid anorexigenic stimuli may be necessary (e.g., offer food in a quiet environment away from dogs, have the owner hand feed in a private area).

Warming the food may help coax an inappetent cat to eat.

In patients with encephalopathic tendencies, where there is concern about feeding high-protein foods, a low-protein meal may be fed. If vomiting is a problem and its frequency precludes feeding, initial testing is limited to a fasting sample. If the result is above normal, then a significant hepatic disorder remains a consideration. However, if the fasting sample is normal, liver disease cannot be ruled out.

Several studies have shown serum bile acid measurements to be a sensitive and specific indicator of hepatic function in the dog and cat. In dogs, fasting serum bile acid concentrations are significantly increased with congenital portosystemic shunts, glucocorticoid-induced hepatopathy, hepatic neoplasia, hepatitis, cholestasis, hepatic necrosis, and cirrhosis. Of these diseases, dogs with glucocorticoid-induced hepatopathy have the lowest increase in concentration of serum bile acids. Therefore marked increase in elevations (i.e., greater than 75 to 100 μmol/L) are unlikely to be caused by glucocorticoid-induced hepatopathy. Although serum bile acid concentrations are a sensitive indicator of hepatic function, they do not distinguish the cause of the disease process. The magnitude of elevation in serum bile acid concentrations is weakly correlated with histologic severity. Furthermore, dogs with intestinal disease and normal hepatic function have normal serum bile acid concentrations. This is important in cases of "reactive hepatopathy" associated with intestinal or pancreatic disease. The determination of 2-hour postprandial concentrations further increases the sensitivity of this test in most diseases and should be done routinely in conjunction with the preprandial sample.

In cats the measurement of fasting serum bile acids concentrations has a specificity approaching 100%. Bile acid concentration is also the most sensitive test for most feline hepatic diseases, although it only approaches 60% to 70%. The value of serum bile acids for detecting hepatic disease is also increased when combined with standard biochemical tests, and visa versa. As in dogs, the magnitude of elevation does not help in the differential diagnosis of hepatobiliary disease.

In detecting portosystemic shunts, serum bile acid concentrations have the best diagnostic accuracy compared with conventional biochemical tests and BSP excretion and sensitivity equal to the ammonia tolerance test. The accuracy is improved when postprandial bile acid concentrations are measured in conjunction with the preprandial sample.

In summary, serum bile acid concentrations are a sensitive and specific indicator of hepatobiliary function and hepatoportal circulation and are a clinically useful tool in the diagnosis of these disorders. Serum bile acid concentrations are especially valuable in anicteric hepatic disease. They are more conveniently measured than blood ammonia concentration because specimen handling is routine. They are more sensitive than BSP retention and do not require the injection of a foreign compound (which is becoming increasingly more difficult to obtain). In my laboratory, when postprandial concentrations exceed 30 to 40 μmol/L in the dog and 20 to 30 μmol/L in the cat, further diagnostic efforts, such as hepatic biopsy, are warranted.

Plasma Ammonia and the Ammonia Tolerance Test

Because ammonia is metabolized primarily in the liver, blood ammonia concentration represents a sensitive test of hepatic function. Ammonia is produced from bacterial action in the colon on substrates such as dietary proteins, sloughed intestinal epithelial cells, and urea, which freely diffuses into the colon from the plasma. Once absorbed into the portal circulation, ammonia is extracted by the liver and converted to urea through the urea cycle enzyme pathway. Normally this extraction process is very efficient, with only a small amount of ammonia escaping into the systemic circulation. The concentration of ammonia in the portal vein is approximately 350 μg/dl in the dog (and approximately 700 μg/dl in the cat), whereas the normal concentration in the systemic circulation is approximately 20 to 120 μg/dl. When there is abnormal hepatocyte function or abnormal portal circulation (as would occur with portosystemic shunting), the liver cannot efficiently extract portal ammonia and systemic plasma levels increase.

Increasing the demand on the liver by increasing portal vein ammonia concentration can increase the sensitivity of plasma ammonia concentration in detecting abnormal hepatic function. This can be done by measuring ammonia concentration in the postprandial state or by administering an oral or rectal ammonia load. The latter provocative test is known as the oral ammonia tolerance test. The test is performed by taking a resting plasma ammonia sample, then administering oral ammonium chloride (NH_4Cl) at a dosage of 45 mg/lb body weight, with a maximum dose of 3 g. Ammonium chloride is available from most chemical reagent suppliers or as the main ingredient of some urinary acidifiers. It is dissolved in 20 to 50 ml tap water and administered via orogastric tube, then flushed with 20 ml water. Alternatively, it can be administered in empty gelatin capsules. A plasma sample is then obtained 30 minutes later for ammonia measurement. A rectal ammonia tolerance test has been described. This is performed by administering 1 ml/lb body weight of a 5% solution of NH_4Cl following cleansing enemas. A plasma sample is then obtained 20 to 40 minutes later. Theoretically, rectal administration has the advantage that vomiting of the orally administered solution is not a problem. However, in my experience, vomiting following oral NH_4Cl administration is rarely a clinical problem, especially when the solution is diluted with water as described above, and does not invalidate the test if it occurs. Often the cause of vomiting is hyperammonemia, and therefore ammonia measurements are diagnostic of hepatic failure. In normal patients, there should be little or no increment in plasma ammonia concentration following administration of ammonium chloride (less than 32% increase).

Sample handling is critical for plasma ammonia determinations. It is important that the venipuncture be rapid and atraumatic. Prolonged stasis of blood can result in ammonia generation. When the sample is obtained, it must be placed in an ammonia-free heparinized tube and immediately placed in an ice bath, then centrifuged as soon as possible (within 30 minutes). Red blood cells elaborate ammonia (they contain two to three times as much ammonia as plasma), and, when the sample is not separated in a prompt manner, falsely elevated concentrations will result. Likewise, hemolysis will result in a falsely increased ammonia concentration. Ideally the sample should be assayed for ammonia as soon as possible (within 2 hours) to eliminate artifacts, because the ammonia concentration can increase or decrease with storage and thus yield unpredictable and unreliable results. Ammonia concentration may increase because of deamination of proteins such as glutamine, breakdown of adenyl pyrophosphate and/or adenylic acid, or hydrolysis of other ammoniogenic substances. Plasma ammonia may decrease during storage because of vaporous loss.

The main clinical usefulness of the ammonia tolerance test is in detecting patients with portosystemic shunts, in assessing hepatic function in anicteric hepatic disease (especially when hepatic enzyme activities may be normal), and in assessing the role of ammonia (and therefore hepatic function) in patients with encephalopathic signs. The test is as sensitive as measuring serum bile acid concentrations in assessing hepatic function and more sensitive than measuring BSP excretion. The ammonia tolerance test has been shown to be virtually 100% sensitive in detecting portosystemic shunts, whereas approximately 10% of dogs with congenital portosystemic shunts can have normal resting ammonia concentrations or normal BSP retention. Its main limitation is the need for meticulous sample handling and the need for the determination to be performed soon after obtaining the sample. In addition, it requires the administration of an exogenous compound (NH_4Cl), which in rare instances can worsen encephalopathy and induce hepatic coma. If the latter complication is anticipated, a resting ammonia determination can be performed first, and the need and safety of NH_4Cl administration can then be determined.

Serum Hepatic Enzyme Activities

The routine use of measuring serum hepatic enzyme activities as an indication of hepatic disease has been made possible by automated biochemistry profiles. It must be pointed out that enzyme activities do not reflect hepatic function. *They reflect either the integrity of the hepatocyte membrane or the patency of the biliary system.* Severe hepatic dysfunction can occur in the face of normal enzyme activities, whereas hepatic function may be near normal despite marked increases in serum enzyme activities. Therefore the limitations and usefulness of hepatic enzymes must be appreciated. Loss of intracellular enzymes (with the exception of certain proteases) does not lead to abnormal function or clinical signs but can be a useful laboratory test for diagnostic purposes. The enzymes that leak into plasma following increased hepatocellular membrane permeability include ALT, AST, SDH, LDH, and OCT. Enzyme activities that increase with biliary obstruction include ALP, GGT, and 5'-nucleotidase.

Serum Alanine Aminotransferase

Serum alanine aminotransferase (SALT; formerly serum glutamic-pyruvic transaminase [SGPT]) is the most liver-specific enzyme in the dog and the cat. It is used to detect hepatocyte membrane damage and necrosis. This enzyme is found only in the cytoplasm. Serum activity increases when there is increased permeability of the hepatocyte membrane, resulting in leakage from the hepatocyte. The extent to which enzyme leakage occurs depends on both the severity and number of cells damaged (i.e., how diffuse the lesion is) but does not indicate the reversibility of the injury or the functional status of the liver. The activity of SALT is most marked with chronic active hepatitis, primary hepatic neoplasia, and hepatic necrosis (see Table 9-1). There is often normal or only mildly increased SALT activity with portosystemic shunts, cirrhosis, and metastatic neoplasia. In rare cases, increased SALT activity can occur with severe muscle disease.

Although the activity of SALT usually parallels the degree of hepatocyte necrosis, there is often poor correlation with the serum enzyme activity and the degree of morphologic change on a light microscopic level, especially during the recovery phase. Likewise, there is often poor correlation between the serum activity of SALT and the degree of hepatocyte dysfunction and clinical signs. For example, there can be severe increases in SALT activity following automobile trauma or certain toxins, yet the patient often shows no signs of hepatic failure and other tests of hepatic function (such as serum bile acids or blood ammonia concentrations) remain normal. In these patients the magnitude of increase in SALT activity reflects the number of hepatocytes affected (i.e., the diffuseness of the lesion), although they maintain their ability to perform other intracellular functions. On the other hand, patients with portosystemic shunts, cirrhosis, or metastatic neoplasia often have normal SALT activity despite severe hepatic failure. In these patients the normal enzyme activity reflects either an intact hepatocyte membrane or, in the case of terminal cirrhosis, intracellular enzyme depletion.

There is often a mild to moderate increase in SALT activity with certain systemic diseases that result in hypoxia (such as right-sided heart failure with secondary ischemic injury to the hepatocyte, severe anemia, or severe pulmonary disease), endotoxemia, or sepsis. There is also a mild to moderate increase in SALT activity with biliary obstruction, probably as a result of the toxic effects of bile acids that diffuse back into the hepatic parenchyma. Pancreatitis and inflammatory intestinal diseases also may result in increased SALT activity. These cases are sometimes referred to as a "reactive hepatopathy."

Serum Aspartate Aminotransferase

AST, like ALT, has high activity in the liver. However, there is also high AST activity in muscle and red blood cells, and serum aspartate aminotransferase (SAST; formerly serum glutamic oxaloacetic transaminase [SGOT]) activity is therefore less specific than SALT activity in detecting hepatocellular leakage. Increased activity of SAST occurs with both hepatocyte and muscle damage, as well as with hemolysis (in vitro or in vivo). AST is found both free in the cytoplasm and within mitochondria of the hepatocyte. With hepatic disease, SAST activity usually parallels that of SALT. Usually the magnitude of increase in SALT activity exceeds that of SAST activity. This may be due to the shorter half-life of SAST and because SAST is also found in the mitochondria of the hepatocyte. Therefore a more severe insult is required to cause mitochondrial damage and thus release of SAST from this site compared with damaging the hepatocellular membrane only. *When the activity of SAST exceeds that of SALT, muscle or red blood cell, rather than the liver, should be considered as the source of the isoenzymes.*

Serum Alkaline Phosphatase

The serum activity of ALP usually increases with biliary stasis, steroid hepatopathy, and bone lesions. ALP is found in many tissues, including the liver, bone, intestine, placenta, and kidney. However, in clinical situations only the isoenzymes found in the liver and in bone are important. This is because the serum half-lives of the other isoenzymes are only 3 to 6 minutes, whereas the half-life of the hepatic isoenzyme is 3 days in the dog. Serum activity of bone ALP increases with osteoblastic activity (and is therefore elevated in young, growing animals), bone tumors, osteomalacia, and hyperparathyroidism.

The serum activity of ALP increases with hepatic disease primarily when there is biliary obstruction (intrahepatic or extrahepatic). Unlike the transaminases (SALT and SAST), ALP is not a leakage enzyme associated with increased hepatocyte permeability. Rather, its production is induced by biliary obstruction, produced by cells lining the bile canaliculi. This increase in production is accompanied by inability to excrete the enzyme through the biliary system, thus resulting in increased serum activity. In addition to primary biliary obstruction, serum ALP activity is often elevated with primary hepatocellular disease of many causes due to swelling of hepatocytes (e.g., associated with inflammation, cloudy swelling, lipid accumulation, neoplastic infiltration) resulting in intrahepatic cholestasis (see Table 9-1). Diseases that are periportal in location tend to cause more marked increases in serum ALP activity than centrilobular disorders, because they tend to affect bile flow through canaliculi more.

In addition to the isoenzyme induced by biliary obstruction, there is also a steroid-induced isoenzyme of ALP. Although this isoenzyme is also produced in the liver, it is a separate entity from that induced by biliary obstruction. The dog is very sensitive to the effects of glucocorticoids in this regard as opposed to the cat. A single injection of a glucocorticoid can increase the serum activity of the steroid-induced isoenzyme of ALP. This increase in activity can last for several weeks with short-acting preparations and for several months with long-acting preparations. The magnitude of increase depends on the dose administered, duration, route, and individual sensitivity. In addition, dogs with spontaneous hyperadrenocorticism (Cushing's syndrome) usually have marked increases in serum ALP activity. Assays are now available to readily distinguish the isoenzyme induced by biliary obstruction from the steroid-induced isoenzyme. These assays generally report the percentage of total ALP activity that is accounted for by the steroid-induced isoenzyme. However, this is not a reliable test to distinguish patients with steroid hepatopathy from those with other hepatopathies because the serum activity of the steroid-induced isoenzyme of ALP is variably increased with many types of hepatic diseases and nonhepatic illness. Alternatively, hepatic biopsy specimen analysis in dogs readily distinguishes steroid-induced hepatopathy from primary hepatobiliary disease of other causes.

Certain drugs will also induce increases in serum ALP activity. The most common drugs to have this effect are glucocorticoids, barbiturates, and anticonvulsant drugs, including phenobarbital, primidone, and phenytoin. These drugs will result in increased serum ALP activity, with or without morphologic changes in the liver or alterations in hepatic function (as documented with hepatic function tests).

Unlike the dog, the activity of ALP is much lower in feline serum. This is because the half-life is much shorter in the cat (6 hours versus 3 days) and less feline ALP is produced secondary to biliary obstruction than in the dog because the feline liver contains only one third the concentration of ALP per gram of liver that the canine liver contains.

Therefore even mild elevations of serum ALP activity in the cat are indicative of marked hepatobiliary disease. The magnitude of increase in serum ALP activity is most marked with feline hepatic lipidosis, almost always exceeding the magnitude of increase in serum GGT activity in this syndrome. Other diseases in the cat that result in increased serum ALP activity include hepatic malignant lymphoma, feline cholangiohepatitis complex, bile duct obstruction, and hyperthyroidism.

Gamma Glutamyltranspeptidase

GGT measurement is now available on chemistry profiles from many commercial laboratories. Its serum activity increases with biliary stasis and steroid hepatopathy. In most cases the activity of serum GGT parallels that of serum ALP and its measurement is of only occasional value in the dog and cat. There is GGT activity in liver, kidney, pancreas, and intestine; however, the half-life of the hepatic isoenzyme is the only one long enough to account for significant serum activity. Therefore elevated serum GGT activity is specific for hepatobiliary disease or hepatic induction from drugs. As with serum ALP, elevations are most marked with biliary obstruction, but activity can also increase with primary hepatocellular disease if it results in intrahepatic cholestasis. The serum activity of GGT may increase earlier in biliary disease than ALP activity. In addition, there is also marked elevation in serum GGT activity with glucocorticoid administration or spontaneous hyperadrenocorticism. Other drugs (such as anticonvulsants) will also increase serum GGT activity.

In the cat, serum GGT activity has a higher sensitivity but lower specificity than serum ALP activity for detection of hepatobiliary disease. *Only in feline hepatic lipidosis does the magnitude of increase in serum ALP activity generally exceed that of serum GGT activity.* In the dog, serum GGT activity is generally more specific but less sensitive than serum ALP activity for the detection of hepatobiliary disease. Thus serum GGT activity has a higher positive predictive value, whereas ALP activity has a higher negative predictive value for evaluating hepatobiliary disease. The diagnostic performance is best when both enzyme activities are evaluated together. In general, serum GGT activity is less influenced by nonhepatic diseases or enzyme-inducing drugs.

Other Biochemical Tests

Many of the tests routinely obtained on automated serum biochemistry profiles give information regarding hepatic function, including determinations of bilirubin, albumin, BUN, and glucose (see Table 9-1).

Serum and Urine Bilirubin

Hepatobiliary excretion of bilirubin requires adequate uptake, conjugation, and secretion by the hepatocyte, as well as a patent biliary system. There must be considerable hepatocellular disease or increase in the bilirubin load (hemolysis) to result in hyperbilirubinemia, because the liver's reserve capacity for bilirubin processing is up to 30 times the normal bilirubin load. Conjugated bilirubin is water soluble and readily excreted by the kidneys. The dog has a very low renal threshold for bilirubin excretion; thus the finding of +1 to +3 bilirubinuria in a concentrated sample is normal. Therefore the concentration of bilirubin in the urine increases before that of the serum. Thus the serum bilirubin concentration is an insensitive indicator of hepatocellular disease, and serum concentrations are not increased until there is marked decrease in hepatic function. Therefore slight elevations in serum bilirubin concentration are significant, suggesting hepatobiliary disease. The exception to this is with artifactual increases in serum bilirubin concentration, as would occur with lipemia or hemolysis. If there is not significant bilirubinuria associated with a serum bilirubin concentration greater than normal, artifact should be considered. The cat has a high renal threshold for bilirubin excretion, and any bilirubin in the urine is abnormal. When serum bilirubin is in the normal range (anicteric hepatic disease), other tests of hepatic function discussed earlier are needed for detection, such as serum bile acid or blood ammonia measurements. *However, when serum bilirubin concentration is elevated, there is no need to run additional function tests if hemolysis can be excluded. In this setting, bilirubin represents an accurate and specific indicator of hepatic function.*

Increased serum total bilirubin concentration can result from prehepatic (hemolysis), intrahepatic (primary hepatocellular disease), or posthepatic (biliary obstruction) causes. The relative amounts of conjugated or unconjugated bilirubin are variable with all three general categories of hyperbilirubinemia because secondary events can change the relative concentrations of the two forms. Therefore their measurement does not aid the clinician in localizing the nature of the lesion. The magnitude of increase in serum bilirubin concentration also is not helpful in localizing the nature of the lesion. Other methods of localizing the cause of hyperbilirubinemia include measur-

ing the hematocrit (to rule out hemolysis) and ultrasonography, laparoscopy, cholecystography, and laparotomy (to distinguish intrahepatic from posthepatic causes).

In general, serum bilirubin concentration increases most markedly with extrahepatic biliary obstruction. Hepatocellular diseases that may result in cholestasis and therefore hyperbilirubinemia include chronic active hepatitis, certain cases of primary neoplasia, feline cholangiohepatitis, feline hepatic lipidosis, and cirrhosis (see Table 9-1). Other hepatic disorders that generally have normal serum bilirubin concentration include portosystemic shunts, hepatic necrosis, steroid hepatopathy, and metastatic neoplasia (see Table 9-1). In general, disorders involving the periportal areas are most likely to result in increased bilirubin concentration.

Serum Albumin

Albumin represents approximately 25% of the proteins synthesized by the liver. Because albumin has a relatively high priority for synthesis, severe hepatocellular disease must exist before serum albumin concentration falls. Hypoalbuminemia resulting from hepatic disease suggests chronic dysfunction. Because the serum half-life of albumin is 7 to 21 days (depending on the disease state and the serum concentration), there must be prolonged hepatic disease before serum concentration decreases. In addition to lack of production occurring with hepatic disease, albumin concentration can drop from protein-calorie malnutrition (sometimes associated with an extremely low protein diet, often used in the therapeutic management of hepatic disease) and from an increased volume of distribution due to ascites, resulting in a dilutional effect on serum albumin concentration. Although serum albumin concentration is an insensitive and nonspecific test of hepatic function, *hypoalbuminemia may be the only change on a serum biochemistry profile in certain cases of hepatic failure (such as cirrhosis and portosystemic shunts), and its presence may justify specific hepatic function tests (e.g., serum bile acid assay), which may subsequently identify hepatic failure.* In one study the presence of hypoalbuminemia in dogs with chronic hepatitis was a predictor of shorter survival time.

Blood Urea Nitrogen

A low BUN concentration may indicate chronic hepatic disease. The liver manufactures urea by extracting portal vein ammonia and converting it to urea through the urea cycle enzyme pathway. With hepatic failure this process fails, and BUN concentration falls. However, because there are many other factors that influence urea metabolism (including renal function, dietary protein concentration, catabolic states, systemic perfusion and hydration status, and GI function), BUN concentration is an insensitive and nonspecific test of hepatic function. However, like serum albumin concentration, a low BUN concentration may be the only abnormality on a serum biochemistry profile and may be an important clue as to the presence of hepatic disease. Subsequent specific hepatic function tests would then be used to document hepatic failure.

Serum Glucose

The liver plays an important role in glucose metabolism. Hepatic failure can result in either preprandial hypoglycemia or postprandial hyperglycemia. In dogs with chronic hepatitis the presence of hypoglycemia is an accurate predictor of early death. When there is abnormal glucose concentration, causes in addition to hepatic disease must be explored. In patients with hypoglycemia associated with hepatic disease, it is usually easy to get the blood glucose concentration into the normal range with intravenous glucose supplementation, as opposed to patients with insulin-producing tumors, in which it can be very difficult despite aggressive intravenous glucose administration.

Radiographic Evaluation of the Liver

Survey Radiographs

Survey radiographs are often informative when evaluating the liver. They give information about the size, shape, position, and radiodensity of the liver. Survey radiographs are also useful to screen for other abnormalities, including ascites, renal calculi (present in some cases of portosystemic shunts), thoracic metastasis, and abdominal lymphadenopathy. Radiographic signs of abnormal hepatic size are listed in Boxes 9-4 and 9-5. Causes of abnormal hepatic size are listed in Boxes 9-6 and 9-7. In addition to hepatic size, abnormalities in hepatic radiodensity can also be determined from survey radiographs. These abnormalities include (1) calcification (cholelithiasis, parasitic cysts, neoplasia, or granulomas), (2) gas accumulation (cholecystitis, gas in the portal veins, hepatic abscess, or necrotic tumors), and (3) inability to visualize hepatic borders (ascites or emaciation). Radiography is reviewed in detail in Chapter 2.

BOX 9-4 | Radiographic Signs of Decreased Hepatic Size

Decreased distance between the diaphragm and stomach

Displacement of the stomach cranially or upright angulation of the stomach axis in the lateral view

Displacement of the stomach to the right in the dorsoventral view

Cranial displacement of the cranial duodenal flexure, right kidney, and transverse colon

Liver and stomach entirely within the chest cavity

BOX 9-5 | Radiographic Signs of Increased Hepatic Size

Extension of the liver margin caudal to the costal arch

Rounding of the caudal margins on the lateral view

Displacement of the stomach caudally and dorsally on the lateral view

Displacement of the stomach caudally and to the left on the ventrodorsal view

Caudal displacement of the cranial duodenal flexure, right kidney, and transverse colon

---

BOX 9-6 | Causes of Radiographic Signs of Decreased Hepatic Size

Cirrhosis
Portosystemic shunt
Acute and subacute necrosis
Hernias (diaphragmatic and peritoneal-pericardial)
Deep-chested breeds (normal)

Evaluation of Hepatic Blood Flow

Along with nuclear scintigraphy and laparotomy, contrast radiography is a reliable method to determine whether there is a portosystemic shunt present. There are several techniques to evaluate hepatic blood flow, including intraoperative mesenteric portography, percutaneous splenoportography, and cranial mesenteric arterial portography.

Intraoperative Mesenteric Portography

The indications to perform intraoperative mesenteric portography are to confirm the existence, number, and location of portosystemic shunts. In

BOX 9-7	Causes of Radiographic Signs of Increased Hepatic Size

Neoplasia (primary or metastatic)
Congestion (right-sided heart failure)
Fatty infiltration
Diffuse inflammation
Hyperadrenocorticism
Storage diseases
Abscess
Hepatic or biliary cyst
Liver lobe torsion
Puppies and kittens (normal)
Deep inspiration (normal)

addition, the residual portovenous flow into the liver can be assessed for prognostic importance. If a portosystemic shunt is identified, surgical correction may be performed during the same anesthetic procedure.

Technique

Intraoperative mesenteric portography is a technique that can readily be performed in general practice, because no special equipment is needed. A mesenteric or jejunal vein is catheterized at laparotomy. A vessel that can eventually be sacrificed is selected, and as large a catheter as possible is used. Once the catheter is secured, an intravenous extension set is attached and the abdomen temporarily closed (with the extension set exiting through the abdominal wall). A total of 0.25 to 0.5 ml/lb body weight of an iodinated radiographic contrast media is injected as rapidly as possible through the extension set. A radiograph is obtained just at the end of the injection. Unless a portable radiographic unit is available, it is usually easiest to perform the laparotomy on the x-ray table. With portosystemic shunting, contrast media passes directly into the systemic venous circulation and bypasses the liver. If the caudal extent of the shunt is cranial to T13, it is probably an intrahepatic shunt; if it is caudal to T13, it is probably an extrahepatic shunt.

Percutaneous Splenoportography

The indications for percutaneous splenoportography are similar to those described for intraoperative mesenteric portography. Splenoportography often yields a lesser quality study but has the advantage of not requiring a laparotomy. This is especially important in a hypoalbuminemic patient that is at risk for wound dehiscence.

Technique

General anesthesia or heavy sedation is required for splenoportography. The spleen is localized by transabdominal palpation, or ultrasound or laparoscopy can be used to aid in needle placement. Approximately 0.25 to 0.5 ml/lb body weight of an iodinated radiographic contrast media is injected directly into the splenic pulp at the rate of 1 to 2 ml/sec. Radiographs are taken immediately and approximately 10 seconds after the end of the injection.

Cranial Mesenteric Arterial Portography

Cranial mesenteric arterial portography is an excellent method of evaluating the entire portal system and evaluating hepatic blood flow. The technique is less invasive than operative mesenteric portography; however, it requires fluoroscopy, serial films, and special injection equipment.

Ultrasonographic Evaluation of the Liver

Ultrasonography is now widely used to evaluate the liver because it is ideally suited for soft tissue imaging. It gives specific information regarding structural abnormalities in the liver and can readily distinguish fluid-filled structures from solid soft tissue structures, including visualization of the gallbladder, hepatic vessels, and adjacent parenchyma. Hepatic ultrasonography is discussed in Chapter 2. Also see the References for additional information regarding basic principles of ultrasound and the ultrasonographic appearance of the liver.

The main reasons I use ultrasonography to evaluate hepatic disease are to distinguish focal from diffuse disease (and thus help determine an appropriate biopsy method) and to distinguish intrahepatic causes of cholestasis from extrahepatic causes of cholestasis (the former being a potentially medically treatable problem, the latter a surgically treatable problem). Additional indications for an ultrasound evaluation of the liver include any abnormality in hepatic function, size, or radiodensity. Diffuse changes in hepatic echogenicity (compared with falciform fat, the renal cortex, and spleen) may suggest certain hepatic diseases. Diffuse hyperechogenicity is seen with fatty change, steroid hepatopathy, fibrosis, and cirrhosis. Hypoechogenicity is seen with passive congestion, lymphoma, and suppurative hepatitis. Ultrasonography can also be a useful method to obtain a biopsy specimen of the liver, because it can be used to guide a biopsy needle into an appropriate portion of the liver. Normal structures and abnormalities detectable by ultrasonography are listed in Boxes 9-8 and 9-9.

Nuclear Scintigraphy to Evaluate the Liver

Nuclear scintigraphy is primarily used to evaluate hepatic blood flow and aids in the detection of portosystemic shunts. Scintigraphy may in some cases localize the shunt and distinguish intrahepatic from extrahepatic shunts. It also represents a noninvasive method of proving the existence of a shunt. It may be followed by more invasive studies, such as mesenteric portography or surgery. Nuclear scintigraphy equipment is primarily available at referral centers.

Technique

Technetium-99m pertechnetate is an inexpensive, available radioisotope that is absorbed across the colonic mucosa. When administered in high concentration into the colon, dynamic imaging during the first 1 to 2 minutes can provide a nuclear angiogram of the portal system. These images in normal dogs result in sequential visualization of the portal vein, liver, and several seconds later the heart and lungs. In patients with portosystemic shunts, heart and lung activity occur before liver activity.

The procedure is well tolerated and does not require sedation. In many cases the study allows distinction between intrahepatic shunts, single extrahepatic shunts, and multiple extrahepatic shunts. Although the study does not give the anatomic detail of radiographic contrast studies, the information is usually specific enough to determine whether the patient is a good operative

candidate. In addition, the radioisotope enters the portal system more caudal to the liver than in angiographic studies, so distal or caudal shunts are not missed. The study can also be performed on cats but may require a higher imaging frequency.

A similar procedure has also been described in dogs using transcolonic ^{123}I–iodoamphetamine (IMP). This is a radiolabeled amine that binds to liver and lungs following absorption from the colon. Imaging within 10 minutes of administration and counting activity in liver and lung allows a direct calculation of portal blood flow that is bypassing the liver. This method is also noninvasive and accurate. However, disadvantages compared with transcolonic administration of ^{99m}Tc pertechnetate are the high expense and relatively long half-life of the radioisotope ^{123}I.

An alternative technique involves analysis of an intravenous injection of radiocolloid. Radiocolloids are removed from the circulation by the RES of the body. It has been shown that the uptake of radiocolloid by the liver is a reflection of hepatic blood flow rather than phagocytic properties of Kupffer's cells. Thus radiocolloid scintigraphy is a sensitive technique to screen for portosystemic shunts. The procedure is safe, does not require sedation, and is relatively rapid. Radiocolloid scintigraphy is performed by injecting 3 to 5 mCi ^{99m}Tc sulfur colloid intravenously and subsequently scanning the organs of the body with a gamma camera. A computer is used to plot activity in the lungs and liver against time.

In normal dogs there is initial activity in the lungs, which rapidly decreases during the initial

---

BOX 9-9　**Abnormalities Detectable by Hepatic Ultrasonography**

Ascites
Hepatic enlargement
Hepatic fibrosis
Neoplasia (focal or metastatic)
Distended gallbladder and biliary tree
Portal or hepatic venous distension
Hepatic cysts
Hepatic abscess
Calcification
Portosystemic shunts
Lipidosis/vacuolar hepatopathy
Nodular regeneration

BOX 9-8　**Normal Structures Detectable by Hepatic Ultrasonography**

Diaphragm
Hepatic parenchyma
Gallbladder
Hepatic and portal veins
Intrahepatic bile ducts (variable)
Cystic duct (variable)
Common bile duct (variable)

passage of the bolus (60 seconds) as the radiocolloid is cleared from the circulation by the spleen and liver. There is subsequent gradual increase in activity in the liver, reflecting uptake of the radiocolloid. In dogs with portosystemic shunts, there is increasing activity in the lungs after the initial passage of the bolus, indicating pulmonary uptake. The rate of hepatic uptake is considerably less than that seen in normal dogs. Unfortunately, there are many indeterminate and false-positive results with this method compared with transcolonic administration of the radioisotope. In normal cats, extrahepatic uptake in the lungs occurs, preventing adequate images of the liver.

Hepatic Biopsy

Hepatic biopsy specimen analysis is the only way to accurately diagnose and classify hepatic disease. Biochemical tests, radiographs, and ultrasonography determine that hepatic disease exists. None of these tests accurately determines the cause or appropriate treatment or predicts prognosis (with the exception of angiography or scintigraphy for detecting portosystemic shunts). Recent advances in biopsy methods and in noninvasive imaging of the liver have made hepatic biopsy a routine and essential tool in the diagnosis and management of patients with hepatic disease. Many types of hepatic diseases are treatable, and a definitive diagnosis allows the clinician to make appropriate clinical decisions with regard to specific treatment, rather than just supportive care. Hepatic biopsy specimen analysis helps determine whether the abnormality is (1) reversible or irreversible, (2) progressive or static, (3) primary hepatic or secondary, (4) treated with specific therapy or only with supportive therapy and whether there is a need for follow-up biopsy posttreatment.

Indications

The most common indication for performing hepatic biopsy is abnormal hepatic function and/or increased serum hepatic enzyme activities of unknown origin. This is usually identified by hepatic function tests (such as serum bile acids or blood ammonia measurements) and serum biochemical profile findings obtained in patients showing signs compatible with hepatic disease or in routine preanesthetic blood work. If clinical illness is attributed to hepatic disease, a biopsy is warranted.

In patients with persistently abnormal serum hepatic enzyme activities, efforts to rule out nonhepatic causes of enzyme elevations should be made first, such as hyperadrenocorticism, diabetes mellitus, congestive heart failure, and feline hyperthyroidism. In an asymptomatic patient, when increased hepatic enzyme activities are detected on routine biochemical profiles, I generally assess hepatic function with serum bile acid measurements. If these are not grossly elevated, the biochemistry profile is repeated in 4 to 6 weeks. If there is a persistent increase in hepatic enzyme activity at this time, hepatic biopsy is justified.

Abnormal hepatic size of unknown cause (either microhepatica or hepatomegaly) is another indication for hepatic biopsy. If hepatomegaly is present, efforts must be made to rule out nonhepatic causes, such as hyperadrenocorticism, diabetes mellitus, and congestive heart failure. Even in the presence of these disorders, it might be clinically indicated to assess hepatic involvement in these multisystem diseases with hepatic biopsy specimen analysis. In many cases of hepatomegaly (with either diffuse or focal enlargement), the purpose of the biopsy is to confirm suspected neoplasia. Recent advances in chemotherapy have made this an important step in proper management.

Finally, hepatic biopsy specimen analysis is important to document the progression of disease. Often multiple or serial biopsies are necessary to document remission (as in certain cases of chronic active hepatitis [CAH] or hepatic malignant lymphoma) and therefore determine appropriate treatment.

Precautions

Most contraindications to hepatic biopsy are relative contraindications and depend on the biopsy method. When these factors are present, the clinician must weigh the potential benefits of obtaining the biopsy (i.e., a definitive diagnosis and the opportunity to begin rational specific therapy) with the risks of the complications that could potentially occur. However, with experience and knowledge of various methods of hepatic biopsy, these risks can be minimized.

The most common contraindication to hepatic biopsy is a coagulopathy. Determining the nature of the coagulopathy is important in minimizing its influence. The most common coagulopathy associated with hepatic disease is DIC. When DIC is present, knowledge of the underlying disease is essential in long-term management, and thus obtaining the biopsy is essential. In this setting I recommend high volumes of intravenous fluids to maintain tissue perfusion in the face of micro-thrombi, platelet function inhibition with aspirin to minimize the hypercoagulable state, and a transfusion with fresh crossmatched whole blood collected in a plastic collection bag (glass activates factor XII) with 125 units of heparin added per 500 ml of blood to activate antithrombin III (to minimize the hypercoagulable state). Methods of obtaining the biopsy that require a minimal incision yet allow control of bleeding, such as laparoscopy-guided or the keyhole method, are preferred.

When there are prolonged clotting times unaccompanied by DIC, there may be decreased clotting factor synthesis or vitamin K deficiency. Vitamin K administration may be helpful in certain situations. In one report vitamin K administration improved PIVKA times in 10 of 23 dogs with hepatic disease and normalized PIVKA times in 12 of 48 cats. It has been my experience that bleeding following hepatic biopsy does not correlate with coagulation tests, including the PIVKA test. Patients with coagulopathies are no more likely to bleed than patients without coagulopathies. In most cases of significant bleeding following hepatic biopsy, there are technical problems. In my experience the rapidity of bleeding and/or necropsy examination suggest that a large vessel has been damaged rather than hemorrhage being due to persistent oozing from needle biopsy sites. The exception to this is that patients with DIC often have significant hemorrhage regardless of technique. Controlled studies in veterinary patients will be necessary to make final conclusions regarding postbiopsy hemorrhage in the patient with a coagulopathy.

An unstable patient that cannot be safely anesthetized is another relative contraindication for performing a liver biopsy. In these patients blind percutaneous or ultrasound-guided biopsy methods may be considered because these can often be done with minimal or no sedation.

Complete biliary obstruction with dilation of intrahepatic bile ducts is a contraindication described in humans because of the potential for bile peritonitis. Theoretically this occurs because there is increased intraductal pressure, and therefore inadvertent duct rupture following biopsy results in bile leaking into the abdominal cavity. In my experience, however, this complication has not been recognized in cases when percutaneous biopsy was performed in animals with biliary obstruction.

Finally, hepatic abscess, cyst, or vascular tumors are contraindications to percutaneous biopsy methods. Unfortunately, it is usually not known that these are present until it is too late, unless an imaging modality such as ultrasonography or laparoscopy is available.

Prebiopsy Considerations

Appropriate biochemical and hepatic function tests must be performed to assess the need for the biopsy and identify concurrent disease. Once the need for hepatic biopsy is determined, several considerations must be made. History, physical examination, laboratory, and ancillary findings determine the overall health status of the patient. This is important in deciding an appropriate anesthetic regime. Certain biopsy methods require minimal to no sedation (blind percutaneous or ultrasound-guided), some require short general anesthetics (keyhole or laparoscopy-guided), whereas others require a long general anesthetic (laparotomy). In addition, patients with extremely low serum albumin concentration are at greater risk for wound dehiscence and therefore biopsy is more appropriately performed with percutaneous methods.

Abdominal radiographs are helpful to assess hepatic size. This information is useful to narrow the list of differential diagnoses and also to help plan the biopsy approach. For example, with microhepatica the transthoracic percutaneous approach may be preferred over the transabdominal percutaneous approach and laparoscopy-guided biopsy may be preferred over ultrasound-guided biopsy. The reverse is true with hepatomegaly. Thoracic radiographs are helpful to rule out metastatic neoplasia.

Coagulation profiles should be performed before hepatic biopsy because of the multitude of abnormalities possible with hepatic disease. These were discussed in detail in the section on pathophysiologic derangements occurring with hepatic disease. Ideally PIVKA time, prothrombin time, partial thromboplastin time, platelet count, and fibrin degradation product determinations should be made before hepatic biopsy. If there are significant cost and time concerns, a less acceptable alternative is the measurement of activated clotting time and toenail bleeding time. The former test assesses the intrinsic and common clotting pathways but is only abnormal when clotting factor activity drops below 10% of normal (whereas partial thromboplastin time is abnormal when clotting factor activity drops below 30% of normal). The management of coagulopathies when obtaining hepatic biopsy was discussed in the section on precautions for hepatic biopsy.

Because chemical restraint is sometimes necessary to insure a safe procedure, the patient should be clipped before sedation. For general anesthesia I prefer isoflurane or sevoflurane induction by face mask or induction chamber. If an injectable anesthetic is desired, I prefer the combination of ketamine and diazepam. Although oxymorphone provides adequate restraint and can be reversed if necessary, excessive panting often occurs, which interferes with the biopsy procedure and therefore is not recommended.

Biopsy Methods

The five basic methods of obtaining a hepatic biopsy are *blind percutaneous, keyhole technique, ultrasound-guided, laparoscopy-guided,* and *laparotomy biopsy.* Each method has certain advantages and disadvantages. Knowledge of these, as well as practice and expertise in each respective method, allow the clinician to select the most appropriate and safest method to obtain hepatic tissue.

Blind Percutaneous Biopsy

The advantages of blind percutaneous biopsy are that it is very rapid, requires minimal sedation, and is low cost. Disadvantages of this method are that there is the potential for inadvertent trauma to other organs, focal lesions may be missed, and detection of bleeding may be delayed.

Equipment

Various biopsy needles can be used for percutaneous biopsy. In general, newer automated needles are preferred. These are spring-loaded needles that are similar in style to manual Tru-Cut (Baxter) or ABC (Monoject) needles. Automated needles can be completely automatic or semiautomatic. Automated cutting needles include the Monopty (Bard), ASAP (Microvasive), and Biopty (Bard) needles. Completely automatic needles thrust the inner obturator (containing the biopsy tray or specimen notch) followed by the outer cutting sheath into the organ in a fraction of a second. These needles can easily be operated with one hand. Because the action is so quick, there is minimal displacement of the organ, a shorter intraparenchymal phase, and much more reliable yield of tissue. This allows the biopsy of the organ to be performed with minimal manual mobilization, allows a smaller diameter needle to be used, and allows a lighter degree of sedation.

Semiautomated cutting needles include the Vet-Core needle (Cook). Semiautomatic needles require manual thrusting of the internal obturator (containing the biopsy tray or specimen notch) into the organ, followed by an automatic thrusting of the outer cutting sheath by the spring-loaded mechanism. These needles have some of the advantages of the completely automatic needles and have the additional advantages of having more control over final needle position and being lighter with a smaller handle. These characteristics also make these needles well suited to computed tomography (CT) guidance because the handle can be let free by the operator for intraprocedural scanning without the weight of the handle causing the needle to move. In addition, the tip of the needle can be precisely localized before the outer cutting sheath is "fired." The older manual cutting needles (Tru-Cut or ABC needles) offer no advantages over these newer needles.

Aspiration needles are generally used to obtain smaller samples that would be suitable for cytologic preparations (rather than histopathologic preparations), or for Menghini and Westcott needles, used to obtain small samples for histopathologic examination (see below). These needles are also well suited to obtain samples of fluid, such as intraparenchymal cysts and gallbladder puncture. Usually these are smaller-gauge needles (20 to 22 gauge) and therefore tend to be less traumatic. Aspiration needles employ suction to obtain fluid or cut the core of tissue. The Menghini needle is especially suited for transthoracic hepatic biopsy but can be used for transabdominal techniques as well. The tip of the needle is slightly oblique and convex and cuts a core of tissue when suction is applied as the needle is rapidly thrust into the liver and immediately withdrawn. The intrahepatic phase should last just a fraction of a second. A sliding screw acts as a depth gauge and prevents the needle from entering too deeply into the parenchyma. For the Westcott needle, suction is used to draw tissue into a specimen notch at the distal end. Gentle back-and-forth movement allows a core of tissue to be cut.

Transthoracic Technique

Because of the short intrahepatic phase, the transthoracic technique is especially suitable for patients in which sedation is too risky or undesirable and in patients with microhepatica, in which the transabdominal technique may be difficult. The patient is given corn oil orally (1 ml/lb body weight) to cause the gallbladder to contract and thus minimize the risk of inadvertent puncture. A Menghini needle is used to obtain the biopsy specimen. The patient is placed in left lateral recumbency, and the right hemithorax clipped and surgically prepared. A local anesthetic is injected subcutaneously at the needle puncture site: just dorsal to the costochondral junction of the fifth through seventh intercostal space (depending on the size of the patient and distance to the diaphragm). Using a No. 11 blade, a skin incision is made to prevent dulling of the biopsy needle. With the stylet of the Menghini needle in place, the needle is "popped" into the pleural space and then directed caudally and parallel to the rib cage until it contacts the diaphragm (respiratory movements will be felt). Care is taken to avoid lacerating the intercostal vessels that lie along the caudal aspect of each rib. Upon making contact with the diaphragm, the needle depth gauge is slid to within approximately 1.5 cm of the skin so that the depth of penetration into the liver is limited to this distance. The stylet is then removed and quickly replaced with a 12-ml syringe filled with 5 to 6 ml of sterile saline. Negative pressure corresponding to approximately 3 ml of fluid volume is produced by drawing on the plunger. At the peak of expiration, the needle is rapidly thrust into the liver (with the distance limited by the depth gauge) and immediately withdrawn from the patient in one swift motion, maintaining negative pressure throughout. This entire step (i.e., the intrahepatic phase) should last only a split second. The core of hepatic tissue should rest within the fluid in the syringe or in the needle. The plunger is removed and the contents poured into culture broth, onto a slide for impression cytologyic study, and/or into a jar containing 10% formalin. The patient is then immediately turned onto its right side for approximately 5 minutes to allow the weight of the liver to control hemorrhage.

Possible complications with this technique include gallbladder puncture (and possible bile peritonitis and pleuritis), pneumothorax, and excessive bleeding. In patients with firm fibrotic livers, this technique may not yield a suitable sample. In this situation a cutting type of needle used with a transabdominal approach may be successful.

Transabdominal Technique (Blind)

The transabdominal technique is especially useful when the size of the liver is normal or large. It has a longer intrahepatic phase than the transthoracic technique if a cutting type of needle is used, and therefore a higher degree of sedation may be necessary in an uncooperative patient. The patient is given corn oil orally (2 ml/kg body weight) to cause the gallbladder to contract and thus reduce the risk of inadvertent puncture. I prefer to use automated cutting type of needles such as the Monopty or ASAP needles. The patient is placed in right dorsal oblique recumbency at a 45-degree angle. In this position the stomach falls down toward the right side. A large area around the xiphoid cartilage is clipped and surgically prepared. A local anesthetic is injected subcutaneously at the needle entry site: just caudal and to the left of the xiphoid cartilage, in the middle of the "V" formed by the xiphoid cartilage and the rib cage. If the needle enters too far cranially, it may inadvertently enter the thoracic cavity. If there is hepatomegaly, the entry site is moved caudally as appropriate for the hepatic size. The skin is incised with a No. 11 blade to prevent dulling of the biopsy needle. The biopsy needle is inserted and advanced just through the body wall and aimed in a craniolateral direction towards the left shoulder. The needle should be advanced during inspiration. The liver should be very close to the body wall, and the needle need not be advanced very far. Penetration of the liver is often not felt. The most common error using this technique is inserting the needle too far and going completely through the liver. Once the liver is entered the biopsy needle is operated to cut the sample. This is done during peak inspiration. The needle is removed after each attempt. The core of hepatic tissue should be resting within the specimen notch of the needle. If the initial attempt fails to obtain hepatic tissue, the needle is redirected based on perceived location of the liver, body conformation (i.e., deep chested), and direction of previous attempts. Tissue is carefully removed with a 25-gauge needle and placed into culture broth, onto a slide for impression cytologic study, and/or into 10% formalin. The patient is immediately placed in sternal recumbency to allow the weight of the liver to control hemorrhage.

Possible complications of this technique include puncture of the stomach, gallbladder rupture (and possible bile peritonitis), puncture of the diaphragm and lung (and possible pneumothorax), and excessive bleeding.

Keyhole Technique

The keyhole technique offers the advantages of providing more guidance of the needle than blind percutaneous biopsy, being relatively rapid, and being low cost. Disadvantages of this method include the requirement for more sedation compared with blind percutaneous biopsy, the possibility of causing inadvertent trauma to other organs, the possibility that focal lesions may be missed, and the possibility that detection of bleeding may be delayed. This technique is especially suitable for individuals who lack the experience to perform a blind percutaneous biopsy.

The keyhole technique and equipment are similar to that described for the blind transabdominal percutaneous biopsy. Under a general anesthetic a small incision into the abdominal cavity is made just caudal to the site of needle introduction. A gloved finger is inserted into the abdomen to palpate the liver and stabilize it for biopsy. The needle is inserted through the same incision or through a separate incision just cranial to the first incision. The finger then guides the needle into the liver, and the biopsy specimen is cut. I prefer an automated cutting needle for this technique because it can be operated with one hand, whereas the Tru-Cut needle would require an assistant to operate the needle. Complications are similar to those described for blind percutaneous biopsy.

Ultrasound-Guided Biopsy

Ultrasound-guided biopsy offers the advantage of providing more guidance to the needle than is possible with blind percutaneous biopsy, is relatively rapid, and requires minimal sedation. Because intraparenchymal lesions can be visualized, biopsy of them can be selectively performed. In addition, other intrahepatic structures such as the gallbladder and portal vessels can be avoided. Disadvantages of ultrasound-guided biopsy include the requirement for expensive equipment and that detection of bleeding may be delayed. As with other biopsy methods, success is operator-dependant. Ultrasound-guided biopsy is easier when the liver is normal or large in size. When there is microhepatica, overlying gas in the stomach often makes visualization of the liver difficult. In this setting, laparoscopy would offer a more appropriate image-guided biopsy method.

Technique

Most dogs require minimal sedation for ultrasound-guided biopsy. I use a low dose of ketamine for cats (10 to 20 mg intravenously) or isoflurane or sevoflurane administered by face mask. A careful ultrasound examination is performed before biopsy. This allows planning of the procedure based on the type of echo pattern, size of the lesion, proximity to other organs, proximity to blood vessels, determination of cystic or solid tissue, and determination of the needle path. For focal liver biopsy the location of the lesion will determine the position of the scan head and needle path. For diffuse lesions the transducer is usually placed just caudal and to the left of the xiphoid and aimed at the left medial or lateral lobes. In patients with extremely small livers, it may be difficult to adequately visualize the needle without stomach gas interfering. In this case placing the patient in a 45-degree right ventral oblique position often helps reduce interference from the stomach. Otherwise the patient is usually placed in dorsal recumbency for most procedures. A rubber trough or V tray assists in positioning. In addition, if the patient is under gas general anesthesia, an assistant compresses the rebreathing bag to hold the patient in deep inspiration. This moves the diaphragm and liver caudally to improve visualization. If a lesion cannot be seen due to overlying gas or bone, changing patient or transducer position usually allows adequate visualization.

The area to be scanned, including the needle entry site, is surgically prepared. The ultrasound transducer is covered with sterile plastic wrap (or a sterile glove) after a small amount of coupling gel is placed on the transducer surface. A biopsy guide may be used if desired, allowing accurate placement of the needle in the same plane as the scan. However, it is sometimes desirable to have the needle enter in a different plane due to overlying structures in the plane of the scan, in which case a biopsy guide cannot be used. Biopsy guides also limit the angle of insertion of the needle, and the entry site is usually 2 to 3 cm from the scan head. Therefore for superficial lesions or those in the center of the scan, a biopsy guide should not be used. Furthermore, when the needle is in a rigid biopsy guide, inadvertent trauma to the organ may result if the patient moves or takes a deep breath.

A small amount of sterile coupling gel or water-soluble lubricant is placed on the skin, and the ultrasound examination is repeated to verify the needle path. A small stab incision is made in the skin at the needle insertion site. Automated needles are generally preferred because they can be easily operated with one hand. Therefore the needle must be loaded before entry into the abdomen. While one hand maneuvers the transducer, the other hand advances the needle into the organ under direct ultrasound visualization. If the needle tip cannot be seen, gentle movement of the transducer should allow visualization. To allow distinction of the needle from other echogenic structures in the image, the needle can be gently moved in and out. Ideally this should be minimal and just enough to move the organ within the abdominal cavity rather than moving the needle within the organ. If a spinal needle is used, moving the stylet in and out of the stationary needle increases the echogenicity and visualization of the needle tip without creating tissue trauma. Occasionally the needle cannot be visualized. Indirect evidence of organ puncture can be used, including movement of the organ or visualization of motion at the organ border. The needle is directed so the trajectory will avoid other structures when it is fired. Care must be taken to prevent going too deep with the needle, or it will be seen to penetrate the diaphragm and enter the thoracic cavity. Once the biopsy specimen is obtained, the needle is removed. The core of liver should be resting within the specimen notch of the needle. A 25-gauge needle is then carefully used to transfer the tissue into culture broth, onto a slide for impression cytologic study, and/or into 10% formalin. The number of biopsy specimens obtained will depend on the coagulation status of the patient, types of diagnostic tests planned, and adequacy of tissue retrieved. After completion of the procedure, an ultrasound examination is performed to check for excessive hemorrhage. External digital pressure or an abdominal compression wrap may be used to control hemorrhage. Possible complications of this technique are similar to those described above for the blind transabdominal percutaneous biopsy.

Laparoscopy-Guided Biopsy

The main advantage of laparoscopy-guided biopsy is the ability to visualize the liver, biliary tree, and other abdominal organs. With experience the gallbladder can be examined, palpated with a blunt probe, and the bile duct traced to its entry into the duodenum. In this manner it can be determined whether there is a common bile duct or cystic duct obstruction. In addition, because focal lesions on the liver can be directly visualized, an appropriate biopsy site can be selected, and other intrahepatic structures such as the gallbladder and portal vessels can be avoided. Hemorrhage can be observed and, when excessive, controlled with direct compression with a blunt probe over the biopsy site, with electrocautery, or with application of gel foam. Compared with laparotomy, there is much less anesthetic time. With experience the operator can

perform a complete laparoscopic examination and obtain multiple biopsy specimens in 10 to 15 minutes in most cases, and because there is only a 1.0-cm incision, there is much less risk for wound dehiscence. Disadvantages of laparoscopy are the requirement for a general anesthetic and the need for expensive equipment. Details of the equipment and techniques for performing laparoscopy are found in Chapter 3.

Potential complications of the procedure include those related to a general anesthetic, excessive bleeding, overdistention of the abdomen with gas, air embolism, and a tension pneumothorax if the diaphragm is inadvertently punctured (as abdominal gas enters the thoracic cavity). In my experience these complications are extremely rare.

Laparotomy Biopsy

Advantages of a laparotomy biopsy include the ability to view the entire abdominal cavity and to treat disease when surgically correctable. Therefore one can visualize and select the biopsy site. If there is excessive hemorrhage, it can be controlled. However, if there is a known coagulopathy, laparotomy is not advised because of the size of the incision and therefore high potential for additional bleeding. In this setting laparoscopy is the preferred method for obtaining the biopsy specimen. Laparotomy offers the additional advantage of being able to obtain large biopsy specimens. Disadvantages of laparotomy biopsy include the requirement for a long general anesthetic and therefore more risk to the patient. In addition, there may be poor wound healing if severe hypoalbuminemia is present and therefore increased risk for dehiscence.

The techniques to obtain hepatic tissue at laparotomy are beyond the scope of this chapter. The reader is referred to surgical textbooks for further information on this subject.

Postbiopsy Monitoring

The most important complication to monitor for following hepatic biopsy is excessive hemorrhage and subsequent hypovolemic shock. Hematocrit and total solid measurements are an unreliable means of identification of hemorrhage, because several hours are necessary for extravascular fluid redistribution to occur following acute bleeding and therefore changes in hematocrit are delayed. By the time the hematocrit drops, it might be too late to begin a life-saving blood transfusion. Therefore clinical monitoring, including assessing mucous membrane color and capillary refill time, is most helpful. Intravenous fluid support and/or blood transfusion may be necessary to treat hypovolemic shock. If the patient has a known coagulopathy before biopsy, crossmatching should be performed and compatible blood made available. *If at all possible, blood transfusion with stored blood should be avoided because it contains a high concentration of ammonia resulting from elaboration from red blood cells.* Therefore fresh blood should be collected in plastic collection bags (platelets stick to glass, and glass activates factor XII and can therefore worsen DIC). In my experience if there are no complications from hemorrhage within 5 hours of the biopsy procedure, the patient is unlikely to experience bleeding problems.

Biopsy Specimen Handling

Hepatic biopsy samples are often quite friable and need to be handled with care to avoid excessive fragmentation. Depending on the biopsy method, the amount of tissue submitted may be small. The pathologist must be familiar with interpreting small samples. Therefore representative sections of the liver must be submitted. A portion of all hepatic biopsy samples should be cultured for both aerobic and anaerobic bacteria. Therefore appropriate culture media should be available. Bacterial infection of the liver can be a primary event or can be secondary to abnormal clearance of portal bacteria associated with abnormal hepatic reticuloendothelial cell function.

A portion of the biopsy sample can be placed on a glass slide to obtain an impression smear for cytologic study before placing the sample in 10% formalin. Several diseases can be readily diagnosed by cytologic examination before histopathologic confirmation, including feline hepatic lipidosis, hepatic malignant lymphoma, hepatic carcinoma, and fungal hepatitis.

In addition to routine hematoxylin-eosin (H & E) staining, copper stains may be helpful, including orcein, rhodamine, rubeanic, or Timm's stains. Use of these stains is indicated in suspected cases of primary copper-storage diseases (as occurs in the Bedlington terrier and West Highland white terrier) or to assess whether chelation therapy will be necessary in cases of chronic active hepatitis (especially in Doberman pinschers). It is recommended that copper stains be requested anytime a hepatic biopsy sample is obtained from any of these breeds.

Biopsy Specimen Interpretation

Controversy exists as to whether fine needle aspirates, needle biopsy specimens, laparoscopic "spoon" biopsy specimens, and surgical wedge biopsy samples give similar results. There appears to be strong institutional bias in regard to this question, usually depending on expertise and experiences of the entire team of clinicians involved (e.g., internist, radiologist, pathologist). My impression is that fine needle aspirates are only helpful for certain conditions, such as to confirm the diagnosis of hepatic lipidosis and certain types of neoplasms (lymphoma and mast cell tumor). However, fine needle aspirates usually fail to define lobular architecture, the location of inflammation within the lobule, degree of fibrosis, degree of cholestasis, vascular pathologic condition, and so on. Fine needle aspirates are also often unreliable in mixed lesions. A recent study comparing fine needle aspirates for cytologic study with surgical biopsy specimens suggested that cytologic examination is unreliable in all categories of hepatic disease in dogs and cats. Needle biopsies may also be limited in their usefulness in some situations as well, depending on the quality and quantity of the biopsy samples obtained. I occasionally receive results of needle biopsy specimen analysis that do not adequately explain the clinical and laboratory features of the patient. It is likely that some of these cases simply have sampling error. Needle biopsy specimens procured via ultrasound guidance are typically obtained from the portion of liver that can be seen best (usually the left medial lobe), with minimal attempts to sample other sites. Geographic diversity and the limited sample size may explain failure in these cases. For example, needle biopsy specimens of regenerative nodules often can be suggestive of a metabolic disorder. Several portal triads need to be included to be of most benefit, often from several areas. A recent study showed only 49% concordance between needle biopsy and surgical biopsy specimen analysis.

Clearly laparoscopic and surgical wedge biopsies give the most information because of the size of biopsy specimens obtained. Caution must be used when obtaining a biopsy sample from the edge of a lobe. There is often an increase in fibrous tissue at the surface due to blending of fibrous tissue of the capsule with portal fibrous tissue. Therefore the center of lobes should be included in sampling with laparoscopic or surgical biopsy procedures. In addition, laparoscopic biopsy allows the sampling of multiple lobes. I typically obtain at least seven "spoon" biopsy specimens with most laparoscopic examinations.

The most common histopathologic abnormalities encountered in the experience of many clinicians are listed in order of frequency in Box 9-10. From a clinical perspective the biopsy specimen analysis has the following purposes:

1. To categorize the disease (inflammatory, neoplastic, degenerative, dysplastic, or metabolic abnormality such as lipidosis or steroid hepatopathy)
2. To establish a specific cause if possible
3. To determine the prognosis
4. To direct institution of appropriate specific therapy

Information that must be determined from hepatic biopsy specimen analysis includes the following:

1. Chronicity (acute or chronic)
2. Severity
3. Involvement of structures within individual lobular units (bile canaliculi, blood vessels and lymphatics, hepatocytes in each major zone of the lobule, or the hepatic capsule)
4. Distribution, severity, and nature of inflammatory cells
5. Degree of degeneration and necrosis
6. Distribution and severity of fibrosis
7. Presence of pigment
8. Vacuolar changes (fat, steroids)
9. Presence of organisms
10. Need for special stains (copper, amyloid, glycogen, or fibrous tissue)

BOX 9-10 Histopathologic Abnormalities Seen in Hepatic Biopsy Specimens (in Order of Frequency)

Vacuolar hepatopathy (steroid hepatopathy)
Chronic active hepatitis (dog)
Hepatic lipidosis (cat)
Cholangiohepatitis complex (cat)
Neoplasia (lymphoma most common)
Focal necrosis with inflammation
Cholestasis
Cirrhosis
Passive congestion (ischemia)
Other

HEPATIC DISEASES

Many diseases of the liver are treatable when a definitive diagnosis is known. However, proper management requires an understanding of the etiology, proper interpretation of diagnostic tests, and an etiologic diagnosis based on hepatic biopsy specimen analysis. This discussion will cover the most commonly encountered diseases of the liver and review specific treatment when appropriate.

Inflammatory Diseases of the Liver

Inflammatory diseases represent one of the most common manifestations of hepatic disease. The liver is often affected with infectious and toxic inflammatory diseases because it has an active reticuloendothelial cell function and plays an important role in detoxifying agents absorbed from the bowel. The liver also receives a large portion of the cardiac output and therefore has potential for systemic hematogenous involvement. The liver also may be involved in noninfectious immune-mediated reactions.

Noninfectious Inflammatory Diseases

Noninfectious inflammatory diseases are among the most common hepatic diseases seen. Unfortunately, the cause is often unclear, and they remain idiopathic entities. In addition to primary inflammatory hepatic disease, the liver can be involved secondary to disease in other organs ("innocent bystander"). Because the liver receives GI products and toxins in portal blood, primary GI disease resulting in mucosal damage can lead to increased absorption of these agents in the portal circulation. These can cause direct damage to the liver (toxic hepatopathy) or incite immunologic reactions leading to inflammation in the liver. It is not uncommon to find elevated hepatic enzyme activities associated with idiopathic inflammatory bowel disease (lymphocytic-plasmacytic enteritis or colitis), viral enteritis (parvovirus, coronavirus), or severe pancreatitis. In this setting, absorption of endotoxins and other toxic products results in hepatic damage and inflammation. These cases are often referred to as a "reactive hepatopathy." Generally there are increases in serum transaminase activities (ALT, AST) but normal concentrations of serum bile acids. In addition, the hepatic abnormalities resolve when the underlying disease is treated.

Drugs can also cause hepatic damage resulting in inflammation, including anticonvulsants and certain antiparasitic drugs (mebendazole, thia-cetarsamide). Finally, metabolic abnormalities such as copper-storage diseases can result in hepatic inflammation. The histologic appearance of all these entities can be very similar. Therefore the clinician must be aware of the many factors that can lead to hepatic inflammation and thoroughly evaluate the patient to manage the disorder appropriately.

Chronic Active Hepatitis, Chronic Hepatitis

CAH is defined as an idiopathic active inflammatory disease of the liver that is chronic in duration. The term has been applied to a proposed specific disease analogous to the disease in humans of the same name or to a description of the pathologic process that results in the histologic appearance characterized by chronic ongoing inflammation. Some clinicians believe that the disorder is not a specific disease but rather a general reaction by the liver to any injury, with the histologic pattern one of nonspecific inflammation as a response to any insult. Others believe that the clinical features, histologic pattern, and response to immune-modulating drugs are similar enough to the disease in humans to warrant the name as a true disease entity.

Several distinct clinical entities can result in chronic hepatitis, including copper-storage diseases (Bedlington terrier, West Highland white terrier, Skye terrier, and possibly the Doberman pinscher), infectious diseases (viral hepatitis, leptospirosis), drugs (anticonvulsants), or idiopathic causes. This discussion will focus primarily on idiopathic causes, although *it must be emphasized that diseases with a known underlying cause must be*

looked for and that not all cases of chronic hepatitis are "steroid-responsive" or "autoimmune."

When an underlying cause for chronic hepatitis cannot be identified, a pathogenesis similar to that described for humans (Figure 9-1) may have merit. Briefly, it is proposed that immunologic factors lead to the perpetuation of inflammation following hepatocyte damage caused by any agent. Following hepatocyte injury, there is a release of hepatic antigens previously not exposed to the systemic immune system (hidden from immune surveillance). This results in an influx of inflammatory cells (primarily lymphocytes and plasma cells), which cause antibody-mediated and complement-mediated cytotoxicity. This results in further hepatocyte injury, and this vicious cycle is perpetuated by these immunologic events and occurs long after the initial insult is gone. At first the reaction occurs near the portal triads, but eventually it extends beyond the limiting plate of hepatocytes (the single-cell–thick layer of hepatocytes surrounding the portal triad) into the hepatic lobule. This eventually results in necrosis and bridging fibrosis (inflammation and fibrosis extending between adjacent portal areas). When the normal hepatic architecture is lost and the fibrotic process becomes diffuse, it is termed cirrhosis. Whether these events occur in the dog as has been proposed in humans, and whether the syndrome seen in dogs is analogous to CAH in human beings, is unknown.

Clinical Features of Chronic Active Hepatitis in Dogs

CAH is represented in approximately 5% to 16% of dogs undergoing hepatic biopsy in one study. The disease occurs primarily in middle-age dogs (average 6 years), with the majority (greater than

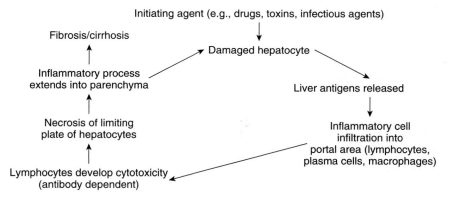

FIGURE 9-1 Pathogenesis of chronic active hepatitis.

75%) occurring in females. There is a marked predisposition in Doberman pinschers, with virtually all cases (greater than 95%) occurring in females of this breed. Because of the finding of marked copper accumulation in the livers of affected Doberman pinschers, it is unclear if the disease seen in this breed is the same as that occurring in other breeds. However, copper is normally excreted in the bile, and it accumulates in hepatocytes with any cholestatic disorder. The finding of high hepatic copper concentrations in two Doberman pinschers with subacute hepatitis (i.e., without evidence of cholestasis) suggests the possibility of a primary copper-storage disease. For the purposes of this discussion, however, the disease seen in the Doberman pinscher breed will be considered with that seen as idiopathic CAH in other breeds because the clinical features are similar. There is also a breed predisposition in American cocker spaniels.

Clinical signs of CAH include those typical of chronic hepatic disease, such as polyuria, polydipsia, weight loss, anorexia, icterus, ascites, abnormal bleeding tendency, depression, disorientation, and seizures. Some patients have a short fulminant clinical course and die within a short period of showing clinical signs. Others are presented with progressive signs of hepatic disease, although signs often wax and wane. A third group of dogs is asymptomatic when presented, with the disease identified from biochemical screening and subsequent hepatic biopsy specimen analysis.

Abnormal laboratory findings include increased serum activity of all hepatic enzymes (including ALT, AST, ALP, and GGT) in virtually all dogs. Most dogs (approximately 75%) have increased serum total bilirubin concentration (mild to marked), and many (approximately 50%) are hypoalbuminemic. Abnormalities in other chemistry values are inconsistent. Hepatic function tests (serum bile acids and plasma ammonia concentrations) are usually abnormal. Clotting times may be abnormal. These test results generally reflect the severity of the disease and stage in which it is detected. In one large series of dogs reported with chronic hepatitis from any cause, low serum glucose concentration and prolonged prothrombin time were the best predictors of early death (within 1 week of presentation). In dogs surviving more than 1 week, hypoalbuminemia was the laboratory change most predictive of shorter survival time. The degree and severity of necrosis and fibrosis were accurate predictors of early

death, and the presence of bridging fibrosis was the histologic change most predictive of shorter survival time in dogs surviving more than 1 week.

Radiographic findings vary with the severity of the disease. Abnormal findings include microhepatica (usually associated with terminal cirrhosis), ascites (associated with portal hypertension and hypoalbuminemia), and, in those cases that undergo angiographic evaluation, there are multiple acquired tortuous portosystemic shunts indicative of chronic portal hypertension.

The histologic appearance is not unique to CAH but can be seen in other inflammatory hepatic diseases. Therefore other inflammatory diseases must be eliminated to suggest the diagnosis of CAH. Histologic features include piecemeal necrosis, bridging necrosis, and active cirrhosis. Piecemeal necrosis refers to a specific pattern that is typical of CAH and characterized by periportal necrosis and inflammation occurring in an irregular fashion surrounding islands of normal hepatocytes. The majority of inflammatory cells are lymphocytes and plasma cells, although there are lesser numbers of neutrophils and macrophages. Accompanying features include bile duct hyperplasia, bile stasis, and regenerative nodules. Eventually there is deposition of fibrous tissue as a sequela to the inflammation and necrosis, eventually connecting adjacent portal triads (bridging necrosis and fibrosis). When normal hepatic architecture is lost and the fibrotic process becomes diffuse, it is termed cirrhosis. In most Doberman pinschers that have been evaluated, copper stains are strongly positive and quantitative measurements of hepatic copper concentration are high. Other breeds have not been studied as extensively for the presence of hepatic copper; however, I have seen several cases in other breeds with high hepatic copper concentrations histologically. The gross appearance of the liver can be normal in early cases. As the disease progresses, the liver becomes shrunken, loses its normal lobular pattern, becomes discolored (brown, red, and yellow mottling), and the surface becomes irregular. Eventually the surface becomes coarsely nodular in texture, reflecting regenerative nodules occurring in a setting of terminal cirrhosis.

Treatment of Chronic Active Hepatitis in Dogs

The treatment of CAH in dogs remains speculative because controlled clinical trials with large numbers of dogs have not been performed. The necroinflammatory response is usually progressive, and most dogs do not go into spontaneous remission. If cirrhosis is present, the likelihood of successfully managing the case is low. Therefore the prognosis is poor in severe cases, and most of these dogs die within several weeks to months despite appropriate treatment. *This emphasizes the need for early detection.*

There are three basic goals in treating dogs with CAH:

1. To arrest inflammation
2. To correct nutritional imbalances and treat hepatic encephalopathy with dietary management
3. To resolve fibrosis

Arresting Inflammation

Though there are no controlled trials using glucocorticoids to treat dogs with CAH, many clinicians have had success using them as part of the therapeutic regimen. In a large study of Doberman pinschers with CAH, however, there was little benefit seen with prednisone alone. In another study of chronic hepatitis in various breeds, dogs surviving more than 1 week that were treated with prednisone had improved survival compared with dogs not treated with prednisone. However, the varieties of hepatic diseases treated and lack of a prospective control group limit the validity of conclusions of that study. Studies in humans show that the combination of low-dose glucocorticoids and azathioprine (Imuran) is as efficacious as high-dose glucocorticoids alone and has fewer side effects. Because of these observations, the combination may be justified in dogs. I have had more success using a combination of prednisone and azathioprine than prednisone alone.

On a theoretical basis, prednisolone is preferred over prednisone in treating dogs with hepatic disease because the latter drug requires hepatic conversion to the former (active) drug. However, studies in humans with CAH have shown the two drugs to have equal efficacy and reach similar blood levels of the active form. Similar studies have not been performed in the dog, although I have found no difference between prednisolone and prednisone in treating dogs with hepatic disease.

The recommended starting dosage of prednisone is 0.5 to 1 mg/lb body weight per day. The starting dosage of azathioprine is 50 mg/m^2 body surface area once daily. Once clinical remission is achieved (usually 3 to 4 weeks), the dose of prednisone is gradually tapered to a low maintenance dose (approximately 0.2 mg/lb body weight).

Likewise, azathioprine is tapered to an alternate-day dosage schedule (at the original dose). I generally taper prednisone first and do not taper azathioprine until the dose of prednisone is low. This is because azathioprine is generally associated with fewer side effects and is better tolerated. A complete blood count (CBC) and platelet count should be obtained 3 and 6 weeks after starting azathioprine and every 2 months thereafter to look for potential myelosuppression. If this is detected, azathioprine should either be tapered or discontinued depending on the magnitude of the cytopenia. During the tapering process, patients are monitored with serum biochemistry profiles for relapses. Often it is difficult to differentiate the effect of prednisone on serum hepatic enzyme activities (especially ALP activity) from the effect of the disease process on serum enzyme activities. In this setting, clinical judgment is used to determine if prednisone should continue to be tapered. Serial bile acid assays and serum bilirubin and albumin concentrations also can be used to monitor the patient. If hepatic inflammation is being adequately controlled by azathioprine, the enzyme activities will decrease as prednisone is tapered. Eventually prednisone is discontinued, and later azathioprine is discontinued.

In cases with cholestasis the use of the hydrocholeretic drug ursodeoxycholic acid (ursodiol; Actigall or Urso) may be helpful. Ursodeoxycholic acid is a naturally occurring dihydroxylated hydrophilic bile acid found in small quantities in normal human bile and in larger quantities in the bile of certain species of bears. One of its uses is for dissolution of radiolucent gallstones. The proposed mechanism of action is that it alters the composition of bile, changing it from cholesterol-precipitating to cholesterol-solubilizing and dispersing cholesterol as liquid crystals in the bile, thus solubilizing the gallstones. In humans, ursodiol dissolves gallstones at the rate of approximately 1 mm/month and works best on radiolucent, non-calcified gallstones less than 20 mm in diameter. Side effects are rare (diarrhea), and there is no influence on either serum total cholesterol or triglyceride concentrations.

The exact mechanisms of its beneficial effects in inflammatory hepatic diseases remain controversial. It is believed that there is a favorable change in the bile acid pool, rendering retained endogenous bile acids less toxic by changing the bile acid pool from the more toxic hydrophobic bile acids to less toxic hydrophilic bile acids. It is also thought that ursodeoxycholic acid has antiinflammatory, immunomodulatory, and choleretic effects (promoting bile flow and decreasing viscosity of bile). The latter mechanism is believed to be mediated through the cholehepatic shunting hypothesis. This proposes that ursodeoxycholate is converted to ursodeoxycholic acid through addition of a hydrogen ion originating from carbonic acid. This leaves a bicarbonate ion to act as an osmotic draw for water to decrease viscosity and promote bile flow. Ursodeoxycholic acid has been used in the management of chronic hepatic diseases in humans, including CAH, primary biliary cirrhosis, and primary sclerosing cholangitis. Significant improvement in symptoms, laboratory parameters, and survival has been reported in many patients undergoing treatment for these diseases.

I have used ursodeoxycholic acid, either alone or in combination with other drugs, in patients with various cholestatic diseases (including dogs with CAH and cats with cholangiohepatitis). The drug is very well tolerated, and in some cases the response can be dramatic. Use of ursodeoxycholic acid should be considered as either primary or adjunctive (in combination with immunosuppressive or antiinflammatory drugs) treatment in patients with chronic liver diseases. It may be the only effective drug in patients in which glucocorticoid therapy or other immunosuppressive drug therapy is contraindicated or ineffective. Ursodeoxycholic acid is also a powerful choleretic agent that can be used to treat sludged bile and cholelithiasis. The drug is supplied in 300-mg capsules and more recently in 250-mg tablets. A safe and effective dose is 6 to 7 mg/lb/day, administered either once daily or divided twice a day. The drug should be given with food. Studies need to be performed to substantiate its efficacy and dosage in the dog and cat.

Vitamin E therapy is also recommended in many types of hepatic diseases, including CAH. Oxidative injury to the liver is now well recognized in several types of inflammatory processes. Free radicals are generated in chronic hepatitis by the injurious effects of certain drugs, toxins, or immunologic injury. These free radicals can damage cellular macromolecules via lipid peroxidation and thus participate in cellular injury and play an important role in initiating and/or perpetuating hepatic injury. Vitamin E reduces oxidant injury to hepatic tissue by providing protection from free radicals. Vitamin E is used at a dosage of 7 units/lb

twice a day. Bile acids are required for fat-soluble vitamin E absorption, and, because they may be reduced with liver disease, a water-soluble formulation should be used. This type of formulation is available at most health food stores.

S-adenosylmethionine (SAMe) is a molecule synthesized by all cells and is critical to intermediary metabolism. It is especially important in the liver, where much of the body's intermediary metabolism occurs. SAMe is derived from the amino acid methionine and initiates three major biochemical pathways (transmethylation, transsulfuration, and aminopropylation). These pathways are involved with major anabolic and catabolic reactions that influence steroid hormone effects, carnitine synthesis, drug metabolism and detoxification, and hepatocyte and red blood cell membrane function. In addition, SAMe is involved in detoxification of toxins and protection against oxidative injury. The latter effect is in large part mediated through glutathione, a metabolite of SAMe through the transsulfuration pathway of metabolism. Glutathione depletion has been documented in approximately 45% of canine and feline hepatopathies. With glutathione depletion, oxidative injury is more likely to result in membrane damage and toxin accumulation, resulting in hepatocellular injury and death. It has been speculated that this could be minimized by supplementation with SAMe. Furthermore, SAMe has aminopropylation metabolites that contribute to antiinflammatory effects.

SAMe is available as a "nutraceutical" that has been studied experimentally and clinically in a variety of species. Oral use became possible when a stable oral salt in an enteric-coated tablet was developed. Nutramax Laboratories, Inc, currently markets it under the trade name Denosyl SD4. Several studies have shown the product to be safe in a variety of species, including dogs and cats.

Potential indications for usage in dogs and cats include hepatic necrosis, inflammatory disorders, cholestasis, drug-induced hepatotoxicity, copper storage hepatopathy, and metabolic disorders such as glucocorticoid-induced hepatopathy and idiopathic feline hepatic lipidosis. In these disorders administration of SAMe is meant to help minimize oxidative injury, protect against free radical damage, protect against the deleterious effect of retained bile acids, enhance bile flow, stabilize hepatocellular membranes, decrease inflammation, and aid in detoxification of endotoxins and other substances absorbed from the portal circulation. Since SAMe has such a diverse spectrum of effects, it may be helpful in a diverse group of hepatopathies. The currently recommended dose is 9 mg/lb divided twice daily for dogs and 90 mg (per cat) once daily for cats. It is rapidly absorbed and is best administered on an empty stomach to maximize absorption. The drug can be safely administered with other drugs used to treat hepatic diseases without toxicity or compromising effects of other drugs, including ursodeoxycholic acid. Controlled studies are needed to substantiate these recommendations and to determine which disorders are most likely to benefit from SAMe administration.

The optimal duration of treatment is unknown and can be quite variable. The decision to discontinue medication should ideally be based on follow-up hepatic biopsy specimen analysis. If there is evidence of ongoing inflammation, therapy should be continued. In the absence of follow-up hepatic biopsy specimen analysis, the decision to discontinue treatment may be arbitrary but should be based on clinical and biochemical information. Patients should be monitored at least monthly for relapses at first. Some patients require long-term (years), low-dose therapy (e.g., prednisone every 48 to 72 hours) to maintain remission.

Possible sources of sepsis should be examined for while these immunosuppressive drugs are being administered. This includes a culture of the original hepatic biopsy specimen, because it is not uncommon to grow bacteria as a secondary event in cases of hepatic failure due to abnormal hepatic reticuloendothelial cell function. Urinary tract infections are also common in dogs receiving prednisone and azathioprine.

It must be emphasized that there are no long-term controlled studies to support these recommendations in treating dogs with CAH. Such studies are needed and should help clarify the most appropriate treatment. Because Doberman pinschers are at increased risk of developing CAH, I recommend that a serum chemistry profile be performed every 6 to 12 months to screen for CAH in this breed so that treatment can be instituted before the development of clinical signs. Certainly owners who wish to provide the very best care should be given this option early in their pet's life.

Dietary Treatment and Correction of Nutritional Imbalances

Goals of dietary therapy are to minimize hyperammonemia, correct amino acid imbalances, and cor-

rect vitamin and mineral deficiencies. Feeding a controlled diet will also reduce the production and absorption of toxins from the small intestine, potential antigens that can worsen CAH. These therapeutic efforts are similar to those used to manage any case of hepatic disease symptomatically. These are discussed in detail in the section on management of hepatic disease.

In cases where there is excess hepatic copper documented by special copper stains or quantitative hepatic copper measurement, efforts must be made to minimize hepatic copper concentration. Drugs such as penicillamine (Cuprimine) and trientine (Syprine) are useful chelators of hepatic copper (enhancing urinary excretion). Supplementation with vitamin C (ascorbic acid) will also increase copper excretion in the urine. Supplementation with zinc acetate, gluconate, or sulfate will limit intestinal copper absorption and deposition in the liver, as well as remove copper from the liver. These drugs will be discussed in detail in the section on copper-storage diseases.

Resolving Fibrosis

Because fibrosis is a common sequela to CAH and its severity an accurate predictor of early death and shorter survival times in those surviving the initial 1 week postdiagnosis period, its management is an important part of managing cases of CAH. The drug of choice to decrease further fibrotic deposition and to dissolve existing fibrous tissue in the liver is colchicine. There are several studies in humans with alcoholic, posthepatitic, and primary biliary cirrhosis that show colchicine to have beneficial effects clinically, biochemically, histologically, and on survival. Colchicine has been used with success in cases of chronic hepatitis with fibrosis or cirrhosis in dogs. Controlled trials are needed to further substantiate these clinical observations.

The mechanism by which colchicine benefits patients with chronic hepatitis with cirrhosis is unclear, although it has antifibrotic and antiinflammatory effects. Its antifibrotic effects are primarily due to inhibition of microtubule assembly within cells by binding to the protein tubulin (thus interfering with collagen synthesis and secretion) and by stimulating collagenase activity (thus enhancing breakdown of existing collagen). Colchicine also interferes with the transcellular movement of collagen, reduces activity of hepatic collagen-processing enzymes, and inhibits proliferation of fibroblasts. Thus colchicine inhibits collagen production and increases collagenase-mediated removal of fibrous tissue. Colchicine also has many antiinflammatory properties. It has long been used as an antiinflammatory agent to treat gout in human beings. Its antiinflammatory effects include inhibition of leukocyte migration and degranulation and decreasing levels of interleukin-1. Because of these many effects, colchicine may be indicated in many diseases in which inflammation and fibrosis are prominent.

The recommended dosage of colchicine in the dog is 0.014 mg/lb body weight once daily. I generally use this drug in conjunction with prednisone, azathioprine, ursodeoxycholic acid, SAMe, and vitamin E. Side effects in the dog are minimal and are dose dependent. They include primarily diarrhea and rarely vomiting. If these side effects occur, the dose should be decreased by 25%. If there is improvement, the dose can often be increased after a few weeks and is subsequently well tolerated. Side effects in humans are also uncommon and usually reversible. They include nausea, diarrhea, abdominal pain, alopecia, bone marrow depression, myopathy, neuropathy, and epistaxis. Controlled studies are needed to define the role of colchicine in managing CAH in dogs.

D-Penicillamine (Cuprimine) has had limited use as an antifibrotic agent in humans. It interferes with collagen cross-linking and maturation and has additional antiinflammatory effects. It may also be effective in lowering hepatic copper concentrations in Doberman pinschers with CAH. The dosage in the dog is 5 to 7 mg/lb three times a day. Unfortunately, the drug has a high incidence of side effects, especially vomiting and anorexia. These often preclude its use.

Feline Cholangitis/Cholangiohepatitis Complex

The term *cholangiohepatitis* refers to a complex of diseases that includes inflammatory changes of the hepatobiliary system. Cholangiohepatitis is one of the most common hepatobiliary diseases of the cat. The diseases are named by the predominant inflammatory cell involved. The most common form is that of lymphocytic-plasmacytic cholangiohepatitis. Other forms include a predominantly neutrophilic infiltration (suppurative cholangiohepatitis), lymphocytic infiltration, and biliary cirrhosis (diffuse fibrosis of the biliary system, thought to be an end stage of a primary inflammatory disease).

Etiology

Despite this being one of the most common feline hepatobiliary diseases, the etiology remains unknown. Because the predominant inflammatory cells are usually lymphocytes and plasma cells, an immune-mediated etiology is suspected. There are also histologic similarities to primary biliary cirrhosis in humans, believed to have an immune-mediated basis. In humans there are abnormalities in cell-mediated and humoral immunity, circulating immune complexes, and antimitochondrial antibodies. These have not been documented in the cat because of the limitation of laboratory techniques for their detection. Additional evidence for an immune-mediated etiology is the marked improvement seen with glucocorticoid treatment in many cats. Although immune-mediated mechanisms may occur in many cats, there are concurrent diseases identified in some cases. These include pancreatitis, inflammatory bowel disease, bile duct obstruction, systemic infection, toxins, and cholelithiasis. In cases of suppurative cholangiohepatitis, it is suspected that bacterial infection may be an underlying cause. *Escherichia coli* or other bacteria are occasionally grown from cultures of hepatic biopsy samples in cases of either neutrophilic or lymphocytic-plasmacytic cholangiohepatitis, which supports this theory. It is unclear whether bacterial growth is a cause or effect of the hepatic disease. As with any cause of hepatic failure, decreased clearance of portal bacteria (such as *E. coli* ascending from the bowel) secondary to abnormal hepatic reticuloendothelial cell function can occur. When evaluating a suspected case of cholangiohepatitis, the clinician should make efforts to rule out other predisposing causes mentioned above. If no other causes are identified, immune-mediated mechanisms should be suspected.

Clinical Features

Cats may be affected with cholangiohepatitis at any age. The suppurative form is more commonly found in male cats and in younger cats, whereas the nonsuppurative form is more commonly found in older cats. There does not seem to be a breed predisposition, although there was a tendency seen in Persian cats in one report. Clinical signs are typical of those seen with hepatic failure in cats. These include anorexia, vomiting, depression, and weight loss. Most affected cats are icteric. Some affected cats have minimal depression and anorexia and have icterus as the main sign. Many cats are febrile. Clinical signs are often acute in onset, although some cats with the nonsuppurative form can have chronic illness. Despite these trends in presentation, none of these features reliably distinguishes the suppurative from the nonsuppurative form of cholangiohepatitis.

Laboratory findings include a marked increase in SALT activity, moderate increases in serum ALP and GGT activity, and usually hyperbilirubinemia. Concurrent bilirubinuria is also seen. Some cats have a mild nonregenerative anemia consistent with anemia of chronic disease. Ultrasound findings are nonspecific but may identify underlying diseases such as pancreatitis and extrahepatic bile duct obstruction.

Definitive diagnosis depends on histologic examination of hepatic biopsy tissue. Cytologic examination is usually not reliable for establishing the diagnosis. The disease is characterized by diffuse involvement of the liver, so random-location hepatic biopsy is adequate for obtaining representative tissue. There is usually a prominent infiltrate of lymphocytes and plasma cells, lymphocytes alone, or predominantly neutrophils in the portal triads (depending on the form of the disease). Portal triad fibrosis, bile duct proliferation, and centrilobular accumulation of bile with bile casts in canalicular areas is also frequently present. Septa of fibrous tissue with a variable lymphocytic infiltrate often link portal tracts and form circumscribed nodules of hepatocytes. It has been suggested that the disease can progress to biliary cirrhosis characterized by bridging portal fibrosis, bile duct proliferation and hyperplasia, and nodular regeneration with minimal inflammation. Aerobic and anaerobic culture of hepatic tissue with or without bile (obtained via cholecystocentesis) should be obtained. Culture is often positive, although it is not always clear if this is a primary or secondary event. In cats with suppurative cholangiohepatitis, the most common organisms cultured (in descending order of prevalence) are *E. coli, Staphylococcus,* α-hemolytic streptococcus, *Bacillus, Actinomyces, Bacteroides, Enterococcus, Enterobacter,* and *Clostridia*. Prior treatment with antibiotics may result in false-negative cultures.

The liver in cats with cholangiohepatitis may appear large with rounded margins. The surface is often irregular and nodular, although it may also be smooth depending on the degree of nodular regeneration. The color is often a mottled red and brown with the normal lobular pattern being completely lost (reflecting distortion of the normal lobular architecture). There may be accentuated lobular markings giving a reticulated appearance (reflecting the prominent portal infiltrate).

Treatment

If an underlying associated disease is identified, this should be aggressively treated. For example, in cases of bile duct obstruction, surgical correction is usually necessary. This may involve biliary decompression if the obstruction can be relieved or rerouting of the bile duct through a cholecystoenterostomy. Concurrent inflammatory bowel disease or pancreatitis should also be considered.

In cases of lymphocytic-plasmacytic cholangiohepatitis, glucocorticoids are the drug of choice. Prednisolone (preferred over prednisone in cats due to the possibility of improved bioavailability of prednisolone in some cats) is instituted at a dosage of 1 to 2 mg/lb body weight twice a day for at least 1 month and subsequently tapered over 2 to 3 months when there is biochemical and clinical remission. If there is positive growth on culture of hepatic biopsy tissue, an appropriate antibiotic is given concurrently. Metronidazole (Flagyl) may also be a useful adjunct to treatment due to its immune modulatory effects. It is administered at a slightly reduced dosage of 3.5 mg/lb two to three times a day because it undergoes hepatic metabolism.

In cats that are refractory to the above immunosuppressive regimen or with the sclerosing form (biliary cirrhosis), low-dose pulse oral methotrexate in combination with prednisolone, metronidazole, SAMe, and ursodeoxycholic acid is used. A total dose of 0.13 mg methotrexate is given at 12-hour intervals for a total of three doses over a 24-hour period. If this dose is well tolerated at 7-day intervals (based on hematologic and clinical evaluation) and there is no biochemical improvement, the first morning dose is doubled to 0.26 mg. Some cats need the dosage interval extended to every 10 days because of GI side effects.

Treatment of the suppurative form of feline cholangiohepatitis involves use of an appropriate antibiotic based on culture results of hepatic biopsy specimens. If culture results are negative, amoxicillin–clavulanic acid (7 mg/lb body weight three times a day) or a quinolone antibiotic is usually a good choice. Metronidazole is effective against anaerobes and can be combined with the antibiotics mentioned above at a dosage of 3.5 mg/lb body weight two to three times a day. Duration of therapy often ranges from 2 to 6 months. In many cases there is only a transient response to antibiotic administration and subsequent concurrent glucocorticoid administration is often necessary. Clinical judgment is used in this situation to determine when glucocorticoids should be started. Some cases, however, are worsened by glucocorticoid administration, emphasizing the need for hepatic biopsy. Glucocorticoids therefore should only be given for the suppurative form as a last resort when antibiotics have failed.

In virtually all cases without extrahepatic bile duct obstruction, the use of the hydrocholeretic drug ursodeoxycholic acid (ursodiol; Actigall or Urso) may be helpful (see discussion of ursodeoxycholic acid in section on chronic active hepatitis). Ursodeoxycholic acid is a naturally occurring dihydroxylated hydrophilic bile acid found in small quantities in normal human bile and in larger quantities in the bile of certain species of bears. The exact mechanisms of its beneficial effects in inflammatory hepatic diseases remain controversial. It is believed that there is a favorable change in the bile acid pool, rendering retained endogenous bile acids less toxic by changing the bile acid pool from the more toxic hydrophobic bile acids to less toxic hydrophilic bile acids. It is also believed that ursodeoxycholic acid has antiinflammatory and immunomodulatory effects. Ursodeoxycholic acid has been used in the management of chronic hepatic diseases in humans, including CAH, primary biliary cirrhosis, and primary sclerosing cholangitis. Significant improvement in symptoms and laboratory parameters has been reported in many patients undergoing treatment for these diseases.

I have used ursodeoxycholic acid, either alone or in combination with other drugs, in patients with various cholestatic diseases (including dogs with CAH and cats with cholangiohepatitis). The drug is very well tolerated, and in some cases the response can be dramatic. Use of ursodeoxycholic acid in feline cholangiohepatitis complex should be considered as adjunctive (in combination with immunosuppressive or antiinflammatory drugs or antibiotics) with any of the histologic forms of the disease. Ursodeoxycholic acid is also a powerful choleretic agent that can be used to treat sludged bile and cholelithiasis. The recommended dose is 6 to 7 mg/lb/day, administered either once daily or divided twice a day. The newer 250-mg tablet form of the drug (Urso) has made dosing more convenient. The drug has minimal side effects, and in my experience it may dramatically improve therapeutic benefit. Studies need to be performed to substantiate its efficacy and dosage in the dog and cat. The use of SAMe also appears helpful for this disease. See section on CAH for detailed description of this drug.

Specific dietary management is generally not critical to a successful outcome; however, nutritional support may be necessary. It is more important that the affected cat eat any balanced diet than any specific diet. A protein-restricted diet is rarely necessary in cats. In most cases, response to therapy is rapid and tube feeding is not necessary. If there is prolonged anorexia, nutritional support should be provided by using an enteral feeding tube (percutaneous endoscopic gastrostomy [PEG] tube, esophagostomy tube, or nasoesophageal tube). Use of feeding tubes is described in Chapter 12.

Vitamin E therapy is also recommended in many types of hepatic diseases, including feline cholangiohepatitis. Oxidative injury to the liver is now well recognized in several types of inflammatory processes. Free radicals are generated in chronic hepatitis by the injurious effects of certain drugs or toxins or by immunologic injury. These free radicals can damage cellular macromolecules via lipid peroxidation and thus participate in cellular injury and play an important role in initiating and/or perpetuating hepatic injury. Vitamin E reduces oxidant injury to hepatic tissue by providing protection from free radicals. Vitamin E is used at a dosage of 100 to 200 units/day. Because bile acids are required for fat-soluble vitamin E absorption and may be reduced with liver disease, a water-soluble formulation should be used. This type of formulation is available at most health food stores.

The prognosis is fair to good unless the disease is histologically advanced. Many patients respond dramatically to glucocorticoid administration, and most can eventually be weaned off medication. However, some cats will relapse and need ongoing or intermittent treatment. Some cats require prednisolone at a dosage of 0.5 to 0.7 mg/lb/day on a long-term basis (months to years) for successful control of the disease process. Fortunately, the long-term side effects of glucocorticoid administration are minimal in the cat.

Hepatic Necrosis and Toxic Hepatopathies

Hepatic necrosis often leads to acute hepatic failure. Because the hepatocyte is exposed to an extensive portal and systemic venous circulation, it is susceptible to injury by a variety of etiologic agents. Hepatic necrosis can occur secondary to other hepatic processes such as inflammation or neoplasia, can be associated with known hepatotoxins, or can occur when no other cause is known. Causes of hepatic necrosis are listed in Box 9-11.

Clinical Features

Clinical signs of hepatic necrosis depend on the degree of severity. Many patients are asymptomatic, with disease detected only by biochemical screening (such as many cases of hepatic trauma), whereas other cases have acute fulminant hepatic failure. In the latter instance, affected patients range from profoundly depressed to comatose, with the degree of hepatic encephalopathy depending on the cause and severity. Vomiting, anorexia, and fever are often seen. Icterus is often seen when there is periportal involvement. The presence of coagulopathies such as DIC reflect the degree of severity and usually manifest with GI bleeding, hematemesis, ecchymoses, and excessive bleeding at venipuncture sites.

Laboratory findings include profound increases in SALT and SAST activity. Increased SALT activity correlates with histologic findings only in the initial period of hepatocellular injury, after which serum enzyme activity may persist or decline in the following days despite the persistence of extensive necrosis. The activities of serum ALP and GGT and serum bilirubin concentration are variable and reflect the degree of cholestasis. The degree of clinical severity is often poorly correlated with measurements. Other variable abnormalities include hypoglycemia and abnormal clotting parameters. Hepatic function tests such as serum bile acids and plasma ammonia concentration are often normal unless there is massive hepatic necrosis and hyperbilirubinemia. Laboratory abnormalities usually overlap those of other diseases such as CAH and primary hepatic neoplasia.

Histologic findings reflect the degree of hepatic necrosis. The pattern of necrosis is differentiated from that seen in CAH by its location within lobules, by the appearance of neutrophils that enter to phagocytize cellular debris, and by the absence of lymphocytes and plasma cells as the predominant inflammatory cells.

Treatment involves withdrawal of known hepatotoxins or treatment of underlying conditions listed in Box 9-11 that are associated with hepatic necrosis. Efforts must be made to look for these disorders associated with hepatic necrosis. Additional treatment measures are aimed at providing optimum conditions for hepatic regeneration and preventing secondary complications of hepatic disease. These measures are discussed in detail in the section on management of hepatic disease.

Approach to Nonspecific Increases in Hepatic Enzyme Activities

Many patients will be detected as having increased serum activities of hepatic enzymes on routine biochemical screening or when presented with clinical illness. The clinician must try to determine if an underlying nonhepatic cause is present, including endocrinopathies (hyperadrenocorticism, diabetes mellitus, and hyperthyroidism) and those disorders listed in Box 9-11. If no obvious underlying cause exists, the clinician must determine whether clinical signs can be attributed to hepatic disease. If these signs are serious enough to cause illness, further work-up with hepatic function tests (bile acids or blood ammonia concentration), ultrasound examination, and/or hepatic biopsy is warranted. If clinical signs are absent or mild, a baseline hepatic function test (generally serum bile acids assay) is run and is used as a monitoring parameter. Unless hepatic function is significantly abnormal, a repeat chemistry profile and hepatic function test are run in 4 to 8 weeks. If these tests are persistently abnormal, hepatic imaging and biopsy are warranted, even in patients that remain clinically normal.

BOX 9-11	Causes of Hepatic Necrosis

Chemicals
Drugs
Aflatoxins
Septicemia
Pancreatitis
Inflammatory bowel disease
Viral agents
Inflammatory hepatic disease (CAH)
Systemic hypoxia
Anemia
Ischemic injury
Excessive copper storage
Heartworm-associated (postcaval syndrome)
Trauma

CAH, Chronic active hepatitis.

Drug-Induced Hepatic Disease

Many drugs have been reported to cause hepatic disease in patients. The most common ones are listed in Box 9-12. Several types of hepatopathies are associated with drug administration, including hepatocellular necrosis, cholestasis, CAH, vacuolar changes (including steroid hepatopathy), and a combination of these processes. Hepatotoxic drugs can be further classified into those causing predictable hepatic damage (intrinsic toxicoses) and those that are idiosyncratic in their potential to cause hepatic damage. Those drugs causing predictable hepatic damage have a high incidence of hepatotoxicity and are usually dose dependent, and their effects can be reproduced in experimental animals. On the other hand, idiosyncratic reactions are characterized by occurring in a small percentage of patients, are are usually not dose dependent, and are to experimentally reproduce. Idiosyncratic toxicosis is the result of an unusual susceptibility of an affected patient to an adverse reaction resulting from metabolic aberration, hypersensitivity, or immune-mediated events. Specific mechanisms of injury are usually unknown when idiosyncratic toxicosis occurs. In general, treatment of drug-induced hepatic disease involves withdrawal of the drug and supportive care. This discussion will concentrate on the most important drug-induced hepatopathies.

Anticonvulsant Drug–Induced Hepatic Injury

Hepatobiliary disease associated with the administration of many anticonvulsant drugs has been described, including phenytoin, primidone, and phenobarbital (either alone or in combination). These drugs often result in elevations in hepatic enzyme activities, but most patients are asymptomatic and tests of hepatic function, including serum bile acids and plasma ammonia concentrations, are often normal. However, significant hepatobiliary disease occasionally develops in patients given seemingly safe doses or when drug doses are increased to toxic levels to maintain seizure control. Toxic blood levels can also develop in patients receiving appropriate doses when hepatic failure from other causes occurs, because these drugs are metabolized and cleared by the liver. Primidone is more hepatotoxic than phenobarbital.

Clinical signs include those typical of hepatic disease, including depression, anorexia, and weight loss, with subsequent development of jaundice and other features typical of hepatoencephalopathy and end-stage hepatic disease. Terminal events often include excellent seizure control because the anticonvulsant drugs are poorly metabolized and thus achieve high blood levels. By the time clinical signs are noticed, hepatic disease is usually advanced (often with the presence of cirrhosis) and the prognosis is poor. However, it has been estimated that clinical signs develop in only 6% to 15% of dogs receiving anticonvulsant drugs long term.

Laboratory abnormalities include variable increases in SALT, SAST, and serum ALP and GGT activities. These changes are most marked in dogs receiving primidone and/or phenobarbital. Increase in SALT activity is usually reversible upon withdrawal of the drug and does not always correlate with morphologic evidence of hepatocellular necrosis. Increase in serum ALP activity is related to increased hepatic synthesis. Because these enzyme abnormalities occur in many asymptomatic dogs without significant hepatic injury, other tests of hepatic function should be used to determine whether there is impending hepatic failure, including serum bile acids, albumin, and plasma ammonia concentrations. Increased total bilirubin concentration and decreased albumin, BUN, glucose, and cholesterol concentrations, although not specific, are common indicators of

BOX 9-12	Drugs Known to Cause Hepatic Disease

Acetaminophen
Anabolic steroids
Anticonvulsant drugs (phenobarbital, primidone, phenytoin)
Antineoplastic drugs (methotrexate, L-asparaginase, 6-mercaptopurine)
Arsenicals (thiacetarsamide)
Carprofen
Diazepam
Diethylcarbamazine
Furosemide
Glucocorticoids
Griseofulvin
Inhalation anesthetics (halothane, methoxyflurane)
Itraconazole
Ketoconazole
Lomustine (CCNU)
Mebendazole
Mitotane (o,p-DDD)
Sulfonamides
Tetracycline
Trimethoprim-sulfadiazine

hepatic failure. If these tests are abnormal, hepatic biopsy or decreasing the dosage of the anticonvulsant may be warranted.

Two distinct forms of hepatotoxic injury are related to anticonvulsant drug treatment. One form is characterized by the development of clinical signs after extended periods of treatment. Histologic findings include diffuse fibrosis, nodular regeneration, and various amounts of necrosis, lipidosis, and inflammation that eventually lead to macronodular cirrhosis. The second form of hepatotoxic injury is metabolic hepatic failure with intrahepatic cholestasis that is distinct in historical, clinical, and histologic features from those associated with cirrhosis. There is a conspicuous absence of a necroinflammatory response versus other forms of drug toxicity or acquired canine hepatic disease unrelated to drug administration.

The prognosis is poor when histologic lesions are severe and hepatic failure has occurred. Treatment involves withdrawal of anticonvulsant drugs if possible or use of alternative anticonvulsant drugs such as potassium bromide. There are no hepatotoxic effects associated with potassium bromide. There is no indication for the use of glucocorticoids unless there is an active inflammatory component. The use of colchicine might be indicated if fibrosis is a prominent feature (see section on chronic active hepatitis). The use of ursodeoxycholic acid may also be indicated due to the presence of a significant cholestatic component in most cases. The use of SAMe may also be helpful. *It should be emphasized that caution should be used when attributing abnormal hepatic function and hepatic failure to anticonvulsant administration because the incidence of this problem is low. Other laboratory and ancillary tests, including hepatic biopsy specimen analysis, may well be justified in these patients.*

Carprofen Toxicity

Carprofen (Rimadyl) is a commonly used non-steroidal antiinflammatory drug (NSAID) to treat canine osteoarthritis (degenerative joint disease). It is estimated that the incidence of severe hepatotoxic reactions from carprofen is 1.4 dogs per 10,000. In one report 21 dogs were described to have hepatocellular toxicosis associated with administration of carprofen. At the time of the report, over 500,000 dogs had received carprofen. No dog in this report had evidence of a previous significant hepatopathy or medical problems predisposing to a hepatopathy. Various other drugs were given to some dogs, with no apparent relationship to developing hepatic toxicosis. Of the 21 dogs, 13 were Labrador retrievers. Dogs ranged from 4 to 15 years old (mean, 9.4 years). Carprofen was administered for alleviation of signs of musculoskeletal pain in all dogs. The amount of carprofen administered ranged from 0.71 to 1.41 mg/lb of body weight (mean, 1.06 mg/lb) orally every 12 hours. The duration of treatment ranged from 3 to 180 days (mean, 31 days). Clinical signs of toxicosis were noticed for 18 dogs between 5 and 30 days (mean and median, 19 days) after initiation of carprofen. Two dogs received carprofen for 60 and 180 days before developing clinical signs. One dog received the drug for 54 days and did not have clinical signs of toxicosis. The drug was discontinued after discovery of hepatic necrosis on a biopsy specimen obtained for evaluation of possible metastatic cancer in this dog. All Labrador retrievers developed clinical signs at an interval of 14 or more days after initiation of carprofen administration (mean and median, 20 days). One of these dogs received carprofen for only 3 days, but clinical abnormalities developed 18 days after the first dose.

Clinical signs associated with toxicosis were predominantly anorexia (17 dogs) and vomiting (16 dogs). Other signs noticed less frequently were lethargy, diarrhea, polyuria, polydipsia, and hematuria. Physical examination revealed icterus in 15 dogs and ascites in 1 dog. The most common laboratory abnormalities were increases in serum activities of ALT (21 of 21 dogs), AST (14 of 15 dogs), ALP (20 of 21 dogs), and serum bilirubin concentration (18 of 21 dogs). Hypoalbuminemia was seen in only 4 of 21 dogs. In addition, urinalyses were performed in 9 dogs. In 7 dogs evidence of renal disease was present (including isosthenuria with azotemia, glucosuria, proteinuria, and evidence of epithelial cells and granular casts). Hemogram, radiographic and ultrasonographic abnormalities were minimal. Histopathologic evaluation (performed in 18 of 21 dogs) revealed varying degrees of vacuolar change, ballooning degeneration, necrosis of hepatocytes, bridging fibrosis, mixed-cellular inflammation, and accumulation of bile pigment.

Fifteen of the dogs were treated. Of these dogs, 12 were hospitalized. These 12 dogs received intravenous fluids and antibiotics. Drugs used to manage GI signs included histamine H_2-receptor antagonists, metoclopramide, sucralfate, and misoprostol. Three dogs were given ursodeoxycholic acid for 14 to 60 days.

Four dogs died or were euthanized within 3 to 5 days after initial examination. One dog with severe hepatic and renal failure also had perforation of the GI tract and diffuse intestinal ulcers documented during necropsy. It is unknown whether the GI tract ulcers and subsequent perforation were directly attributable to carprofen use or indirectly attributable to hypoperfusion, ischemia, or uremia. The other 17 dogs fully recovered from drug-induced hepatic disease. All 13 Labrador retrievers recovered from the hepatic injury. The mortality rate for the other breeds was 50%. For surviving dogs, vomiting resolved 1 to 5 days after supportive care was instituted and carprofen was discontinued. Inappetence was the primary persistent clinical sign, which resolved 6 to 20 days after carprofen was discontinued. Carprofen administration was discontinued but was repeatedly reinstituted and discontinued during a 1-month period for 1 dog. Clinical signs resolved after discontinuance and reappeared in association with drug administration. Laboratory evaluations were performed on all surviving dogs 3 to 4 weeks after onset of clinical signs. All dogs were markedly improved with regard to hepatic variables. Values determined 3 months after diagnosis of the toxic condition for 8 dogs were within reference ranges or only slightly increased. Fifteen of 17 surviving dogs were healthy 60 days after the episode of toxicosis. The other 2 dogs had unrelated problems.

The results of this study suggest that the drug reaction to carprofen is idiosyncratic and host-dependent in nature. Progression of the condition did not appear to correlate with the dose of carprofen, magnitude of hepatic enzyme activities, or histopathologic severity of hepatic lesions. It is also noteworthy that renal lesions were detected in a number of dogs, a well-documented side effect of other NSAIDs. Although prescreening hematologic and serum biochemical analyses may not yield results that can be used to predict dogs that will have adverse reactions to carprofen, evaluation of renal and hepatic function before administration of the drug is recommended. Dogs with renal and hepatobiliary abnormalities may be poor candidates to receive this drug, or extra caution should be used if carprofen is to be used in these dogs. In addition, serum biochemistry analysis should be obtained approximately 3 to 4 weeks after starting carprofen to detect patients with developing hepatic or renal disease. Owners should be informed of the clinical signs of drug intolerance and instructed to immediately discontinue the drug if these signs develop.

Mebendazole-Induced Hepatic Disease

Mebendazole (Telmintic) is an anthelmintic drug that is useful for its effects against ascarids, hookworms, and whipworms. Though generally considered to be a safe drug, acute hepatic necrosis associated with mebendazole administration to dogs has been reported. In addition to this report, 45 additional cases of adverse drug reactions associated with mebendazole administration have been reported to the U.S. Food and Drug Administration. Based on these reports and extensive safety studies in normal animals and in induced hepatic disease, it is unclear whether mebendazole is an intrinsic (predictable) or idiosyncratic hepatotoxin. The fact that toxicity is of low incidence, difficult to reproduce experimentally, and apparently not dose related suggests that mebendazole is an idiosyncratic toxin, whereas the presence of toxicity in several members of one kennel suggests that mebendazole is an intrinsic hepatotoxin.

Regardless of the mechanism of toxicity, I recommend that mebendazole not be used. Safer and more effective anthelmintics with a similar antiparasitic spectrum such as fenbendazole (Panacur) or febantel (Drontol Plus) are recommended.

Copper-Storage Hepatopathy
Pathophysiology

The abnormal accumulation of copper in hepatocytes as a result of a metabolic defect in copper metabolism has been documented in the Bedlington terrier, West Highland white terrier, Skye terrier, and possibly the Doberman pinscher breed. These disorders are similar (but not identical) to Wilson's disease in humans. Once excessive copper accumulates in hepatocytes, it results in progressive hepatocyte destruction. The disease in these breeds must be distinguished from other causes of secondary hepatic copper accumulation. Copper is normally excreted through the biliary tract. Therefore copper can accumulate in the liver with any cholestatic disorder, including CAH or cirrhosis. In dogs with a primary copper-storage disease, copper accumulates in the liver before the development of hepatic damage or cholestasis.

Once copper is ingested, 40% to 60% is passively absorbed in the proximal small intestine, with the remainder lost in the feces. Some ingested copper is bound to the copper transport protein, metallothionein. This portion is lost in the feces. Unbound copper is absorbed from the intestine and enters the portal circulation, where it is bound to albumin and another copper transport protein, transcuprein. Copper is then transported to the liver. Within hepatocytes, copper is bound to cytosolic metallothionein and stored in lysosomes. Copper can then undergo two fates: it can be excreted in bile or bound to the copper transport protein ceruloplasmin for transport to peripheral tissues. Of these steps, the most important step that regulates copper homeostasis is biliary excretion. In dogs with abnormal copper storage, copper accumulates within the lysosomes of hepatocytes. While in the lysosomes, copper is innocuous. Once the lysosomal storage capacity is exhausted, copper breaks into the cytoplasm, where it is toxic to the hepatocytes. Excessive hepatic copper can alter hepatic membrane permeability and interfere with normal hepatocyte transport of proteins and triglycerides, and eventually these hepatocytes undergo cellular lysis and necrosis. This can result in massive release of copper from damaged hepatocytes, which when taken up in the circulation can lead to a hemolytic crisis.

In Bedlington terriers the disease is an autosomal recessive disorder. The specific defect in copper metabolism is thought to be excessive copper binding by an abnormal metallothionein in the liver, which sequesters copper in the liver (lysosomes) and reduces biliary excretion. The excess copper accumulation can be detected as early as 6 months of age and progresses with time. It is unclear whether a subset of Doberman pinschers with CAH have a primary copper-storage disease or whether the abnormal hepatic copper concentration is secondary to the cholestasis associated with the active hepatitis. One report, however, documented increased hepatic copper concentrations in two Doberman pinschers with subacute hepatitis in which cholestasis was not present histologically, leading to the speculation that a genetic defect in copper metabolism might be the primary cause of hepatic inflammatory disease in some Doberman pinschers. The disease in West Highland white terriers differs from the copper-storage disease in Bedlington terriers by comparatively lower concentrations of hepatic copper. West Highland white terriers can generally tolerate up to 2000 µg/g (ppm) of copper. West Highland white terriers rarely accumulate excess copper throughout their lifetime. By 6 months of age a West Highland white terrier has reached its upper limit of excess copper, and some dogs with excess hepatic copper will return to normal by 1 year of age. In the Skye terrier excessive copper accumulation in the liver appears to be related to cholestasis, thought to result from a disorder of intracellular bile metabolism and abnormal bile secretion.

Although Wilson's disease in humans is similar to the disease in affected Bedlington terriers, there are several important differences. Wilson's disease often leads to copper accumulation and subsequent damage in other tissues, including the brain. These manifestations are not seen in the dog. In addition, the concentration of ceruloplasmin in humans with Wilson's disease is low, whereas the concentration of unbound copper is variable but may be high. In affected Bedlington terriers, serum copper and ceruloplasmin concentrations are normal.

Clinical Features

The disease is an autosomal recessive inherited defect. In studies in which large numbers of Bedlington terriers have been screened by liver biopsy for abnormal copper storage, approximately 50% to 80% of dogs have been affected. Recent genetic studies by VetGen, LLC, suggest that only 30% of Bedlington terriers tested are homozygous clear of the disease, 39% are homozygous affected, and the remainder (31%) are heterozygous carriers.

The copper-storage disease of Bedlington terriers can be categorized into three general groups. In the first group, affected dogs are usually young adults. They have a short, fulminant course of acute hepatic necrosis and failure with a high mortality rate. These dogs are usually icteric, anorectic, and vomiting, and they may undergo a hemolytic crisis because of copper toxicity from rapid lysis of hepatocytes. Most dogs die despite supportive measures. Sometimes a stressful event such as whelping or showing precipitates the onset of signs.

In the second group, affected dogs are usually middle-age or older. There is usually an insidious deterioration of their general condition, characterized by chronic weight loss, anorexia, intermittent vomiting, and a general unthriftiness. On presentation many dogs have hallmarks of chronic end-stage hepatic disease, including icterus and ascites.

In the third group, affected dogs are asymptomatic and the disease is detected by biochemical screening (usually with increased SALT activity) and documented by hepatic biopsy specimen analysis. It is thought that dogs in this group represent a prestage of the first two groups. In affected dogs of all groups, hepatic copper concentration can be elevated as early as a few months of age. Progressive increases in copper concentration usually occur until 5 to 6 years of age (if the patient survives), at which time levels slowly decline, although they never completely return to normal.

The most consistent laboratory abnormality is increased SALT activity, usually occurring once hepatic injury has taken place. The SALT activity usually correlates with the severity of the disease histologically, although enzyme depletion may occur with terminal cirrhosis. Serum ALP activity and serum bilirubin concentration are variable, reflecting the degree of cholestasis. A presumptive diagnosis should be considered in any Bedlington terrier with increased SALT activity, although the disease needs to be confirmed with hepatic biopsy specimen analysis. It must be pointed out that a normal SALT level does not rule out the disease, and Bedlington terriers get other forms of hepatic disease.

The diagnosis is confirmed with quantitative measurements of hepatic copper from hepatic biopsy specimens. Normal hepatic copper concentrations range from 91 to 377 $\mu g/g$ (ppm) of liver on a dry weight basis, although there is marked variability among dogs of various breeds. Formalin-fixed hepatic tissue is suitable for quantitative measurement. Dogs having values above this range are considered affected, and most affected dogs have hepatic concentrations from 5 to 50 times above normal. The disease can also be documented by histochemical staining for copper with rubeanic acid, Timm's, rhodanine, or orcein stains (most pathologists use rubeanic acid). In affected livers, granules of copper can be seen with these stains and are qualitatively estimated. The measurement of copper-64 excreted in stool following intravenous injection has also been advocated as a noninvasive method of detecting affected dogs. Histologic findings vary from normal (with the exception of excess copper accumulation) to varying severities of chronic hepatitis. The disease progresses from focal hepatitis and necrosis to features identical to those described for CAH. Eventually the disease progresses to micronodular and macronodular cirrhosis. The gross appearance of the liver reflects the histologic severity, ranging from normal to a fine or coarse

nodular surface, with regenerative nodules reflecting end-stage liver disease.

Recently VetGen, LLC, began offering a genetic test for copper toxicosis of the Bedlington terrier breed. This test uses a linked marker that has two alleles, or marker types, called 1 and 2. It was found that over 90% of dogs that were 1/1 marker type were homozygous normal (clear of the disease) and over 90% of dogs that were affected with the disease were 2/2 marker type. Most 1/2 dogs are carriers with the 2 allele usually associated with the copper toxicosis disease allele. The finding of such a strong genetic disequilibrium allows this to be potentially a valuable test. In interpreting the results, if the dog is a 1/1, it is more than 90% likely that it is homozygous normal (clear of disease). If the dog is a 2/2, it is 72% likely that it is affected (over 90% of affected dogs are 2/2, but 72% of 2/2 are affected; 24% are carriers). If the dog is a 1/2, VetGen data indicate the dog has a 95% chance of being a carrier. This test may be helpful in making recommendations to breeders. If only 1/1 and 1/2 dogs are chosen for breeding, the 2 gene could be eliminated in subsequent generations. *However, breeders should still allow liver biopsy specimens to be obtained in 1/1 dogs to be used for breeding for the near to intermediate future because it is currently the only way to detect the small number of affected dogs associated with the 1 allele.* VetGen provides a collection kit for DNA using a soft cheek brush. This test can be completed before puppies are purchased at an early age.[*]

Treatment

Early detection is essential. Therefore, because of the high incidence in the breed, it is strongly recommended that Bedlington terriers undergo biochemical screening two to three times per year. Ideally a liver biopsy should be performed at 1 year of age. Once a positive diagnosis is established, treatment depends on the stage of the disease. In affected dogs, specific therapy involves the administration of drugs that chelate copper and increase urinary excretion, as well as efforts to decrease copper absorption. Traditionally, the drug of choice has been D-Penicillamine (Cuprimine). The recommended dosage for dogs is 4.5 to 7 mg/lb two times a day. The drug should ideally be given before meals to maximize its effect. In this manner, penicillamine will remove approximately 1000 $\mu g/g$ (ppm) of copper per year. When

---

[*]VetGen can be contacted at (800) 483-8436 (3728 Plaza Dr, Suite 1, Ann Arbor, MI 48108).

given with meals the efficacy decreases by approximately half. Common side effects include anorexia and vomiting. Further dividing the dosage into three to four daily doses and/or administering it with food often minimizes these signs. Unfortunately, these side effects may be intolerable in some dogs and necessitate discontinuation of the drug. It usually takes several years for hepatic copper concentrations to decrease to normal, and therapy must be continued for life. In addition to chelating copper, D-Penicillamine has antifibrotic properties, stabilizes lysosomes, and has immune-modulating effects that might also be of benefit in managing this disease.

More recently tetramine cupruretic agents (2,2,2-tetramine; 2,3,2-tetramine) have been evaluated and have been shown to be effective decoppering agents, lowering hepatic copper and increasing urinary excretion. These drugs are also better tolerated than D-Penicillamine. Trientine (Syprine; 2,2,2-tetramine) is my drug of choice. It has cupruretic effects similar to those of D-Penicillamine (i.e., removing approximately 1000 µg/g [ppm] of copper per year), although it may attack a different copper pool. The recommended dose is 7 to 14 mg/lb two times a day. Side effects are minimal in dogs compared with those caused by D-Penicillamine. Trientine is often used first or in patients that experience side effects with D-Penicillamine. Trientine is not always readily available, but many pharmacists will order it or it can be ordered directly from the manufacturer (Merck). 2,3,2-Tetramine is an experimental drug that has been shown to be a potent copper chelator. It is not yet commercially available.

Additional measures to reduce hepatic copper concentrations include supplementing the diet with zinc (0.7 to 1.15 mg/lb zinc gluconate three times a day, 0.3 mg/lb zinc sulfate three times a day, or 100 mg elemental zinc as zinc acetate two times a day). Zinc induces increased concentration of intestinal metallothionein, which then binds ingested copper to intestinal epithelial cells, thus preventing copper absorption. As these cells are sloughed, copper is subsequently lost in the feces. In addition, zinc will enhance removal of copper from hepatocytes. Zinc lowers hepatic copper indirectly by affecting multiple areas of copper equilibria and by displacing copper in target tissues. Zinc also induces hepatic metallothionein, which will then bind to and sequester excessive copper into an innocuous form compared with free copper. The rate of removal of hepatic copper

is relatively slow. For this reason dogs with severe or fulminant hepatitis secondary to copper accumulation are not candidates for zinc therapy alone. For these patients zinc is commonly combined with a chelating agent such as trientine. One study demonstrated marked improvement in hepatitis and hepatic copper concentrations in three Bedlington terriers and three West Highland white terriers treated with zinc acetate as the sole decoppering agent. The advantages of zinc for treatment include efficacy, low cost, and minimal side effects. With any of the above types of zinc supplements, it is important to measure serum zinc levels. The goal is to achieve plasma zinc concentrations of 200 to 600 µg/dl. After a 3- to 6-month loading period, the dose is decreased to approximately half of the original dose. Serum zinc levels are then measured every 4 to 6 months. If the serum concentration drops below 150 µg/dl, the dose is increased to the original dose. To be effective, zinc must be given separately from food by at least 1 hour because some food constituents such as phytates can bind zinc and diminish its efficacy. If zinc causes vomiting, it may be mixed in a tablespoon of tuna fish (in oil) to minimize nausea.

Vitamin C also might be useful because it decreases copper absorption and increases copper excretion in the urine. In addition, dogs with hepatic insufficiency are deficient in ascorbic acid. Ideally vitamin C should be given with meals. The recommended dosage is 12 mg/lb/day. Dogs should also be fed a diet low in copper concentration. Some commercial diets low in copper include Hill's Prescription Diet l/d, Purina Fit & Trim, Purina HiPro, Wayne, ANF, Pedigree, Nutro Natural Choice, and Precise. Diets high in copper include Iams Eukanuba, Science Diet, and Blue Seal Natural. Homemade diets that do not contain excess copper should include meats, poultry, fish, and dairy products. Foods with excessive copper should be excluded from the diet. These include eggs, liver, shellfish, organ meats, beans/legumes, mushrooms, chocolate, nuts, and cereals. Mineral supplements containing copper should also be avoided. Other treatment measures are supportive and symptomatic. These are discussed in detail in the section on management of hepatic disease.

Infectious Inflammatory Diseases

Primary infections involving the liver are rare causes of hepatitis in dogs and cats. It is not uncommon, however, to culture bacteria as a secondary event in noninfectious hepatic diseases due to decreased hepatic reticuloendothelial cell function. In addition to bacterial pathogens, parasitic and fungal infections can involve the liver.

Bacterial Hepatobiliary Infections

Because the liver plays a central role in processing portal products, receives an extensive arterial blood supply, has an important reticuloendothelial cell function, and has a direct connection to the intestine via the biliary tract, it is subject to infection by several routes, including hematogenous (portal or arterial) and ascending via the biliary system. However, bacterial infection of the liver only occurs under unusual circumstances, including patients receiving immunosuppressive drugs, and patients with hyperadrenocorticism, diabetes mellitus, severe enteritis, biliary stasis, septicemia, decreased hepatic blood supply, and devitalization or necrosis of hepatic tissue. When the source of infection originates from the bowel, treatment is aimed at bacteria normally found in the gut. In one study in cats with suppurative cholangiohepatitis, bacteria cultured from hepatic biopsy specimens (in descending order of prevalence) were *E. coli, Staphylococcus,* α–hemolytic streptococcus, *Bacillus, Actinomyces, Bacteroides, Enterococcus, Enterobacter,* and *Clostridia.* In another study of 14 dogs with hepatic abscesses, *E. coli, Clostridium* sp., *Klebsiella pneumoniae, Enterococcus* sp., *Staphylococcus epidermidis,* and *Staphylococcus intermidius* were the most common bacteria isolated. Many patients have polymicrobial infections.

Clinical Findings

Bacterial cholangiohepatitis or hepatic abscesses usually cause persistent fever and anorexia. Hepatomegaly is variable, as is abdominal pain or other signs of peritonitis. There may be other signs of systemic infection, including lymphadenopathy, or signs of infection of other organs such as pneumonia, endocarditis, urinary tract involvement, or enteritis. Other risk factors include biliary obstruction, inflammatory bowel disease, and pancreatitis.

Laboratory findings usually include increased activities of SALT and SAST. If there is involvement of the biliary system, there will be increased activities of serum ALP and GGT and possibly increased bilirubin concentration. There may be a neutrophilic leukocytosis and hyperglobulinemia (especially with chronic infection). Coagulopathies may be present.

Radiographic findings are usually normal; however, radiolucent areas within the liver or biliary system and/or gallbladder may be seen

secondary to gas-forming bacteria. Radiopaque choleliths may also be seen. Ultrasound imaging may detect discrete abscesses if present, seen as multiple hypoechoic, hyperechoic, heterogenous, or anechoic areas within the liver. In cases of cholecystitis, ultrasonographic findings include a thickened gallbladder wall with sludge within the lumen.

A definitive diagnosis is made by hepatic biopsy. If discrete abscesses are suspected from radiographic or ultrasonographic findings, blind percutaneous biopsy methods are contraindicated. Aerobic and anaerobic cultures of the liver should be obtained whenever hepatic biopsy is performed. False-negative cultures can be obtained with prior antibiotic treatment.

Treatment involves an appropriate antibiotic based on hepatic biopsy specimen culture. If culture results are negative despite gross and histopathologic findings suggestive of bacterial infection, the antibiotic choice depends on the suspected route of infection. If the GI tract is the origin, antibiotic use should include coverage against anaerobes and gram-negative organisms. Good combinations include a fluoroquinolone and ampicillin or metronidazole. Fluoroquinolones have excellent gram-negative activity and are effective orally administered drugs for treatment of hepatobiliary bacterial infections. Ampicillin and metronidazole are indicated for anaerobic infections. Single-agent amoxicillin–clavulanic acid (Clavamox) is also a good choice due to this agent's broad spectrum of activity. Clindamycin is also very active against anaerobes and enters the liver in high concentrations. However, it should not be used with bile duct obstruction or severe impairment of hepatic function. Antibiotics must be administered for several months. If discrete abscesses are present, ultrasound imaging can guide an end point for therapy. Antibiotics are given for at least 1 month following resolution of ultrasound lesions.

If discrete abscesses are present, surgical intervention for drainage or resection may be necessary. Likewise, if severe cholecystitis is present, cholecystectomy may be indicated. Concurrent medical treatment with appropriate antibiotics is also indicated. In one study of 14 cases there was a high survival rate in those dogs that underwent surgical treatment for hepatic abscesses.

Cholestasis has also been associated with extrahepatic bacterial infections in dogs and cats. Typical findings include hyperbilirubinemia with variable increases in serum hepatic enzyme activities. Histologically there is bile pigment accumulation in hepatocytes with variable inflammatory changes.

Parasitic Hepatobiliary Infections

Parasitic infections of the liver and biliary tract are rare but are more common in certain geographic areas such as the southeastern United States. Cats are most frequently infected with trematode parasites because of their propensity to ingest intermediate hosts (land snails, fish, reptiles, and amphibians). Parasites reported to infect the liver and biliary system include *Platynosomum, Heterobilharzia, Cytauxzoon, Opisthorchis, Amphimerus, Metorchis,* and *Clonorchis.*

Clinical signs of fluke infestation are usually associated with extrahepatic biliary obstruction. Many cats with fluke infestation are asymptomatic; thus the detection of the presence of flukes may not mean that they are the causative agent for the observed signs. The diagnosis is established by detecting eggs in the feces or by histologic examination of hepatic biopsy tissue. The drug of choice for treatment of flukes is praziquantel (Droncit) at a dosage of 2.3 mg/lb body weight two times a day for 3 days. Nitroscanate (Lopatol) at a single dose of 45 mg/lb may also be effective. Some cats require corticosteroids for treatment of concurrent eosinophilic cholangiohepatitis.

Fungal Infections of the Liver

Systemic mycoses, including histoplasmosis, blastomycosis, and coccidioidomycosis, can affect the liver. Hepatic involvement usually reflects systemic involvement and is one of many tissues affected. The significance of hepatic involvement is that it often represents an easy means of detection of the offending organism. Hepatic enzyme elevations suggest hepatic involvement and may justify hepatic biopsy. This is often the least invasive means of establishing a definitive diagnosis. Histopathologic examination reveals a granulomatous hepatitis with the offending organism usually seen with special stains. Fungal culture of hepatic tissue is usually not necessary but may be helpful.

Noninflammatory Diseases of the Liver

Important noninflammatory diseases of the liver include vascular anomalies (portosystemic shunts, portal vein hypoplasia), metabolic derangements (feline hepatic lipidosis, steroid hepatopathy,

glycogen-storage diseases), hepatic amyloidosis, urea cycle enzyme deficiencies, abnormal iron storage, and hepatic neoplasia. This discussion will review the more common of these disease entities.

Portosystemic Shunts

Portosystemic shunts (portal vascular anomalies, portacaval shunts, portosystemic vascular anastomoses) can occur as a congenital anomaly or as an acquired entity secondary to chronic portal hypertension. In the latter circumstance, elevated portal blood pressure leads to opening of fetal blood vessels that shunted portal blood away from the liver into the systemic circulation. These vessels normally close at birth. They act as a reservoir to handle the increased pressure load. Unlike congenital portosystemic shunts, these shunts are usually multiple, extremely tortuous, and variable in their extrahepatic location. The most common cause for acquired portosystemic shunting is cirrhosis. The remainder of this discussion will concern congenital portosystemic shunts.

Etiology of Congenital Portosystemic Shunts

Normally blood leaving the stomach, intestines, spleen, and pancreas enters the portal vein and flows through the liver before entering the hepatic vein and the systemic venous circulation. Portal blood thus contains absorbed nutrients, intestinal hormones (which are tropic to the liver), and bacterial products and toxins. In the fetus the function of the liver for processing these products is minimal, and thus there are vessels to shunt blood away from the liver into the systemic venous circulation. Normally these vessels close shortly after birth, allowing the establishment of hepatic circulation. When any of these vessels remain patent after birth, portosystemic shunting occurs. The cause of these anomalies is unknown. When blood is diverted away from the liver, hepatic atrophy results because of the lack of tropic factors present in portal blood (especially insulin and glucagon).

There are several types of congenital portosystemic shunts seen in dogs and cats. These include (but are not limited to) the following:

1. Patent ductus venosus with or without a hypoplastic portal system
2. Major solitary portal–caudal vena caval anastomosis
3. Portal vein atresia, associated with the development of multiple portal–caudal vena caval anastomoses

4. Major solitary portal-azygous shunt
5. Portal-azygous shunt with discontinuation of the prerenal segment of the caudal vena cava
6. Left gastric vein to caudal vena cava
7. The development of intrahepatic arterioportal fistula.

Approximately one fourth of congenital portosystemic shunts are intrahepatic in both dogs and cats, with most associated with a patent ductus venosus. Single extrahepatic shunts, with a major solitary portal–caudal vena caval shunt being the most common, constitute 50% of portosystemic shunts. Most intrahepatic shunts are found in large-breed dogs (Doberman pinscher, golden retriever, Labrador retriever, Irish setter, Samoyed, and Irish wolfhound), whereas most extrahepatic shunts are seen in small-breed dogs (miniature schnauzer, Yorkshire terrier, miniature poodle, and dachshund). Dogs with intrahepatic shunts may develop clinical signs at an earlier age than dogs with extrahepatic shunts, possibly due to a larger volume of blood flow through intrahepatic shunts. Approximately 2% of portosystemic shunts seen in small animals occur in cats.

The severity of clinical signs depends on the volume and location of the shunt. Clinical signs result from impairment of hepatic function, leading to hepatic encephalopathy. The most important factors that lead to encephalopathy are the accumulation of blood ammonia and other gut-associated encephalopathic toxins that are normally metabolized and cleared by the liver. With portosystemic shunting, ammonia and other toxins increase in the blood, leading to encephalopathy. In addition, increased benzodiazepine-like substances and amino acid derangements (increased aromatic amino acids) occur with portosystemic shunts, contributing to encephalopathic signs.

Clinical Signs

Most cases are diagnosed in patients less than 1 year of age; however, there have been cases in patients as old as 10 years at the time of diagnosis. There is no sex predilection. Clinical signs in patients with portosystemic shunts are highly variable. Because of the diverse nature of signs, the clinician must maintain a high index of suspicion in any young patient with unexplained signs compatible with a shunt to avoid missing the diagnosis. Clinical signs often change throughout the day or week. There may be an exacerbation of signs after feeding, reflecting ammonia generation from

dietary substrates; however, this finding seldom occurs in most cases.

The most common clinical signs are chronic depression, retarded growth, and weight loss. Most dogs are stunted in appearance and "poor doers." Additional clinical signs include chronic GI signs (vomiting, diarrhea), anorexia, polydipsia/polyuria, and neurologic signs. It is often the neurologic signs that are most suggestive of a shunt, and approximately 90% of cases have some degree of neurologic dysfunction related to hepatic encephalopathy. Neurologic signs are often variable and wax and wane over time, including depression, incoordination, behavioral changes (often aggressive), amaurotic blindness, seizures, dementia, and stupor. An additional abnormality is intolerance of anesthetic agents (often seen during routine neutering in the first year of life). Any young patient that has persistence of any of these signs (especially neurologic or behavior changes) should be suspected of having a portosystemic shunt. *In the cat, ptyalism is a common sign, as are central nervous system (CNS) and GI signs. Any young cat with ptyalism and/or CNS signs should be evaluated for the presence of a portosystemic shunt.*

Laboratory Findings

Routine hemograms and serum chemistry profiles may be normal. Often there will be a mild nonregenerative microcytic anemia, and target cells may be seen. Most patients have conspicuously normal (or mildly increased) serum hepatic enzyme activities despite hepatic failure. This is because the principal lesion is one of atrophy and lack of portal blood supply. Cholestasis and hepatocellular necrosis and leakage are not features of this disease. Approximately 50% of patients will have mild hypoalbuminemia (reflecting decreased albumin synthesis or increased volume of albumin distribution if ascites is present), and many patients (70%) have decreased BUN concentrations (reflecting decreased synthesis from ammonia). Virtually all patients have normal serum bilirubin concentrations. A fasting hypoglycemia may be seen.

Because many of these changes are nonspecific, hepatic function tests must be performed to document hepatic failure. Serum bile acid measurements and the ammonia tolerance test are the most sensitive tests to detect the presence of a portosystemic shunt, being abnormal virtually 100% of the time.

Approximately one third to half of dogs with portosystemic shunts have ammonium biurate crystals in the urine. These form because of the increased concentration of uric acid in the urine as a result of decreased hepatic conversion to allantoin and increased urine concentration of ammonia associated with hyperammonemia. When the urine is acidic and supersaturated with these substrates, crystallization and precipitation can occur. In addition to crystals in the urine, calculi can form in the kidney or less commonly in the bladder. These stones usually are composed of ammonium acid urate or uric acid. Often the presence of renal calculi is an important clue that a portosystemic shunt is present in a young patient. If calculi are removed and crystallographic analysis identifies that uric acid stones are present, the patient should be evaluated for the presence of a portosystemic shunt.

Radiographic Findings

The most reliable methods of confirming the presence of a portosystemic shunt are contrast radiography and nuclear scintigraphy. Plain radiographic findings are usually indicative of microhepatica, best determined by upright angulation of the stomach on a lateral projection. Because puppies and kittens normally have large livers relative to their body size, this finding should increase the index of suspicion of a portosystemic shunt. The diagnosis can then be confirmed by evaluating hepatic blood flow with contrast radiography or nuclear scintigraphy.

There are several techniques to evaluate hepatic blood flow, including intraoperative mesenteric portography, percutaneous splenoportography, and cranial mesenteric arterial portography. Intraoperative mesenteric portography is the most practical technique to be applied in general practice. In addition to identifying the shunt, mesenteric portography can also assess the residual portovenous flow into the liver for prognostic importance. Following an injection into a mesenteric or jejunal vein, radiographic contrast medium normally flows into the portal vein and arborizes into the liver. In patients with a portosystemic shunt, contrast medium will bypass the liver and be seen in the caudal vena cava or azygous vein. If the caudal extent of the shunt is cranial to T13, it is probably an intrahepatic shunt, whereas if the caudal extent of the shunt is caudal to T13, it is probably an extrahepatic shunt. Once a shunt is identified on the angiographic study, one can proceed with surgical correction during the same surgical procedure. Alternatively, the patient can be allowed to recover from the anesthetic procedure used to obtain the angiogram and a second procedure is then performed later (2 to 4 weeks or longer) to correct the shunt. I prefer the latter approach in small patients that are under anesthesia for a long time for the angiogram because of the potential for hypothermia and prolonged anesthetic recovery.

Portosystemic shunts can also be identified with ultrasonographic guidance or nuclear scintigraphy (see section on nuclear scintigraphy to evaluate the liver). If the latter diagnostic method is used, mesenteric portography may still be necessary to locate the shunt if it is not readily seen during exploratory laparotomy.

Pathologic Findings

Histopathologic findings in patients with portosystemic shunts include diffuse hepatic atrophy, lobular collapse, and proliferation of small hepatic arterioles. Atrophy is characterized by close proximity of the portal triads, compressed hepatic cords, and inconspicuous portal veins. These findings are usually diagnostic of a congenital vascular anomaly, and hepatic biopsy specimen analysis represents another method (in addition to radiographic findings) to obtain a diagnosis. However, these changes may be difficult to distinguish from portal vein hypoplasia without a macroscopic shunt (formerly known as hepatic microvascular dysplasia; see section starting on p. 334). The latter disorder has clinical and histopathologic features of a portosystemic shunt but has normal findings on mesenteric portography and/or nuclear scintigraphy. Degenerative changes in the brain suggestive of hepatic encephalopathy include leukopolymicrocavitation at the gray-white matter junction, spongiform degeneration, and cortical necrosis.

Surgical Treatment

The treatment of choice for single portosystemic shunts is surgical ligation, because long-term medical management is palliative rather than curative. Before surgical intervention, medical management may be necessary to stabilize the patient. Emergency treatment of hepatic encephalopathy includes cleansing enemas, oral antibiotics or lactulose administration (see section on management of acute hepatic failure). Surgical correction of multiple portosystemic shunts is usually not successful because underlying portal hypertension and hepatic pathologic abnormalities persist. (See the References or surgical textbooks for detailed descriptions of surgical techniques.)

As a general rule small-breed dogs have extrahepatic shunts and large-breed dogs have intrahepatic shunts. Single extrahepatic shunts are usually

readily identified at surgery and can thus be isolated and attenuated or occluded (depending on portal pressure). Surgical manipulation of intrahepatic shunts is much more difficult, whereas extrahepatic shunt ligation is more adaptable to general practice. Most extrahepatic shunts are found terminating in the caudal vena cava between the left phrenicoabdominal and renal veins.

Once the shunt vessel is isolated, correction can be made by gradual occlusion using an ameroid constrictor (see below) or by occlusion with cellophane banding on suture material. If suture is used, portal pressures must be measured to determine whether complete occlusion is possible. This is readily done by placing a 3½ or 5 Fr feeding tube into a mesenteric vein and threading it into the portal vein. This is then connected to a saline manometer to measure pressure, with the zero level standardized at the level of the femoral triangle or heart. Normal portal pressure is 10 to 15 cm H_2O (8 to 12 mm Hg), and most patients have normal or decreased portal pressure before shunt manipulation. If a shunt is completely ligated, fatal acute portal hypertension can develop. This results from splanchnic congestion and stasis of blood, with the rapid development of endotoxic shock. During shunt attenuation with a silk suture, portal pressure should not exceed 20 to 23 cm H_2O (18 to 21 mm Hg) or 11 cm H_2O (8 mm Hg) above baseline. The silk ligature is placed as close to the vena cava as possible and gradually tightened while measuring portal pressure. Observing splanchnic viscera for signs of stasis, including blanching of the bowel, hypermotility of the small bowel, and distended and pulsating jejunal arteries is also important. Monitoring central venous pressure may also be helpful to predict the presence of portal hypertension. With increased portal resistance and decreased portal venous flow, central venous pressure drops because of decreased venous return and splanchnic venous pooling.

To avoid the need to measure portal venous pressure and still allow complete occlusion of the shunt, attenuation can be accomplished with an ameroid constrictor.* This is a device that is shaped like a miniature donut that has a small opening allowing it to be placed around the shunt. It can be subsequently locked to prevent its removal after placement around the shunt vessel.

The constrictors come in various inner diameters (3.5, 5.0, or 6.0 mm) so that they can be used on various-sized shunt vessels. The constrictor is made of hygroscopic casein material that is porous, surrounded by a metal outer ring. As the porous material is gradually saturated with peritoneal fluid, it expands. Because the outer metal ring prevents outward expansion, there is inward expansion, gradually occluding the central hole, which has the shunt vessel in it. In this manner the shunt is gradually occluded, usually over a period of 4 to 8 weeks. Because there is gradual occlusion, there is no need to measure portal pressures. As the shunt is occluded the hepatic vasculature becomes more perfused, thus acting to prevent portal hypertension. In general there is complete occlusion of single extrahepatic shunts using the ameroid constrictor in approximately 80% to 90% of cases.

Manipulation of intrahepatic shunts is technically more difficult. Several techniques have been described for attenuation of intrahepatic shunts. See the References and surgical literature for details. If possible, the shunt can be isolated before its entry into the liver or as it leaves the liver before entering the caudal vena cava. Otherwise the shunt is looked for by incising the prehepatic vena cava after occluding hepatic and vena caval blood flow and located by noting the abnormal irregular margins of the shunt vessel as it enters the vena cava from the inside. Alternatively, the shunt can be located by a transportal approach following vascular occlusion. If the shunt cannot be occluded completely without causing portal hypertension, a novel approach has been described that involves complete intrahepatic shunt closure along with the surgical creation of a portacaval shunt using an external jugular vein graft. An ameroid constrictor is placed around the graft to permit its gradual closure.

Dogs that have mild to moderate portal hypertension (20 to 23 cm H_2O) following shunt manipulation usually have normal portal pressure within several weeks of surgery. These dogs often have ascites secondary to the transient portal hypertension, which disappears in 1 to 3 weeks as portal pressure drops. Often the silk ligature used to partially occlude a shunt will cause a reaction that results in gradual complete occlusion of the shunt over time.

A biopsy of the liver is always performed for histopathologic evaluation and occasionally for bacterial culture. If there are cystic or renal calculi

---

*Research Instruments and Mfg, Corvallis, Ore.

concurrent with the portosystemic shunt, they can be removed during the procedure for shunt correction if the patient is stable and the anesthetic time is not excessive. Otherwise a second surgery is performed several weeks later to remove the urinary calculi. A follow-up mesenteric portogram and hepatic biopsy can be performed at this time to evaluate the shunt correction.

Postoperative monitoring is important to detect signs of severe portal hypertension, including abdominal pain, hemorrhagic diarrhea, and endotoxic shock leading to death. Fortunately, the use of an ameroid constrictor or intraoperative monitoring of portal pressure makes this an unusual complication. Hypoglycemia may occur if the patient is not eating, necessitating intravenous glucose supplementation. Intravenous crystalloids or colloids (if there is significant hypoalbuminemia) are essential in the immediate postoperative period. Status epilepticus and generalized motor seizures can occur following shunt attenuation. These are usually first observed 3 days postoperatively. The etiology of the seizures is unknown, but one theory is that there may be stimulation of brain receptors for benzodiazepines associated with the presence of the shunt. Following ligation of the shunt, seizures may result from withdrawal of benzodiazepine-like substances (documented to be present in portal blood of dogs with portosystemic shunts) following shunt ligation. The prognosis is poor in my experience despite control of status epilepticus. The role of prophylactic anticonvulsant drugs such as potassium bromide needs to be defined.

Medical management of chronic hepatic disease should continue as needed to manage signs of encephalopathy; however, most patients are asymptomatic shortly after surgical shunt correction. Patients should be evaluated 1, 3, and 6 months after surgery with serum biochemical and hepatic function tests (e.g., bile acids assay). Persistent abnormal function suggests incomplete shunt closure, concurrent portal vein hypoplasia, or the development of multiple extrahepatic shunts if portal hypertension results. If an ameroid constrictor or partial ligation is used to attenuate the shunt, nuclear scintigraphy (or mesenteric portography) is performed 2 to 3 months after surgery to evaluate for complete closure. If there is evidence of incomplete shunt closure, nuclear scintigraphy is repeated 4 to 5 months following surgery. If there is still evidence of incomplete closure and the patient is still symptomatic, a second surgery

could be performed for complete shunt closure. In one study 50% of dogs undergoing partial shunt closure developed complications associated with continued or renewed portosystemic shunting in a 4-year follow-up period despite excellent short-term results. This suggests that a second surgery should be considered in these dogs.

Prognosis

The prognosis for medical management of congenital portosystemic shunts is poor. Most patients have progressive hepatic atrophy, and eventually signs of hepatic encephalopathy become refractory to medical management. Occasionally a patient will live to an old age (with or without medical therapy), although later in life such patients often have urate urinary calculi or signs of hepatic encephalopathy. These cases are uncommon, however.

The prognosis for single extrahepatic shunts with surgical correction is excellent, unless severe portal hypertension persists (which is unusual). Clinical improvement is often seen shortly after surgical correction. Hepatic biopsy specimen analysis obtained several months after surgical correction may be normal if there is no concurrent portal vein hypoplasia. The results of surgical ligation of extrahepatic portosystemic shunts in cats seem to be worse than in dogs, with only approximately 50% to 60% of cats having a favorable outcome.

The prognosis for intrahepatic shunts is more guarded due to the technical difficulties of the surgical correction and inability to completely attenuate the shunt without developing portal hypertension. Success depends in large part on the skill and experience of the surgeon.

Portal Vein Hypoplasia Without a Macroscopic Shunt (Formerly Hepatic Microvascular Dysplasia)

Portal vein hypoplasia without a macroscopic shunt (formerly referred to as HMD) refers to a microscopic pathologic malformation of the hepatic microvasculature. It is characterized by small intrahepatic portal vessels, portal endothelial hyperplasia, portal vein dilation, random juvenile intralobular blood vessels, and central venous mural hypertrophy and fibrosis. It is thought that these lesions allow abnormal communication between portal and systemic circulation. It is important to note that portal vein hypoplasia can occur as an isolated disease or in conjunction with macroscopic portosystemic shunts. In one large study

58% of dogs and 87% of cats with portal vein hypoplasia also had concurrent congenital portosystemic shunts. Dogs and cats with portal vein hypoplasia can have clinical signs similar to those of portosystemic shunts, including neurologic and GI abnormalities, as well as urate urolithiasis. Portal hypertension does not usually develop in dogs and cats with portal vein hypoplasia.

Breeds of dogs affected with portal vein hypoplasia are similar to those with congenital portosystemic shunts, including Yorkshire and Cairn terriers (a hereditary mechanism has been described in this breed). Reports of dogs with portal vein hypoplasia suggest that clinical signs and clinicopathologic features are similar to those of portosystemic shunts, although often not as severe. A recent study of 42 cases comparing dogs with portal vein hypoplasia alone and dogs with portal vein hypoplasia concurrent with portosystemic shunts revealed that dogs with portal vein hypoplasia alone were older and had higher values for mean corpuscular volume (MCV) and serum total protein, albumin, creatinine, cholesterol, BUN, and blood glucose concentrations. In addition, dogs with portal vein hypoplasia alone had lower preprandial and postprandial bile acid concentrations. The most discriminating variables for the two groups were postprandial bile acid concentrations, MCV, and serum albumin and cholesterol concentrations. However, there is a large overlap in values, suggesting that patients with presenting clinical findings of a congenital vascular anomaly must undergo an imaging study (nuclear scintigraphy or mesenteric portography) to detect patients with macroscopic portosystemic shunts, because these are amenable to surgical therapy. Further definition of portal vein hypoplasia requires hepatic biopsy. A surgical wedge biopsy or laparoscopic "spoon" biopsy is preferred because they provide more hepatic lobules for evaluation.

Treatment for portal vein hypoplasia is supportive because there is no macroscopic shunt to attenuate. Dietary measures and agents used to treat hepatic encephalopathy are described in the section on management of chronic hepatic disease. Many dogs remain asymptomatic with dietary therapy alone, although the prognosis is variable.

Steroid Hepatopathy

Steroid hepatopathy can result from excessive endogenous (hyperadrenocorticism) or exogenous (iatrogenic administration) amounts of glucocorticoids. It represents one of the most common causes of increased serum hepatic enzyme activities and the most common diagnosis on hepatic biopsy specimen analysis in dogs. Steroid hepatopathy occurs only rarely in the cat. The etiology of changes in the liver induced by glucocorticoids is unknown. The likelihood that an individual patient will develop steroid hepatopathy following glucocorticoid administration is variable and depends on individual sensitivity, type, route, and duration of administration of the glucocorticoid. Some patients show minimal changes in serum hepatic enzyme activities and morphologic changes in the liver even after chronic glucocorticoid administration, whereas other patients have increased serum hepatic enzyme activities and morphologic changes that persist for weeks after a single dose of a glucocorticoid. Changes can persist for several months after a single injection of a long-acting glucocorticoid or after chronic administration of oral glucocorticoids. Changes can also occur after topical or ocular administration of glucocorticoids.

Clinical Findings

Clinical signs of steroid hepatopathy range from asymptomatic to those associated with glucocorticoid excess. These signs include polyuria, polydipsia, polyphagia, endocrine alopecia, distended abdomen, and lethargy. There are usually no signs specifically related to hepatic failure with the exception of lethargy in severe cases. Hepatomegaly is often identified on abdominal palpation and on abdominal radiographs.

Laboratory Findings

There are usually mild to moderate increases in SALT and SAST activities, and marked increases in serum ALP and GGT activities in dogs with steroid hepatopathy. These increases are variable. Occasionally the magnitude of elevation in serum activities of the transaminases (ALT and AST) exceeds the magnitude of elevations of serum ALP and GGT activities. Serum albumin and bilirubin concentrations are usually normal (when these are abnormal, other causes should be looked for). Often the laboratory abnormalities seen with primary nonhyperbilirubinemic hepatobiliary disease and with steroid hepatopathy are similar. The presence of increased serum bilirubin concentration virtually eliminates steroid hepatopathy from the differential diagnosis of primary hepatobiliary disease.

The increase in serum ALP activity is attributed to an isoenzyme that is different from that induced by biliary stasis. This isoenzyme, also produced in the liver, is referred to as the steroid-induced isoenzyme of ALP. Laboratory methods are available to distinguish the steroid-induced isoenzyme from that induced by biliary stasis. However, the steroid-induced isoenzyme of ALP is variably elevated with many primary hepatobiliary diseases and therefore measurement of its activity is not a useful test to determine the presence of steroid hepatopathy. Though there is not a specific isoenzyme of GGT induced by glucocorticoids, it is important to note that the magnitude of increased serum GGT activity induced by glucocorticoids often parallels that of ALP and that serum GGT activity cannot be used to distinguish steroid hepatopathy from primary hepatobiliary disease.

Results of hepatic function tests, including serum bile acids and blood ammonia concentrations, are variable with steroid hepatopathy. Serum bile acids can be normal or slightly to moderately elevated (less than 75 to 100 µmol/L). Marked increases in serum bile acids are unlikely to result from steroid hepatopathy, and other hepatobiliary diseases should be considered. Blood ammonia concentration and the ammonia tolerance test results are usually normal with steroid hepatopathy.

Histopathologic Findings
Histopathologic abnormalities are usually highly suggestive for steroid hepatopathy. There is usually marked vacuolization and ballooning of hepatocytes in a centrilobular or diffuse distribution. The vacuoles are thought to be due to glycogen deposition. There might also be a variable degree of hepatic necrosis.

Diagnosis
If laboratory and clinical signs are compatible with steroid hepatopathy or the patient is asymptomatic, steroid hepatopathy should be ruled out before hepatic biopsy. This can be done with a history of glucocorticoid administration or appropriate laboratory tests such as the adrenocorticotropic hormone (ACTH) stimulation or low-dose dexamethasone suppression tests. If the diagnosis is still uncertain, hepatic imaging with ultrasound (usually revealing hyperechoic and sometimes mottled parenchyma) and biopsy are warranted. Biopsy specimen analysis usually readily distinguishes steroid hepatopathy from other hepatic diseases. Hepatic biopsy specimen analysis is another method of diagnosing hyperadrenocorticism when other laboratory tests are inconclusive.

Treatment
Treatment includes elimination of the source of excess glucocorticoids. If the source is exogenous administration, corticosteroids should be discontinued if their administration is not necessary or decreased by at least 50% if their ongoing use is considered important. If clinical signs such as lethargy are present and persist, alternative immune-modulating drugs may be substituted if appropriate (such as azathioprine, cyclophosphamide, or cyclosporine). Hyperadrenocorticism should be treated if clinically indicated. The laboratory and morphologic changes in the liver seen with steroid hepatopathy are completely reversible when the source of excess glucocorticoids is removed.

Feline Hepatic Lipidosis Syndrome
Feline hepatic lipidosis is a common condition in cats that results in intrahepatocyte accumulation of triglycerides because of abnormalities in lipid metabolism and is associated with severe hepatic dysfunction. In the dog and cat, accumulation of fat in hepatocytes can be associated with a number of causes, including endocrine, nutritional, metabolic, and toxic abnormalities. These causes are listed in Box 9-13. In these instances there is a known underlying cause. In the syndrome referred to as feline hepatic lipidosis, there is no known underlying cause and the disease occurs as an idiopathic entity. This discussion will be confined to this syndrome.

BOX 9-13	Causes of Lipid Accumulation in the Liver

Nutritional
    Prolonged overnutrition
    Starvation
    Obesity
    Deficiency of essential nutrients (lipotrophic agents)
    Protein deficiency
Endocrine disorders
    Diabetes mellitus
Toxins
    Drugs
    Bacterial endotoxins
    Chemicals
    Plants
Hypoxia
Idiopathic
    Feline hepatic lipidosis syndrome

Etiology

In some cases an underlying disease is associated with feline hepatic lipidosis, although the majority of cases are idiopathic. The most common underlying diseases identified are pancreatitis, inflammatory bowel disease, and cholangiohepatitis. The etiology of idiopathic feline hepatic lipidosis is unknown. Theories proposed are based on the liver's role in triglyceride metabolism. Triglycerides accumulate in the liver when the rate of hepatic uptake or synthesis exceeds the rate of removal. Sources of triglycerides include de novo synthesis in the liver and from fatty acids in the systemic circulation (derived from dietary sources and from adipose stores). Once in the hepatocyte, fatty acids are esterified to triglycerides and phospholipids or oxidized within the liver. Triglycerides are released from hepatocytes primarily as very-low-density lipoproteins (VLDLs).

When the ability of the liver to excrete or oxidize triglycerides is exceeded by triglyceride supply, triglycerides will accumulate in the hepatocyte. Therefore hepatic lipid accumulation can result from (1) excessive hepatic triglyceride synthesis, (2) impaired fatty acid oxidation within the hepatocyte, (3) impaired fatty acid transport from the liver as VLDL, and (4) changes in the nutritional or hormonal status or toxic influences on hepatocellular functions that adversely affect triglyceride metabolism. In addition to the possibility that excessive triglyceride storage is damaging to the hepatocyte, excessive hepatic triglyceride accumulation may indicate an abnormality in cellular metabolism that may also affect other cell functions.

It is not known how these mechanisms are involved in the pathogenesis of feline hepatic lipidosis. Anorexia in previously obese cats is an important feature of this disorder and may initiate fatty deposition in the liver. During starvation, free fatty acids increase because of release from adipose tissue. Obesity probably predisposes to this process. There is excessive mobilization of fatty acids, which are subsequently incompletely metabolized in the liver, leading to accumulation within hepatocytes. Some cats have an underlying systemic disease that initiates the anorexia and is concurrent with hepatic lipidosis, although in most cases an underlying disorder is not identified. It has also been proposed that cats with hepatic lipidosis are diabetic or prediabetic, although this is speculative and there is little evidence for this. It is possible that an insulin-resistant state would result in continued release of fatty acids from adipose tissue and subsequent accumulation in the liver.

It is not known what metabolic or hepatocellular derangements prevent triglyceride removal from the liver, although some metabolic and ultrastructural abnormalities have been identified. In ultrastructural studies, cats with hepatic lipidosis have hepatocellular organelles and nuclei displaced to the cell periphery, resulting in compression of the lumen of bile canaliculi. This contributes to cholestasis and bile acid retention. There is also a unique abnormality in that there is a relative paucity of peroxisomes (rather than the up-regulation expected in circumstances of increased fatty acid oxidation), organelles important in the preprocessing of long-chain fatty acids before their presentation for mitochondrial oxidation. Peroxisomes take on an increased role in circumstances of mitochondrial dysfunction. Unlike mitochondria (which are dependent on carnitine), peroxisomal fatty acid oxidation and transport is facilitated but not dependent on carnitine. Peroxisomes are also involved in bile acid synthesis, and subsequent peroxisome dysfunction has lead to abnormal bile acid profiles in cats with hepatic lipidosis. Thus these defects in peroxisomes and increased dependency on peroxisomal oxidation may increase "oxidative stress" on hepatocytes.

There is also speculation that there is a relative carnitine deficiency, resulting in hepatocellular triglyceride accumulation in cats with hepatic lipidosis. It has been shown that plasma, urine, and hepatic tissue carnitine concentrations are normal (or elevated) in cats with hepatic lipidosis. However, it is possible that there may be inadequate carnitine for the quantity and rate of mitochondrial oxidation and disposal of accumulating acetyl CoA. Furthermore there is increased urine concentration of short-chain acyl-carnitines in cats with hepatic lipidosis, reflecting an increased production or carnitine-facilitated removal from the liver. This could allow a route for elimination of excess fatty acids from the liver. Finally, there is evidence that carnitine supplementation to cats with hepatic lipidosis improves recovery rates.

Previous theories have been disputed as well. Orotic acid is a toxin capable of inducing hepatic lipidosis in other species by impaired phospholipid synthesis and VLDL transport from the liver. Arginine deficiency (seen in cats with hepatic lipidosis) can lead to orotic acid accumulation because arginine is essential for normal urea cycle function, and impaired urea cycle function is associated with production of orotic acid precursors. However, attempts to produce hepatic lipidosis in cats with orotic acid administration were unsuccessful, and urine orotic acid concentrations are normal in cats with hepatic lipidosis. Vitamin B_{12} deficiency has also been speculated to be associated with hepatic lipidosis. In one description of 96 cats with hepatic lipidosis, vitamin B_{12} deficiency was not documented. In that series, inspection of plasma and urine for unusual fatty acids reflecting site-specific impaired mitochondrial oxidation did not reveal unique moieties, suggesting no obvious defect in a particular mitochondrial enzyme.

Clinical Features

As mentioned earlier, most cats with hepatic lipidosis are obese. There is usually a period of anorexia followed by signs typical of hepatic failure. In some cases a known illness, stressful event (e.g., boarding, travel), or diet change may cause the initial period of anorexia. In most cases, however, no initiating cause is known. When hepatic lipidosis occurs, clinical signs include inappetence, weight loss, vomiting, and jaundice. Physical examination findings include obesity with evidence of dorsal muscle wasting, jaundice, and possible hepatomegaly.

Laboratory and Radiographic Findings

Laboratory findings include marked elevations in serum hepatic enzyme activities, especially ALP and to a lesser extent the transaminases (SALT, SAST). Because the half-life of ALP is very short in the cat (6 hours), activity of this enzyme is only increased in the serum with severe hepatobiliary disease. In *hepatic lipidosis the activity of ALP is usually markedly elevated and often higher than in any other form of hepatic disease in cats*. Hepatic lipidosis is also the most common hepatobiliary disease in the cat to result in a magnitude of increased ALP activity exceeding that of serum GGT activity. Serum total bilirubin concentration is usually increased and reflects the degree of intrahepatic cholestasis. Coagulation abnormalities (especially elevated PIVKA times) are also common, occurring in almost 50% of cats in one study. However, overt bleeding (including from hepatic biopsy sites) is rare in my experience. Hypokalemia was present in 25% to 30% of affected cats and was found to be a negative prognostic factor. Postprandial serum bile acid concentrations are almost always abnormally elevated. Hypophosphatemia was present in 10% to 15% of cats in one report. Oral alimentation may result in a further decline in serum phosphorus concentration, resulting in clinical manifestations such as hemolytic anemia. Radiographs usually reveal normal hepatic size or hepatomegaly.

Ultrasonographic Findings

Ultrasonographic findings are almost always abnormal in feline hepatic lipidosis. Findings include overall increased echogenicity of hepatic parenchyma compared with falciform fat. In one study this finding was seen in 100% of cats with hepatic lipidosis. However, other studies have also found this relationship in diseases other than hepatic lipidosis, making this a nonspecific finding. In addition, there is increased beam attenuation by the liver, and borders of hepatic vessels are difficult to visualize. Other underlying disorders, such as pancreatitis, may also be detected with an ultrasound examination.

Pathologic Findings

The diagnosis of feline idiopathic hepatic lipidosis is based on histologic findings and the absence of other concurrent diseases that are known to cause lipid accumulation in the liver (see Box 9-13). Typical histopathologic features are a diffuse lobular fatty infiltration within individual hepatocytes. The lipid accumulation is usually macrovesicular in nature, although it can be microvesicular in some cats. Usually there is evidence of intrahepatic cholestasis. The diagnosis can often be made by analysis of fine needle aspiration of the liver or impression smear made of hepatic biopsy specimens. Cytologic features include vacuolated hepatocytes with minimal inflammation. However, cytologic examination cannot exclude the presence of concurrent diseases such as cholangiohepatitis and lymphoma.

Grossly the liver in cats with hepatic lipidosis is usually large, friable, and has slightly rounded margins with a smooth surface. The color is usually yellow with an accentuated lobular pattern.

Treatment

If precipitating causes of the anorexia can be identified, they should be addressed. These include environmental influences such as diet changes and boarding. If concurrent diseases are identified, such as cholangiohepatitis, inflammatory bowel disease, or pancreatitis, they should be treated.

The goal of treatment is to reverse the metabolic changes that resulted in mobilization of free fatty acids occurring during starvation. This is usually accomplished with aggressive force-feeding. In mild cases, methods to stimulate voluntary oral intake may be effective. Heating food and adding seasoning and salt substitutes to food may

be helpful. However, tube feeding seems to be necessary in most cases. This is best accomplished with a PEG tube (No. 18 to 20 Fr), esophagostomy tube (No. 18 to 20 Fr), or nasoesophageal tube (No. 5 Fr). My preference is to place a PEG tube in most cases, often when the cat is under general anesthesia for the hepatic biopsy procedure if analysis of an impression smear of the biopsy sample is suggestive of hepatic lipidosis. This avoids the stress of a second anesthetic procedure. However, there are some cats that are clearly not stable enough to undergo an anesthetic procedure for placement of a feeding tube. In these cases, cats often never recover completely from the procedure. In these patients it is usually much safer to obtain a biopsy specimen under local anesthesia or to rely on cytologic analysis of a fine needle aspirate. This is then followed by placement of a nasoesophageal tube with the cat awake. This allows administration of a liquid nutritional formula (such as CliniCare [Pet-Ag]) on a temporary basis. Constant administration with an infusion pump or gravity flow (versus bolus feeding) is also helpful if vomiting is a problem during the initial few days of treatment. These cats often have electrolyte disturbances such as hypokalemia and should also be stabilized with appropriate intravenous fluids (non–lactate-containing fluids supplemented with potassium chloride or potassium phosphate). When the cat is more stable, a PEG or esophagostomy tube is then placed for long-term use at home. These large-bore tubes are preferred because they are more comfortable to the cat than nasoesophageal tubes and allow the owner to feed blended cat food at home.

The total calorie intake should be 28 to 36 kcal/lb body weight per day. If a large-bore tube is used, a balanced commercial cat food gruel (e.g., Hills Feline p/d [674 kcal per can] or c/d [604 kcal per can]) can be used as the feeding solution. These are generally diluted 1:1 with water, to make a gruel containing approximately 0.75 kcal/ml. They can also be diluted 1:2 with water to make a gruel containing approximately 1.0 kcal/ml. Restricted protein diets are not indicated unless there are overt signs of hepatic encephalopathy present (such as ptyalism). Initially feeding is started at one half the calculated amount for the first 24 to 48 hours. The calculated daily requirement is divided into four to six feedings per day initially. Eventually most cats tolerate the necessary volume in three to four feedings per day. The volume should not exceed 14 ml/lb body weight at any feeding. Attempts are made to gradually increase the feeding volume to maintenance over the first 3 to 5 days.

Antiemetics may be necessary to prevent vomiting during the first few days (or longer) of treatment in many cases. The drug of choice is metoclopramide (Reglan). This is given at a dosage of 2.5 to 5 mg 30 minutes before feeding. In most cases it works when given through the feeding tube (a liquid form is available for this purpose). Occasionally subcutaneous administration or constant intravenous infusion may be necessary. Other strategies to control vomiting include the addition of other antiemetics such as prochlorperazine (Compazine), chlorpromazine, or ondansetron. Other strategies are to administer a liquid enteral formula (CliniCare) by constant infusion or to decrease the amount of water added to the cat food gruel to decrease the volume administered and still provide the same amount of calories. When diluted with one part water to two parts food, the gruel contains 1.0 kcal/ml.

Various dietary supplements have been proposed to be helpful in treating cats with idiopathic hepatic lipidosis. Carnitine supplementation seems to improve survival rates and shorten recovery times. In one report (n = 57) supplementation with L-carnitine (250 to 500 mg/day) was advocated based on the possibility that there is a relative carnitine deficiency. Compared with historical controls, cats that received L-carnitine had a recovery rate of 81% compared with a recovery rate of 37% in cats that did not receive L-carnitine. Cats that received L-carnitine and gastrostomy tube feedings had a recovery rate of 89% (cats that did not receive L-carnitine but had gastrostomy tube feedings had a recovery rate of 29%). In this report, taurine supplementation (250 to 500 mg/day) was also advocated because many cats with hepatic lipidosis have decreased serum taurine concentrations. Taurine is important because this amino acid is used for obligatory bile acid conjugation in the cat and may modify the injurious potential of retained bile acids and increase their renal excretion. Thiamine should also be provided (100 mg by injection or orally two times a day for 3 days) if there is evidence of thiamine deficiency (ventral neck flexion). Vitamin E may be helpful to minimize oxidative hepatic injury. SAMe administration (9 mg/lb/day) may also help speed recovery. Vitamin K supplementation is used if overt bleeding is detected or suspected. If there is prolonged recovery (rare), ursodeoxycholic acid may be beneficial to help stabilize peroxisomes and because cholestasis is usually present (see earlier section on use of ursodeoxycholic acid in cats with cholangiohepatitis). In most cases ursodeoxycholic acid is not necessary because most cats recover or die before this drug can alter the outcome or provide hepatoprotection. Supplementation with L-citrulline (to promote ureagenesis and minimize synthesis of orotic acid) and choline (required for phospholipid synthesis in VLDL production) have also been empirically recommended.

Low-dose insulin therapy is indicated only if the cat is overtly diabetic. There is no evidence that arginine supplementation is helpful in this disease. Lipotropic agents containing methionine have no therapeutic benefit and are contraindicated because they can result in the production of encephalopathic toxins (mercaptans). Use of glucocorticoids and anabolic steroids should likewise be avoided.

Prognosis

The prognosis is fair to good in most cases. I have been successful in treating approximately 80% to 90% of cats, with the recovery rate dependent on how stable the cat is at the time of presentation, the aggressiveness of force-feeding, and the ability to control vomiting. Virtually all cats recover if they survive beyond the first few days. The earlier they are treated, the higher the recovery rate. Spontaneous recovery is rare. Force-feeding may need to be prolonged (3 to 12 weeks). Most owners are able to manage gastrostomy or esophagostomy tube feeding at home during this period. Once there is normalization of biochemical parameters, tube feeding is gradually decreased and the cat should be coaxed to eat on its own. Once the cat is eating completely on its own without any tube feedings for 1 to 2 weeks, the tube is pulled. There is no evidence that affected cats are prone to recurrences following initial recovery or that there is residual hepatic damage. To prevent hepatic lipidosis, nutritional support should be provided to obese cats that stop eating because of other diseases.

Diseases of the Gallbladder and Bile Duct

Disorders of the gallbladder and bile duct are uncommon in small animals. Clinical signs depend on whether there is obstruction to the flow of bile or infection of the extrahepatic biliary system.

Bile Duct Obstruction

Etiology

Causes of common bile duct obstruction are listed in Box 9-1. Because the extrahepatic bile duct goes through the pancreas before it enters the duodenum, disease in the area of the pancreas can result in obstruction. Though pancreatitis is the most common cause of bile duct obstruction, most cases of pancreatitis do not result in bile duct obstruction.

Clinical Findings

Many patients with bile duct obstruction are symptomatic for their underlying disease (for example, patients with pancreatitis often have vomiting and abdominal pain). Signs associated with bile duct obstruction include weight loss, jaundice, anorexia, acholic feces, and vomiting. If the cause of the obstruction is not inflammatory in nature, clinical signs are often surprisingly mild. Often jaundice is the first sign observed.

Laboratory findings include elevations in serum hepatic enzyme activities. Often the serum activities of the cholestatic enzymes (ALP and GGT) are disproportionately elevated compared with serum activities of the transaminases (ALT and AST). However, this is not a consistent finding and many cases of intrahepatic cholestasis have similar biochemical profiles. Serum total bilirubin concentration is also elevated to a variable degree depending on the degree of obstruction. The relative amounts of direct (conjugated) and indirect (unconjugated) bilirubin are variable and often indistinguishable from changes seen with intrahepatic cholestasis. *Therefore laboratory findings identify hepatobiliary disease but do not aid in distinguishing intrahepatic from posthepatic causes of cholestasis. This is currently best accomplished with ultrasonography.* Ultrasonographic findings include common and intrahepatic bile duct distention, as well as gallbladder enlargement. These changes take several days to occur following obstruction. Dilation progresses from common bile duct to peripheral intrahepatic bile ducts over a period of 5 to 7 days following bile duct obstruction. Enlarged intrahepatic bile ducts can be distinguished from portal vessels by their tortuosity, irregular branching pattern, and abrupt and variable changes in lumenal diameter. In addition, the cause of obstruction (such as neoplasia) is often identified on an ultrasonographic examination.

Hepatobiliary scintigraphy has also been used to distinguish extrahepatic biliary obstruction from intrahepatic disease. Following injection of ^{99m}Tc-diisopropyl iminodiacetic acid (disofenin) into patients with unobstructed biliary tracts, there is nuclear activity in the intestine within 3 hours. There is failure to visualize the intestine with nuclear imaging by 3 hours in patients with biliary obstruction. In one study, this method was 83% sensitive and 94% specific (91% accurate) in diagnosing extrahepatic biliary obstruction. Finally, hepatic biopsy often suggests the presence of extrahepatic biliary obstruction.

Treatment

Treatment of bile duct obstruction depends on the underlying etiology (see Box 9-1). In most cases, specific medical therapy is not possible and symptomatic care or surgery is necessary. Approximately 80% of patients with pancreatitis that results in bile duct obstruction will eventually resume normal bile flow without surgical intervention if given appropriate supportive care and enough time. In these cases obstruction is probably associated with acute edema and inflammation around the bile duct. When this resolves, bile duct patency returns. Therefore if pancreatitis is suspected as the cause of biliary obstruction, supportive care is warranted in the initial period. If there is no biochemical or clinical improvement within 2 weeks, patency is unlikely to spontaneously occur and surgical intervention is warranted. During this period, nutritional support with jejunostomy tube feeding or total parenteral nutrition (TPN) may be required. There is no specific medical therapy for bile duct obstruction caused by pancreatitis.

Surgical treatment is usually necessary for most other causes of bile duct obstruction. Surgery is intended to establish patency of the extrahepatic biliary system with the intestine. The procedure used depends on the location of the obstruction, the degree of distention of the common bile duct and gallbladder, the presence of concurrent cholecystitis, and the underlying disease. The most common procedures performed are cholecystojejunostomy or cholecystoduodenostomy. If the gallbladder is infected and the common bile duct is large enough, a cholecystectomy and choledochoenterostomy is indicated. A detailed description of these procedures is beyond the scope of this chapter. The reader is referred to the surgical literature for more information. Recurrent cholangitis and/or cholecystitis can be sequelae to biliary-enteric anastomoses; however, this is seldom a clinical problem if a large enough stoma is created. Clinical signs include depression, fever, and vomiting. Empirical antibiotic administration is usually effective in controlling these episodes.

Cholelithiasis and Choledocholithiasis

Etiology

Choleliths are rare in dogs and cats, and the etiology is unknown. Most theories implicate bile stasis, infection, and changes in bile composition. Choleliths in dogs and cats have been reported to contain primarily cholesterol and bilirubin. Relative percentages of these components are variable, and mixed stones often occur. Additional components include calcium, magnesium, and oxalates. If choleliths are analyzed by methods used for cystic calculi, cholesterol and bilirubin contents will not be determined.

Clinical Findings

Cholelithiasis is usually asymptomatic unless associated with cholecystitis or obstruction of bile flow. In one report approximately 75% of choleliths were discovered at necropsy and were not associated with clinical signs. When clinical signs are present, they are often intermittent. When cholecystitis is present, there is often fever, abdominal pain, and vomiting. When bile duct or cystic duct obstruction occurs, jaundice and other signs of extrahepatic biliary obstruction are seen. Physical examination findings usually reflect the degree of abdominal pain and jaundice.

Laboratory findings may be normal or similar to those seen with extrahepatic biliary obstruction, including increased serum activities of hepatic enzymes and bilirubin concentration.

Radiographic findings depend on whether choleliths are calcified. In most cases there is not enough calcium in the stones to make them radiopaque. However, when they are calcified, they are seen in the area of the gallbladder or rarely in the area of the common bile duct. Ultrasonography is the modality of choice in detecting choleliths, because the gallbladder is readily seen on an ultrasonographic examination. Choleliths appear as a hyperechoic area with a hypoechoic acoustic shadow. It can also be determined by ultrasonography whether there is gallbladder and biliary duct distention. A thickened gallbladder wall with inspissated bile suggests the presence of cholecystitis.

Treatment

Surgical intervention is usually the treatment of choice unless the patient is asymptomatic. Usually the procedure of choice is cholecystectomy, especially if there is concurrent cholecystitis. An alternative is cholecystotomy and stone removal. If there is common bile duct obstruction that cannot be relieved, a cholecystoenterostomy or choledochoenterostomy will be necessary. At surgery bile should be cultured aerobically and anaerobically, so an appropriate antibiotic can be administered to manage concurrent cholangitis and cholecystitis. Additional therapeutic methods used to manage choleliths in humans include endoscopic removal, chemical dissolution, and extracorporeal shock wave lithotripsy. These methods have not been evaluated in small animals. A high-protein, low-cholesterol diet might be helpful to prevent recurrences.

Cholecystitis
Etiology
Cholecystitis is rare in the dog and cat. Predisposing factors include cholelithiasis, bile stasis, ascending biliary tract infection, and bacteremia with secondary cholangitis and cholecystitis. Cholecystitis is most commonly associated with complete or partial bile duct obstruction. Necrotizing cholecystitis often results in either chronic or acute gallbladder rupture with secondary bile peritonitis.

Clinical Findings
In mild cases, signs may be intermittent and include vomiting, fever, and abdominal pain. In acute necrotizing cholecystitis, signs include vomiting, anorexia, abdominal pain, and fever. Many of these patients will show signs of shock, including increased heart rate, pale mucous membranes, poor capillary refill, and weak pulses. When gallbladder rupture occurs, signs of bile and septic peritonitis will result.

Laboratory findings in severe cases include a neutrophilic leukocytosis with a left shift, hypoproteinemia, hypoglycemia, and increased BUN concentration. These changes are associated with sepsis and endotoxic shock. In addition, there are usually increased serum hepatic enzyme activities and increased serum bilirubin concentration if there is biliary obstruction. Abdominal paracentesis may reveal evidence of septic or bile peritonitis.

Radiographic findings include decreased abdominal detail if there is leakage of bile and peritonitis. If choleliths are present, they may be seen radiographically if they are calcified. Some cases have gas in the gallbladder (emphysematous cholecystitis) if there is a gas-forming organism involved (usually *Clostridium* spp. or *E. coli*). Ultrasonographic findings include gallbladder and biliary duct distention, cholelithiasis, thickening of the gallbladder wall, and inspissated bile.

Treatment
In mild cases treatment involves an appropriate antibiotic based on results of bile culture. In these patients the prognosis is fair. In severe cases, including those with necrotizing or emphysematous cholecystitis, the treatment of choice is cholecystectomy. In many cases the gallbladder is ruptured at the time of surgery. In this situation cholecystectomy and exploration of the abdomen for stones that escaped the gallbladder are required. Patency of the bile duct must be established and treated appropriately with diversion procedures if necessary. In cases without gallbladder rupture, it is still advisable to remove the gallbladder because it will be easier to treat the infection if the source is removed. Aerobic and anaerobic cultures of bile, calculi, and the gallbladder wall are mandatory to determine appropriate antimicrobial therapy. Pending culture results, a combination of an aminoglycoside or quinolone and ampicillin is recommended. In one large study the most common bacteria isolated were *E. coli*. Other bacteria cultured included *Klebsiella* sp., *Clostridium* sp., and *Pseudomonas* sp. Aggressive fluid support is also mandatory.

Prognosis
The prognosis is guarded to poor in severe cases. Early diagnosis and surgical intervention is the key for successful therapy. Death is usually attributed to sepsis, shock, peritonitis, and stress of anesthesia. Therefore patients that show signs compatible with cholecystitis should have the diagnosis aggressively pursued with serial abdominal paracentesis, ultrasonography, peritoneal lavage, abdominal radiography, and serial hemograms. When the diagnosis is suggested, surgical exploration should not be delayed.

Hepatic Neoplasia
Incidence
The liver is frequently affected with primary or metastatic neoplasia. Primary tumors account for 0.6% to 1.3% of all neoplasms in the dog. Metastatic tumors occur at least twice as frequently as primary tumors. Hepatic neoplasia occurs less frequently in the cat with the exception of malignant lymphoma and myeloproliferative diseases. The prevalence of hepatic neoplasia in the cat is 1.5% to 2.3%. The most common primary hepatic neoplasms in the dog in order of

frequency are hepatoma, hepatocellular carcinoma, cholangiocarcinoma (bile duct carcinoma), fibroma, fibrosarcoma, hemangioma/hemangiosarcoma, leiomyoma, osteosarcoma, and hamartoma. The most common metastatic tumors in the dog that involve the liver are lymphoma and hemangiosarcoma. Other important primary sites are the mammary glands, adrenal gland, pancreas, bowel, bone, lung, and thyroid gland. Metastasis to the liver can occur via the portal vein, hepatic artery, lymphatics, or by direct extension. Spread from the portal circulation is most common. In the cat, malignant lymphoma and myeloproliferative diseases are the most common metastatic tumors. Nonhematopoietic hepatic neoplasms in cats include benign bile duct adenomas, bile duct adenocarcinomas, and hepatocellular carcinoma. Most hepatic tumors, with the exception of lymphoma, are seen in older patients. Hepatic neoplasia is reviewed in detail in Chapter 11.

Clinical Signs

Clinical signs of hepatic neoplasia depend on the extent of involvement. In many cases of primary neoplasia, especially hepatic adenomas and adenocarcinomas, signs are not seen until the tumor is very advanced. When symptomatic, patients show signs typical of other hepatic diseases, including anorexia, lethargy, vomiting, polyuria, and polydipsia. If there is involvement of the biliary system by direct involvement (cholangiocarcinoma) or by impingement of an extrahepatic bile duct, jaundice may be seen. In many cases hepatomegaly can be detected on physical examination. Clinical signs of metastatic neoplasia involving the liver tend to be more severe earlier in the disease, because more of the liver is usually affected. In addition to signs typical of hepatic failure, patients may also show signs typical of their primary tumor location.

Treatment and Prognosis

The treatment of hepatic neoplasia depends on the type of tumor and extent of involvement. Hepatomas and hepatocellular carcinomas grow very slowly and are often localized to a single lobe of the liver. They are often amenable to surgical resection and have good long-term prognosis. Up to 75% of the liver can be resected without significant hepatic dysfunction, and regeneration usually occurs within 6 to 8 weeks. Less commonly, hepatocellular carcinomas are nodular or diffuse. In these cases the prognosis is poor. Cholangiocarcinomas are usually widespread and either massive or diffuse. They are currently untreatable, usually rapidly progressive, and highly metastatic and have a grave prognosis.

Metastatic tumors are only treatable with chemotherapy. Lymphoma is the most responsive tumor to chemotherapy. Various protocols have been described, and most consist of various combinations of prednisone, cyclophosphamide (Cytoxan), vincristine (Oncovin), doxorubicin (Adriamycin), and L-asparaginase (Elspar). The reader is referred to veterinary oncology literature for details of these protocols. The prognosis with hepatic involvement is similar to that of multicentric involvement. In cats with well-differentiated lymphocytic lymphoma of the liver, the prognosis is better in my experience, with survival times usually between 1.5 and 2 years or longer when treated with a combination of prednisone and chlorambucil (Leukeran). Hemangiosarcoma can also be palliated with chemotherapy (using doxorubicin plus dacarbazine, or the combination of vincristine, doxorubicin, and cyclophosphamide). In humans hepatic arterial infusions of chemotherapeutic agents or embolization agents (such as iodinated poppyseed oil) using a pump delivery system or via angiography procedures are more efficacious than systemic administration for certain tumors, allowing higher regional drug concentrations. These methods have not been evaluated extensively in small animals.

■ MANAGEMENT OF HEPATIC DISEASE

Many types of hepatic disease are managed with specific treatment modalities. Examples of disorders with specific treatments are listed in Table 9-2. In addition to specific treatment, many patients with hepatic disease require general supportive care to manage the acute and chronic aspects of the derangements seen with hepatic failure. This discussion will concern therapeutic efforts common to the management of hepatic disease in general. Refer to the discussion of specific hepatic diseases for appropriate specific therapy.

Management of Acute Hepatic Failure

The cornerstone of treating acute hepatic failure includes elimination of the inciting cause (such as drugs or toxins), providing optimal conditions for hepatic regeneration, preventing complications, and reversing derangements that occur with

TABLE 9-2	Examples of Hepatic Diseases With Specific Treatments
Disease	**Treatment**
Extrahepatic biliary obstruction	Surgery
Bacterial hepatitis	Appropriate antibiotic
Chronic active hepatitis	Antiinflammatory drugs, others (see text)
Portosystemic shunt	Surgery
Feline hepatic lipidosis	Aggressive force-feeding
Hepatic lymphoma	Chemotherapy
Copper-storage diseases	Copper-chelating agents
Steroid hepatopathy	Exogenous: reduce or discontinue corticosteroids
	Endogenous (hyperadrenocorticism): mitotane

hepatic failure. The important derangements that may be seen include dehydration and hypovolemia, hepatic encephalopathy, hypoglycemia, acid-base and electrolyte abnormalities, coagulopathies, gastric ulceration, sepsis, and endotoxemia.

Dehydration, Hypovolemia, and Electrolyte Disturbances

Many patients with severe hepatic disease have vomiting, diarrhea, and anorexia. Therefore dehydration can readily occur. In addition, patients with ascites already are using all of their circulatory reserve function to maintain intravascular volume and tissue perfusion. When additional fluid losses (such as vomiting or diarrhea) occur, hypovolemic shock can result. In addition to volume depletion, these patients frequently have electrolyte and acid-base disturbances. Patients with hepatic disease frequently have hypokalemia in addition to total body potassium depletion. In addition to other deleterious effects, hypokalemia contributes greatly to the severity of hepatic encephalopathy. Often potassium supplementation makes an enormous difference in the treatment of these patients. The most common acid-base disturbance with hepatic disease is alkalosis, although other disturbances can be seen. If prerenal azotemia occurs, excess urea will diffuse into the colon, where it becomes a substrate for ammonia production and thus worsens encephalopathy. Appropriate fluid therapy will minimize this deleterious effect.

To manage these derangements, aggressive intravenous fluid therapy is often needed. The fluid of choice may be determined by measurement of serum electrolyte and arterial blood gas levels. If arterial blood testing is not available, the serum bicarbonate concentration can be estimated from the serum total CO_2 concentration. However, these values are usually not available

immediately. In general the fluid of choice is half-strength saline (0.45%) with 2.5% dextrose, supplemented with potassium chloride. Potassium chloride should be added at the rate of 30 mEq/L of fluids until serum potassium concentration is known, at which time the concentration can be adjusted. Ringer's solution or normal saline (0.9%) are acceptable alternatives, but their higher sodium content makes them less desirable because many patients with hepatic disease have excessive sodium retention and their administration can exacerbate ascites. Lactated Ringer's solution should be avoided because lactate must be converted to bicarbonate in the liver. Care must also be taken not to administer fluids too aggressively because patients with hepatic disease cannot efficiently excrete a salt and water load in response to volume expansion, thus exacerbating ascites and portal hypertension. Diuretics such as furosemide should be given with caution because these can exacerbate hypovolemia, prerenal azotemia, hypokalemia, and metabolic alkalosis.

Acute Hepatic Encephalopathy

The approach to managing acute hepatic encephalopathy involves reducing the formation and absorption of encephalopathic toxins from the intestinal tract, avoidance of drugs that exacerbate encephalopathy (e.g., tranquilizers, anticonvulsants, anesthetics), controlling GI hemorrhage, and appropriate dietary management. Factors that precipitate metabolic changes that can lead to encephalopathy are listed in Box 9-14. These factors must be avoided or treated if possible.

Decreasing Encephalopathic Toxins

The therapeutic efforts designed to reduce formation and absorption of encephalopathic toxins are primarily directed towards reducing ammonia absorption, although other encephalopathic toxins are also important, including benzodiazepine-like

BOX 9-14	Factors That Precipitate Metabolic Changes Leading to Hepatic Encephalopathy

Increased dietary protein intake
Gastrointestinal hemorrhage
Diuretic administration
Sedative or barbiturate administration
Uremia
Infection or endotoxemia
Constipation
Large intestinal bacterial overgrowth
Methionine administration

substances, mercaptans, short-chain fatty acids, and aromatic amino acids. Because ammonia is produced primarily in the colon from bacterial action on dietary amines (proteins) and urea (which diffuses from the systemic circulation into the colon), efforts at lowering blood ammonia concentration are aimed at interrupting this process. This can be done in several ways. First, food is withheld initially to prevent dietary proteins from reaching the colon. In addition, large-volume (25 ml/lb body weight) cleansing enemas are used to decrease bacterial numbers. The enema solution should be composed of normal saline solution with betadine solution added to make a 10% solution to further decrease colonic bacterial numbers. Alternatively, gentamicin can be added (0.45 mg/lb body weight) to the saline solution to kill urease-producing bacteria. Saline also has the advantage of lowering colonic pH. This has the effect of converting freely absorbable ammonia (NH_3) to the nonabsorbable ammonium ion (NH_4^+). Enemas should be retained as long as possible and repeated often (up to every 2 hours) as necessary to manage neurologic manifestations of encephalopathy and hepatic coma.

Lactulose (Cephulac) administration is another useful adjunct to decrease ammonia absorption. Lactulose is a disaccharide that undergoes minimal absorption in the stomach and small intestine, reaching the colon unchanged. There it is metabolized by bacteria, resulting in the formation of low molecular weight acids that acidify the colonic contents. This has the effect of converting ammonia (NH_3) to the ammonium ion (NH_4^+), thus trapping it in the colon and preventing its absorption. In addition, the metabolic by-products of lactulose induce an osmotic catharsis and there-

fore lower colonic bacterial numbers. The initial dose of lactulose is 0.5 ml/lb body weight. It can be given by several routes. The oral route is preferred. In stuporous patients it can be administered via orogastric tube. Alternatively, it can be given mixed with a saline enema. In conscious patients the liquid is given orally by syringe. In the acute situation it can be given up to every 2 to 4 hours. In the long-term management of chronic hepatic encephalopathy, it is given at the above dose orally three times a day. The dose can be titrated by noting the consistency of the feces, because excessive amounts of lactulose will cause diarrhea. Ideally the feces should be loose to slightly liquid.

Orally administered antibiotics can also be helpful in decreasing colonic bacterial numbers. Because ammonia-generating bacteria in the colon are primarily gram-negative and anaerobes, appropriate antibiotics include an oral fluoroquinolone or aminoglycoside (which undergo minimal intestinal absorption) plus metronidazole (Flagyl) or ampicillin. Amoxicillin-clavulanate (Clavamox) is also a good choice as a single agent. My first choice is either amoxicillin-clavulanate alone or the combination of a fluoroquinolone and ampicillin. When an aminoglycoside is used, I have had more success with orally administered gentamicin (using the injectable product given orally at a dosage of 1 mg/lb body weight three times a day) than neomycin (9 mg/lb body weight three times a day), although the latter is an acceptable alternative. Metronidazole is given at a dosage of 2.7 to 4.5 mg/lb body weight two to three times a day. This drug is also systemically absorbed and may be useful for anaerobic sepsis. This can occur with hepatic failure because of abnormal hepatic reticuloendothelial cell function and resultant decreased clearance of bacteria absorbed into the portal circulation.

Drugs That Exacerbate Encephalopathy

Drugs that can depress the CNS should be avoided because of their potential to exacerbate hepatic encephalopathy because these patients have increased cerebral sensitivity to CNS depressants. In addition, drugs that are cleared by the liver have prolonged activity as a result of decreased hepatic clearance. Analgesics, tranquilizers, sedatives, anesthetics, and barbiturates should be avoided if possible. If sedation is necessary, these drugs should be used in decreased dosages. If a convulsive state is present, diazepam is the safest drug to use to control seizure activity. If analgesia is required, I have had the fewest problems with meperidine (Demerol). This drug is used at a lower dose than in patients with normal hepatic function.

Controlling Gastrointestinal Hemorrhage
GI hemorrhage must also be controlled. Patients with hepatic disease are prone to GI hemorrhage because gastrin concentration may be increased (due to decreased hepatic clearance and increased secretion stimulated by excess bile acids), resulting in gastric hyperacidity, and because microthrombi in the mucosal microcirculation (if DIC is present) result in inability to handle back-diffused hydrogen ions. In addition, patients with hepatic disease often have coagulopathies that exacerbate any bleeding tendency. The result of GI hemorrhage is increased ammonia production because blood is a substrate for bacterial conversion to ammonia (100 ml of blood yields 15 to 20 g of protein). In addition, GI hemorrhage leads to hypovolemia, shock, and hypoxia. These effects also exacerbate encephalopathy as discussed above.

A bland diet with minimal residue is helpful to minimize potential inflammation in the bowel. In addition, specific drug therapy is indicated, including drugs that inhibit gastric acid secretion. The drugs of choice are histamine H_2-receptor antagonists. These drugs include ranitidine (Zantac), famotidine (Pepcid), and cimetidine (Tagamet). I prefer using ranitidine parenterally at a dosage of 1.0 mg/lb body weight two times a day subcutaneously or intramuscularly in the acute stages, whereas the drug can be administered orally at the same dosage and frequency for chronic maintenance. For cats oral famotidine (2.5 mg one to two times a day) is the best choice. The dose of cimetidine is 2.5 mg/lb body weight four times a day intravenously, subcutaneously, intramuscularly, or orally.

I also frequently combine ranitidine with sucralfate (Carafate). The latter drug has local protective effects at sites of GI erosions or ulcers. It forms a complex with proteins in the ulcer crater and provides a barrier to the penetration of gastric acid. In addition, recent evidence has demonstrated it to have protective effects for normal gastric mucosa by stimulating the production of the protective prostaglandin E_1 and by stimulating normal epithelial cell turnover (a protective effect). Sucralfate is given at a dosage of 0.5 to 1.0 g orally three to four times a day. It has a very wide safety margin because it is not absorbed. The dose for cats is 0.25 g orally three to four times a day.

Another drug that might have potential for managing GI ulceration is misoprostol (Cytotec), a synthetic prostaglandin E_1 analogue. It has been approved for use in humans and has also undergone clinical evaluation in veterinary medicine as a prophylactic agent for NSAID-induced ulcers. It acts by stabilizing the protective mucous layer in the stomach, increases epithelial cell turnover, and inhibits gastric acid secretion. I have used it on a limited basis at a dosage of 1 to 2.5 µg/lb body weight orally three to four times a day in the dog. Therapeutic trials are needed to further define its role in managing GI hemorrhage in animals with hepatic disease.

It is important to note that blood transfusion should be avoided unless absolutely necessary. Red blood cells have a high ammonia content. And, once blood is stored, ammonia is released. Storage of blood for 1 day results in the elaboration of 170 µg ammonia per 100 ml blood; after 4 days, 330 µg per 100 ml; and after 21 days, 900 µg per 100 ml. It is not uncommon to see clinical deterioration shortly after blood is administered to patients with hepatic failure. If blood administration is necessary, freshly collected blood must be used. Ideally plastic blood collection bags should be used because platelets stick to glass and glass activates factor XII and can exacerbate DIC.

Dietary Management
Dietary management is important in the acute and chronic stages of hepatic failure. In the acute stages, food restriction is important to minimize dietary substrates for ammonia production in the colon. Most encephalopathic patients are anorectic, so this is not a problem. Once acute encephalopathy is controlled, dietary management is important. This involves protein restriction, small frequent meals, and the careful selection of ingredients in the diet. These factors will be discussed in detail in the section on management of chronic hepatic disease.

Hypoglycemia

Many patients with severe hepatic failure are hypoglycemic because of inadequate gluconeogenic enzymes and depletion of glycogen stores. Hypoglycemia can significantly worsen hepatic encephalopathy in addition to its other deleterious effects. It has been shown that hypoglycemia is an accurate predictor of early death in patients with hepatitis. Glucose supplementation will correct hypoglycemia, prevent catabolic processes, and may lower CNS and blood ammonia concentrations. It is usually easy to restore normal blood glucose concentration with intravenous glucose supplementation in patients with hepatic failure, whereas it is more difficult to maintain euglycemia with other causes of hypoglycemia such as insulin-producing tumors. Glucose can be supplied in the intravenous fluids up to a concentration of 5% to 10%. It is rare that higher glucose concentrations will be necessary to maintain euglycemia.

Coagulopathies

The causes of coagulopathies associated with severe hepatic disease are numerous (see section on pathophysiologic derangements occurring with hepatic disease), and appropriate management depends on identifying the cause. The most common coagulopathy seen is DIC. Appropriate treatment includes aggressive intravenous fluids to maintain tissue perfusion and treatment of the underlying hepatopathy if possible. Additional treatment measures include inhibition of platelet function with aspirin, and clotting factor and antithrombin III replacement with a fresh whole blood transfusion (collected in a plastic collection bag to prevent activation of factor XII) along with heparin therapy (110 units/lb body weight subcutaneously three times a day). Heparin can also be added to the transfused blood at a concentration of 125 units/500 ml blood to activate antithrombin III. If there is antithrombin III depletion and it is not supplied in the form of a fresh blood transfusion, heparin therapy will be deleterious.

If the cause of the coagulopathy is from abnormal clotting factor production, a fresh whole blood or plasma transfusion is indicated. As mentioned above, stored blood should be avoided due to its high ammonia content. In some instances, vitamin K deficiency causes abnormal clotting ability. This can be corrected by administering vitamin K_1 orally or subcutaneously. Even if this does not correct abnormal clotting times, it is a therapeutic measure that does little harm and is sometimes worth trying.

Sepsis and Endotoxemia

Patients with severe hepatic disease are prone to systemic and hepatic infection due to abnormal hepatic reticuloendothelial cell function. Because the liver is responsible for clearing bacterial products from the portal blood, therapy is directed primarily against intestinal flora. The main concern is with gram-negative enteric bacteria and anaerobes, as well as endotoxins. If sepsis is strongly suspected, multiple blood cultures (both aerobic and anaerobic) are indicated. If hepatic biopsy is performed, a culture of the specimen should always be obtained. If an organism can be cultured, appropriate antibiotic therapy can be employed. Otherwise patients should be placed on antibiotics empirically. In most patients with severe hepatic disease, prophylactic antibiotics are indicated.

Appropriate choices for empiric antibiotic use are based on activity against intestinal flora, degree of hepatic clearance, and toxicity. Drugs requiring hepatic inactivation should be avoided, whereas drugs excreted by the liver should be beneficial, although they must be used with caution. Drugs with good activity against anaerobes include metronidazole (2.7 to 4.5 mg/lb body weight two to three times a day), penicillins, and cephalosporins. Often these drugs are combined with a quinolone or an aminoglycoside such as gentamicin to combat gram-negative organisms. These drugs can be given systemically for septicemia or orally to kill intestinal bacteria (because aminoglycosides are not absorbed when given by this route). Oral amoxicillin-clavulanate (Clavamox) is a good broad-spectrum single-agent antibiotic.

Tetracycline is concentrated in the bile and may be useful for biliary tract infections. However, it should be used with caution to avoid excessive blood levels and toxicity. Quinolone antibiotics (enrofloxacin, orbifloxacin, marbofloxacin) also have promise for use with hepatic disease because they have excellent activity against aerobic intestinal flora and reach high concentrations in the liver.

Antibiotics that should be avoided include chloramphenicol, lincomycin, sulfonamides, erythromycin, clindamycin, chlortetracycline, and hetacillin. These drugs are either inactivated by the liver, require hepatic metabolism, or can cause hepatotoxicity.

Methods used to control endotoxin absorption include nonabsorbed orally administered antibiotics (aminoglycosides) and cholestyramine. The latter drug binds to bile acids and endotoxins and prevents their absorption into the portal circulation.

Other Therapeutic Modalities

Additional therapeutic measures to treat acute hepatic coma include the intravenous administration of branched-chain amino acids. Because amino acid derangements (mainly increased aromatic amino acids) contribute to hepatic encephalopathy, normalization of amino acid ratios may be helpful. By administering branched-chain amino acids, fewer aromatic amino acids enter the CNS, because they compete for a common carrier to get across the blood-brain barrier. However, there is conflicting evidence as to their effectiveness in managing hepatic coma. The high cost of these solutions will also limit their use. The use of conventional amino acid solutions or protein hydrolysates should be avoided because use of these solutions leads to a high serum ammonia concentration.

The use of the dopamine agonist L-dopa has also been proposed to treat acute hepatic coma. It is thought that this and similar drugs act to favorably alter neutrotransmitter concentrations in the brain. The use of benzodiazepine-receptor antagonists (such as flumazenil) has also been suggested in the management of patients with hepatic encephalopathy. Elevations in the activity of the inhibitory neurotransmitter gamma-aminobutyric acid (GABA) seem to be mediated by increased brain concentrations of benzodiazepine-receptor agonists in patients with hepatic encephalopathy. Clinical trials in dogs with hepatic coma are needed before these drugs can be recommended for routine clinical use.

Management of Chronic Hepatic Disease

If a specific disease is identified by hepatic biopsy, specific therapy should be instituted if possible (see Table 9-2). However, supportive care will be necessary to treat the patient during the acute and chronic phases of hepatic disease. Often ongoing care is essential because many hepatic diseases cannot be readily reversed and are progressive. In addition, a long time is often required for definitive therapy to be effective. *The goals of therapy in chronic hepatic disease are to (1) slow the progression of the disease, (2) ameliorate existing clinical signs and hepatic encephalopathy, (3) support hepatic regeneration, and (4) reduce the need for specific hepatic functions.*

Nutritional Management

Nutritional therapy represents the cornerstone for long-term management of chronic hepatic disease and is the most effective way to minimize signs of hepatic encephalopathy. The basis for these recommendations stems from knowledge of the pathophysiology of hepatic encephalopathy.

Limitation of dietary protein concentration is one of the most important aspects of an appropriate diet. Because ammonia is produced in the colon by bacterial action on dietary peptides, a low-protein diet will decrease substrates for ammonia production. Ideally the protein source should be of high biologic value and of high digestibility. These features will minimize the amount of protein reaching the colon and allow the protein that is absorbed to be used for the body's synthetic functions. It is recommended that 1 g of protein be fed per 20 kcal. If too little protein is fed, there will not be enough nitrogen for the liver's synthetic functions, including synthesis of albumin and clotting factors. In addition, a protein deficiency causes catabolism of body proteins, leading to negative nitrogen balance and a cachectic state. This can also result in excess ammonia production. It is also necessary to supply an adequate amount of nonprotein calories to support protein synthesis and decrease gluconeogenesis and body protein catabolism.

In addition to the quantity of protein, it is helpful to feed a protein source that is high in branched-chain amino acids and low in aromatic amino acids because amino acid derangements (especially high concentrations of aromatic amino acids) contribute to the pathogenesis of hepatic encephalopathy. Milk proteins are higher in branched-chain amino acids and lower in aromatic amino acids than meat sources and thus are preferred protein sources. Fish proteins are intermediate in amino acid concentrations. Red meat should be avoided because it is the protein source most likely to precipitate encephalopathy (which resulted in the term "meat intoxication" for hepatic encephalopathy). Dogs with experimentally produced hepatic failure do better when fed milk proteins than when fed other protein sources. I have also seen clinical improvement with cottage cheese as the main protein source compared with commercial low-protein diets (k/d or u/d Prescription Diet [Hill's Pet Products]). Researchers have described two appropriate homemade diets. An additional low-protein diet with cottage cheese as the main protein source is listed in Box 9-15. If a commercial diet is used, dry 1/d Prescription Diet (Hill's Pet Products) is preferred. Alternatively, various diets intended for renal failure are acceptable.

Easily digested carbohydrates should be the major source of energy. Rice is the most highly digestible carbohydrate source and therefore the

BOX 9-15	Low-Protein, Low-Copper, and Low-Salt Diet for Management of Chronic Hepatic Disease*

4 oz cottage cheese (or cooked meat if cottage cheese will not be consumed)
1 cup cooked rice (or potato)
1 cup cooked green beans
1 tbsp corn oil
2 tsp calcium phosphate
Salt-free, copper-free, vitamin-mineral supplement
Ascorbic acid (see text)
Zinc gluconate or sulfate (see text)
Flavor with salt substitute or onion or garlic powder

*Contains 35 g protein/lb, 600 kcal/lb, 1 g protein/17 kcal.

preferred nutrient in this regard. Potatoes are an acceptable alternative. Increased intestinal bacterial numbers can result from poorly digested carbohydrate sources because bacterial growth in the colon is supported by fermentation of polysaccharides and other foodstuffs that are not absorbed in the small intestine. This results in increased ammonia production. Feeding a low-residue diet (see Box 9-15) will also minimize turnover of epithelial cells, a major source of nitrogen to the colon. As mentioned earlier, providing adequate calories as carbohydrates will minimize catabolism of body proteins and amino acids to meet energy needs. In addition, profound negative energy balance can be an inciting factor in the development of feline hepatic lipidosis.

Because free fatty acids are encephalopathic toxins, dietary efforts should be made to decrease their formation and absorption. Dietary fat is not a source of short-chain fatty acids that may exacerbate encephalopathy. Rather, microbial fermentation in the bowel of carbohydrates (and to a lesser extent amino acids) leads to production of short-chain fatty acids. This underscores the need for a highly digestible diet. Some fat is needed in the diet to provide essential fatty acids, and, in addition to its value as an energy source of nonprotein calories, fat enhances the palatability of the diet. Fat malabsorption (steatorrhea) and fat-soluble vitamin malabsorption is seldom a clinical problem, with the exception being in

cases of prolonged bile duct obstruction. Vitamin therapy (see following discussion) is often helpful, however. Finally, fasting will mobilize fatty acids in the body. Therefore frequent meals are helpful.

Certain B vitamins are converted to their active form and stored in the liver. Therefore supplementation with a good-quality multiple vitamin preparation is helpful. Fat-soluble vitamins require normal bile secretion for absorption. However, it is rare to get malabsorption of fat-soluble vitamins unless there is prolonged bile duct obstruction. Because intestinal bacteria produce vitamin K, prolonged antibiotic use can result in malabsorption of this vitamin.

Vitamin C (ascorbic acid) supplementation is also recommended. The liver produces an important part of the dog's daily requirement of ascorbic acid, and dogs with experimentally induced hepatic disease have marked decreases in ascorbic acid concentrations (as low as 10% of normal). Supplementation with ascorbic acid will also increase copper excretion in the urine. Copper will accumulate in hepatocytes with cholestatic disorders and primary copper-storage diseases, and its presence is toxic to hepatocytes. Therefore ascorbic acid should be given at a dosage of 11 mg/lb body weight per day to maintain normal plasma concentrations.

Potassium supplementation is also helpful in some cases of chronic hepatic disease, because many patients are hypokalemic. Signs of hepatic encephalopathy are exacerbated by hypokalemia, and supplementation frequently improves clinical signs. Serum potassium concentration measurement is necessary to determine whether supplementation is necessary. Potassium chloride tablets or granules (Tumil-K) can be given, or an elixir (1.3 mEq/ml) can be given at a dosage of 0.05 to 0.11 ml/lb body weight three times a day.

Minerals that can be harmful should be avoided. Copper can be hepatotoxic and accumulate in the liver in patients with hepatic disease. Therefore a copper-free vitamin preparation should be used. Zinc inhibits the absorption of copper and its deposition in the liver. Therefore supplementation with zinc is recommended for certain hepatic diseases. The dosage is 0.7 to 1.14 mg/lb body weight three times a day of zinc gluconate, and 0.3 mg/lb body weight three times a day of zinc sulfate.

Sodium retention is frequently a problem in chronic hepatic disease, leading to the presence of ascites. Therefore a low-sodium diet is recommended (see Box 9-15).

Lipotrophic agents that contain methionine should *not* be administered. This amino acid is a precursor to mercaptans, a group of potent encephalopathic toxins. Methionine administration can significantly worsen signs of encephalopathy. Therefore lipotrophic drugs containing methionine have no place in the management of hepatic disease and are contraindicated.

Summary of Nutritional Management

In summary, the nutritional management of chronic hepatic disease should include the following considerations:

1. Calories from protein should be moderately restricted, and ingredients that are of high biologic value and highly digestible should be used.
2. Protein sources with high branched-chain/aromatic amino acid ratios are preferred. Cottage cheese is an ideal protein source in this regard.
3. A palatable energy-dense diet in amounts sufficient to meet energy needs is necessary to avoid negative energy balance.
4. Carbohydrates supply most nonprotein calories but should be from highly digestible sources.
5. Sodium and copper should be restricted.
6. Supplementation with zinc, ascorbic acid, and a salt- and copper-free vitamin-mineral supplement may be helpful.
7. These considerations must be present in a highly digestible, low-residue diet and should be fed in small, frequent meals.

Other Drugs to Manage Chronic Hepatic Encephalopathy

As previously discussed, lactulose is effective in decreasing ammonia absorption by decreasing colonic bacterial numbers and lowering colonic pH. For chronic administration, lactulose is given at an initial dosage of 0.5 ml/lb body weight three times a day. The dosage is titrated to yield two to three loose to slightly liquid bowel movements per day. Oral antibiotics will also decrease ammonia absorption by decreasing colonic bacterial numbers.

Inflammation and Fibrosis

The presence of active inflammation and fibrosis in patients with hepatic disease may justify the use of glucocorticoids and antifibrotic drugs such as colchicine and D-Penicillamine. See the section on

treatment of chronic active hepatitis for a detailed discussion of these drugs.

Ascites

Ascites can be an important complication of chronic hepatic disease. See the section on pathophysiologic derangements occurring with hepatic disease for a detailed discussion of the pathogenesis of ascites.

Emergency treatment of ascites is rarely necessary. Occasionally, however, the volume of ascitic fluid is high enough to result in respiratory distress because of compression of the diaphragm, limiting inspiratory efforts. In these patients, paracentesis may be helpful. The only other reasons to withdraw fluid from the abdominal cavity are to make it easier to perform percutaneous hepatic biopsy, laparoscopy, abdominal radiographs, and for diagnostic fluid analysis and cytologic examination. Otherwise, paracentesis is of no therapeutic value. The risks of paracentesis are hypovolemic shock, iatrogenic infection, protein depletion, and perforation of abdominal viscera. Patients with ascites are already using their maximum cardiac and circulatory reserve to maintain tissue perfusion. When a large volume of fluid is rapidly removed, fluid shifts from the intravascular to extravascular compartment and can precipitate hypovolemic shock. Although this is rare in my experience, it is recommended that if paracentesis is necessary, fluid should be withdrawn slowly and intravenous fluid support should be available if necessary.

Dietary salt restriction, diuretics, and aldosterone-inhibiting drugs are used in the long-term control of ascites. Diuretics should be administered with caution to avoid dehydration. Patients with hepatic failure are already using their maximum circulatory and cardiac reserve to maintain perfusion when ascites is present. Because one of the main causes of sodium retention in patients with hepatic disease is excessive aldosterone activity, aldosterone-inhibiting drugs are used first. I recommend spironolactone at a dosage of 0.5 mg/lb body weight two times a day initially. If this dose is ineffective, it is doubled to 1 mg/lb body weight two times a day. Spironolactone will also not exacerbate hypokalemia. Loop diuretics such as furosemide (Lasix) are also effective. Furosemide should be used with caution because it can cause excessive urinary fluid loss that will result in hypovolemia before it improves ascites and also exacerbate hypokalemia and alkalosis. Furosemide is used at a dosage of 0.5 to 1 mg/lb body weight two to three times a day. Serum electrolytes must be measured periodically in addition to clinical assessment.

If ascites persists, enalapril or benazepril is added at a dosage of 0.125 to 0.25 mg/lb one to two times a day. These drugs are angiotensin-converting enzyme (ACE) inhibitors that decrease activity of the renin-angiotensin-aldosterone system. Dietary salt restriction is of prime importance to minimize sodium retention. Appropriate low-salt diets include those listed in Box 9-15, in the References, and Prescription Diet 1/d (Hill's Pet Products).

REFERENCES

Allen L et al.: Clinicopathologic features of dogs with hepatic microvascular dysplasia with and without portosystemic shunts: 42 cases (1991-1996), *J Am Vet Med Assoc* 214:218, 1999.

Aronson LR et al.: Endogenous benzodiazepine activity in the peripheral and portal blood of dogs with congenital portosystemic shunts, *Vet Surg* 26:189, 1997.

Berry W, Reichen J: Bile acid metabolism: its relation to clinical disease, *Semin Liver Dis* 3:330, 1983.

Biller DS, Kantrowitz B, Miyabayashi T: Ultrasonography of diffuse liver disease, *J Vet Intern Med* 6:71, 1992.

Birchard SJ, Sherding RG: Feline portosystemic shunts, *Comp Cont Educ Pract Vet* 14:1295, 1992.

Boothe HW et al: Use of hepatobiliary scintigraphy in the diagnosis of extrahepatic biliary obstruction in dogs and cats: 25 cases (1982-1989), *J Am Vet Med Assoc* 201:134, 1992.

Brewer GJ et al.: Use of zinc acetate to treat copper toxicosis in dogs, *J Am Vet Med Assoc* 201:564, 1992.

Breznock EM, Whiting PG: Portacaval shunts and anomalies. In Slatter DH, ed,: *Textbook of small animal surgery*, vol 1, Philadelphia, 1985, WB Saunders.

Center SA: Feline liver disorders and their management, *Comp Cont Educ Pract Vet* 8:889, 1986.

Center SA, Erb HN, Joseph SA: Measurement of serum bile acids concentrations for diagnosis of hepatobiliary disease in cats, *J Am Vet Med Assoc* 207:1048, 1995.

Center SA, Magne ML: Historical, physical examination, and clinicopathologic features of portosystemic vascular anomalies in the dog and cat, *Semin Vet Med Surg* 5:83, 1990.

Center SA, Slater MR, Manwarren T: Diagnostic efficacy of serum alkaline phosphatase and gamma-glutamyltransferase in dogs with histologically confirmed hepatobiliary disease: 270 cases (1980-1990), *J Am Vet Med Assoc* 201:1258, 1992.

Center SA et al.: Bile acid concentrations in the diagnosis of hepatobiliary disease in the dog, *J Am Vet Med Assoc* 187:935, 1985.

Center SA et al.: Bile acid concentrations in the diagnosis of hepatobiliary disease in the cat, *J Am Vet Med Assoc* 189:891, 1986.

Center SA: Hepatic lipidosis in the cat. Proceedings of the fourth annual Veterinary Medicine Forum, American College of Veterinary Internal Medicine, Washington, DC, 13, 1986.

Center SA: S-adenosylmethionine (SAMe): an antioxidant and anti-inflammatory nutraceutical. Proceedings of the eighteenth American College of Veterinary Internal Medicine Forum; 2000, 550-552.

Center SA: S-adenosylmethionine (SAMe), glutathione (GSH), & Vitamin B12 rescue therapy in cats with hepatic lipidosis. Proceedings of the seventh International Veterinary Emergency and Critical Care Symposium (IVECCS); 2000, 230-235.

Farrar ET, Washabau RJ, Saunders HM: Hepatic abscesses in dogs: 14 cases (1982-1994), *J Am Vet Med Assoc* 208:243, 1996.

Feldman EC, Ettinger SJ: Percutaneous transthoracic liver biopsy in the dog, *J Am Vet Med Assoc* 169:805, 1976.

Fraser CL, Arieff AI: Hepatic encephalopathy, *N Engl J Med* 313:865, 1985.

Gagne JM et al.: Clinical features of inflammatory liver disease in cats: 41 cases (1983-1993), *J Am Vet Med Assoc* 214:513, 1999.

Grooters AM, Sherding RG, Johnson SE: Hepatic abscesses in dogs, *Comp Cont Educ Pract Vet* 17:833, 1995.

Hardie EM, Kornegay JN, Cullen JM: Status epilepticus after ligation of portosystemic shunts, *Vet Surg* 19:412, 1990.

Hardy RM: Diseases of the liver. In Ettinger SJ, ed: *Textbook of veterinary internal medicine, vol 2, Diseases of the dog and cat*, Philadelphia, 1983, WB Saunders.

Hardy RW: Copper-associated hepatitis in Bedlington terriers. In Kirk RW, ed: *Current veterinary therapy VIII*, Philadelphia, 1983, WB Saunders.

Hardy RW: Hepatic biopsy. In Kirk RW, ed: *Current veterinary therapy VIII*, Philadelphia, 1983, WB Saunders.

Hardy RW: Chronic hepatitis in dogs: a syndrome, *Comp Cont Educ Pract Vet* 8:904, 1986.

Hunt GB, Bellenger CR, Pearson MRB: Transportal approach for attenuating intrahepatic portosystemic shunts in dogs, *Vet Surg* 25:300, 1996.

Jones BD, Hitt M, Hurst T: Hepatic biopsy, *Vet Clin North Am* 15:39, 1985.

Kershenobich D et al.: Colchicine in the treatment of cirrhosis of the liver, *N Engl J Med* 318:1709, 1988.

Kobilk PD et al.: Use of transcolonic [99m]technetium-pertechnetate as a screening test for portosystemic shunts in dogs, *J Am Vet Med Assoc* 196:925, 1990.

Komtebedde J et al.: Long-term clinical outcome after partial ligation of single extrahepatic vascular anomalies in 20 dogs, *Vet Surg* 24:379, 1995.

Lamb CR, White RN: Morphology of congenital intrahepatic portacaval shunts in dogs and cats, *Vet Rec* 142:55, 1998.

Lowseth LA et al.: Detection of serum alpha-fetoprotein in dogs with hepatic tumors, *J Am Vet Med Assoc* 199:735, 1991.

MacPhail CM et al.: Hepatocellular toxicosis associated with administration of carprofen in 21 dogs, *J Am Vet Med Assoc* 212:1895, 1998.

Magne ML, Withrow SJ: Hepatic neoplasia, *Vet Clin North Am* 15:243, 1985.

Neer TM: A review of disorders of the gallbladder and extrahepatic biliary tract in the dog and cat, *J Vet Intern Med* 6:186, 1992.

Nyland TG, Gillett NA: Sonographic evaluation of experimental bile duct ligation in the dog, *Vet Radiol Ultrasound* 23:252, 1982.

Nyland TG, Hager DA: Sonography of the liver, gallbladder, and spleen, *Vet Clin North Am* 15:1123, 1985.

Schermerhorn T et al.: Characterization of hepatoportal microvascular dysplasia in a kindred of cairn terriers, *J Vet Intern Med* 10:219, 1996.

Strombeck DR: *Small animal gastroenterology*, Davis, Calif, 1979, Stonegate Publishing.

Strombeck DR, Miller LM, Harrold D: Effects of corticosteroid treatment on survival time in dogs with chronic hepatitis: 151 cases (1977-1985), *J Am Vet Med Assoc* 193:1109, 1988.

Strombeck DR, Schaeffer MC, Rogers QR: Dietary therapy for dogs with chronic hepatic insufficiency. In Kirk RW, ed: *Current veterinary therapy VIII*, Philadelphia, 1983, WB Saunders.

Taboada J, Meyer DJ: Cholestasis associated with extrahepatic bacterial infection in five dogs, *J Vet Intern Med* 3:216, 1989.

Tams TR: Hepatic encephalopathy, *Vet Clin North Am* 15:177, 1985.

Thornburg LP et al.: Hepatic copper concentrations in purebred and mixed-breed dogs, *Vet Pathol* 27:81, 1990.

Twedt DC, Hunsaker HA, Allen KGD: Use of 2,3,2-tetramine as a hepatic copper chelating agent for treatment of copper hepatotoxicosis in Bedlington terriers, *J Am Vet Med Assoc* 192:52, 1988.

Vogt JC et al.: Gradual occlusion of extrahepatic portosystemic shunts in dogs and cats using the ameroid constrictor, *Vet Surg* 25:495, 1996.

White RN et al.: A method for controlling portal pressure after attenuation of intrahepatic portacaval shunts, *Vet Surg* 25:407, 1996.

Wilson SM, Feldman EC: Diagnostic value of the steroid-induced isoenzyme of alkaline phosphatase in the dog, *J Am Anim Hosp Assoc* 28:245, 1992.

Yeager AE, Mohammed H: Accuracy of ultrasonography in the detection of severe hepatic lipidosis in cats, *Am J Vet Res* 53:597, 1992.

Youmans KR, Hunt GB: Experimental evaluation of four methods of progressive venous attenuation in dogs, *Vet Surg* 28:38, 1999.

10

Diseases of the Pancreas

Kenneth W. Simpson

Disease of the exocrine pancreas is most often a consequence of inflammation, which may be acute or chronic, or a reduction in pancreatic mass and exocrine secretion. Neoplasia is less common and is discussed in Chapter 11.

◼ PANCREATITIS

From a clinical perspective pancreatitis can be broadly categorized as acute, recurrent acute, or chronic. It can be further classified according to its effect on the patient as mild or severe, nonfatal or fatal, and also by the presence of sequelae such as abscess formation. Histologically, acute pancreatitis is characterized by findings that range from pancreatic edema to necrosis, variable infiltrates of mononuclear and polymorphonuclear cells, and local changes such as peripancreatic fat necrosis and thrombosis. Acute pancreatitis may resolve or persist and can be complicated by secondary infection and pseudocyst or abscess formation (Figure 10-1). Although it is tempting to equate mild acute pancreatitis with pancreatic edema, and severe or fatal pancreatitis with pancreatic necrosis, this relationship has not been critically examined in patients with naturally occurring pancreatitis, because the pancreas is rarely visualized or a biopsy performed in patients with mild, self-limiting pancreatitis. Chronic pancreatitis is char-

acterized by fibrosis and low-grade mononuclear inflammation and may be a sequela of recurrent acute pancreatitis or a subclinical disease process that may present as diabetes mellitus or exocrine pancreatic insufficiency (EPI).

Etiology and Pathogenesis

The etiology and pathogenesis of spontaneous pancreatitis is poorly understood. The major factors that have been implicated (by association) as causes of acute pancreatitis in the dog and cat and the experimental evidence to support their involvement are summarized in Table 10-1.

Acute pancreatitis has only recently been considered a significant disease entity in cats. It is my impression that pancreatitis in cats seems to be more chronically active and severe than in the majority of dogs. Although pancreatitis in cats has been diagnosed as the sole or predominant disease entity in cats at necropsy, it has also been variably associated with diseases in other organs, for example, the liver (cholestasis, cholangiohepatitis, hydropic change, severe lipidosis), the kidney (mild to severe nephritis), the endocrine pancreas (diabetes mellitus), the lungs (pulmonary thrombosis), and the intestine (inflammation, ulceration). Effusions have also been noted in the pleural and peritoneal cavity. Whether these nonpancreatic abnormalities arise as

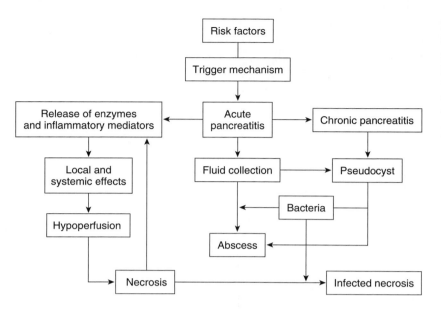

FIGURE 10-1

Schematic diagram of the progression of acute pancreatitis. (From Simpson KW, Lamb CR: Acute pancreatitis in the dog, In *Practice: J Vet Postgrad Clin Study* 17:328, 1995.)

TABLE 10-1	Factors Associated With the Development of Acute Pancreatitis in Dogs and Cats	
Potential Etiology	**Clinical**	**Experimental**
Hyperlipidemia	Lipemia	High-fat diet
	Abnormal lipid profiles	IV free fatty acids
	Lipodystrophy	
Diet	Dietary indiscretion	Fat >> protein diet
	Obesity	Ethionine supplementation
Bile reflux	Concomitant biliary disease (? cats)	Bile infusion
Hypercalcemia	Ca infusion	Ca infusion
	? Hyperparathyroidism	
Corticosteroids	? Hyperadrenocorticism	Increased CCK sensitivity
	? + Disk surgery?	Pancreatic duct hyperplasia
Drug related	Organophosphates	Organophosphates
	L-Asparaginase	
	Azathioprine, various	
Ischemia/reperfusion	Post-GDV	Ex vivo pancreas
Hereditary predisposition	? Miniature schnauzer, miniature poodle, terriers, nonsporting dogs	
Infectious agents	Cats: liver flukes, *Toxoplasma,* FIP	
Endocrinopathies	? Hypothyroidism, diabetes mellitus	

IV, Intravenous; *CCK,* cholecystokinin; *GDV,* gastric dilatation volvulus; *FIP,* feline infectious peritonitis.

a consequence of pancreatitis or are associated with disease processes that cause pancreatitis or are unrelated to pancreatitis is unclear at this time.

Irrespective of the initiating cause, pancreatitis is generally believed to occur when digestive enzymes are activated prematurely within the pancreas. Experimental pancreatic hyperstimulation with cholecystokinin (CCK, or its analogue, cerulein), dietary supplementation with ethionine, and obstruction of the pancreatic duct lead to the formation of large intracellular vacuoles in acinar cells. Vacuole formation is thought to be a consequence of the uncoupling of exocytosis of zymogens and abnormal intracellular trafficking of digestive and lysosomal enzymes. These subcellular alterations are considered to precipitate the intracellular activation of digestive enzymes. Edematous pancreatitis induced by CCK hyperstimulation in dogs is characterized by a rapid but self-limiting burst of trypsinogen activation. It is of note that pancreatic necrosis in humans is associated with persistent trypsinogen activation, so it may be the ability of the pancreas to limit trypsinogen activation that stops edematous pancreatitis from progressing to necrotizing pancreatitis.

Pancreatic hyperstimulation may also be of direct relevance to naturally occurring pancreatitis in dogs and cats. CCK is normally released by cells in the duodenum in response to intraluminal fat and amino acids and coordinates and stimulates pancreatic secretion and gallbladder contraction during digestion. It is possible that high-fat diets exert their effects via the excessive release of CCK and that hypercalcemia, organophosphates, and high levels of circulating glucocorticoids also facilitate or cause pancreatic hyperstimulation; however, this is not proven.

Often pancreatic inflammation is a self-limiting process, but in some patients reduced pancreatic blood flow and leukocyte and platelet migration into the inflamed pancreas may cause progression to pancreatic necrosis. Secondary infection may arise by bacterial translocation from the intestine. Release of active pancreatic enzymes and inflammatory mediators from the inflamed pancreas, such as tumor necrosis factor-α (TNF-α), interleukin-1 (IL-1), and phospholipid platelet activating factor (PAF), amplifies the severity of pancreatic inflammation and adversely affects the function of many organs (systemic inflammatory response). Derangement in fluid, electrolyte, and acid-base balance also results (Figures 10-2 and 10-3). *It is the development of multisystemic abnormalities that separates mild from severe, potentially fatal pancreatitis.*

Further study of the cellular mechanisms governing enzyme secretion and activation, leukocyte and platelet recruitment to the pancreas, bacterial translocation, and the development of the systemic inflammatory response in pancreatitis will hopefully provide information that will be useful in treating acute pancreatitis in the patient population in the future.

Diagnosis

There is currently no single specific test for pancreatitis in dogs and cats, and diagnosis is based on a combination of compatible clinical, clinicopathologic, and imaging findings. Laparoscopic or surgical biopsy may be required to confirm a diagnosis and to distinguish inflammation from neoplasia.

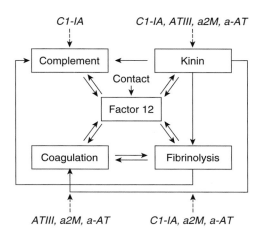

FIGURE 10-2 The complex interactions of the complement, kinin, fibrinolytic, and coagulation pathways following activation of factor XII by contact or trypsin. Inhibitors are shown in italics. *ATIII,* Antithrombin III; *a2M,* alpha₂-macroglobulin; *a-AT,* alpha₁-antitrypsin; *C1*-1A, complement fragment *C1*-1A. (Modified from Lasson A: Acute pancreatitis in man: a clinical and biochemical study of pathophysiology and treatment, *Scand J Gastroenterol* 99:1, 1984.)

Clinical Findings
Signalment and History

Dogs. Middle-age to old dogs (more than 5 years of age) that are overweight appear to be at higher risk. Miniature schnauzers, Yorkshire and Silky terriers, nonsporting breeds, and perhaps miniature poodles may be at increased risk of developing pancreatitis. There is no clear sex predisposition. Endocrinopathies such as hypothyroidism, diabetes mellitus, and hyperadrenocorticism may also be risk factors. The history may reveal a recent episode of dietary indiscretion or drug administration. Common clinical signs include lethargy, anorexia, hunched stance, vomiting (with or without blood), diarrhea (with or without blood), increased respiratory rate, and enlarged abdomen. Some dogs have a history of icterus preceded by vomiting.

Cats. Acute pancreatitis has been reported in cats from 4 weeks to 18 years of age. Domestic short and long hair cats are most commonly affected. Siamese cats have been overrepresented in some series. No sex bias has been demonstrated. A small number of cases have been associated with trauma, *Toxoplasma gondii,* pancreatic and liver flukes, feline infectious peritonitis (FIP), and lipodystrophy. Usually there are no obvious associated factors.

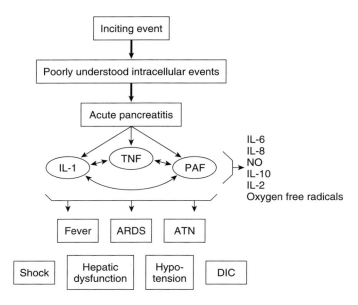

FIGURE 10-3 Inflammatory mediators in acute pancreatitis. Regardless of the inciting event (e.g., alcohol or gallstones), many poorly understood intracellular events lead to the development of acute pancreatitis. The progression of pancreatitis depends on several inflammatory mediators (interleukin [IL]-1, tumor necrosis factor [TNF], and platelet activating factor [PAF] are believed to be the most important). Other mediators (e.g., IL-6, IL-8, and nitric oxide [NO]) are produced, but they are markers of disease severity or regulatory proteins and are not mediators of disease progression. IL-1, TNF, and PAF stimulate the production of each other and mediate distant organ dysfunction such as adult respiratory distress syndrome (ARDS), hepatic dysfunction, shock, and death. *DIC,* disseminated intravascular coagulation; *ATN,* acute tubular necrosis. (From Denham W, Norman J: The potential role of therapeutic cytokine manipulation in acute pancreatitis, *Surg Clin North Am* 79:767, 1999.)

The most common clinical findings in cats with acute pancreatitis are lethargy, anorexia, and weight loss. Vomiting, diarrhea, constipation, icterus, dehydration, ascites, and dyspnea are more variably present. Vomiting is not as prominent a sign of pancreatitis in cats as it is in dogs. Polyuria and polydipsia have been encountered in some cats with diabetes mellitus and pancreatitis. The duration of clinical signs until presentation varies from less than 3 days to 12 weeks.

Physical Examination

Dogs. Physical findings in dogs with acute pancreatitis are highly variable and range from depression, to mild dehydration with signs of abdominal pain, to acute abdominal crisis with shock (tachycardia, prolonged capillary refill time, tacky mucous membranes, hypothermia), petechiation, icterus, and ascites. An abdominal mass is palpated in some dogs.

Cats. In cats dehydration and hypothermia have been most commonly observed. Icterus may also be present. Abdominal pain is infrequently elicited. The presence of a palpable cranial abdominal mass or abdominal pain has been reported in a quarter to

a third of cats in some clinical series and in cats with experimental and trauma-induced pancreatitis.

Diagnostic Approach and Differential Diagnosis

Dogs. The differential diagnosis of acute pancreatitis in dogs is usually centered around the problems of vomiting and abdominal pain (Box 10-1).

In vomiting dogs the initial approach is to distinguish self-limiting from more severe causes of vomiting on the basis of physical findings and a minimum database (e.g., packed cell volume, total protein, blood urea nitrogen [BUN; e.g., Azostick], urinalysis, plasma concentrations of sodium and potassium). Where vomiting is associated with systemic signs of illness, or is persistent, the clinician has to differentiate metabolic, polysystemic, infectious, toxic, and neurologic causes from intraabdominal causes. This is usually achieved on the basis of combined historical and clinical findings coupled with a minimum database and the evaluation of hematology and serum chemistry profile, urinalysis, and abdominal radiography. Measurement

BOX 10-1 Differential Diagnosis of Pancreatitis in Dogs

CAUSES OF ABDOMINAL PAIN
Gastric
Dilatation/volvulus, ulceration
Intestinal
Obstruction, intussusception, rupture, torsion, enteritis
Pancreatic
Pancreatitis
Hepatic
Acute hepatitis, ruptured bile duct, hepatic neoplasia
Splenic
Torsion, ruptured neoplasm
Urogenital
Nephritis, pyelonephritis, ruptured bladder, ureteral/urethral calculi, pyometra, prostatitis
Peritoneum
Primary or secondary peritonitis (e.g., chemical: bile and urine, septic: ruptured viscus)
Pseudoabdominal Pain
Discospondylitis, prolapsed disk

CAUSES OF VOMITING
Intraabdominal
Gastric
Gastritis, ulceration, neoplasia, outflow obstruction, foreign bodies, motility/functional disorders
Intestinal
Inflammatory bowel disease, neoplasia, foreign bodies, intussusception, torsion, rupture, bacterial overgrowth, functional disorders
Non-Gastrointestinal (Non-GI)
Pancreas: pancreatitis, pancreatic neoplasia
Liver: cholangiohepatitis, biliary obstruction
Genitourinary: pyometra, nephritis, nephrolithiasis,
Urinary: obstruction, prostatitis
Peritonitis
Metabolic/Endocrine
Uremia, hypoadrenocorticism, diabetic ketoacidosis, hepatic encephalopathy, hypercalcemia, septicemia
Drugs
Digoxin, erythromycin, chemotherapy, apomorphine, xylazine
Toxins
Strychnine, ethylene glycol, lead
Dietary
Indiscretion, intolerance, allergy
Neurologic
Vestibular disease, encephalitis, neoplasia, raised intracranial pressure
Infectious
Distemper, parvovirus, infectious canine hepatitis, leptospirosis, *Salmonella*

of serum amylase or lipase activity is often reported on routine serum chemistry profiles. Additional procedures such as ultrasonography, abdominal paracentesis, or pancreatic lipase immunoreactivity (PLI) assay are usually performed on the basis of these initial test results and help to distinguish pancreatitis from other intraabdominal causes of vomiting.

Where abdominal pain is the major finding, localizing abnormalities such as abdominal distention are rapidly pursued with radiography, ultra-

sonography, and paracentesis. Concurrently, supportive treatment is provided on the basis of physical findings and a minimum database while awaiting the results of hematology, serum chemistry profile, and urinalysis findings. *Abdominal pain can arise from any intraabdominal structure. Musculoskeletal disorders such as discospondylitis and prolapsed disks can be hard to distinguish from abdominal causes of pain.*

It is of note that diarrhea, which was bloody in some cases, was a more frequent sign than vomiting in dogs with experimental acute pancreatitis. Acute pancreatitis and its complications (infection, pseudocyst or abscess formation) should also be considered in the differential diagnosis of icterus and pyrexia. Some dogs with pancreatitis exhibit few localizing clinical signs. Diagnosis in these patients requires a high index of suspicion and use of versatile diagnostic tests such as ultrasonography.

Cats. In cats, lethargy, anorexia, and weight loss are the usual presenting complaints. Where encountered, localizing signs or findings such as vomiting, icterus, diarrhea, abdominal pain, abdominal mass, polyuria, or polydipsia should be pursued. Because the antemortem diagnosis of acute pancreatitis is rarely made, its overall significance as a cause of these problems is unclear at this time.

Where vomiting is present, it is approached by pursuing localizing findings such as abdominal pain or masses and by ruling out infectious, parasitic, metabolic, and gastrointestinal (GI) causes. Hyperthyroidism should be ruled out in older cats by determination of serum total thyroxine (T_4) concentration. Elevated levels of hepatic enzymes, hyperbilirubinemia, hyperglycemia, and glucosuria are frequently encountered in cats with acute pancreatitis, so pancreatitis should be strongly considered in these cats.

The diagnostic approach to feline icterus is first to rule out prehepatic causes and then to pursue hepatic or posthepatic causes. The association of acute pancreatitis and hepatic lipidosis of increased mortality, cholangiohepatitis, and inflammatory bowel disease has been demonstrated in some studies. A high index of suspicion should be adopted for pancreatitis in cats with hepatic, biliary, or intestinal disease. Cats with a confirmed diagnosis of hepatic lipidosis and that have a peritoneal effusion should also be strongly suspected of having pancreatitis.

Pancreatitis may be the cause of diabetes mellitus in some cats, but the true association between these diseases is unclear. One study suggests that cats with pancreatitis and diabetes mellitus are very sensitive to insulin. Transient euglycemia and reduced insulin requirements after removal of a pancreatic abscess suggest that pancreatic inflammation or infection can exacerbate diabetes mellitus in cats. Transient diabetes mellitus has also been reported in a cat that was suspected of having pancreatitis.

Where a high index of suspicion for pancreatitis is present, ultrasonography and enzymology (assay of feline PLI) should initially be employed to help to detect pancreatitic inflammation. Pancreatic biopsy is required to achieve a definitive diagnosis.

Clinicopathologic Findings

Hematology

Dogs. Hematologic findings are highly variable, ranging from mild neutrophilia and slightly increased hematocrit, through marked leukocytosis with a left shift, to thrombocytopenia, anemia, and leukopenia with a degenerative left shift. If thrombocytopenia is detected, blood clotting tests (one stage prothrombin time [OSPT], activated partial thromboplastin time [APTT], fibrin degradation products [FDP or D-dimer]) are performed to determine if the patient has disseminated intravascular coagulation (DIC). Where available, the measurement of antithrombin III is useful in the early diagnosis of DIC.

Cats. A mild anemia that may be nonregenerative and a leukocytosis that is usually not accompanied by a left shift are the most common findings in cats with pancreatitis.

Serum Biochemistry

Dogs. Serum biochemical abnormalities are variable and include azotemia (prerenal and renal), increased levels of liver enzymes (alanine aminotransferase [ALT], aspartate aminotransferase [AST], alkaline phosphatase [AP]), hyperbilirubinemia, lipemia, hyperglycemia, hypoproteinemia, hypocalcemia, metabolic acidosis, and variable alterations (usually decreased) in sodium, potassium, and chloride.

Cats. Increased levels of ALT, AP, bilirubin, cholesterol, and glucose and hypokalemia and hypocalcemia are most common. Azotemia is variably present.

Urinalysis

Urinalysis enables azotemia to be characterized as renal or prerenal. Transient proteinuria occurs in some dogs with acute pancreatitis, possibly as a consequence of pancreatic enzyme-mediated glomerular damage. The absence of white cell casts or bacteria helps to rule out pyelonephritis as a cause of abdominal pain. The presence of glucosuria or ketonuria should prompt consideration of diabetes mellitus.

Pancreas-Specific Enzymes

Classically elevations in serum amylase and lipase activity have been used as indicators of pancreatic inflammation in dogs. However, these tests are not very accurate because dogs with nonpancreatic disorders may have elevated enzyme activities. This may occur because both amylase and lipase are normally present in other organs and their serum activities may increase with nonpancreatic disorders, including intestinal obstruction (amylase), corticosteroid administration (lipase), and renal disease (both enzymes). Dogs with confirmed pancreatitis may also have normal amylase and lipase activity. For example, in two recent case series of dogs with histologically confirmed pancreatitis, lipase was normal in 28 dogs (61%) and amylase was normal in 31 dogs (47%). This may be due to exhaustion of enzymes, thrombosis of pancreatic vessels, the presence of inhibitors, alterations in activity, and perhaps increased clearance. *In cats it seems fair to state that measuring total amylase and lipase activity is of no utility for diagnosing pancreatitis.*

These limitations have stimulated the development of assays for enzymes considered pancreatic in origin. TLI is one candidate. This species-specific immunoassay measures circulating trypsinogen in healthy individuals and trypsinogen and trypsin in those with pancreatitis.

In dogs, circulating TLI is abolished by pancreatectomy and extremely low concentrations occur in EPI. Experimental and clinical studies have documented high concentrations of TLI in dogs with acute pancreatitis. TLI is therefore considered a useful indicator of pancreatic mass and potentially inflammation. Nonpancreatic diseases such as renal disease and possibly corticosteroids may increase circulating TLI. It is important to note that the utility of TLI assay for the diagnosis of spontaneous pancreatitis in dogs has not been thoroughly evaluated, and I have observed both normal and subnormal concentrations in dogs with pancreatitis.

A TLI test has also been developed for cats. Cats with EPI and some cats with spontaneous pancreatitis have abnormal concentrations of TLI. Increased application of this test indicates that high TLI concentrations may occur in the face of normal pancreatic histologic findings in cats with inflammatory bowel disease or lymphoma (Table 10-2). The reason for this is unclear. Nonpancreatic diseases such as renal disease and possibly corticosteroids may increase circulating TLI in cats.

At the present time it seems fair to conclude that the TLI assay is highly accurate for differentiating EPI from small intestinal disease. It appears less accurate in detecting pancreatitis. This is not surprising because pancreatitis is a very dynamic disease, which may influence the synthesis, secretion, elimination, and activity of circulating marker enzymes such as TLI. The tissue specificity of TLI makes it an attractive alternative to amylase and lipase activity tests in dogs, and it is presently the only useful indicator in the cat. The recent development of assays that measure pancreas specific lipase in dogs and cats (cPLI and fPLI) has yielded promising initial results in helping to diagnose pancreatic inflammation and may in time prove to be a useful diagnostic aid.

Radiography

Radiographic findings in cats and dogs with acute pancreatitis may include loss of serosal detail, increased opacity in the right cranial quadrant of the abdomen, displacement of the duodenum ventrally and/or to the right, dilated hypomotile duodenum, and caudal displacement of the transverse large intestine (see Chapter 2). Punctate calcification is occasionally identified in dogs with longstanding pancreatitis; it indicates saponification of mesenteric fat around the pancreas.

Although radiographic signs often are absent and are nonspecific, radiography remains a useful diagnostic method for pancreatitis largely because it may enable detection of other abnormalities that can cause similar signs (e.g., gastric foreign body or intestinal obstruction). Radiography is a logical first-choice imaging modality for patients with vomiting or abdominal pain. Negative or equivo-

TABLE 10-2	Evaluation of Pancreatic Disease in Cats With Subnormal Serum Concentrations of Cobalamin				
	Pancreatic Ultrasonography		Pancreatic Histopathology		
Trypsin-like Immunoreactivity	Normal	Abnormal	Normal	Abnormal	
Normal (17-49 µg/L)	3	3	0	2	
Increased (>49 µg/L)	8	6	3	4	
Decreased (<17 µg/L)	1	1	ND	ND	

Modified from Simpson KW et al.: Subnormal concentrations of serum cobalamin (vitamin B_{12}) in cats with gastrointestinal disease, *J Vet Intern Med* (submitted).

cal radiographic findings may be followed up with ultrasonography or an upper GI contrast study.

Thoracic radiographs may enable the detection of pleural fluid, edema, or pnemonia, which has been associated with pancreatitis in dogs and cats.

Ultrasonography

The use of ultrasound for detecting pancreatic lesions is perhaps one of the most significant advances in the diagnosis of acute pancreatitis in dogs and cats. Ultrasonographic findings include enlarged, hypoechoic pancreas, cavitary lesions such as abscess or pseudocyst, dilated pancreatic duct, swollen hypomotile duodenum, biliary dilation, and peritoneal fluid. A recent study of dogs with fatal acute pancreatitis indicated that ultrasound supported a diagnosis of pancreatitis in 23 of 34 dogs. Findings in cats are also encouraging (Figure 10-4, see Table 10-2) but emphasize that a normal ultrasound examination may be present in approximately 60% of cats with pancreatitis. The clinician should also be careful to consider differential diagnoses other than pancreatitis, for example, pancreatic neoplasia, pancreatic edema (associated with hypoproteinemia or portal hypertension), and enlarged peripancreatic structures, which can have an ultrasonographic appearance identical to pancreatitis. Fine-needle aspirates of cavitary lesions may be useful to distinguish abscess from pseudocyst.

Abdominal Paracentesis

Examination of peritoneal fluid may aid the detection of various causes of acute abdominal signs such as pancreatitis, GI perforation, or ruptured bile duct. The accumulation of fluid in the abdomen or the pleural cavity has been variably encountered in cats with acute pancreatitis. Effusion in the abdomen or chest was present in 17 of 40 cats in one study, in the abdomen of 5 of 5 cats with hepatic lipidosis and pancreatitis, and in the abdomen of 2 of 8 cats in another.

Prognostic Indicators

Stratifying the severity of pancreatitis is useful when deciding how aggressive to be with medical and nutritional support and in offering a prognosis. Severe pancreatitis requires aggressive support and carries a guarded prognosis, whereas mild pancreatitis often responds to short-term symptomatic therapy and has a good prognosis. Clinical and clinicopathologic criteria can be used to predict the severity of acute pancreatitis. The presence of shock or abnormalities such as oliguria, azotemia, icterus, markedly elevated levels of transaminases, hypocalcemia, hypoglycemia, hypoproteinemia, acidosis, leukocytosis, falling hematocrit, thrombocytopenia, and DIC should be considered likely indicators of severe pancreatitis in the dog and cat.

The measurement of components of the systemic inflammatory response such as TNF-α, C-reactive protein, and IL-6 may also yield information about the severity of pancreatitis in dogs and cats and in the future might lead to the administration of specific antagonists of this response.

Indicators that are potentially useful in the diagnosis and prognosis of pancreatitis include assay of trypsinogen activation peptide (TAP), trypsin complexed with inhibitors, and phospholipase A_2. TAP has been shown to accurately predict severity in humans with pancreatitis. This peptide is released when trypsinogen, a pancreas-specific enzyme, is converted to its active form and rapidly accumulates in the urine and plasma of dogs and cats with experimental acute pancreatitis. Phospholipase A_2 is elevated in dogs with severe pancreatitis. Further validation of these markers is required before clinical application.

Morphologic assessment of severity is accomplished in humans by use of contrast-enhanced computed tomography (CE-CT). Where lack of pancreatic perfusion is encountered (i.e., necrosis), fine-needle aspiration is used to distinguish infected from sterile necrosis. Substantially reduced mortality has been achieved by the detection and surgical treatment of humans with infected necrosis. The lack of availability of CT has restricted veterinary application to date, but a recent study of cats with pancreatitis failed to demonstrate any benefit of CE-CT. Where a diagnosis of infected necrosis is being considered, the relative accessibility of the canine and feline pancreas to ultrasound-guided needle aspiration holds the potential of the adoption of a similar approach.

Treatment

Medical treatment is based on maintaining or restoring adequate tissue perfusion, limiting bacterial translocation, and inhibiting inflammatory mediators and pancreatic enzymes. Surgical treatment consists principally of restoring biliary outflow, removing infected necrotic pancreatic tissue, or coping with sequelae such as pseudocysts. No

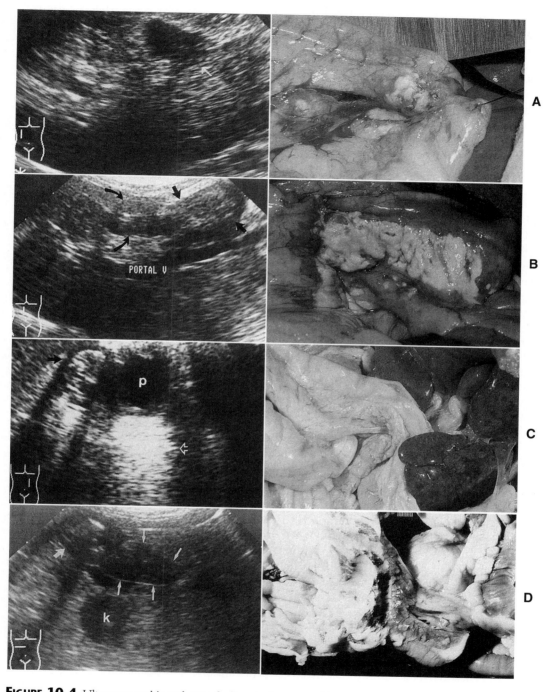

FIGURE 10-4 Ultrasonographic and gross findings in four cats with pancreatitis. **A,** A hypoechoic mass *(arrow)* visualized in the right cranial abdomen corresponded to an abscess in the right limb of the pancreas. **B,** A large mass of complex echogenicity *(arrows)* detected in the right cranial abdominal quadrant was consistent with acute necrotizing pancreatitis with saponification of fat detected at surgery. **C,** A cystic mass *(p)* with distal acoustic enhancement *(open arrow)* was identified in the region of the left pancreatic lobe. Necropsy confirmed biliary obstruction and cystic dilation of the pancreatic duct secondary to pancreatitis. **D,** A hypoechoic structure *(small arrows)* medial to the duodenum *(large arrow)* and ventral to the cranial pole of the right kidney *(k)* was confirmed at necropsy to be an inflamed pancreas. (From Simpson KW et al.: Antemortem diagnosis of pancreatitis in 4 cats, *J Small Anim Pract* 35:93, 1994.)

studies have critically evaluated treatment modalities in dogs or cats with naturally occurring pancreatitis.

Initial Management

The initial medical management of dogs and cats with acute pancreatitis is invariably initiated before a diagnosis is confirmed and is based on the presenting clinical findings and the results of an initial database. Where dehydration or hypovolemia are encountered, these are supported with intravenous fluid therapy. Lactated Ringer's solution or 0.9% NaCl are common first choices. Potassium and glucose should be supplemented where necessary. The type of fluid should be tailored on the basis of electrolyte and pH measurements to restore normal electrolyte levels and acid-base balance. For example, dogs with a history of vomiting that are mildly dehydrated are usually given crystalloids such as lactated Ringer's solution at a rate that will provide maintenance and replace both deficits and ongoing losses over a 24-hour period. Dogs with signs of shock require more aggressive support. The volume deficit can be replaced with crystalloids at an initial rate of 30 to 45 ml/lb/hr, then tailored to maintain tissue perfusion and hydration.

Plasma (10 ml/lb intravenously) or colloids (e.g., degraded gelatin or hetastarch at 5 to 10 ml/lb/day intravenously) may be indicated in the presence of hypoproteinemia or shock. Colloids such as dextran 70 and hetastarch may also have antithrombotic effects that help maintain the microcirculation.

Insulin therapy is initiated in diabetic patients. Stress hyperglycemia has to be differentiated from diabetes mellitus in cats.

Where vomiting is a problem, oral intake is restricted, and antiemetics (metoclopramide or chlorpromazine) and gastric acid reduction with an H_2-receptor antagonist (e.g., famotidine at 0.25 mg/lb intravenously twice a day) are prescribed when vomiting is persistent or severe. Patients with persistent or severe vomiting are at risk for development of esophagitis (see Chapter 4). H_2-receptor antagonist therapy will help in management of both esophageal and gastric erosive conditions. Chlorpromazine is an excellent antiemetic drug that helps provide mild sedation along with its effects of reducing nausea and vomiting. Ondansetron (Zofran) is a potent antiemetic drug that may be more effective in controlling severe and frequent vomiting in dogs and cats when chlorpromazine or metoclopramide is not considered to be effective enough. Ondansetron is administered at 0.05 mg/lb slowly intravenously two to three times a day.

Prophylactic broad-spectrum antibiotics (e.g., amoxicillin with or without enrofloxacin, depending on severity) may be warranted in patients with shock, fever, diabetes mellitus, or evidence of breakdowm of the GI barrier.

Analgesia is an important aspect of caring for patients with pancreatitis. It can be provided using injectable opioids such as buprenorphine (0.0023 to 0.0045 mg/lb subcutaneously every 6 to 12 hours), oxymorphone (0.023 to 0.05 mg/lb in cats, 0.05 to 0.1 mg/lb in dogs intramuscularly or subcutaneously every 1 to 3 hours), or morphine (0.05 to 0.2 mg/lb in cats subcutaneously or intramuscularly, 0.2 to 0.5 mg/lb in dogs subcutaneously or intramuscularly every 6 hours). It may be necessary to administer low-dose sedation with acepromazine (0.005 mg/lb intramuscularly) to patients that become dysphoric after opioids. It should be borne in mind that buprenorphine is a partial agonist and may antagonize the administration of more potent analgesics in patients with severe pain. A transdermal fentanyl patch (Duragesic) applied to a clipped, clean area of skin is a good way of providing a longer duration of analgesia in dogs (5 to 30 lb, 25 μg/hr patch; 30-60 lb, 50 μg/hr patch; 60 to 120 lb, 75 μg/hr; every 72 hours) and cats (25 μg/hr patch every 118 hours). Adequate fentanyl levels are not attained for between 6 and 48 hours after application (it takes somewhat longer in some dogs than in cats), so another analgesic should be administered in the short term (morphine, oxymorphone). In cats effective levels are reached by 6 to 12 hours and in some by 3 to 4 hours. It is emphasized that each patient should be treated as an individual. Careful monitoring for ongoing signs of pain is very important, and some patients will require more aggressive analgesic therapy than others. Without question, however, analgesic therapy is warranted in patients that have acute pancreatitis. Nonsteroidal analgesics are generally not used in patients with acute pancreatitis because of concerns for GI ulceration, renal failure, and potential hepatotoxicity.

Steroids in Cats With Pancreatitis, and Management of Concurrent Diseases

The high frequency of intercurrent hepatic and intestinal disease in cats with pancreatitis must be taken into consideration when formulating a treatment plan. Treatment with amoxicillin and metronidazole should be initiated if cholangio-hepatitis is present. Dietary support is broadly similar in hepatic lipidosis and pancreatitis, though jejunostomy tube feeding may be theoretically indicated in the latter. The principal dilemma arises in cats with pancreatitis and inflammatory bowel disease. Should corticosteroids be used? In my experience the use of corticosteroids in cats with pancreatitis and inflammatory bowel disease has enabled resolution of diarrhea and weight gain without exacerbating pancreatitis. Subnormal cobalamin concentrations are frequently present in cats with pancreatitis and GI disease, and cobalamin should be supplemented parenterally (1 mg subcutaneously every 14 days). There is a possibility of adverse effects of chemotherapeutic agents, such as methotrexate and chlorambucil, in the treatment of cats with pancreatitis and intestinal lymphoma or sclerosing cholangitis. Serum folate level should be evaluated before initiating chemotherapy and supplemental folic acid administered if indicated.

Specific Therapy

Once a diagnosis of pancreatitis is confirmed, potentially more specific therapy can be employed. The majority of dogs with acute pancreatitis respond to fluid therapy and nothing by mouth for 48 hours. Hence, specific therapy is usually reserved for dogs that do not respond to fluid therapy or those with signs of multiorgan system involvement or DIC. Pancreatitis in cats seems to be more chronically active and severe than in dogs; thus cats with a confirmed diagnosis of pancreatitis generally need more support than the majority of dogs.

The specific treatment of pancreatitis has evolved along two lines:

1. Stopping further pancreatitis from occurring
2. Limiting the local and systemic consequences of pancreatitis

Therapies aimed at inhibiting pancreatic secretion (e.g., glucagon, somatostatin) or the intracellular activation of proteases (e.g., gabexate mesilate), which have been of benefit in ameliorating the severity of experimental pancreatitis, have shown little benefit in the treatment of patients with spontaneous pancreatitis. This lack of success is probably related to the timing of therapy in relation to the development of pancreatitis. Experimental therapy is usually initiated before or shortly after the induction of pancreatitis, whereas most clinical patients are not presented until 24 to 48 hours after the onset of pancreatitis. Support for this hypothesis is provided by the efficacy of somatostatin and gabexate mesilate in reducing pancreatitis in humans undergoing elective procedures, such as endoscopic retrograde cholecystopancreatography, that are associated with pancreatitis.

The lack of success with inhibiting the progression of spontaneous pancreatitis has led to increased emphasis on damage limitation: ameliorating the effects of inflammatory mediators or pancreatic enzymes on the patient and maintaining pancreatic perfusion.

Coagulation abnormalities should be pursued, and treatment with parenteral vitamin K can be assessed. If a coagulopathy (e.g., DIC) or hypoproteinemia is present, or if the patient's condition is deteriorating, fresh frozen plasma (5 to 10 ml/lb) may be beneficial in alleviating the coagulopathy and hypoproteinemia and restoring a more normal protease-antiprotease balance. The administration of heparin (35 to 70 IU/lb three times a day) may be potentially useful in ameliorating DIC, promoting adequate microcirculation in the pancreas, and clearing lipemic serum. In experimental pancreatitis, isovolemic rehydration with dextran has also been shown to promote pancreatic microcirculation in dogs. A dopamine infusion had a protective effect when administered to cats within 12 hours of induction of experimental pancreatitis. Therapy to abrogate the systemic inflammatory response with antagonists of PAF (e.g., lexipafant), IL-1, and TNF-α holds promise for the future.

Oral pancreatic enzyme extracts have been reported to reduce pain in humans with chronic pancreatitis, though this is controversial. They are less likely to be effective in dogs because they do not appear to have a protease-mediated negative feedback system.

Dietary Management

Our ability to make precise recommendations for dietary management of acute pancreatitis is limited by the absence of controlled studies of the dietary management of this syndrome.

Dogs. In dogs suspected of having acute pancreatitis, oral intake is usually withheld for the initial 48 hours and then gradually reintroduced if tolerated. The rationale for giving nothing by mouth even when vomiting is absent is to "rest the pancreas" by decreasing pancreatic stimulation. Because fats and amino acids are potent stimulators of pancreatic enzyme secretion, their effects are initially avoided by feeding a diet high in carbohydrate and then gradually increasing fat and protein content during the recovery period (the first and second weeks after the onset). Continued fat restriction is usually recommended for dogs that have had pancreatitis and is based on clinical and experimental observations that suggest an association between high-fat meals, hyperlipidemia, and a "high plane" of nutrition and pancreatitis. The protein content of the diet may also be important because dogs fed a choline-deficient ethionine-supplemented diet or a protein-restricted high-fat diet develop pancreatitis.

Alternative strategies of minimizing pancreatic stimulation include total parenteral nutrition (TPN) and feeding distal to the CCK-releasing part of the intestine via a jejunostomy tube, but these options are usually reserved for dogs with persistent vomiting or severe pancreatitis. Recent studies in humans indicate that acute pancreatitis may be exacerbated by the early administration of TPN (before 5 days) and that enteral nutrition, administered via a nasojejunostomy tube, can attenuate the systemic inflammatory response and may decrease complications. Feeding tube placement is discussed in Chapter 12.

Cats. In contrast to dogs, where vomiting and abdominal pain predominate, pancreatitis in cats is usually associated with anorexia and weight loss. The presence of anorexia and weight loss in cats with pancreatitis may be a significant contributing factor to their poor prognosis. Prolonged fasting (more than 3 days) to avoid pancreatic stimulation may only serve to compound malnutrition. The clinician is faced with the dilemma of having to provide nutritional support to prevent or reverse malnutrition and hepatic lipidosis and fasting the patient to prevent pancreatic stimulation. The surgical or endoscopic placement of a gastrostomy or esophagostomy tube may circumvent anorexia where vomiting is not a problem. Current dogma suggests that a diet that limits pancreatic stimulation and provides adequate nutrients should be fed. However, this ideal may be difficult to achieve because cats are physiologically adapted to diets that are high in fat and protein, and most balanced cat foods contain between 30% and 60% fat on an energy basis. I have had success when feeding commercial maintenance or intestinal diets through a gastrostomy tube.

As discussed above, the endoscopic or surgical placement of a jejunostomy tube and feeding a liquid diet distal to the duodenum and TPN are other solutions to providing balanced nutrition and minimizing pancreatic secretion that may prove useful in refractory cases.

Patient Monitoring

Patients with suspected or confirmed pancreatitis should be carefully monitored to enable early detection of shock or other systemic abnormalities. Minimal monitoring for stable patients includes regular assessment of vital signs and fluid and electrolyte balance. In those with systemic abnormalities, monitoring should be more aggressive and may include vital signs, weight, hematocrit, total protein concentration, fluid intake and output, blood pressure (central venous and arterial), levels of electrolytes and glucose, acid-base status, platelets, and coagulation status. Monitoring amylase, lipase, or TLI on an intermittent sequential basis may also help to support resolution or progression of pancreatic inflammation.

Ultrasound-guided fine-needle aspiration of the pancreas may enable infected pancreatic necrosis to be detected. Ultrasonography may also enable detection of delayed consequences of acute pancreatitis such as pancreatic abscessation, pseudocyst formation, and biliary obstruction.

Surgical Intervention

Surgery is potentially indicated to remove devitalized tissue in patients with infected pancreatic necrosis and to investigate and relieve persistent biliary obstruction. The removal or drainage of abscesses is another indication for surgery. Resection or surgical drainage of pancreatic pseudocysts is not always necessary because these can resolve spontaneously or following percutaneous drainage. Pancreatitis that is recurrent or is unresponsive to treatment may also require surgery to confirm a diagnosis and to exclude pancreatic cancer.

Surgery has often been necessary to confirm an antemortem diagnosis of acute pancreatitis in cats. The increased application of ultrasonography and measurement of TLI has led to a reduced dependency on surgery in cats with high TLI and sonographic abnormalities. However, it should be stressed that cats with pancreatitis often have concomitant abnormalities in other organ systems (e.g., liver and intestine), and biopsy of these organs and the pancreas may be indicated to optimize diagnosis and treatment. Transient euglycemia and reduced insulin requirements were noted after the removal of a pancreatic abscess in one cat, suggesting that surgical intervention may be beneficial in these cases.

Prognosis

Dogs. The prognosis for dogs with mild acute pancreatitis is good. Severe or recurrent pancreatitis is associated with a guarded prognosis.

Cats. The prognosis for acute pancreatitis in cats must always be considered guarded. Where extensive hepatic lipidosis is present or suppurative pancreatitis is diagnosed, the prognosis is poor.

| EXOCRINE PANCREATIC INSUFFICIENCY

EPI is characterized by a lack of effective pancreatic exocrine secretions in the small intestine. It is most often a consequence of the severe reduction in pancreatic mass caused by pancreatic acinar atrophy, or chronic pancreatitis, but may occur secondary to excessive secretion of gastric acid (increased destruction and decreased activity of pancreatic enzymes by acid) or severe protein malnutrition (decreased synthesis of pancreatic enzymes). Pancreatic hypoplasia and concomitant diabetes mellitus have also been rarely documented in dogs.

Pancreatic acinar atrophy (PAA) is probably the most common cause of EPI in the dog, whereas chronic pancreatitis is the most common cause in the cat. The precise cause of PAA has not yet been determined (Box 10-2). A familial predisposition to PAA has been reported in German shepherd dogs, collies, and English setters. Histologically, canine PAA closely resembles the pancreas of CBA/J mice in which ultrastructural and biochemical studies suggested that pancreatic atrophy was a consequence of the premature activation of trypsinogen and chymotrypsinogen within the zymogen granule. However, it is impossible to determine the cause of atrophy in a pancreas with end-stage disease, so prospective studies of the development of canine PAA have been conducted. The initial study demonstrated that subcellular pancreatic abnormalities (characterized by fusion of zymogen granules and proliferation of endoplasmic reticulum) and a decrease in TLI preceded the development

---

BOX 10-2	**Potential Etiologies of Pancreatic Acinar Atrophy in Dogs**

Hereditary
   German shepherd dogs, collies, English setters
Primary acinar problem
   Pancreatic secretory trypsin inhibitor deficiency
Nutritional
   Selective malabsorption
   Vitamin or mineral deficiency (e.g., E or B_{12})
Decreased trophic stimuli
   Abnormal cholecystokinin (CCK) release
Immune destruction
   Cell-mediated, antipancreatic antibodies
Apoptosis

---

of gross pancreatic atrophy, reduced pancreatic protease secretion, and diarrhea in one dog. However, a subsequent investigation in dogs with subclinical EPI, detected by assay of circulating TLI, has shown that atrophy is preceded by a marked lymphocytic infiltration, suggesting an autoimmune basis for the disease. Studies that have examined the possibility that decreased CCK release or antipancreatic antibodies play a role in the genesis of PAA have yielded no evidence to support their involvement in the development of PAA.

Pathophysiology

The extensive loss of exocrine pancreatic mass (approximately 90%), whether by atrophy or chronic inflammation, is required before signs of EPI are evident. The major signs of EPI are diarrhea, weight loss, and an ensuing ravenous appetite. These signs can be attributed to decreased intraduodenal concentrations of pancreatic enzymes, bicarbonate, and various other factors with resultant malassimilation of fats, carbohydrates, and proteins. Abnormalities in levels of fat-soluble vitamins and cobalamin have been documented in dogs and cats with EPI and may contribute to their clinical condition. Increased susceptibility of the enterocyte to damage by bacteria or their products and potentially an increase in small intestinal flora have been observed in dogs with EPI. Other abnormalities encountered in dogs with EPI include alterations in glucose homeostasis (subclinical glucose intolerance), pancreatic and GI regulatory peptides (e.g., vasoactive intestinal polypeptide, gastric inhibitory polypeptide), and the regulation of small intestinal mucosal growth, enzyme synthesis, and enzyme degradation. The clinical significance of these abnormalities is unclear. The marked maldigestion of nutrients in EPI may lead to the development of protein–calorie malnutrition, which can further compromise residual pancreatic function, intestinal absorption, and metabolic homeostasis.

Diagnosis

A diagnosis of EPI is usually made on the basis of compatible historical and clinical findings and by ruling out infectious, parasitic, metabolic, and anatomic causes of small bowel diarrhea and demonstrating a subnormal circulating concentration of TLI (species-specific TLI: less than 2.5 μg/L in dogs, less than 8 μg/L in cats).

Clinical Findings

Dogs and cats with EPI usually have a history of chronic small bowel diarrhea (large volume, cowpat consistency) and weight loss (mild to extreme), which is often associated with a ravenous appetite. Poor hair coat and marked muscle loss are observed in some patients. Although pancreatic acinar atrophy is prevalent in young German shepherd dogs, it is important to note that many other breeds are affected by EPI. Young dogs diagnosed with EPI are usually suspected to have pancreatic acinar atrophy, whereas older dogs and cats with EPI probably have a higher incidence of chronic pancreatitis.

Clinicopathologic Tests

Results of routine hematologic and biochemical studies are usually unremarkable in cats with EPI. Modest increases in ALT concentration and a decrease in cholesterol concentration are observed in some dogs. Serum concentrations of cobalamin are usually subnormal in both dogs and cats with EPI. Serum concentrations of folate may be high in dogs with EPI. Serum folate concentrations are decreased in some cats as a consequence of concommitant inflammatory bowel disease or intestinal lymphoma. Serum concentrations of vitamin E are often markedly reduced in dogs with EPI. Vitamin K–sensitive coagulopathies have been reported in cats with EPI. The presence of hyperglycemia and glucosuria should prompt consideration of diabetes mellitus secondary to chronic pancreatitis or pancreatic hypoplasia.

Tests of Pancreatic Function or Mass

The analysis of feces for proteolytic activity (film digestion, azocaesin assay) and the indirect estimation of intestinal chymotrypsin activity (BT-PABA test) for the diagnosis of EPI have been largely superseded by the development of an assay that determines the concentration of TLI in serum. Serum TLI is considered to be derived solely from the pancreas and can be used as an indicator of pancreatic mass or inflammation. In dogs and cats with EPI caused by atrophy or chronic inflammation, the amount of TLI that leaks from the pancreas into the circulation is reduced and a subnormal TLI concentration can be demonstrated. Healthy dogs usually have a fasting (overnight fast) TLI concentration greater than 5.0 μg/L, whereas dogs with EPI caused by reduced pancreatic mass have fasting concentrations less than 2.5 μg/L. Preliminary information in cats suggests that healthy cats have a fasting TLI concentration greater than 17 μg/L, whereas cats with EPI have fasting concentrations less than 8 μg/L. When the TLI concentration is between 2.5 and 5.0 μg/L in dogs and 8 and 17 μg/L in cats, the patient may be normal or may have partial EPI and the test should be repeated after ensuring adequate fasting. Patients with persistently intermediate TLI concentrations are likely to have partial EPI that may progress to complete EPI.

The BT-PABA test and fecal azocaesin digest test are likely to be the best means of diagnosing EPI that is secondary to the destruction of pancreatic enzymes by hypersecretion of gastric acid.

Treatment

Exogenous Pancreatic Enzymes

Powdered pancreatic extracts (dog: 0.12 to 0.2 g/lb body weight per meal or 2 tsp/45-lb body weight per meal or 2.5 g/300-g food; cat: 1 tsp per meal two times a day) are far superior to enteric-coated tablets, granules, and capsules. Preincubating enzymes with food is not advantageous. Raw chopped pancreas (dog: 0.7 to 1.4 g/lb body weight per meal; cat: 30 to 90 g per meal two times a day) is an effective treatment when available and can be stored frozen for at least 3 months. In patients that show a good response the dose of pancreatic extract or pancreas can be gradually decreased to the smallest amount that maintains remission.

Diet

In clinical practice a good response has been observed when patients with EPI are fed either a normal maintenance diet or a highly digestible fat-restricted diet that is supplemented with pancreatic enzymes. The outcome in terms of survival of dogs with EPI is reported to be similar in dogs with EPI fed maintenance diets and those fed modified diets.

Highly digestible fat-restricted diets are theoretically attractive due to the limited digestive capabilities of patients with EPI. Clinical studies in dogs have shown highly digestible diets to be beneficial in reducing fecal volume, borborygmi, and flatulence but have no clear effects on fecal consistency, appetite, or coprophagy. Studies in dogs with experimental EPI suggest that it is fat digestibility, rather than the amount of fat, that is important and have demonstrated an inverse correlation between fat digestibility and fecal water content. However, further controlled trials are necessary to determine if feeding a fat-restricted highly digestible diet is warranted on a routine basis. Fat-restricted, highly digestible diets may be useful in the treatment of dogs with EPI that show poor weight gain in response to initial treatment with enzyme therapy and a maintenance diet. Dietary supplementation with medium-chain triglyceride oil (2 to 4 ml per meal) may also be beneficial in these patients.

Vitamin Supplementation

Cobalamin deficiency can have a myriad of effects on the body, so the provision of supplementary cobalamin (cyanocobalamin, vitamin B_{12}) is prudent. It has recently emerged that dogs and cats do not have the capacity to store large quantities of cobalamin in their bodies and can become rapidly depleted when normal homeostasis is disrupted by EPI or intestinal disease. Studies in dogs indicate that the parenteral administration of a single dose of cyanocobalamin (1 mg subcutaneously) is enough to prevent recurrence of metabolic abnormalities for up to 1 month. Cats may require supplementation every 2 weeks to maintain normal serum concentrations of cobalamin. Dogs with EPI may also have to be supplemented with Vitamin E (400 to 500 IU orally once a day for 1 month). A vitamin K–responsive coagulopathy has been reported in cats with EPI, and it seems sensible to examine the vitamin K status of dogs with EPI that have laboratory evidence of a coagulopathy.

Treatment Failures
Confirm EPI

Review the patient's history, physical examination, and laboratory findings to ensure that EPI is a likely cause of the diarrhea. If the TLI test results do not fit the patient, then resubmit the test and/or evaluate pancreatic function by measuring fecal proteolytic activity.

Inadequate Enzyme Supplementation

Ensure that the enzyme supplement being administered is appropriate (non–enteric-coated powder), current, and being fed at the correct dose. A new batch, change of preparation, or increased amounts may produce a response. In dogs if a response is not being achieved with a dose of 0.2 g/lb of non–enteric-coated powdered extract or 1.4 g/lb body weight per meal whole pancreas, consider other reasons for treatment failure. Some dogs and cats develop aversions to the enzyme supplement, and raw pancreas may have to be used if attempts to disguise the taste are unsuccessful. Rarely some dogs develop a stomatitis related to the enzyme supplement.

Hyperacidity

Lipase is the most acid-sensitive enzyme, and its activity may be enhanced by decreasing gastric acid secretion. In dogs a treatment trial with cimetidine (2.5 to 5 mg/lb orally two times a day) may reveal whether the enzyme supplement is being inactivated. This problem has not been studied in cats with EPI.

Antibiotic-Responsive Diarrhea/"Bacterial Overgrowth"

Small intestinal bacterial overgrowth has been diagnosed in dogs with EPI when a cut-off value greater than 5 (log 10 colony-forming units [CFUs] per milliliter) of duodenal juice is applied. The bacterial flora of dogs with EPI created by pancreatic duct ligation increases after the induction of EPI but returns towards baseline after supplementation with pancreatic enzymes. These observations suggest that increases in bacterial numbers in EPI are a consequence of increased substrate availability secondary to EPI. The bacterial counts in this experimental study (6.4 [log 10 CFUs per milliliter]) were within the range for healthy dogs, and antimicrobials were not needed to control clinical signs. Most dogs with spontaneous EPI respond to treatment with enzyme supplementation and do not require antibiotics. However, some dogs need and respond to antibiotic therapy. In those dogs it is likely that the balance between intestinal damage and repair is altered by EPI: increased degradation of microvillar enzymes by the increased (relatively) bacterial flora versus decreased degradation by pancreatic enzymes in the face of decreased synthesis of microvillar enzymes.

The abnormal flora cannot be predicted accurately by serum concentrations of cobalamin and folate, so a trial with an antibiotic such as oxytetracycline (9 mg/lb orally two times a day for 28 days) may be undertaken in dogs that are unresponsive to enzyme and dietary manipulation. Antibiotic-responsive diarrhea has not been reported in cats with EPI.

Small Intestinal Disease

Some dogs and cats with EPI have small intestinal disease causing malabsorption despite adequate enzyme supplementation. Results of routine hematologic and biochemical studies are almost always normal in uncomplicated EPI, so abnormalities such as hypoproteinemia (which may indicate a protein-losing enteropathy) should be pursued. Dogs and cats with EPI that respond poorly to the above treatment modifications and have no evidence of extraintestinal disorders usually require further investigation of the small intestine. Further evaluation that should be considered includes checking the serum folate level, ultrasound, and endoscopy with intestinal biopsy.

REFERENCES

Pathogenesis of Pancreatic Disease

Denham W, Norman J: The potential role of therapeutic cytokine manipulation in acute pancreatitis, *Surg Clin North Am* 79:767, 1999.

Karne S, Gorelick FS: Etiopathogenesis of acute pancreatitis, *Surg Clin North Am* 79:699, 1999.

Ruaux CG et al.: Tumor necrosis factor-alpha at presentation in 60 cases of spontaneous canine acute pancreatitis, *Vet Immunol Immunopathol* 72:369, 1999.

Simpson KW: Current concepts of the pathogenesis and pathophysiology of acute pancreatitis in the dog and cat, *Compendium for Continuing Education for the Practicing Veterinarian* 15:247, 1993.

Simpson KW et al.: Cholecystokinin-8 induces edematous pancreatitis in dogs which is associated with a short burst of trypsinogen activation, *Dig Dis Sci* 40:2152, 1995.

Weiss DJ, Gagne JM, Armstrong PJ: Relationship between inflammatory hepatic disease and inflammatory bowel disease, pancreatitis, and nephritis in the cat, *J Am Vet Med Assoc* 209:1114, 1996.

Westermarck E et al.: Sequential study of pancreatic structure and function during development of pancreatic acinar atrophy in a German shepherd dog, *Am J Vet Res* 54:1088, 1993.

Wiberg ME, Saari SAM, Westermarck E: Exocrine pancreatic atrophy in German shepherd dogs and rough-coated collies: an end result of lymphocytic pancreatitis, *Vet Pathol* 36:530, 1999.

Diagnosis and Treatment of Acute Pancreatitis

Akol KG et al.: Acute pancreatitis in cats with hepatic lipidosis, *J Vet Intern Med* 7:205, 1993.

Bruner JM et al.: High feline trypsin-like immunoreactivity in a cat with pancreatitis and hepatic lipidosis, *J Am Vet Med Assoc* 210:1757, 1997.

Hess RS et al.: Clinical, clinicopathologic, radiographic, and ultrasonographic abnormalities in dogs with fatal acute pancreatitis: 70 cases (1986-1995), *J Am Vet Med Assoc* 213:665, 1998.

Hess RS et al.: Evaluation of risk factors for fatal acute pancreatitis in dogs, *J Am Vet Med Assoc* 214:46, 1999.

Hill RC, Van Winkle TJ: Acute necrotizing and acute suppurative pancreatitis in the cat: a retrospective study of 40 cases (1976-1989), *J Vet Intern Med* 7:25, 1993.

Johnson SE: Fluid therapy for gastrointestinal, pancreatic, and hepatic disease. In DiBartola SP, (ed): *Fluid therapy in small animal practice,* Philadelphia, 1992, WB Saunders.

Karanjia ND et al.: Assay of trypsinogen activation in the cat experimental model of pancreatitis, *Pancreas* 8:189, 1993.

Kitchell BE et al.: Clinical and pathologic changes in experimentally induced acute pancreatitis in cats, *Am J Vet Res* 47:1170, 1986.

Lamb CR et al.: Ultrasonography of pancreatic neoplasia in the dog: retrospective review of 16 cases, *Vet Rec* 137:65, 1995.

Lucena R et al.: Effects of dexamethasone administration on serum trypsin-like immunoreactivity in healthy dogs, *Am J Vet Res* 60:1357, 1999.

Macintire DK: The acute abdomen: differential diagnosis and management, *Semin Vet Med Surg (Small Anim)* 3:302, 1988.

Murtaugh RJ: Acute pancreatitis: diagnostic dilemmas, *Semin Vet Med Surg (Small Anim)* 2:282, 1987.

Ruaux CG, Atwell RB: A severity score for spontaneous canine acute pancreatitis, *Aust Vet J* 76:804, 1998.

Ruaux CG, Atwell RB: Levels of total alpha-macroglobulin and trypsin-like immunoreactivity are poor indicators of clinical severity in spontaneous canine acute pancreatitis, *Res Vet Sci* 67:83, 1999.

Salisbury SK et al.: Pancreatic abscess in dogs: six cases (1978-1986), *J Am Vet Med Assoc* 193:1104, 1988.

Saunders HM: Ultrasonography of the pancreas. In Kaplan PM, ed: *Problems in veterinary medicine,* vol 3, Ultrasound, Philadelphia, 1991, WB Saunders.

Simpson KW, Lamb CR: Acute pancreatitis in the dog, *In Practice: J Vet Postgrad Clin Study* 17:328, 1995.

Simpson KW et al.: Antemortem diagnosis of pancreatitis in four cats, *J Small Anim Pract* 35:93, 1994.

Steinberg WM, Schlesselman SE: Treatment of acute pancreatitis: comparison of animal and human studies, *Gastroenterlogy* 93:1420, 1987.

Steiner JM, Medinger TL, Williams DA: Development and validation of a radioimmunoassay for feline trypsin-like immunoreactivity, *Am J Vet Res* 57:1417, 1996.

Diagnosis and Treatment of Exocrine Pancreatic Insufficiency

Boari A, Williams DA, Famigli-Bergamini P: Observations on exocrine pancreatic insufficiency in a family of English setter dogs, *J Small Anim Pract* 35:247, 1994.

Hall EJ et al.: A survey of the diagnosis and treatment of canine exocrine pancreatic insufficiency, *J Small Anim Pract* 32:613, 1990.

Simpson JW et al.: Long term management of canine exocrine pancreatic insufficiency, *J Small Anim Pract* 35:133, 1994.

Steiner JM, Williams DA: Feline exocrine pancreatic disorders, *Vet Clin North Am Small Anim Pract* 29:551, 1999.

Westermarck E, Wilberg A, Juntilla J: Role of feeding in the treatment of dogs with pancreatic degenerative atrophy, *Acta Vet Scand* 31:325, 1990.

Williams DA, Batt RM: Sensitivity and specificity of radioimmunoassay of serum trypsin-like immunoreactivity for the diagnosis of canine exocrine pancreatic insufficiency, *J Am Vet Med Assoc* 192:195, 1988.

Williams DA, Batt RM, McLean L: Bacterial overgrowth in the duodenum of dogs with exocrine pancreatic insufficiency, *J Am Vet Med Assoc* 191:201, 1987.

11

ONCOLOGIC DISEASES OF THE DIGESTIVE SYSTEM

Nicole F. Leibman
Victoria S. Larson
Gregory K. Ogilvie

Exciting advances have been made in the diagnosis and treatment of tumors of the gastrointestinal (GI) tract. Without a doubt, as our knowledge base expands regarding diagnostic techniques and the biologic behavior of neoplastic disease, so do our options for methods of diagnosis and treatment. Perhaps just as important is our general awareness that cancer medicine has a tremendous emotional impact on everyone involved, including the owners and the entire veterinary health care team. When approaching the dog or cat with cancer, we must be cognizant that the myths and misperceptions that our clients and the veterinary health care team carry with them can alter judgment and bring us to false conclusions about the management of the disease. Similarly, we must realize that although the veterinary health care team is key in providing medical and surgical care for the patient,

cancer is a disease that has an emotional impact for all people involved. Therefore the myths associated with cancer must first be dispelled through appropriate education, then the veterinary health care team can proceed to meet the nonmedical needs of the client, along with the medical needs of the patient. The next step, which is predicated on the success of these first two steps, is to provide compassionate care to enhance quality of life first and length of life second. Quality of life can be enhanced in part by meeting all the needs of the patient, including providing adequate pain and nausea control and meeting the patient's changing nutritional needs. Fully understanding the cancer we are facing can enhance both length and quality of life. *This understanding is best achieved by first, obtaining a tissue sample from the disease in question (making an accurate tissue diagnosis); second, determining the extent of the disease (staging the cancer); and third, assessing the condition of the patient.*

ORAL TUMORS

Oral tumors represent 6% of all neoplasms in the dog and are the fourth most common neoplasm in dogs. Cancer of the mouth and pharynx occurs more frequently in dogs than in cats. Male dogs may be at greater risk for developing an oral tumor than female dogs. Most oral tumors occur in geriatric patients. *Malignant melanomas, nontonsillar squamous cell carcinomas, and fibrosarcomas are the three most common oral tumors in dogs. Squamous cell carcinoma occurs anywhere in the oral cavity and is by far the most common oral tumor that occurs in the cat.* Metastasis due to oral tumors is rare with the exception of melanomas, high-grade sarcomas, and tonsillar squamous cell carcinomas in both the dog and cat.

Before obtaining a biopsy specimen or attempting surgical resection of an oral tumor, the clininician should confirm the general good health of all dogs and cats with a complete blood count, biochemical profile, total thyroxine (T_4) level, and urinalysis. Thoracic radiographs should be obtained to rule out macroscopic pulmonary metastases. Fine-detail radiographs of the affected area may provide information on the aggressiveness of the tumor. Any local lymphadenopathy should be further investigated by fine-needle aspiration or biopsy performed at the same time as tumor biopsy. In a small percentage of cases, tumor metastasis can be demonstrated in lymph nodes that are not enlarged. Therefore the recommendation is to aspirate and potentially perform a biopsy of the regional lymph nodes in every case. The parotid and medial retropharyngeal lymph nodes should be evaluated. A fine-needle aspirate may in fact provide useful information regarding metastatic disease secondary to malignant oral tumors. The surgical approach for lymph node staging of oral and maxillofacial neoplasms in dogs has been described.

The first surgical excision is the most likely to result in tumor control; therefore appropriate planning is essential. The tumor should not be scraped or peeled from underlying bone, as recurrence is certain and the tumor bed will be enlarged. A definitive aggressive first surgery, such as maxillectomy or mandibulectomy, should be performed in cases where the tumor involves bone. Prompt diagnosis followed by aggressive treatment often results in improved survival and local tumor control.

Specific oral tumors in dogs and cats, the staging of these tumors, and their treatment options are discussed below.

CANINE EPULIDES

Background

Greater than 40% of all oral tumors are of dental or periodontal origin. There are three types of epulides: fibromatous epulides, ossifying epulides, and acanthomatous epulides. All arise from the periodontal ligament; therefore they are intimately related to the dental arcade. Fibromatous epulides and ossifying epulides are benign, whereas acanthomatous epulides may act aggressively by destroying bone and surrounding tissue. Other terms that have been used to describe acanthomatous epulis include *adamantinoma* and *ameloblastoma,* although ameloblastoma may be a distinct tumor seen in young dogs. Most of these tumors are considered benign, although acanthomatous epulides can be locally aggressive.

Epulides affect both sexes at equal rates. Although most affected dogs are middle-age, the age range is wide. Epulides have been documented in dogs as young as 1 year and as old as 15 years of age. Although boxers may be predisposed to developing gingival hyperplasia, this breed does not seem to be at excessive risk for developing epulides.

Clinical Parameters

Dogs with epulides often have malodorous breath, facial swelling, or a lump on the gums. Fibromatous and ossifying epulides are slow-growing, discrete masses that rarely exceed 2 cm in diameter. They are firm gingival tumors covered by oral epithelium. They may be single or multiple but are always discrete and located near teeth. Ossifying epulis differs from fibromatous only in osteoid production.

Acanthomatous epulis is a more rapidly progressive tumor that has a high epithelial component and infiltrates readily into bone. It is usually found in the mandible but may also occur in the maxilla.

Clinical Work-up

On first presentation, epulides may look like other oral tumors; therefore a biopsy of the tumor, aspirates or biopsies of regional lymph nodes, radiographs of the affected bone, chest radiographs, and blood work are warranted. Fibromatous and ossifying epulides are not invasive; therefore high-detail radiographs of the affected bone are unlikely to identify changes in bone. Such radiographs may be helpful in assessing the degree of the specific bony destruction caused by acanthomatous epulides. In one series of 39 dogs with acanthomatous epulis, radiographic changes in bone were primarily osteolytic in 23 dogs and osteoblastic in only 8 dogs. More than 50% of the bone must be replaced by tumor before lysis is evident radiographically; therefore radiographs should not be relied on for surgical margins. Computed tomography (CT) may assist in delineating the margins of tumor involvement more accurately. Technetium-99m nuclide scans tend to overestimate tumor margins by imaging peripheral reactive bone.

Therapeutic Approach

Local gingival excision of an epulis is unlikely to be curative for most cases. These tumors arise from the periodontal ligament and can recur from subgingival tumor tissue. Surgery can be curative if surgical margins include the affected tooth root, as with mandibulectomy or maxillectomy. If normal bone is included in a wide surgical excision, the procedure should be curative. With larger tumors, however, tumor-free margins may be difficult to obtain. In a series of 37 dogs treated with surgery for acanthomatous epulis, there was just 1 local recurrence and all dogs were alive at 1 year. Cryosurgery has been used for treatment of epulides, but it is difficult to penetrate bone using this modality and therefore recurrence is common. Cryotherapy should not be used if it will delay more definitive treatments.

Radiation therapy is a very effective treatment for acanthomatous epulis. In one report of 39 dogs that received between 20 and 70 Gy of orthovoltage radiation therapy on a Monday, Wednesday, Friday schedule, 27 of the dogs had a complete remission. The majority (30 of 39) received 35 to 50 Gy. Twelve dogs did not have a complete regression of visible tumor. Regrowth occurred in only 3 dogs at 8, 18, and 24 months after radiation. Two of these dogs had tumors that responded to reirradiation. Overall survival ranged from 1 month to 102 months, with a median of 37 months. These dogs did not have surgery before radiation therapy. Possible adverse

effects of orthovoltage radiation are osteonecrosis and malignant transformation of the original epulis at the site of radiation. Malignant transformation occurred in 7 dogs at a median of 47 months after radiation therapy. One can reasonably hypothesize that some of these tumors may have been initially misdiagnosed as epulides. In another series of 37 dogs with acanthomatous epulis, progression-free survival for 3 years was 80% after cobalt-60 radiation therapy. These dogs were treated with megavoltage radiation to a total of 48 Gy delivered over 4 weeks on an alternate-day schedule of 4-Gy fractions. Most of the tumors recurred within the field rather than at the margins. Malignant tumor formation at the site of previously irradiated acanthomatous epulides was reported as a complication in 4 of 32 dogs treated in one study.

In one dog an acanthomatous epulis regrew 6 weeks after receiving 50 Gy of orthovoltage radiation therapy. This dog had almost complete regression of the tumor after 10 doses of doxorubicin (30 mg/m^2 intravenously every 3 weeks) and cyclophosphamide (50 mg/m^2 orally daily for 4 days every week) and had stable disease for at least 20 months after starting chemotherapy.

In one study four dogs with acanthomatous epulides were given bleomycin intralesionally. The dose given was 5 mg weekly. Tumors disappeared within 3 to 10 weeks, and no adverse effects were noted. No tumor recurrence was noted for these dogs.

When considering therapy for acanthomatous epulis, the age of the patient should be considered. In younger dogs, surgery may be offered as the treatment of choice owing to the risk, albeit low, of radiation-induced tumorigenesis. For geriatric dogs, radiation-induced malignant transformation may be less of a concern due to the protracted course of this phenomenon. Alternatively, radiation can be considered for the first course option with a reasonable probability of being successful with surgery for the second option, should radiation fail.

Ameloblastomas have been reported in young dogs. These tumors also arise from odontogenic tissue, but they are distinct from acanthomatous epulides. Two dogs younger than 1 year of age with ameloblastoma were treated with surgery; tumors recurred in both dogs within 6 months. A second surgery resulted in a cure for one of these dogs, with no recurrence 105 months after surgery.

ODONTOGENIC TUMORS IN CATS

Background

In one study fibromatous epulis was the third most common feline oral tumor, accounting for 29 of 371 oral tumors (7.8%). Epulides occur in middle-age to older cats. Fibroameloblastoma is a rare tumor that typically affects cats younger than 1 year of age. These tumors are different from the epulides in that they histologically resemble embryonic connective tissue of the dental pulp. These tumors are benign and grow by expansion rather than invasion. Complete surgical excision can be challenging with large tumors.

Clinical Parameters

Cats with oral tumors, including odontogenic tumors, often have malodorous breath, dysphagia, anorexia, oral bleeding, ptyalism, and, in advanced cases, facial deformity. Weight loss may be a common concurrent problem.

Clinical Work-up

Cats with oral tumors should have a biopsy performed, as well as blood work, thoracic radiographs, evaluation of regional lymph nodes via aspiration or biopsy, and fine-detail intraoral radiographs of the affected area. Thoracic radiographs rarely show evidence of metastasis from feline odontogenic tumors because of their typically benign behavior but should be performed as part of a thorough staging scheme for oral tumors.

Therapeutic Approach

The treatment of choice for feline fibroameloblastomas is surgical excision. One must remove a "cuff" of normal bone around the tumor, which requires removal of part of the mandible or maxilla in most cases. Surgery can be curative if adequate surgical margins are obtained. Seven cats with fibroameloblastoma were treated with surgery in one report; one had recurrence of the tumor 42 months later. Four cats had complete tumor control 6, 7, 24, and 36 months after surgery. One cat had tumor recurrence and was tumor-free 5 years after a second surgery. The seventh cat was lost to follow-up. There is no known published literature on treatment for fibromatous epulis in cats,

but a prognosis similar to that of dogs should be expected after surgery or radiation therapy.

ORAL MALIGNANT MELANOMA IN DOGS

Background

Melanoma is the most common oral malignancy found in the dog. *Unlike cutaneous melanomas, which are often benign, melanomas of the oral cavity in dogs are very aggressive and commonly metastasize to local lymph nodes and lungs.* Oral melanomas are often poorly responsive to conventional therapy. Although some oral melanomas may appear histologically benign, these tumors may behave very aggressively. Oral malignant melanomas are most common in poodles, dachshunds, Scottish terriers, golden retrievers, standard and miniature schnauzers, Doberman pinschers, and Irish and Gordon setters.

In three studies totaling 193 dogs with oral melanoma, there were 94 male and 99 female dogs. This is a disease of old dogs. In one study the median age of affected dogs was 11 years; ages ranged from 4 to 16 years.

Clinical Parameters

Most oral melanomas originate in the gingiva, but these tumors can also arise from the palatine, labial, and buccal mucosa.

Clients may present dogs for an oral mass or more frequently for persistent halitosis, bleeding from the mouth, and (occasionally) dysphagia. Tumors may be quite large, ranging in volume up to 64 cm^3 in one study. Although masses are frequently pigmented, amelanotic tumors can occur. Oral melanomas are friable and invasive within the soft tissues of the mouth.

Clinical Work-up

Dogs with oral tumors of any type should be staged using blood work, radiographs of the lesion, a metastasis evaluation of the thorax, and cytologic or histopathologic examination of the lesion and regional lymph nodes. The metastatic rate is very high for oral melanoma, but the time to metastasis varies. At diagnosis, fine-needle aspiration of the mandibular lymph nodes (both ipsilateral and contralateral), as well as any enlarged node, should be performed for cytologic examination. It is important to remember that nodes that are palpably within normal parameters can still demonstrate metastatic disease. The surgical approach for lymph node evaluation has been previously published. In one study, only 5 (12%) of 41 dogs had metastatic disease in regional lymph nodes at the time of diagnosis. Aspiration cytologic findings that are suspicious should be confirmed by surgical biopsy. Thoracic radiographs may indicate pulmonary metastasis at the time of diagnosis. Pulmonary metastasis, however, frequently occurs late in the course of the disease or may be a micrometastasis at the time of diagnosis and therefore undetectable by radiography. In one study, only 3 (7%) of 41 dogs had evidence of pulmonary metastasis at diagnosis, but at the time of death, metastatic rate for this tumor approximated 80%. Melanoma may also spread systemically, and metastasis has been reported to kidney, myocardium, brain, and other sites.

Metastasis due to melanoma probably occurs early in the course of this disease (during clinical stages I and II, indicating small, localized disease); however, metastases are often not detected until long after the primary melanoma is resected. The growth rate of metastases may vary, and it is this variation, rather than the time that metastasis occurs, that determines survival time.

Some investigators have found that the World Health Organization (WHO) staging system provides prognostic information, but an alternative staging system has been proposed that includes the WHO criteria and also uses the mitotic index from histopathologic results and location within the oral cavity. This staging system also offers prognostic information.

Current recommendations for staging oral melanoma therefore include a complete blood count, biochemical profile, urinalysis, lymph node evaluation by cytologic examination or biopsy, thoracic radiographs, and tumor measurements, as well as anatomic location and evaluation of mitotic index as determined by histopathologic findings.

Prognostic Factors

Some studies have demonstrated significantly longer survival for dogs with stage I (small) tumors (median, 511 days) than for dogs with stage II or III tumors (median, 164 days) (Table 11-1). Small melanomas were also associated with longer survival times in another study.

One study found that the location of the tumor was not prognostic, but two other studies indicated that tumors of the rostral mandible and the caudal maxilla had longer remissions and survival after surgery. Another study found longer survival times for dogs with tumors that had fewer than three mitotic figures per high-power field.

Therapeutic Approach

Surgery is the treatment of choice for oral melanoma and should consist of mandibulectomy or maxillectomy. Radiation has a role in local tumor control. Chemotherapy with platinum compounds, perhaps combined with liposome-encapsulated muramyl-tripeptide-phosphatidylethanolamine (L-MTP-PE, not yet commercially available) immunotherapy, may offer the best adjunctive treatment for metastatic disease.

Although metastatic rate with oral melanoma is high, metastases frequently are not observed until late in the course of disease, occasionally more than 1 year after local therapy. Most dogs therefore are euthanized because of progression or recurrence of local disease. Surgery should be aggressive from the outset; it may prolong survival and provide palliation. Aggressive local therapy should include resection of underlying bone. In one early study 34 of 49 dogs had local recurrence of tumor, and 33 dogs developed metastases. The recurrence rate of 84% probably reflects the less aggressive nature of the surgery, because more recent studies reported local recurrence rates of less than 15% for melanomas treated by mandibulectomy to 48% for tumors treated by maxillectomy. Both mandibulectomy and maxillectomy are tolerated well by dogs, with median hospitalization times ranging from 2 days for simple excision to 8 days for total hemimandibulectomy. Eighty-five percent of owners in one study who decided to treat their dogs with mandibulectomy or maxillectomy were very satisfied with the outcome. In three studies, dogs treated with aggressive surgery had a median survival time of 7.3 to 9.1 months, compared with seven dogs that did not have surgery and survived a median of 2 months. *Mandibulectomy or maxillectomy should be the first surgery used to treat oral melanoma in dogs. Less aggressive surgeries do not prolong survival and make subsequent surgery more difficult.*

Surgical excision was used to treat five dogs with melanoma of the tongue and achieved local control in three dogs, with survival times ranging from 3 months to 45 months (median, 19 months). Only one dog developed metastases.

TABLE 11-1	Clinical Stages of Canine Oral Melanoma (World Health Organization)			
	Criteria			
Clinical Stage	**Tumor**	**Node**	**Metastasis**	**Percentage of Dogs**
Stage I	<2 cm	−	−	43
Stage II	2–4 cm	−	−	44
Stage III	>4 cm or any bone invasion	+	−	13
Stage IV	Any	Any	+	Not available

T: PRIMARY TUMOR

T_1 Tumor in situ or ≤2 cm maximum diameter (volume ≤8 cm^3)
T_2 Tumor 2-4 cm maximum diameter (volume 8-64 cm^3)
T_3 Tumor >4 cm maximum diameter (volume >64 cm^3)

MITOTIC INDEX

(a) ≤3 per high power field
(b) >3 per high power field
Oral cavity or oropharyngeal location
(1) Rostral mandible/caudal maxilla
(2) Other

N: REGIONAL LYMPH NODES

N_0 No evidence of regional node involvement
N_1 Histologic evidence of regional node involvement
N_2 Fixed nodes

M: DISTANT METASTASIS

M_0 No evidence of distant metastasis
M_1 Distant metastasis (including distant nodes)

STAGE GROUPING

	T	N	M
I	T_1a^1	N_0	M_0
II	T_1a^2, any T_1b, T_2a^1	N_0	M_0
	Any T	N_1	M_0
III	T_2a^2, any T_2b or T_3	N_0	M_0
	Any T	N_2	M_0
	Any T	Any N	M_1

Within 6 months of surgery the majority of patients will have developed metastatic disease. However, metastases may not be visible for longer than 1 year after surgery. After metastases develop, dogs may still survive for an extended period of time, depending on the growth rate. Dogs may tolerate pulmonary metastatic disease with very little apparent effect on their quality of life.

Radiation therapy has been used and certainly has a role in the treatment of melanoma, particularly for small tumors. In one study 33 dogs with melanoma were treated with 48 Gy of ^{60}Co

teletherapy. Five dogs had local recurrence. One dog had regional lymph node metastasis, and 14 developed distant metastasis. Dogs with rostrally located tumors and dogs with smaller tumors had longer remissions. Median progression-free survival was estimated to be 14 months. In another study, dogs were treated with 48 Gy over 4 weeks on an alternate-day schedule with 4-Gy fractions. In 8% of the dogs, severe acute reactions were recognized (tumors other than melanoma were also included). After completion of radiation, dogs with malignant melanoma in this study were 2.6 times more likely than dogs with squamous cell carcinoma to develop tumor progression. Dogs with larger or more invasive tumors had a worse prognosis. In another study 36 dogs with oral melanomas were treated with 36 Gy given in four fractions of 9 Gy at 7-day intervals. In 25 of the 36 dogs, complete remission was achieved and median survival for these dogs was 37 weeks. None of the dogs in this study suffered severe acute effects, and most died of metastatic disease. Local control of oral melanoma (53% complete response) has been achieved with coarse fractionation using three 8-Gy fractions.

A review of the literature would lead to the conclusion that chemotherapy has demonstrated very little effect on survival times in dogs with oral melanoma. Drugs such as dacarbazine (DTIC) (1000 mg/m^2 intravenously every 3 weeks), doxorubicin (30 mg/m^2 intravenously every 3 weeks), and melphalan (0.23 mg/lb intravenously every 4 weeks) have not had repeatable success. Platinum compounds may be more efficacious; cisplatin (60 mg/m^2 intravenously every 3 weeks) provided partial response for a dog with metastatic disease, and carboplatin (300 mg/m^2 intravenously every 3 weeks) appears to have some efficacy, although the response rate is still probably less than 30%. Intralesional chemotherapy with cisplatin in purified bovine collagen matrix material has been used successfully to treat oral melanomas. Dogs were treated with an average of 20 mg of cisplatin delivered over an average of 5.2 treatments. Dogs with complete responses had a mean survival of 54 weeks, whereas those having a partial response had a mean survival of 14 weeks.

Immunotherapy has a role in treating melanoma in many species. Cimetidine, which appears to have an immunomodulating effect by inhibition of suppressor T cells, has been shown to cause regression of melanoma in some horses, although its role in the treatment of the disease in dogs is not defined. Immunotherapy with interleukin-2 has been beneficial in treating humans with melanoma. Combined with tumor necrosis factor, this treatment might be useful for dogs. This combination was administered to 13 dogs with measurable oral melanoma. Five dogs showed reduction in tumor size, although only two had durable responses. One of these dogs had a complete remission for more than 3 years.

Immunotherapy with heat-inactivated *Corynebacterium parvum* (0.045 mg/lb intravenously per week) was used as an adjunct to surgery in 42 dogs. *C. parvum* activates and increases production of

macrophages, which enhances the antibody response. Improved survival over surgery alone has been reported when oral melanoma was treated with a combination of surgery and *C. parvum*. Immunotherapy with *C. parvum* was found to benefit dogs with small tumors (stage I). L-MTP-PE, a more specific macrophage activator, improves survival in dogs treated after surgery for oral melanoma, with a median survival of 346 days. L-MTP-PE was administered to 24 dogs after surgery, and 26 dogs received a placebo. Only 8 (33%) of the L-MTP-PE dogs had died at an interim analysis, whereas 14 (54%) of the placebo group had died.

Granulocyte-macrophage colony-stimulating factor (GM-CSF) transfected vaccines using autologous tumor cells have been used in dogs with melanoma. Direct intratumoral injection of GTM-CSG plasmid DNA induced partial or complete tumor regression and prolonged survival times compared with historical controls.

ORAL MELANOMA IN CATS

Background

Oral melanoma is very rare in cats. They occur in older cats with no apparent sex or breed predisposition.

Clinical Parameters

Cats with oral melanoma show signs of drooling and facial swelling. Tumors occur in the gingiva, palate, and mandible. These tumors may be pigmented.

Clinical Work-up

Any oral tumor requires staging by blood work, radiographs, and local lymph node evaluation. Metastasis of oral melanoma in cats is common, although it sometimes is late to occur.

Therapeutic Approach

Three cats with oral melanomas were treated with surgical excision. All three died as a result of metastatic disease within 5 months of surgery. Oral melanoma is an aggressive neoplasm, and, without therapy adjunctive to surgery, a poor prognosis should be given. Radiation therapy has been shown to be effective in controlling localized disease. Some believe that carboplatin is an effective drug for control of this tumor; however, there have not been any published studies to confirm this.

ORAL SQUAMOUS CELL CARCINOMA IN DOGS

Background

The second most common oral malignancy in dogs is squamous cell carcinoma. It is usually found in the gingival tissue, although the tongue and tonsils are frequently affected. Tumors of the tonsil behave very differently from other squamous cell carcinomas and are considered separately in this chapter.

Squamous cell carcinoma usually occurs in older dogs; the average age is 9 years. There is no apparent breed or gender predilection, although one study of squamous cell carcinoma of the tongue found that 43% of affected dogs had a white hair coat and 30% were poodles. *Papillary squamous cell carcinoma* occurs in dogs as young as 2 months of age and is a progressive disease with a high rate of lytic bone involvement. *Dogs with this type of tumor are almost always less than 2 years of age* (Figure 11-1).

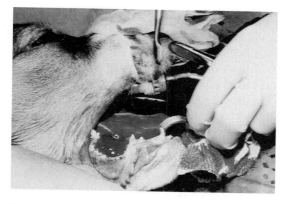

FIGURE 11-1 An intraoperative biopsy of a 7-week-old puppy with dramatic osteolysis of the underlying mandible due to an oral papillary squamous cell carcinoma. Radiation therapy resulted in a cure. She died 13 years later of unrelated causes. Oral papillary squamous cell carcinoma is a curable disease by either surgery or radiation therapy.

Clinical Parameters

Most oral squamous cell carcinomas occur within the rostral portion of the mouth, and the majority occur in the maxilla. However, in one study the most common area for these tumors was the tonsils. Affected dogs show the same signs as do dogs with other oral tumors. The most common signs are drooling, halitosis, and (occasionally) dysphagia. Most dogs have shown signs for 3 months or less, but some dogs may show signs for 6 months to 1 year before diagnosis.

Clinical Work-up

Biopsy is required to differentiate squamous cell carcinoma from amelanotic melanoma, ulcerated fibrosarcoma, or other less common tumors. Staging should be performed as previously described for other oral tumors. Squamous cell carcinoma is highly invasive, and high-detail radiographs of the skull often reveal extensive bony lysis. Bony lysis alone should not be relied on for surgical margins or radiotherapy field size, because this underestimates tumor size. CT or MRI scanning is often helpful in planning radiation therapy and/or surgical excision.

Gingival squamous cell carcinoma rarely metastasizes. Regional lymph nodes are frequently enlarged at diagnosis, and, as for all oral tumors, they should be aspirated and/or biopsy should be performed on them (even if they are not enlarged) for cytologic or histopathologic examination; however, these nodes are usually reactive. In one study 11 of 33 dogs had lymphadenopathy, and only 3 of these dogs had metastatic disease. After therapy, regional lymph node metastasis is still uncommon; however, metastasis was documented in 5 (21%) of 24 dogs in three case series. In contrast, squamous cell carcinoma of the tongue seems more aggressive; 9 (43%) of 21 dogs in one study developed metastasis to lymph nodes, lung, or bone.

Prognostic Factors

One study reported that dogs with maxillary tumors had a longer average response to radiation therapy (12 months) than did dogs with mandibular (3.4 months) or soft tissue tumors (1.8 months). Eight dogs that were younger than 6 years of age lived for a median of 58 months after radiation; older dogs lived for a median of 6 months. Dogs with rostrally located tumors live longer than dogs with caudal tumors, whereas dogs with tumors that extend both rostrally and caudally have significantly shorter survival times. Therefore larger tumors with larger radiation fields are associated with shorter survival. Megavoltage radiation therapy in dogs with nontonsillar squamous cell carcinoma was associated with shorter median survival in dogs older than 9 years of age compared with younger dogs (median survival, 315 versus 1080 days, respectively).

Therapeutic Approach

Rostral gingival squamous cell carcinoma has a generally low metastatic rate, which makes this malignancy a good candidate for local therapies such as surgery and radiation. Aggressive surgery is necessary to obtain adequate surgical margins. Maxillectomy and mandibulectomy have been used to treat this tumor. From several different reports, median survival ranged from 9 to 18 months. Recurrence was more frequent than metastasis after surgery. *Incomplete surgical resection is commonly associated with recurrence, which emphasizes the importance of early diagnosis and obtaining wide surgical margins by mandibulectomy or maxillectomy at the first surgery.* Adjunctive radiation therapy may also be useful.

In 33 dogs, orthovoltage radiation therapy without surgery was used to treat oral squamous cell carcinoma to a total dose of approximately 40 Gy. Overall average survival was approximately 14 months; however, the size and location of the tumor, as well as the age of dog, influenced these figures. Recurrence was noted in 15 dogs, metastasis in 3, and serious complications (e.g., bone necrosis) from radiation in 2 dogs. In another study 39 dogs with squamous cell carcinoma were treated with 48 Gy of ^{60}Co teletherapy delivered over 4 weeks on an alternate-day basis. Twelve dogs had local recurrence, 1 dog developed metastases to regional lymph nodes, and 2 dogs had distant metastases. Dogs with rostrally located tumors and dogs with smaller tumors had longer remissions. Median progression-free survival was approximately 13.6 months. In another study dogs with nontonsillar squamous cell carcinoma had a median survival of 450 days after megavoltage radiation therapy.

Surgery combined with radiation gives the best control for gingival squamous cell carcinoma, and postsurgical radiation should be considered for dogs with large tumors or for dogs with tumors that have tumor-present margins on surgical histopathologic examination. One dog treated in this way had no evidence of disease 16 months after treatment.

Squamous cell carcinoma of the tongue is a more aggressive tumor than gingival squamous cell carcinoma. Metastatic disease in this location often determines survival. Unless wide surgical margins are obtained, recurrence is common. Complete removal of the tongue is indicated in some cases and, surprisingly, dogs adapt to this well. In one study five dogs with small tumors were treated with surgery alone and had a median survival time of 8 months. Three of these dogs had local recurrence.

Recurrence of tongue tumors is also common after radiation therapy. Larger tumors in 10 dogs were treated with radiation therapy, and the dogs survived for a median of 4 months; 9 of 10 had recurrence. The 1 dog that received radiation after surgery survived 26 months with no recurrence.

A combined modality approach for larger tumors of the tongue seems warranted for local control, although metastasis occurs in approximately 50% of the cases. Chemotherapy, with or without radiation, should be considered for these tumors as an adjuvant to surgery. Chemotherapeutic agents that have been reported to be of some help in these cases include cisplatin, carboplatin, mitoxantrone, and piroxicam.

Papillary squamous cell carcinoma in young dogs is an aggressive disease. Conservative surgery alone is unlikely to be curative because of the high rate of bone involvement and the young age of the patient. Radiation therapy has a good success rate, although disruption of normal bone growth in young dogs may produce facial malformations. Radiation therapy to a total dose of 40 Gy was used to treat three puppies with this disease. There was no evidence of disease in any dog 10, 32, and 39 months after treatment.

Chemotherapy is rarely indicated for rostral gingival squamous cell carcinoma in dogs due to the low metastatic rate for this tumor. Chemotherapy may be indicated for squamous cell carcinoma of the tongue, tonsil, and caudal location of the mouth because of the high metastatic rate of such tumors. Subcutaneous bleomycin treatment, as well as doxorubicin, cyclophosphamide, and chlorambucil treatment, failed to induce responses in two dogs with oral squamous cell carcinoma. Cisplatin has caused responses in dogs with metastatic subungual squamous cell carcinoma; however, no responses occurred in five dogs with oral squamous cell carcinoma (including one tongue and one tonsillar tumor). In another report, cisplatin caused a partial response in three of five dogs with oral squamous cell carcinoma for 2, 10, and 15 weeks, respectively. Cisplatin or carboplatin has yet to be fully evaluated for oral squamous cell carcinoma; however, it may be useful in combination therapy for this disease. Mitoxantrone (5 to 6 mg/m^2 every 3 weeks) caused responses in four (45%) of nine dogs with squamous cell carcinoma of various sites, including the oral cavity, for between 6 and 21 weeks. Mitoxantrone chemotherapy in combination with surgery was effective in controlling squamous cell carcinoma of the tongue in dogs in another study.

Oral piroxicam (0.14 mg/lb once daily) may be helpful in alleviating clinical symptoms and in tumor control. Toxicities associated with the use of this drug include GI and renal. A biochemical profile should be performed before the use of this drug, and if clinical signs associated with GI upset occur, the drug should be discontinued.

TONSILLAR SQUAMOUS CELL CARCINOMA IN DOGS

Background

Tonsillar squamous cell carcinoma is a more aggressive tumor than either gingival or lingual squamous cell carcinoma. The median age of dogs with this disease is 9 to 11 years. There appears to be a male predisposition. No breed predisposition has been described. Occasionally, tonsillar squamous cell carcinoma may occur bilaterally.

Clinical Parameters

Dogs with tonsillar squamous cell carcinoma usually present with dysphagia, anorexia, and pain. Owners may have noticed a cervical swelling, which is usually lymph node metastasis rather than primary tumor. Most dogs have shown these signs for 1 month or less, although some dogs may show signs for up to 3 months before presentation.

Clinical Work-up

All dogs with oral tumors should have a thorough examination of both tonsils and aspiration cytologic examination of the local lymph nodes, which

may confirm metastatic carcinoma, in addition to a complete blood count, biochemical profile, urinalysis, and skull, thoracic, and abdominal radiographs or ultrasound. Occasionally dogs with this disease may be seen for a cervical swelling, and upon oral examination a tonsillar swelling is noted. If no diagnosis can be reached, biopsy of the tonsil and the regional lymph node is warranted. Thoracic radiographs should be taken, although metastasis is unlikely to be seen at the time of diagnosis. If treatment is undertaken, radiographs should be repeated at regular intervals to screen for metastasis. In view of the high reported rate of intraabdominal metastases in one study, abdominal radiographs and ultrasonography should be performed before any definitive treatment. Abdominal imaging may also be useful for monitoring the patient for metastases after treatment.

Tonsillar squamous cell carcinoma commonly metastasizes to the local lymph nodes. In one study all 22 dogs had lymphadenopathy, as well as infiltrative primary tumors, at the time of diagnosis. Despite early spread to the lymph nodes, pulmonary metastases are rarely noted at diagnosis. After treatment 9 (33%) of 27 dogs had evidence of distant metastases. In two earlier studies 77 (85%) of 91 dogs with tonsillar squamous cell carcinoma had metastasis to regional lymph nodes at necropsy. Systemic metastases were less common; they occurred in the lung, spleen, liver, and thyroid gland. In a smaller group of dogs, metastasis to the spleen and liver occurred more often than to the lungs.

Therapeutic Approach

Surgery alone is rarely effective in the treatment of tonsillar squamous cell carcinoma due to a high metastatic rate, which manifests early in the course of the disease. A combination of surgery and radiation provided good local control at radiation doses of 35 Gy to 42.5 Gy; six of eight dogs showed a complete response, and one dog showed a partial response. Recurrence was seen in only two of the seven responding dogs, although metastatic disease to the spleen, liver, bone, and lungs was seen or suspected in all seven. Survival ranged from 44 to 631 days, with a median of 109 days.

In another study, dogs were treated with a combination of surgery, orthovoltage radiation therapy, and chemotherapy that alternated doxorubicin (30 mg/m^2 intravenously every 3 weeks) with cisplatin (60 mg/m^2 intravenously every 3 weeks). Of 6 dogs receiving this protocol, 5 achieved a complete response, with a median survival of 240 days. Four of these dogs developed tumor recurrence and metastatic disease. In comparison, 16 dogs had no response to treatment with this chemotherapy protocol (or combinations of doxorubicin, vinblastine, cisplatin, and cyclophosphamide) when it was administered without radiation therapy. Median survival for these 16 dogs was 105 days. Piroxicam may be a good option for analgesia and also because it has anticancer effects.

Aggressive surgery and radiation therapy, combined with doxorubicin and cisplatin chemotherapy, provide the best therapeutic results for this tumor; even then, tumor progression is difficult to control. The prognosis for dogs with tonsillar squamous cell carcinoma is poor.

ORAL SQUAMOUS CELL CARCINOMA IN CATS

Background

Neoplasia of the oral cavity represents 10% of all tumors diagnosed in cats, and approximately 90% of these are malignant. *Squamous cell carcinoma is the most common oral tumor in cats* (Figure 11-2). This tumor accounts for approximately 60% of all oral tumors. The average age of a cat with this disease is 11 to 12 years of age; however, cats as young as 3 years of age may be affected. No gender or breed predilection has been noted.

Most oral squamous cell carcinomas in cats occur at the base of the tongue and involve the frenulum (Figure 11-3). This area should be routinely examined in older cats, especially when they are anesthetized for dental or any other procedure that requires sedation or anesthesia. Some speculation has led to the thought that extensive grooming habits of the cat possibly cause the species to contact carcinogens on its hair coat, thereby predisposing the tongue to development of neoplasia.

Clinical Parameters

Cats with oral squamous cell carcinoma most commonly present for a mass or facial asymmetry. Squamous cell carcinomas are characterized by mucosal ulceration, necrosis, and severe suppurative inflammation. Cats with this tumor may pre-

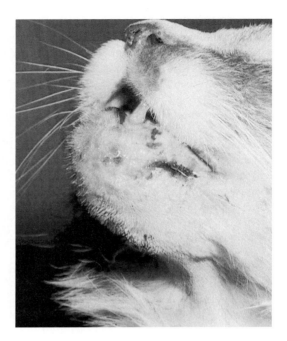

FIGURE 11-2 Squamous cell carcinoma is the most common oral tumor in the cat and one of the three most common oral tumors in the dog. Bone involvement can suggest a more favorable outcome. This 12-year-old spayed female cat had a mandibulectomy, followed by radiation therapy and mitoxantrone chemotherapy. An esophageal feeding tube was placed during this therapy and removed 2 weeks after radiation therapy was discontinued. Her tumor was controlled for 18 months, when metastases were identified. Quality of life was excellent, according to her caregivers.

sent with dysphagia, halitosis, anorexia, nasal discharge, sneezing, pawing at the mouth, changes in eating habits, oral hypersensitivity, loose teeth, weight loss, and drooling of ropelike saliva. In some cats a small mass is found initially in conjunction with a thorough oral examination during anesthesia for routine dentistry. There may be no symptoms whatsoever at this early stage. *In the early stages, differentiating squamous cell carcinoma from gingival proliferation and dental disease may be difficult, so a biopsy should be performed on any oral mass in an older cat, even in absence of the above symptoms.*

The mandible and maxilla are equally distributed as far as frequency of site that is affected. Bone invasion is common with gingival tumors. Some squamous cell carcinomas arise primarily within the mandible, causing enlargement of the jaw as a result of bony proliferation. These tumors should be differentiated from deep-seated osteomyelitis

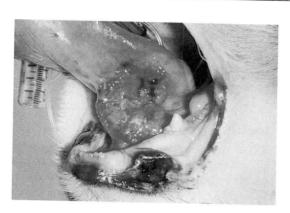

FIGURE 11-3 Sublingual squamous cell carcinoma is a difficult tumor to treat; however, most patients can be made more comfortable with good analgesia and nutritional support, such as assisted tube feeding. Piroxicam (Feldene) is a nonsteroidal antiinflammatory agent and potent analgesic and has been reported to have anticancer effects against selected tumor types. Although its efficacy against sublingual squamous cell carcinoma has yet to be documented in the dog and cat, it is one treatment option for patients that have normal renal function.

generated by severe dental disease and from other malignant tumors, such as osteosarcoma.

Clinical Work-up

Staging of any cat with an oral tumor should be performed as previously described in the dog. High-detail radiography of the skull provides information on bony lysis caused by gingival tumors. As stated previously, however, radiographic appearance of lysis does not occur until more than 50% of the bone has been demineralized; therefore radiography is a poor indicator of tumor margins. Biopsy is required for definitive diagnosis and should be considered in any old cat with severe gingival disease. Common differential diagnoses include eosinophilic granuloma and fibrosarcoma.

Metastasis is rare, although mandibular lymph nodes may be involved and should be evaluated by cytologic or histopathologic examination. Although lymphadenopathy is usually assumed to signal possible metastatic disease, two studies found that less than 50% of cats with enlarged lymph nodes had histologic evidence of metastatic disease. Lymph node metastasis was seen in 8 of 59 cats in these two studies. Metastatic disease may occur late in the course of the disease, or perhaps metastases are slow to progress. This is further supported by 1 cat that had no evidence of metastatic

progression 16 months after lymph node metastasis was detected.

Therapeutic Approach

In five cats with squamous cell carcinoma of the mandible, resection alone was not very successful in maintaining a remission. Recurrence occurred in four cats within 5 to 12 months of surgery despite aggressive surgical technique. These tumors were all large (between 2 and 4 cm in diameter), and all invaded bone. In another study, surgery alone resulted in a median survival of 6 weeks for seven cats. Small tumors, particularly those located rostrally on the mandible, may be more amenable to complete surgical excision.

Radiation therapy used alone for the treatment of this disease has also not been rewarding. Radiation therapy (orthovoltage, 52 Gy) was used to treat 11 cats with oral squamous cell carcinoma. Treatment included ethanidazole, which is a hypoxic cell sensitizer that was injected intratumorally. Eight cats were evaluated for response. Four died from complications of therapy, which included tissue necrosis and ischemia of the tongue, between 45 and 341 days after radiation (median, 114 days). The other 4 cats had tumor recurrence at 125 to 331 days after radiation (median, 170 days). No cats were alive 1 year after treatment. Overall median survival was 132 days. In another study, radiation alone or in combination with chemotherapy or with hyperthermia resulted in a median survival of 10 weeks for 45 cats.

Combination treatment, with mandibulectomy followed by external beam radiation to a dose of 40 Gy to 45 Gy starting 10 to 15 days after surgery, has demonstrated more success. Six of seven cats had tumor recurrence between 3 and 36 months after treatment (median, 12.5 months). One cat died but showed no evidence of disease 14 months after completing radiation therapy.

Placement of a gastrostomy tube by endoscopy or an esophagostomy tube at the time of surgery may prolong survival and definitely facilitates nutritional supplementation in cats undergoing surgery or radiation therapy for oral squamous cell carcinoma (Figure 11-4). The tube allows enteral feeding of the cat during recovery while allowing the mouth to heal. Gastrostomy tubes can remain in place after surgery until the cat is able to eat normally. Placement of gastrostomy tubes and recommendations for providing enteral nutrition are described in Chapter 12.

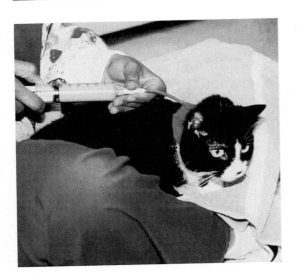

FIGURE 11-4 Esophageal and gastric assisted tube feeding are two vital tools for enhancing quality and length of life in dogs and cats with tumors of the gastrointestinal system. Fluid therapy, medical therapy, and nutritional support can all be achieved through these tubes. They are easy to place and maintain. This cat is being fed via an esophagostomy tube. (Photo courtesy Dr. K.L. Mitchener.)

Because lack of success has often been experienced with other treatment modalities, trials with chemotherapeutic agents have been attempted. Mitoxantrone at doses up to 6.5 mg/m^2 intravenously every 3 weeks caused 1 complete remission and 3 partial remissions for 21 to 60 days in 32 cats. In another study, 7 cats received mitoxantrone (5 mg/m^2 intravenously every 3 weeks) during and following megavoltage radiation therapy. Radiation was delivered as a "shrinking field," whereby the tumor and mandibular lymph node received 39.6 to 46.2 Gy, the mandible received 49.5 to 51 Gy, and the gross tumor received 59.4 to 61.2 Gy in daily 3-Gy fractions. The median survival for these cats was 180 days. Thirty percent of the cats were alive 1 year after radiation therapy. Complete remission has been reported in 2 cats with squamous cell carcinoma after treatment with carboplatin. Oral piroxicam therapy (0.14 mg/lb orally every other day) may be of benefit for clinical symptoms and as an antineoplastic agent.

The best therapy for oral squamous cell carcinoma in cats has not been determined. A combination of surgery, radiation therapy, and chemotherapy probably offers the best chance of success. Preoperative radiation and chemotherapy may cause tumor shrinkage and allow surgical margins to be more easily attained.

ORAL FIBROSARCOMA IN DOGS

Background

The third most common oral malignancy in the dog is fibrosarcoma. These tumors generally occur in older dogs; however, these tumors may occur in young dogs more commonly than melanoma or squamous cell carcinoma. The average age of dogs with oral fibrosarcoma is 7 years, although these tumors have been reported in dogs as young as 6 months of age. There does not seem to be any breed predilection, although 4 of 10 affected dogs in one study were golden retrievers. There is an apparent male predilection for developing oral fibrosarcoma, although this is not consistent in all studies.

Clinical Parameters

Fibrosarcomas are just as likely to arise from the maxilla as from the mandible. These tumors most commonly originate from the gingival tissue. Tumors are usually large, with diameters of greater than 4 cm. Dogs may be asymptomatic, or they may have ptyalism, anorexia, oral bleeding, and facial deformity.

Clinical Work-up

Dogs with any oral tumor should be staged using blood work, thoracic radiographs, lymph node evaluation, and fine-detail skull radiographs. Fibrosarcomas frequently invade bone and may extend much farther than is obvious by external viewing. In addition, all soft tissue sarcomas have "tendrils" of tumor cells that extend deep into normal surrounding tissues, making complete excision very difficult without wide margins.

Before surgery, particularly when the tumor involves maxilla, high-detail skull radiographs or a CT scan should be obtained to gain a better appreciation of tumor borders. Due to the fact that radiographs usually underestimate tumor margins, CT scanning is a more accurate method of assessing fibrosarcoma margins. A CT scan provides a spatial assessment of the tumor that may be useful for planning surgery, as well as either presurgical or postsurgical radiation therapy. CT scanning may also indicate whether complete surgical removal is impossible, thereby protecting the patient from a poorly planned procedure.

Occasionally a tumor may be termed a fibroma, which implies that the process is benign. Fibromas of the oral cavity should be treated as aggressively as fibrosarcomas. A recent report described 25 dogs with tumors that were histologically labeled as either fibromas, nodular fasciitis, or granulation tissue. Although all of these lesions were considered benign, they invaded bone and metastasized in 5 of the dogs. Bony invasion should be interpreted as a sign of malignancy regardless of the pathology report.

Fibrosarcoma is rarely metastatic at the time of diagnosis. However, mandibular lymph nodes should be palpated and always subjected to fine-needle aspiration or biopsy. Young dogs apparently have more aggressive tumors than old dogs. In eight series totaling 107 dogs, metastasis was reported in 23 (21%) dogs. In most cases metastasis was to regional lymph nodes; it is rare for oral fibrosarcoma to metastasize to lungs. Thoracic radiographs should, however, be performed before definitive surgery. Metastases often appear many months after surgery, and it is possible that earlier reports with less effective therapies may have underestimated the metastatic rate, because dogs died from inadequate local tumor control before metastasis occurred.

Therapeutic Approach

Complete surgical excision is the treatment of choice for fibrosarcoma of the oral cavity. Tumor-present margins lead to rapid recurrence. Radical surgical techniques such as maxillectomy and mandibulectomy are well tolerated by dogs and are necessary to obtain adequate surgical margins. In five series, totaling 54 dogs treated for oral fibrosarcoma with aggressive surgery, the median survival was 12 months and ranged from 1.5 weeks to 33 months. Early and aggressive management of maxillary and mandibular fibrosarcoma in large purebred dogs with histologically low-grade yet biologically high-grade tumors should be a standard approach.

Even after mandibulectomy or maxillectomy, local recurrence was a problem in 20 of 54 dogs (37%). Tumor recurrence varied with each study, however, from 20% to nearly 60% and occurred soon after surgery in studies with the highest rates of recurrence. In 3 dogs in one study, recurrence was treated by a second surgery (2 dogs) or surgery plus radiation therapy (1 dog) for second remissions of 2 months, 15 months, and 2 years, respectively.

In one study, pretreatment with 50 to 56 Gy of radiation seemed to improve control rates, although few dogs were involved in this study. Control of fibrosarcoma improves only at high doses of 50 Gy or more. Of 17 dogs treated with 40.0 to 54.5 Gy of orthovoltage, 4 died during or soon after radiation therapy. Survival times in the remaining 13 dogs ranged from 2 months to more than 27 months, with a median survival of 6 months. Tumors recurred in 12 dogs at a mean time of 3.9 months after radiation was complete. In another study, radiation therapy without surgery was able to control tumor growth in 3 of 13 dogs. Megavoltage radiation may be more efficacious than orthovoltage in controlling oral fibrosarcomas. Twenty-eight dogs with fibrosarcoma were treated with 48 Gy of ^{60}Co teletherapy. Nine dogs had local recurrence as the first cause of failure, and 4 dogs developed distant metastasis as the first cause of failure. Dogs with rostrally located tumors and dogs with smaller tumors had longer remissions. Median progression-free survival was estimated to be 26.2 months. Clinical stage was important in predicting time to failure. Radiation alone, or combined with hyperthermia, results in a median survival of over 18 months for biologically high-grade, histologically low-grade, fibrosarcomas.

When used in combination with radiation, interstitial hyperthermia provides better local control rates than those achieved by radiation alone. Ten dogs that received between 32 and 48 Gy of orthovoltage also received interstitial hyperthermia to a temperature of either 50° C or 43° C for 30 seconds. Complete remissions were obtained in 9 of 10 dogs, and overall median survival was 12.9 months, which is comparable to survival times for dogs that undergo surgery. Tumors recurred in 4 dogs between 38 days and 378 days after radiation. Complications of this combined modality include fistula formation and sepsis following tissue necrosis.

Chemotherapy has had little application in the treatment of oral cavity fibrosarcomas, although doxorubicin has been noted occasionally to produce objective responses in soft tissue sarcomas. Low doses of doxorubicin (10 mg/m^2 intravenously every 7 days) appear to act as a "radiation sensitizer" and improve tumor response at lower radiation therapy dosages.

Intratumoral injections of cisplatin and bovine collagen matrix were given every week during a 48-Gy course of ^{60}Co teletherapy to five dogs with oral fibrosarcoma. Complete remission was seen in three dogs, and partial remission was seen in one dog, for a median duration of 14 weeks. There was tumor recurrence in three of these dogs. In these and other dogs treated with radiochemotherapy, recurrences often took place at the periphery of the chemotherapy site but still within the radiation field, implying that the combination is synergistic or additive in its effect on the tumor.

The treatment of choice for oral fibrosarcoma probably involves combined surgery and radiation therapy to dosages that exceed 50 Gy. Intralesional chemotherapy is investigational but may improve tumor control.

ORAL FIBROSARCOMA IN CATS

Background

The second most common oral tumor in cats is fibrosarcoma. There is no obvious breed or gender predilection. Fibrosarcoma is most common in old cats that average 10 years of age.

Clinical Parameters

Feline fibrosarcoma is found mostly in the oral gingivae but has no obvious site predilection. The lesion may be ulcerated, causing halitosis and drooling, and is difficult to distinguish clinically from squamous cell carcinoma.

Clinical Work-up

Staging procedures should be performed as discussed for squamous cell carcinoma. Fibrosarcomas cause tissue destruction and occasionally invade bone or muscle. On histopathologic examination these fibrosarcomas often have a high mitotic index; however, metastatic potential appears low.

Therapeutic Approach

Two cats were treated with hemimandibulectomy or premaxillectomy and were free of disease 11.5 months and 24 months after surgery, respectively. In another two cats treated with hemimandibulectomy, one cat had recurrence in 2 months, and one cat failed to eat and was euthanized. A gastrostomy tube should be placed in all cats undergoing oral surgery.

Vincristine (0.5 mg/m^2 intravenously per week) caused complete regression of an oral fibrosarcoma in one cat when treated for 30 weeks. Other chemotherapy for this tumor has not been described, although doxorubicin reportedly causes regression of fibrosarcoma at other sites in cats.

Oral piroxicam (0.14 mg/lb every other day) may be of benefit in these cats.

Because of the encouraging results of radiation therapy in cats with other soft tissue sarcomas (including fibrosarcoma), this modality in combination with surgery may offer the best chance of tumor control in cats, as it does in dogs. Doxorubicin or carboplatin have been employed with variable results.

LESS COMMON ORAL TUMORS IN THE DOG

Other reported oral malignancies in the dog include osteosarcomas (Figure 11-5), intraosseous carcinomas, neurofibrosarcomas, anaplastic sarcomas, chondrosarcomas, myxosarcomas, invasive nasal tumors, mast cell tumors, hemangiosarcomas, lymphomas, and transmissible venereal tumors.

In one report the overall 1-year survival rate for dogs with mandibular osteosarcomas treated with combination modalities was 53%. Dogs treated

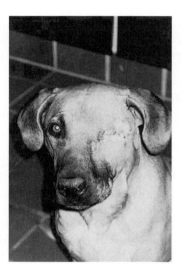

FIGURE 11-5 This 5-year-old male Rhodesian Ridgeback had a maxillectomy to include the orbit and eye for an oral osteosarcoma, followed by radiation therapy to the surgery area beginning 1 week after surgery. Chemotherapy with cisplatin and doxorubicin was continued after radiation was completed. At the time of this picture, several months after the completion of radiation therapy, he was free of disease and absolutely asymptomatic for any adverse effects of therapy. This case is a good example of how many modes of cancer therapy can be used in concert to benefit the patient and control or cure the disease.

with surgery alone had a 1-year survival rate of 71%. Histologic grade was demonstrated to be important for survival.

SALIVARY GLAND TUMORS IN DOGS

Background

Salivary gland tumors are usually seen in older dogs with no obvious gender predilection. Poodles are at higher risk for developing this disease than other breeds.

Carcinomas are the most common tumor type, although salivary glands are occasionally invaded by fibrosarcomas or mast cell tumors. Enlargement of the salivary gland in a dog is more likely to be an inflammatory process than a tumor.

Clinical Parameters

Patients most commonly have a swelling or mass in the neck; however, signs may also include anorexia, dysphagia, and pain on opening the mouth.

Clinical Work-up

The clinical work-up for salivary gland tumors should include a complete blood count, biochemical profile, T_4 levels, urinalysis, and cytologic evaluation of the tumor. Local lymph node metastasis may occur; therefore lymph nodes should always have a biopsy or a fine-needle aspiration. Although pulmonary metastases are rare, thoracic radiographs should always be performed as part of a thorough staging scheme. In one study only 8% of the dogs had metastatic disease at time of diagnosis.

The mandibular glands were more likely to be affected than the parotid glands. In many cases, tumor was dispersed throughout the salivary tissue in the submucosa of the oral cavity, tongue, and oropharynx. Surgical excisional biopsy is warranted for localized tumors; however, more diffuse tumors may require incisional biopsy before a definitive procedure.

Therapeutic Approach

Surgical excision in two dogs resulted in local recurrence within 6 months. One of these dogs and two other dogs received 45 Gy of orthovoltage radiation to the surgical site, and none of the three dogs had developed local recurrence or

metastasis 12, 25, and 40 months after treatment. Radiation therapy should be considered as an adjunct to surgery for salivary gland tumors. In another group of dogs treated with either surgery, surgery and radiation, or surgery and chemotherapy, the median survival was 550 days. The dogs that were treated with surgery and chemotherapy had shorter survival times than the other two groups. Presumably these dogs had more progressive disease and hence were treated with chemotherapy. In another study six dogs with salivary gland adenocarcinoma were treated with surgery alone, and median survival was 74 days with a range of 42 to 300 days. All of the dogs in this report died of pulmonary metastases.

SALIVARY GLAND TUMORS IN CATS

Background

Most salivary gland tumors are carcinomas. *In contrast to dogs, enlargement of a salivary gland in cats is more likely to signal a tumor than inflammation or any other condition.* The median age of affected cats is 10 years, and there is no gender predilection. Siamese cats are at higher risk for developing salivary gland tumors; 7 (26%) of 27 cats were Siamese in one survey.

Clinical Parameters

Cats usually have a mass in the cervical region, which may be accompanied by other signs, such as anorexia, dysphagia, and salivation due to secondary infections and ulceration.

Clinical Work-up

Most reported cats have regional lymph node metastases, and one cat developed lung metastases 5 months after surgery. Careful palpation of regional lymph nodes followed by fine-needle aspiration or biopsy of enlarged nodes, as well as blood work, urinalysis, and thoracic radiographs, should precede any definitive treatment for these tumors. In one study, median survival for cats with this disease was 516 days. Staging was not shown to be prognostic in cats, and a low mitotic index was associated with a poorer prognosis. There was no difference in surgery alone versus surgery with chemotherapy or surgery with radiation.

Therapeutic Approach

Cats treated with surgery alone had recurrence or metastasis within 6 months in one study. There are no reports of adjunctive radiation therapy, but limited success in dogs suggests that this therapy may be worthwhile to reduce the risk of local recurrence. There are no reports of chemotherapy for this tumor; however, carboplatin and doxorubicin have been used with favorable results by some.

ESOPHAGEAL TUMORS IN DOGS

Esophageal neoplasia is uncommon in the dog except for osteosarcoma and fibrosarcoma associated with the helminth parasite *Spirocerca lupi*. Primary esophageal neoplasias are extremely uncommon and include squamous cell carcinoma, scirrhous carcinoma, undifferentiated carcinoma, adenocarcinoma, and leiomyoma, which is the most common. Canine esophageal tumors are often metastatic, having arisen from the thyroid or mammary gland.

Clinical signs associated with esophageal neoplasia include dysphagia, regurgitation, ptyalism, inappetence, progressive weight loss, fetid breath, debilitation, and respiratory signs, which may be secondary to aspiration pneumonia. Clinical investigation includes survey and contrast thoracic radiography and esophagoscopy. Definitive diagnosis of esophageal tumors requires a biopsy, either surgical or endoscopic, and an official diagnosis by a pathologist. Standard therapy historically has involved medical management for esophageal dysfunction and surgical removal when possible. Primary esophageal neoplasia in the canine generally warrants a guarded to poor prognosis. Newer options include laser therapy and photodynamic therapy (PDT). PDT is used relatively routinely in humans, most commonly with localized and minimally invasive carcinomas. PDT employs a photosensitizer and laser light to destroy malignant tissues.

With laser therapy, treatment begins centrally around the residual lumen, proceeding toward but not to the wall. Initial tissue changes are coagulative, and then vaporization occurs with ongoing thermal damage. After several days the superficial necrotic tissue is removed, and laser therapy is then performed a few centimeters distal to the site treated several days earlier. Treatment progresses every several days until the lumen is opened through the entire length of neoplastic tissue. Management of *S. lupi* is discussed in Chapter 4.

STOMACH TUMORS IN DOGS

Background

The most common tumor of the stomach in dogs is gastric adenocarcinoma, which is emphasized in most reports. Leiomyoma, leiomyosarcoma, lymphoma, and adenoma are also found, less commonly.

Most carcinomas occur in the lower two thirds of the stomach, particularly in the pylorus region. The lesser curvature is not usually affected, except in Belgian shepherds. Most affected dogs are old, and there appears to be a male predominance.

Belgian shepherds in Italy (of the Groenendael type) and rough collies are apparently at high risk for gastric adenocarcinoma. Although gastric carcinomas can be experimentally induced in dogs by various compounds, there are no epidemiologic studies to support a role for these compounds in naturally occurring disease.

Gastric leiomyomas are benign tumors of the stomach and are strongly associated with age in the dog.

Clinical Parameters

Gastric tumors are consistently associated with vomiting, weight loss, and inappetence. Vomiting is often chronic and rarely associated with eating. Hematemesis occurs in up to 50% of dogs. Other signs include polydipsia, abdominal pain, melena, and anemia. Occasionally ascites occurs as a result of carcinomatosis. Clinical signs, such as vomiting, are often chronic for 2 weeks to 18 months before presentation; the median duration is 2 months.

There are reports of dogs presenting with metastatic testicular adenocarcinoma, with the primary tumor originating from the stomach.

Leiomyomas are often discovered as incidental findings during necropsy, surgery, or endoscopy in geriatric dogs. Leiomyomas may be identified from a history that reveals chronic vomiting, acute gastric distention, or intermittent severe GI bleeding.

Dogs with gastric leiomyosarcoma may present with clinical signs associated with hypoglycemia, such as weakness, seizures, or coma.

Clinical Work-up

Gastric adenocarcinomas often involve a large area of the stomach wall, making them unresectable. These tumors arise in the mucosa, but most extend to or through the serosa. Ulceration is common and often deep and craterlike, causing hematemesis or melena. Contrast radiography, particularly with fluoroscopy, may give indications of gastric tumor, but these indications are rarely definitive. Endoscopy can determine the location of most tumors, except when neoplasia is diffusely infiltrative, and may reveal tumor ulceration (Figure 11-6). Although endoscopy can be definitive, it can also be inconclusive. Multiple endoscopic biopsy specimens should be obtained, and deep biopsy specimens should be taken if the mucosa is not obviously involved (Figure 11-7). Endoscopy is ideal for evaluating the stomach itself, but ultrasonography should be used to assess epigastric lymph nodes and other abdominal viscera for evidence of metastasis. Ultrasonography or laparoscopy can also be used to define the borders of localized tumors and to identify ulcerations and diffuse infiltration. In one report the use of ultrasonography in the diagnosis of canine gastric neoplasia was evaluated prospectively in a series of six cases that were subsequently confirmed as having adenocarcinoma by cytologic or histologic examination or both. These investigators found that gastric neoplasia was associated with mural thickening, loss of normal wall sonographic layers, and altered motility. Ultrasound findings were consistent with tumor localization obtained by other diagnostic methods that were employed. Fine-needle aspirations of the masses were successful in two out of three cases in which they were performed. Ultrasound-guided microcore biopsy can have a high diagnostic sensitivity. When the aforementioned modalities are unsuitable, exploratory laparotomy or laparoscopy can be used to obtain biopsy specimens from affected sites. A therapeutic excisional biopsy may be possible for small localized tumors via exploratory laparotomy; however, incisional biopsy should be performed on larger tumors.

Gastric adenocarcinoma often metastasizes, particularly to perigastric lymph nodes and viscera. Extension of gastric adenocarcinoma through the serosa creates an intense scirrhous reaction in the mesentery and omentum, which may cause ascites.

Histology of gastric adenocarcinomas varies, and "intestinal" types of tumors (e.g., papillary, aci-

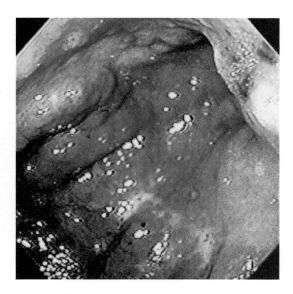

FIGURE 11-6 Endoscopic view of a gastric carcinoma resulting in a mild "cobblestone" effect to the mucosal surface. Note the ulcers in the upper right-hand portion of the image. This dog's only clinical sign was intermittent vomiting. A partial gastrectomy was performed, and the vomiting and endoscopic abnormalities resolved. (Photo courtesy Dr. David Twedt.)

nar, or solid) are less common than diffuse types (e.g., undifferentiated or glandular). No differences in biologic behavior have been ascribed to these different tumor types. *All gastric adenocarcinomas are aggressive malignancies.*

Therapeutic Approach

The advanced stage of gastric adenocarcinomas at diagnosis, their diffuse nature, and their high rate of metastasis usually make surgery unsuccessful. Most tumors are too large or invasive for complete resection. Wide resection often requires gastroduodenostomy (Billroth type I procedure); however, most dogs die within 4 months of surgery from local recurrence and metastases. Earlier diagnosis occasionally allows successful surgical resection and long-term freedom from recurrence and metastasis. There is a report of long-term survival after total gastrectomy for gastric adenocarcinoma in a dog. In this dog the esophagus was anastomosed to a remnant of the antrum, leaving the pylorus intact, and a splenopexy was performed. Another long-term survival case is illustrated in Chapter 1 (see pp. 22-33).

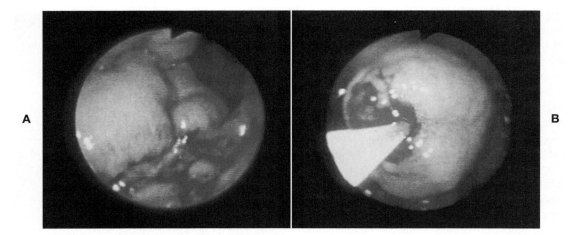

FIGURE 11-7 Gastric adenocarcinoma in a dog. **A,** Lower gastric body with an area of superficial ulceration seen in the lower field. **B,** Close-up view of a mass in the midgastric body. The mass was rigid and had a very dense wall (suggestive of neoplasia). Biopsy of masses such as this one should be performed as deeply as possible. If only superficial tissue is obtained, the endoscopist may fail to retrieve neoplastic cells. The first four attempts to perform a biopsy of the mass yielded very small tissue samples, but on the fifth attempt the biopsy instrument advanced inside the mass. A number of large tissue samples were then obtained, and the diagnosis of adenocarcinoma was confirmed. Biopsy samples were also obtained from the ulcerated area shown in **A.** (Courtesy Dr. Todd R. Tams. From Tams TR, ed: *Small animal endoscopy*, ed 2, St. Louis, 1999, Mosby.)

Photodynamic therapy with rhodamine dye was not successful in treating an unresectable tumor. Results of chemotherapy for adenocarcinoma have not been reported.

A technique using gastrotomy and submucosal resection was evaluated for removal of leiomyomas and other benign masses from the cardiac region of the stomach. There were no postoperative complications in the six dogs that underwent the procedure, and excision was incomplete in two of the dogs.

STOMACH TUMORS IN CATS

Stomach tumors are rare in cats. Most that do occur are lymphoma (Figure 11-8). Adenocarcinomas and leiomyosarcomas are rare. Gastric thickening is common in cats with gastric lymphoma and is often substantial enough to be detected on palpation. Ultrasound-guided biopsy or fine-needle aspiration facilitates diagnosis. Endoscopic biopsy is useful in superficial lesions but is not as helpful for submucosal lymphoma. Most are detectable via endoscopy (given proper endoscopic biopsy instrumentation and good technique). Lymphoma is rarely confined to the stomach and is best treated with chemotherapy. Responses of cats with GI lymphoma to chemotherapy are surprisingly good despite previous reports, especially if they are small cell lymphomas.

INTESTINAL TUMORS IN DOGS

Background

In dogs, adenocarcinomas are the most common tumor in the intestine and the stomach. Leiomyosarcomas are less common than adenocarcinoma and occur more frequently in the intestine than in the stomach (Figure 11-9). Intestinal leiomyomas are uncommon. All reported cecal tumors have been of smooth muscle origin (i.e., leiomyosarcoma or leiomyoma). Epithelial and smooth muscle tumors both occur in other areas of the intestinal tract. Lymphoma may be found anywhere within the GI tract but is usually associated with systemic disease. In one study of 144 dogs with lymphoma, 6.9% had GI involvement.

Intestinal tumors generally occur in older dogs. The median age is 11 to 12 years, although the average age of dogs with lymphoma is younger. There are no obvious breed predilections. Males are more frequently affected by intestinal tumors than females, although this trend is most marked for adenocarcinoma and is less obvious for smooth muscle tumors.

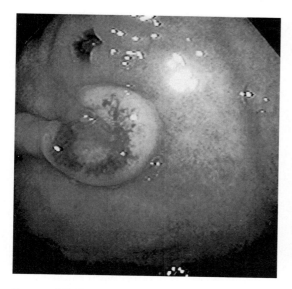

FIGURE 11-8 Ulcer and thickening of the pylorus of a 4-year-old, FeLV-negative cat with a history of intermittent vomiting, diarrhea, and weight loss. Endoscopic biopsy specimens were used to confirm the presence of small cell lymphoma. Vincristine, chlorambucil, and prednisone therapy was used to resolve all endoscopic abnormalities and clinical signs for a 2-year period. (Courtesy Dr. David Twedt.)

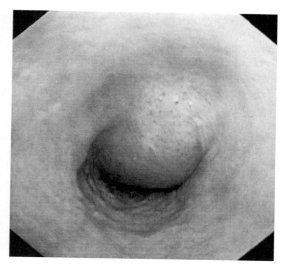

FIGURE 11-9 Small intestinal duodenal tumor causing partial obstruction of the bowel, vomiting, and diarrhea in a 10-year-old poodle. Resection of this leiomyosarcoma resulted in immediate resolution of clinical signs. Doxorubicin chemotherapy was initiated to treat any microscopic metastatic disease. The dog did extraordinarily well, and the owners were very happy with the patient's 2-year, disease-free interval. (Courtesy Dr. David Twedt.)

Clinical Parameters

Clinical signs give very little indication as to the type of neoplasm in a dog with an intestinal tumor. Symptoms may, however, direct the clinician to a particular area of the intestinal tract. For example, vomiting is most often associated with tumors of the duodenum or jejunum, whereas weight loss and diarrhea are usually seen in dogs with jejunal or ileal tumors. Tenesmus or hematochezia most often occurs with colonic or rectal tumors. Distal rectal tumors are mostly palpable as a single pedunculated mass; tumors located rostrally are more likely to be multiple ("cobblestone appearance") or appear as an annular constriction. Dogs with rectal leiomyomas may be asymptomatic, presumably owing to slow growth of these tumors; however, these tumors may become very large (up to 12 cm in one study). Anorexia, depression, and lethargy may accompany tumors in any location. Hypochromic anemia is a less common sign; it may be due to melena and iron deficiency. Ascites, abdominal pain, and peritonitis from intestinal rupture may occur; the last condition is mainly seen with cecal leiomyosarcomas. Clinical signs have often been present for weeks to months, although dogs that are vomiting are usually presented by their owners more rapidly.

On physical examination an abdominal mass may be palpated, particularly if the tumor is in the upper small intestine. Rectal examination may reveal a stricture, mass, or irregular rectal wall in more than 60% of affected dogs.

Clinical Work-up

In addition to routine blood work and urinalysis, thoracic and abdominal radiographs, endoscopy, and ultrasonography should be used to image the tumor and to identify metastasis. Plain radiographs may help delineate an abdominal mass and may also reveal other abnormalities, such as gas-filled and fluid-filled dilated loops of bowel, which are suggestive of obstruction. Pneumoperitoneum may indicate tumor rupture or a septic peritonitis. Contrast radiography most often shows an "apple-core" lesion for tumors of the small intestine but also may show irregular filling defects or leakage caused by perforation. Ultrasonography is a noninvasive and rapid means of identifying intestinal tumors and provides a guide for obtaining biopsy specimens, as well as a method of staging for abdominal metastases. Ultrasonography is the staging method of choice for dogs with intestinal tumors.

Endoscopy can be used to obtain biopsy specimens, which may provide a definitive diagnosis for duodenal or colonic and rectal tumors; however, multiple biopsy specimens should be taken, because lesions deep to the mucosa may escape detection, and tumors that create ulcerated lesions may be obscured by inflammatory changes (Figure 11-10). In one study, endoscopic biopsy of intestinal lymphoma was confounded by the presence of inflammatory infiltrates in nearly 50% of the dogs. Endoscopy of the entire large bowel is particularly important when a distal rectal tumor is palpated, because dogs may have additional proximal lesions that could otherwise remain undetected and continue to cause clinical signs after surgery. Biopsy of small intestinal tumors often requires exploratory laparotomy, but biopsy of rectal tumors may be performed via proctoscopy or by prolapsing the rectum manually or with stay sutures.

Metastasis is more commonly described for intestinal adenocarcinoma than for leiomyosarcoma, and the most common sites of metastasis are the regional lymph nodes. In 22 (71%) of 31 dogs with small intestine adenocarcinoma, there was evidence of metastases to regional lymph nodes. In contrast, metastasis occurred to liver and lung in only four (13%) of these 31 dogs. Leiomyosarcoma

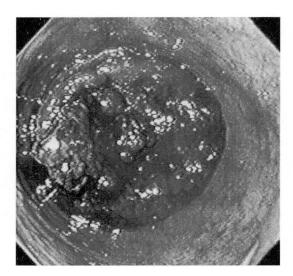

FIGURE 11-10 Colonic carcinoma of a 7-year-old castrated male dog with a 5-week history of straining to defecate. Results of blood work, abdominal and chest radiographs, and abdominal ultrasound were normal. Colonoscopy was used to obtain a diagnosis of colonic carcinoma. Resection of the colon resulted in control of this tumor for 24 months. (Courtesy Dr. David Twedt.)

does not usually metastasize; metastases occur in less than 30% of affected dogs, often long after definitive surgery. Metastasis of colorectal adenocarcinoma is considerably less common. There was no evidence of metastasis in 78 dogs with this disease even after long survival times following surgery.

Carcinoid is a term used to describe intestinal tumors of neuroendocrine derivation that may be hormonally active. Of five reported intestinal carcinoids, all had metastases to regional lymph nodes and liver at the time of diagnosis and there were additional sites of metastasis in two dogs.

Prognostic Factors

In one study of colorectal adenocarcinomas, dogs with annular tumors had the shortest average survival (1.6 months). Dogs with tumors that comprised multiple "cobblestone" nodules had an average survival of 12 months. Dogs with a single pedunculated polyp had the longest survival (32 months) after surgery. These prognostic factors are probably related to the ease with which complete surgical excision may be performed.

In one group of dogs with adenomatous polyps or carcinoma in situ of the colon and rectum, malignant transformation was documented in 18% of the cases. Higher rates of recurrence and malignant transformation occurred in dogs with multiple masses or diffuse disease and in dogs initially diagnosed with carcinoma in situ.

Diffuse intestinal lymphoma carries a poor prognosis in dogs. Prognostic factors for GI lymphoma are those that have been previously described for multicentric lymphoma.

Therapeutic Approach

There is little information regarding survival after surgical resection of small intestinal adenocarcinomas. Four dogs with small intestinal tumors that had not metastasized at the time of surgery had survival times of 3 days, 6 months (two dogs), and 2 years. In another study five dogs with surgically treated cancer of the small intestine had an average survival of 55 days. In another study, dogs with surgically treated epithelial tumors had a mean survival of 6.9 months and local recurrence was the cause of death in all dogs. In one study, dogs with large intestinal adenocarcinoma treated only with fecal softeners had a mean survival of 15 months.

Surgical excision of intestinal or cecal leiomyosarcoma carries a better prognosis. Thirteen (57%) of 23 dogs with leiomyosarcoma survived the perioperative period and had median survivals of 8 to 13 months (ranging from 2 months to 7 years). Only 3 of these 13 dogs developed metastases. One dog had evidence of metastasis at the time of surgery and without explanation survived 3 years without adjuvant therapy. Cecal rupture may occur and lead to death in some dogs as a result of peritonitis. Perioperative mortality was 60% in 10 dogs in one study. Four dogs survived for 19 months, 28 months, 36 months, and 48 months. Two of these dogs died due to recurrence (28 months) or metastases (36 months).

The median survival after surgical resection of colorectal leiomyoma was 26 months. Only one of five affected dogs died from tumor-related causes. Colorectal adenocarcinomas have a low rate of metastasis, and treated dogs may have long survival times following diagnosis. Of multiple treatment modalities, local excision gave the longest average survival (22 months) with the lowest complication rate. Recurrence after local excision of a solitary mass occurred in 11 (52%) of 21 dogs. In contrast, radical surgical excision of annular colorectal adenocarcinoma resulted in wound dehiscence and septic peritonitis in all four dogs treated.

Cryosurgery prolonged survival in 11 dogs with colorectal adenocarcinoma (average survival of 24 months). Recurrence was similar to that after local excision; however, additional complications, including stricture (5 of 11 dogs), rectal prolapse, and perineal hernia followed treatment. Other techniques, such as electrocoagulation and neodymium: yttrium-aluminum-garnet (Nd:YAG) laser-assisted surgery, provide control similar to that of local excision.

Radiation therapy using a single high dose (15 Gy to 25 Gy) of orthovoltage teletherapy may provide reasonable control for recurrent distal rectal adenocarcinomas. In six dogs, median tumor control duration was 6 months and no complications were reported. One dog treated with radiation therapy suffered a rectal perforation and died from peritonitis 2 months after treatment.

Results of chemotherapy have not been reported for intestinal tumors in dogs. Doxorubicin has been suggested by some as a good adjunctive therapy. Few data exist quantitating its efficacy.

Surgery is indicated in obstructive intestinal lymphoma or when bowel perforation has occurred. Chemotherapy protocols for lymphoma can be employed as adjuvant therapy or as the major form of therapy in diffuse disease (Tables 11-2 to 11-5).

For the dog the longest remission and survival times have been reported with the University of Wisconsin-Madison protocol noted in Table 11-5. This protocol is complex but gratifying because of consistently improved responses. The University of Wisconsin-Madison *short* canine lymphoma protocol appears in Table 11-4. Diffuse GI canine lymphoma is associated with a variable response to chemotherapy, although solitary or nodular lymphoma does respond better.

INTESTINAL TUMORS IN CATS

Background

Adenocarcinoma is by far the most common non-hematopoietic tumor of the intestinal tract in cats; sarcomas are rarely described. Intestinal adenocarcinoma is more common in cats than in dogs. The majority of intestinal adenocarcinomas occur in the small intestine of affected cats. The ileum or jejunum is most often affected, whereas the duodenum is rarely involved. Adenocarcinoma of the large intestine is less common and usually involves the colon, although the cecum and rarely rectum may be affected.

Intestinal adenocarcinoma primarily affects old cats; the mean age of affected cats is 10 to 11 years, although they may be as young as 2 years of age. The vast majority of affected cats are Siamese, which constitute 152 (68%) of 225 reported cases. Other purebreds are rarely affected. In one study all 22 adenocarcinomas of the large intestine occurred in domestic short hairs, although no other study addressed this association. Cats with colonic adenocarcinoma typically are older, with a mean age of 16 years. There seems to be no gender predilection for intestinal adenocarcinoma with the exception of one report in which male cats predominated. Feline leukemia virus (FeLV) is unlikely to play a role in this disease. Only two studies reported the FeLV status of affected cats; all 28 cats studied tested negative for FeLV antigenemia.

Although benign tumors of the intestinal tract are rare and the duodenum is not usually affected, 18 cats with adenomatous polyps of the duodenum have been described. Signalment was similar to that in cats with adenocarcinoma in that older, primarily Oriental-breed cats are most often affected. The cats in this study were predominantly castrated males. Most cats were tested for FeLV and feline immuno-

TABLE 11-2	Efficacy of Chemotherapy for the Treatment of Lymphoma*				
Drug	**Species**	**No. of Animals**	**Overall Response Rate (%)**	**Complete Response Rate (%)**	**Median Response Duration (Days)**
SINGLE-AGENT THERAPY					
Mitoxantrone	Dogs, cats	44	41	30	127
Epirubicin	Dogs	35	82	74	143
Idarubicin	Cats	13	—	—	—
Actinomycin D	Dogs, cats	12	85	70	42
Doxorubicin	Dogs	21	85	76	190
COMBINATION THERAPY					
LVPCD	Dogs	55	91	84	252
CVP	Dogs	—	89	75	180
CVPD	Dogs	46	87	83	210
VLCM	Dogs	147	94	—	140
VLCMP	Cats	103	82	62	—
CVP	Cats	38	94	79	321
VCM	Cats	62	—	52	112

L, L-Asparaginase; V, vincristine; P, prednisone; C, cyclophosphamide; D, doxorubicin; M, methotrexate.
*From Ogilvie GK: Chemotherapy. In Withrow SJ, MacEwen EG, eds: *Small animal clinical oncology*, Philadelphia, 1996, WB Saunders.

TABLE 11-3	CVP Chemotherapy Protocol for Dogs and Cats															
		Weeks														
Drug	**Dose (mg/m²)**	**1**	**2**	**3**	**4**	**5**	**6**	**7**	**8**	**9**	**10**	**11**	**12**	**13**	**52**
Cyclophosphamide	250 PO	X			X			X			X			X	X
Vincristine	0.75 IV	X	X	X	X			X			X			X	X
Prednisone*	30 PO	>	>	>	>		>		>		>		>		>

PO, Orally; IV, intravenously.
*Prednisone is given daily for the first 21 days, then every other day thereafter. Note that maintenance is continued on a 3-week schedule for at least 1 year.

deficiency virus (FIV), and all had negative results. All polyps occurred within 1 cm of the pylorus.

For colonic neoplasia in particular, one study found that adenocarcinoma followed by lymphoma, mast cell disease, and neuroendocrine carcinoma were the most common tumors found in this location.

Clinical Parameters

The most common presenting clinical signs for cats with alimentary lymphoma are as follows: vomiting, diarrhea, and interestingly a large portion of cats will present with only weight loss and anorexia. Some cats actually have increased appetite because of poor absorption of nutrients through the tumor of the intestinal tract. Most cats have a palpable abdominal mass. The World Health Organization's classification scheme for lymphoma appears in Table 11-6.

The most frequent presenting signs in cats with intestinal adenocarcinoma reflect involvement of the proximal small intestine. In decreasing order of frequency, vomiting, weight loss, and anorexia predominate. Hematochezia is occasionally described in cats with colonic or rectal tumors. Clinical signs often have been present for a considerable time (median, 2 months, but up to 2 years). Cats with tumors involving more proximal intestinal tract tend

TABLE 11-4	University of Wisconsin–Madison Protocol—Short Canine Lymphoma Protocol Treatment		
		Date	Dose
Week 1	Vincristine, 0.5-0.7 mg/m² IV	_____	_____
	L–Asparaginase, 400 U/kg SQ	_____	_____
	Prednisone, 2 mg/kg PO sid.	_____	_____
Week 2	Cyclophosphamide, 250 mg/m² IV	_____	_____
	Prednisone, 1.5 mg/kg PO sid.	_____	_____
Week 3	Vincristine, 0.5-0.7 mg/m² IV	_____	_____
	Prednisone, 1.0 mg/kg PO sid.	_____	_____
Week 4	Doxorubicin, 30 mg/m² IV	_____	_____
	Prednisone, 0.5 mg/kg PO sid.	_____	_____
Week 6	Vincristine, 0.5-0.7 mg/m² IV	_____	_____
Week 7	Cyclophosphamide, 250 mg/m² IV	_____	_____
Week 8	Vincristine, 0.5-0.7 mg/m² IV	_____	_____
Week 9	Doxorubicin, 30 mg/m² IV	_____	_____
Week 11	Vincristine, 0.5-0.7 mg/m² IV	_____	_____
Week 13	Cyclophosphamide, 250 mg/m² IV	_____	_____
Week 15	Vincristine, 0.5-0.7 mg/m² IV	_____	_____
Week 17	Doxorubicin, 30 mg/m² IV	_____	_____
Week 19	Vincristine, 0.5-0.7 mg/m² IV	_____	_____
Week 21	Cyclophosphamide, 250 mg/m² IV	_____	_____
Week 23	Vincristine, 0.5-0.7 mg/m² IV	_____	_____
Week 25	Doxorubicin, 30 mg/m² IV	_____	_____
If in complete remission at week 25, all therapy stops and monthly reevaluations are instituted.			

IV, Intravenously; *SQ,* subcutaneously; *PO,* orally.

TABLE 11-5	University of Wisconsin-Madison Canine Lymphoma Protocol

CYCLE 1 INDUCTION

Week 1:Vincristine 0.7 mg/m² IV; L-asparaginase 400 IU/kg IM; and once daily prednisone, 2 mg/kg PO
Week 2: Cyclophosphamide, 200 mg/m² IV, and once daily prednisone, 1.5 mg/kg PO
Week 3:Vincristine, 0.7 mg/m² IV, and once daily prednisone, 1.0 mg/kg PO
Week 4: Doxorubicin, 30 mg/m² IV, and once daily prednisone, 0.5 mg/kg PO
Week 6:Vincristine, 0.7 mg/m² IV
Week 7: Cyclophosphamide, 200 mg/m² IV
Week 8:Vincristine, 0.7 mg/m² IV
Week 9: Doxorubicin, 30 mg/m² IV

CYCLE 2

If in complete remission at week 9, continue treatment at 2-week intervals alternating vincristine 0.7 mg/m² IV, chlorambucil (Leukeran) 1.4 mg/kg PO, vincristine 0.7 mg/m², and methotrexate 0.8 mg/kg IV. Doxorubicin 30 mg/m² is substituted for every second methotrexate treatment. This cycle continues through week 25.

CYCLE 3

If in complete remission at week 25, continue treatment sequence outlined in Cycle 2, but now at 3-week intervals. This cycle continues through week 51.

CYCLE 4

If in complete remission at week 51, continue with treatment sequence outlined in Cycle 2, but now at 4-week intervals. Doxorubicin is no longer substituted for methotrexate. All treatment is discontinued at week 156.

IV, Intravenously; *IM,* intramuscularly; *PO,* orally.

TABLE 11-6	World Health Organization's Classification for Lymphoma

Stage I. Involvement limited to a single node or extranodal site, or lymphoid tissue in a single organ, including cranial mediastinum and excluding bone marrow

Stage II. Involvement of many lymph nodes in a regional area, a resectable gastrointestinal tract tumor or extranodal site with regional lymph node involvement

Stage III. Generalized lymph node involvement, nonresectable intraabdominal disease or epidural tumor

Stage IV. Liver and/or spleen involvement associated with stages I-III

Stage V. Manifestation in the blood and involvement of bone marrow involvement with stages I-IV

Each stage is subclassified into:
a. Without systemic signs, or
b. With systemic signs

to present more rapidly (1 month) than cats with tumors of the lower small intestine (3.5 months) or large intestine (4.5 months), presumably because owners more easily perceive the clinical signs of vomiting and anorexia.

On physical examination, affected cats with intestinal tumors are often cachectic and usually dehydrated and an abdominal mass is frequently palpable. Peritoneal carcinomatosis is common and may produce marked ascites.

Cats with intestinal mast cell tumors have a history of vomiting, diarrhea, and anorexia. These cats usually have a palpable abdominal mass that can be localized with ultrasound and rarely have circulating mast cells.

Cats with duodenal adenomatous polyps usually present with a history of acute or chronic vomiting. Vomitus will contain blood only in the acutely affected cat.

Clinical Work-up

In addition to survey abdominal and thoracic radiography, cats with intestinal tumors should have abdominal ultrasonography performed, because metastatic disease is usually abdominal. A complete blood count and biochemical panel, urinalysis, viral serologic study, bone marrow aspiration (lymphoma

and mast cell disease), and biopsy of lymphomatous tissue (lymphoma) should be performed on all cats with suspected intestinal tumors.

Intestinal adenocarcinomas in cats spread by intramural (rather than intraluminal) extension and thus generate an annular ("napkin ring") constriction rather than a mass lesion. Constriction of the intestinal tract causes obstruction. Abdominal radiographs may confirm the presence of a palpable abdominal mass, and plain or barium contrast radiographs may reveal evidence of obstruction of the small intestine (Figure 11-11). Osseous metaplasia may cause the intestinal tumor to mineralize. Endoscopy may help identify lesions of the upper intestinal tract (although duodenal tumors are rare) or of the rectum and colon. Ultrasonography provides a simple and reliable method to perform a biopsy on intestinal tumors in cats, as well as to image abdominal structures for evidence of metastasis. Because of the localized and obstructive nature of the lesion, however, exploratory laparotomy followed by a resection and anastomosis is often both diagnostic and therapeutic.

Ascites from peritoneal metastases is common, and cytologic examination of ascitic fluid may reveal malignant cells. Different histopathologic descriptions have been used to classify intestinal adenocarcinomas as tubular, mucinous, or undifferentiated, but the prognostic significance of these subclassifications is negligible. *All types have a high metastatic rate.*

Metastasis occurs to the peritoneum, mesentery, omentum, and regional lymph nodes in approximately 50% of affected cats with intestinal adenocarcinoma. Less common sites of metastasis are the liver, spleen, uterine stump or uterus, urinary bladder, and other areas in the intestinal tract. Metastasis to the lung is rarely reported.

Cats with suspected mast cell disease or lymphoma should have a similar staging regimen performed. Both of these diseases warrant bone marrow evaluation, as well as a similar work-up as described for adenocarcinoma. Retroviral status should always be evaluated. On thoracic radiographs it may be possible to appreciate a mediastinal mass or pleural effusion. Lymphadenopathy, GI thickening, and hepatomegaly may be observed on abdominal ultrasound. Ultrasound-guided biopsy, particularly in cats with GI tract involvement of lymphoma, has proven to be efficacious in obtaining diagnostic samples. Endoscopy can be used to obtain superficial biopsy specimens and is diagnostic in many cases. However, surgical full-

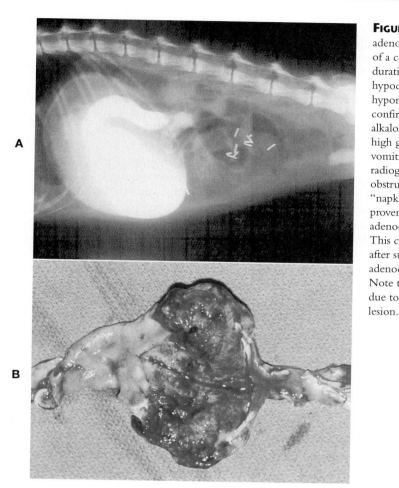

FIGURE 11-11 Intestinal adenocarcinoma in a cat. **A,** Radiograph of a cat with explosive vomiting of short duration. A biochemical profile revealed hypochloremia, hypokalemia, and hyponatremia, and blood gas levels confirmed the presence of a metabolic alkalosis. These findings are classic for a high gastrointestinal obstruction and vomiting of acidic gastric contents. The radiograph shows a high duodenal obstruction. Surgical removal of a "napkin ring" lesion, histologically proven to be an intestinal adenocarcinoma, resolved the problem. This cat remained free of disease 2 years after surgery. **B,** Intestinal adenocarcinoma of the cat noted in **A.** Note the proximal intestine was dilated due to the "napkin ring" obstructive lesion.

thickness biopsy specimens may be necessary for a definitive diagnosis.

In one series 65% of cats with intestinal mast cell tumors had metastases to regional lymph nodes, spleen, liver, lung, or bone marrow.

Anemia in cats with lymphoma is common but is usually low grade and characterized as normocytic and normochromic, which is compatible with anemia of chronic disease. Occasionally a moderate to severe anemia may be present due to GI blood loss secondary to lymphoma. Anemia is rarely a consequence of bone marrow involvement. Lymphocytosis requires evaluation of lymphocyte morphology and could indicate bone marrow involvement and a worse prognosis for remission.

Complete response rates to chemotherapy are as follows: stage I (93%), stage II (48%), stage III (52%), stage IV (42%), and stage V (58%). Cats with stage I and II disease have median survival times of 7.6 months compared with 3.2 months for cats with stage III and IV disease and 2.6 months for those in stage V.

Cats that are positive for the FeLV antigen have shorter survival times, but viral status does not influence response to therapy. In another study, response to therapy, FeLV status, and clinical substage were predictive of outcome. FeLV-negative cats that achieve a complete response following induction therapy are likely to have durable (greater than 6 months) responses, particularly when doxorubicin is included in the chemotherapy protocol.

Therapeutic Approach

Nutritional support is a crucial prerequisite for the successful management of intestinal tumors. Whenever chemotherapy or surgery is indicated, assisted tube feeding with esophageal, gastrostomy, or jejunostomy tubes is a must.

Resection of the intestinal mass is the only reported primary treatment for intestinal adenocarcinoma in cats, and there is only one report of a cat that was treated with adjuvant therapy. That cat received levamisole (2.3 mg/lb orally 3 days per week) for 2 months and lived 28 months before developing widespread metastases. The contribution of this treatment to survival is doubtful, because similar long survival times have been reported following surgery alone. Early studies that included some cats that died perioperatively had median survival times of 5 weeks and 10 weeks, respectively; however, both studies included some cats that lived for 2 years. In more recent studies the average survival ranged from 6 to 15 months and some cats lived more than 4 years. These figures are significant because seven cats with confirmed lymph node metastasis at the time of surgery lived for an average of 12 months, and two cats with carcinomatosis lived 4.5 and 28 months. *The finding of metastatic disease at surgery should not be a disincentive to treat cats surgically for intestinal adenocarcinoma.*

Resection of duodenal adenomatous polyps is predictably associated with a good surgical outcome, although anorexia is a postoperative complication in more than half of feline patients.

Chemotherapy is the mainstay of treatment for cats with alimentary lymphoma. Generally cats with lymphocytic lymphoma do substantially better than cats with large or intermediate lymphoblastic lymphoma. Single agents that have been used include prednisolone, cyclophosphamide, and chlorambucil. Varying responses have been seen with the use of each of these drugs, and in one report a cat had a complete response to cyclophosphamide for 14 months. The use of vincristine alone has produced long-term responses. L-Asparaginase, idarubicin, and mitoxantrone have been used with varying responses.

Combination chemotherapy, for example, the cyclophosphamide, vincristine, prednisone (CVP) protocol (see Table 11-3), still provides the basis for most chemotherapy protocols for feline lymphoma. In one study, median survival of 27 cats with alimentary lymphoma treated with vincristine (0.75 mg/m^2 intravenously weekly for 4 weeks, then every 3 weeks thereafter), cyclophosphamide (300 mg/m^2 orally every 3 weeks), and prednisolone (0.9 mg/lb/day) was 50 days. Although most cats responded poorly to chemotherapy, 9 cats achieved a complete remission. Survival times were not influenced by extent of GI involvement, sex, FeLV status, hematocrit, serum total protein concentration, and clinical stage. Response to therapy is probably the single most important prognostic factor for cats with GI lymphoma.

In another study 14 cats with alimentary lymphoma were treated with vincristine, cyclophosphamide, and methotrexate. The protocol was as follows: week 1, vincristine (0.01 mg/lb) administered intravenously; week 2, cyclophosphamide (4.5 mg/lb) administered intravenously; week 3, vincristine, same as week 1; week 4, methotrexate (0.36 mg/lb) administered intravenously. The median survival of these cats was 2.75 months.

In a different study 21 cats with alimentary lymphoma were treated with combination chemotherapy consisting of prednisolone, L-asparaginase, vincristine, cyclophosphamide, doxorubicin, and methotrexate (see protocol at end of this section). Median survival for these cats was 40 weeks, and overall median duration of first remission was 20 weeks. The only significant prognostic factor associated with duration of first remission was whether cats had a complete response following induction chemotherapy. Duration of first remission was significantly associated with survival time. Cats tolerated this protocol well.

In another study 38 cats with lymphoma were treated with induction COP chemotherapy. After induction, cats were randomized to receive either maintenance COP chemotherapy or single-agent doxorubicin. The median remission duration for the cats continuing on COP chemotherapy was 83 days, which was significantly shorter than the median remission for the cats that received doxorubicin as maintenance, which was 281 days. Therefore doxorubicin should be considered an efficacious agent for the maintenance treatment of cats with lymphoma. It is, however, a drug that is poor at inducing a complete remission. There was minimal toxicity noted in the cats in this report. It should be noted that the dose of prednisolone used in this study was 40 mg/m^2 daily and the doxorubicin dose used was 25 mg/m^2 every 3 weeks. The other drug dosages used are as printed above.

Finally, another study involved 67 cats with GI lymphoma that were treated with chemotherapy. Twenty-nine cats with lymphocytic lymphoma were treated with chlorambucil and prednisolone. The chlorambucil dosage we use is the total cumulative dosage of 6 mg/m² body surface area (BSA). This works out to 2 mg every other day or on a Monday-Wednesday-Friday every week basis, depending on how small the cat is. The rule is to *never* break a tablet. The prednisolone dose is 0.5 to 1 mg/lb/day. Complete remission was obtained in 69% of these cats, with a median disease-free interval of 16 months. The cats with lymphoblastic lymphoma of the GI tract treated with the same chemotherapy did not do nearly as well, with a survival time of only 2.7 months and a complete remission rate of 18%.

Obtaining clean margins at surgery seems to increase survival time in cats with malignant colonic neoplasia. Data from this particular study indicate that survival time of cats with colonic lymphoma may not be affected by chemotherapy. Cats with an unidentified colonic mass should have a subtotal colectomy to increase survival time. Cats with colonic adenocarcinoma should have surgery, and adjunctive chemotherapy, using doxorubicin, should be considered as well.

Intestinal mast cell disease is best treated with large surgical resection. Prednisolone may have some efficacy. The following combination chemotherapy has demonstrated some success: week 1, vinblastine (2 mg/m²) administered intravenously every 3 weeks; week 2, cyclophosphamide (300 mg/m²) administered orally over 3 to 5 days every 3 weeks; and oral prednisolone (0.54 mg/lb) administered daily.

Supportive therapy is very important for cats with GI neoplasia. Often these cats will require feeding tubes. For patients with frequent vomiting a jejunostomy tube may be necessary; otherwise an esophagostomy or gastrostomy tube may be appropriate. Subcutaneous fluid administration, antiemetics (metoclopramide at 0.09 to 0.18 mg/lb orally three times a day and ondansetron at 0.23 to 0.45 mg/lb orally one to two times a day), and appetite stimulants (cyproheptadine at 0.9 to 1.8 mg/lb orally two to three times a day) may be necessary for use in conjunction with chemotherapy. A complete blood count should always be performed 1 week after cyclophosphamide and doxorubicin administration, because both of these agents can be myelosuppressive. If the segmented neutrophil count is less than 1000 cells/μl, the next dose should be decreased by 10% to 25%. Doxorubicin-induced cardiotoxicity and cyclophosphamide-induced hemorrhagic cystitis are rare in the cat.

ADENOCARCINOMA OF THE APOCRINE GLANDS OF THE ANAL SAC IN DOGS

Background

Anal sac adenocarcinoma overwhelmingly occurs in old, female dogs, whether they are intact or spayed. There appears to be no breed predisposition; however, one European study reported that five of eight affected dogs were long-haired and shorthaired German pointers.

A characteristic feature of this tumor is production of a parathyroid hormone–related protein that causes hypercalcemia and hypophosphatemia.

Clinical Parameters

Affected dogs are often presented to veterinarians because of an unrelated problem, because the owner notices a swelling in the perineum, or because there is dyschezia, tenesmus, or a ribbonlike stool shape. Tenesmus may be due either to the primary tumor or to sublumbar lymphadenopathy, which may be palpable rectally. Signs may be present for up to 1 year before presentation. In 40% to 60% of dogs in several reported series the tumor was an incidental finding on rectal examination or was found only after hypercalcemia had been identified. *This emphasizes the importance of including a rectal palpation in routine physical examinations.* The tumor mass is usually between 1 and 10 cm in diameter; smaller primary masses that are difficult to palpate may be present. Because the tumor may be bilateral, it is important to palpate both anal sacs.

Other clinical signs are pruritus, ulceration and bleeding, decreased appetite, weight loss, and weakness or paresis. Polydipsia and polyuria are common in hypercalcemic dogs. *The identification of hypercalcemia on a biochemical profile warrants careful palpation of the anal sacs.*

Clinical Work-up

If anal sac adenocarcinoma is suspected in a dog, a routine blood chemistry profile should be performed to identify hypercalcemia and any secondary renal damage. Definitive diagnosis is made by surgical biopsy, although a high index of suspicion for this disease should follow detection of a perianal mass in an old, female dog with hypercalcemia.

Abdominal ultrasonography should be performed in addition to routine abdominal and thoracic radiographs, because abdominal metastases are much more common than thoracic.

Paraneoplastic hypercalcemia is common in dogs with apocrine gland adenocarcinoma of the anal sacs and may occur in both males and females. In one study, serum calcium was elevated in 25% of the affected dogs to an average of 14.6 mg/dl. In another study 90% of dogs with anal sac adeno-carcinoma had elevated serum calcium levels, to an average of 16.1 mg/dl. Hypophosphatemia occurred concurrently with hypercalcemia in some but not all of the affected dogs.

This neoplasm is highly malignant and metasta-sizes early in the course of the disease to the sub-lumbar and iliac lymph nodes. In one study approximately 50% of the dogs developed lymph node metastases; in two other studies 94% of the dogs had metastases to the above-mentioned sites. Abdominal radiographs are useful in identifying sublumbar lymphadenopathy, but ultrasonography may be more accurate than radiographs or digital rectal palpation in disclosing the extent of lymph node involvement.

Less frequent sites of metastasis are the lungs, which may show a nodular or diffuse pattern ra-diographically, and (rarely) the lumbar vertebrae, liver, and kidneys. Metastasis may occur when the primary tumor is very small, and clinical signs relating to the primary tumor may not be obvious.

Prognostic Factors

In one study, hypercalcemic dogs had a median survival of 6 months after surgical excision of the tumor, compared with 11.5 months for normocal-cemic dogs. Dogs with metastases detected at sur-gery predictably had shorter median survival times (6 months) than did dogs without metastases (15.5 months).

Therapeutic Approach

Ideally, hypercalcemia should be controlled before and during definitive therapy. Surgical excision of the primary tumor is often difficult because of the large size of these tumors and their invasive growth characteristics. Local recurrence occurs in approximately 25% of dogs. Even with incomplete surgical excision, however, most dogs that are hypercalcemic become normocalcemic after sur-gery. Hypercalcemia presumably reflects some

critical tumor mass, because even dogs with metas-tases may not show recurrence of hypercalcemia until those metastases become large.

Complications of surgery reflect the difficulties encountered in any surgical procedure involving the perineal area. Fecal incontinence can follow surgery in up to 20% of dogs and may be perma-nent. Wound infection can occur and cause sepsis.

Local recurrence is a problem with some dogs, and others develop recurrence in the regional lymph nodes. If the sublumbar nodes are enlarged at diagnosis, it may be possible to remove them surgically; however, tumor-invaded nodes are fre-quently friable and invade around the vessels and nerves in this area. The nodes were well-encapsulated in 80% of dogs treated surgically in one study, but they were also well vascularized; thus the surgeon should be prepared to encounter bleeding. In this study, complications during lymph node surgery caused the death of one third of the dogs; almost one third of the survivors developed transient uri-nary incontinence, presumably as a result of neu-rologic trauma. Overall, 6 of 27 dogs died within 2 weeks after undergoing surgery for removal of either the primary tumor or its metastases. Median survival for the remaining dogs was 8.3 months; the range of survival was 6 weeks to 39 months. Five dogs were still alive at 14 months after sur-gery. This moderate success rate was corroborated in another study in which 50% of the dogs died between 2 and 22 months after surgery, with an average survival of 8.8 months. In another report the median survival of dogs with this disease treated with surgery alone was 295 days.

Chemotherapy might be promising as adjuvant therapy for this tumor, but relatively little has been reported. Three dogs treated with doxorubicin and cyclophosphamide, either alone or in combination with prednisolone, vincristine, and L-asparaginase (for concurrent lymphoma), had survival times of 1, 2, and 14 months. Another tumor did not re-spond to treatment with melphalan and cyclophos-phamide. Anecdotally cisplatin has caused complete regression of metastatic lesions in some dogs with this disease. Recent investigations suggest that sur-gical excision of the primary tumor and sublum-bar lymph nodes followed by intraoperative and external beam radiation therapy combined with chemotherapy (e.g., doxorubicin) provides clinical remission times of more than 1 year. In another report, dogs with this disease were treated with several different chemotherapeutic agents and median survival was 245 days.

Dogs with anal sac adenocarcinoma should be treated surgically in an attempt to achieve complete excision of the primary mass. Sublumbar lymph nodes should be removed if they are enlarged, although this is a technically demanding surgery. Adjuvant radiation therapy and chemotherapy using cisplatin should be considered, although the roles of adjuvant therapies are still being defined.

HEPATIC AND PANCREATIC NEOPLASIA

Nonhematopoietic Primary Liver Tumors in Dogs

Background

Primary hepatic neoplasia is uncommon in the dog. When neoplasia is found in the liver, it is more likely to be due to metastasis. The most common histologic types of primary liver tumors include hepatocellular adenoma, hepatocellular carcinoma, bile duct (cholangiocellular) carcinoma, and hepatic carcinoid. Tumor types found less frequently include bile duct cystadenoma, cholangioma, fibroma, fibrosarcoma, hemangioma, hemangiosarcoma, leiomyosarcoma, liposarcoma, myxosarcoma, and osteosarcoma. One study evaluated 110 liver tumors and found that slightly more than 50% were primary hepatocellular carcinomas, with bile duct carcinomas and cystadenomas seen less frequently. Liver carcinomas (hepatocellular or bile duct) affect older dogs with a mean age between 10 and 12 years, whereas hepatic carcinoids occur in younger patients with a mean age of 8 years. In a series of 18 dogs with primary hepatocellular carcinomas, males were affected more often. Another series found that female dogs were more likely to have a bile duct carcinoma.

Clinical Parameters

Dogs with liver tumors often have nonspecific signs of illness. However, the most common signs associated with a primary liver tumor include a palpable abdominal mass localized to the region of the liver, anorexia, weight loss, depression, weakness, vomiting, and ascites. Less often, polyuria and polydipsia, pyrexia, poor hair coat, ataxia, diarrhea, or central nervous system signs due to hepatoencephalopathy or hypoglycemia may occur.

Clinical Work-up

Hematologic abnormalities can be helpful in assessing the patient with a liver mass. Abnormal platelet function, hypoproteinemia, hypoglycemia, elevated liver enzyme levels (especially aspartate aminotransferase [AST], alanine aminotransferase [ALT], and alkaline phosphatase [ALP]) and less commonly hyperbilirubinemia have been reported in dogs with liver tumors. In one study all dogs with hepatocellular carcinomas had elevated levels of ALT and ALP. These parameters were less frequently elevated in dogs with metastatic disease. The use of fasting serum bile acid concentrations does not provide compelling evidence of neoplasia. An enzymatic kit to detect alpha fetoprotein was used to distinguish different liver tumor types before biopsy. Levels of alpha fetoprotein were highest in dogs with cholangiocarcinoma and hepatocellular carcinoma; however, this assay is probably best used in conjunction with a complete blood count, biochemical profile, urinalysis, diagnostic imaging of the chest and abdomen, and biopsy of the lesion.

Abdominal radiography, contrast procedures, and ultrasonography are most commonly employed to confirm a diagnosis of liver cancer. Other useful imaging methodologies include hepatoscintigraphy, CT, and magnetic resonance imaging (MRI). A radiographic finding that supports a diagnosis of a hepatic mass is a right cranioventral abdominal mass that displaces the gastric shadow to the left and displaces the small intestine caudally. In some instances, peritoneal fluid from ascites or carcinomatosis may obscure radiographic detection of the mass.

Ultrasonography is more precise than radiography in detecting the site of origin of an abdominal mass and also enables the examination of hepatic parenchyma, biliary system, perihepatic structures, and portal and hepatic vascular supply. A hepatic tumor may appear as a large, well-circumscribed mass extending from the liver margins with an echogenicity that is usually more mixed than normal liver (see examples in Chapter 2). Hepatic tumors may also be found in multiples or of homogeneous echogenicity. Areas of edema, necrosis, fibrosis, neovascularization, hemorrhage, and inflammation all contribute to the variable appearance of liver tumors on ultrasound. Differentiating between histologic type and benign versus malignant neoplasms is usually not possible with ultrasound examination alone. For this reason, hepatic aspiration or biopsy is commonly required to make a definitive diagnosis. Prebiopsy evaluations should include a review of the patient's overall status, risk for hemorrhage or impaired wound healing, and liver size. A very ill patient may not be a good anesthetic candidate, in which case less-invasive biopsy techniques with the use of local anesthetic would be a better choice. A coagulation profile including prothrombin time (PT), partial thromboplastin time (PTT), fibrin degradation products (FDPs), fibrinogen content, and platelet count should identify those patients at increased risk for hemorrhage. At a minimum, packed cell volume (PCV), total solids (TS), estimate of platelet count, buccal mucosa bleeding time (BMBT), and activated clotting time (ACT) should be performed.

Techniques for obtaining neoplastic material include fine-needle aspiration (percutaneous, blind), keyhole biopsy (percutaneous, blind), ultrasound-guided fine-needle aspiration or biopsy, transthoracic biopsy, laparoscopic biopsy, or exploratory celiotomy. See the References for hepatic aspiration and biopsy techniques. One study found a poor correlation between cytologic and histologic findings for liver disease, with an agreement of only 44% for hepatic tumors in particular. Ultrasound-guided biopsy with a 14-gauge Tru-Cut biopsy instrument usually provides a definitive diagnosis and is the procedure of choice for diffuse lesions, zonal lesions that involve all hepatic lobules or acini, or focal lesions defined by ultrasound. However, with lesions other than those mentioned, wedge liver biopsy samples taken during laparotomy provide the pathologist with the best specimen for evaluation and allow the surgeon to examine the liver during the procedure as well.

Staging of liver tumors should be performed with chest radiographs and abdominal ultrasound to detect hepatic lymphadenopathy, other organ involvement, or lesions in multiple lobes. Of 49 dogs with hepatocellular carcinoma, 30 (61%) were initially diagnosed to have a solitary mass in only one liver lobe, but 24 of the 30 (80%) actually had lesions in other lobes. A solitary liver mass was the most common presenting sign for hepatocellular carcinoma in other studies. Regardless of histologic type, metastasis is common for liver tumors. In a study of 57 dogs with liver tumors, metastasis to the regional lymph nodes (14 dogs), lungs (14 dogs), or peritoneal surfaces (7 dogs) occurred in 35 (61%) cases. In another study, spread to the lungs was less common and occurred in only 2 of 13 dogs with hepatocellular carcinoma and bile duct carcinoma. Large, solitary hepatocellular carcinomas are less likely to metastasize than are multiple lesions. Thirteen of 14 dogs (93%) with multiple or diffuse lesions had metastasis, whereas 11 of 30 dogs (37%) with solitary liver masses had evidence of metastasis. The size of a liver mass has little influence on prognosis, although it is speculated that large lesions that have not led to the demise of the patient are more likely to behave in a less aggressive fashion. Further, the degree of invasion and presence of metastasis are more likely to be prognostic indicators than size. Predictably dogs with solitary liver tumors are probably the best candidates for surgical resection and control of disease, whereas dogs with multiple lesions have a less favorable prognosis.

Treatment

Up to 75% of the liver can be resected with negligible compromise to liver function, and complete regeneration occurs within 6 to 8 weeks. Several techniques are described in the literature, including partial lobectomy, complete lobectomy, and partial hepatectomy. The most commonly used procedures are partial and complete lobectomies. For benign liver masses—such as hepatocellular adenoma, cholangioma, fibroma, and bile duct cystadenoma—surgical excision has the greatest potential for definitively controlling disease.

Surgery is also the treatment of choice for dogs with hepatocellular carcinoma that involves one or two liver lobes (Figure 11-12). In a report of 18 dogs with solitary hepatocellular carcinoma, 16 were resected with single lobectomies and 2 by partial hepatectomy. At the time of publication in that study, 8 dogs had died with a mean survival time of 306 days (range, 1 to 548 days), and 10 dogs were still alive with a mean survival time of 377 days (range, 195 to 1025 days).

The success of treatment for other types of hepatic neoplasms is less defined. In a report of two dogs with bile duct carcinoma and adenocarcinoma treated with partial hepatectomy, both dogs had survival times of 6 months. A hepatic mesenchymoma treated by excision recurred 4 months after surgery in another dog.

It is unknown whether chemotherapy is valuable as an adjunctive treatment; however, many drugs have been used (5-fluorouracil [5-FU], cisplatin, actinomycin D, and mitoxantrone). Occasional responses have been seen with doxorubicin in humans with hepatocellular carcinoma.

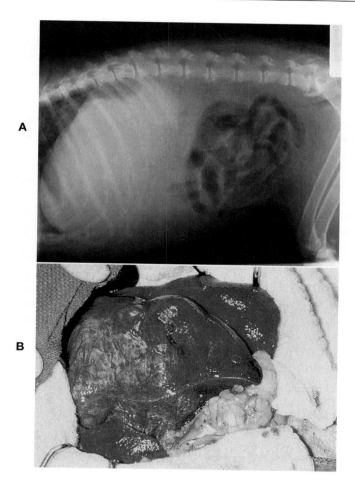

FIGURE 11-12 Hepatic carcinoma in a dog. **A,** Radiograph of a 7-year-old, mixed breed, female dog with a tumor of the liver. The mass was identified on an annual physical examination. The biochemical profile was completely normal, suggesting slow growth of the tumor and incomplete involvement of the liver. Resection resulted in a cure of this condition. **B,** The tumor was a low-grade hepatic carcinoma localized to one liver lobe. This tumor was removed, and the dog was noted to be free of the tumor and all evidence of clinical signs relating to this disease for at least 2 years.

Hematopoietic Liver Tumors in Dogs

Background

Lymphoma is the most common hematopoietic tumor with liver involvement in the dog, followed by a variety of myeloproliferative neoplasias and mast cell tumors.

Clinical Parameters, Work-up, and Treatment

Clinical signs result from the infiltration and disruption of liver function. Diagnosis and treatment for these tumors are similar to that which is described in the section on tumors of the GI tract.

Metastatic Liver Tumors in Dogs

Background

Hemangiosarcoma, islet cell carcinoma, pancreatic carcinoma, and fibrosarcoma are the most common tumor types that metastasize to involve the liver. Less commonly osteosarcoma, transitional cell carcinoma, mammary carcinoma, intestinal carcinoma, nasal carcinoma, pheochromocytoma, and thyroid carcinoma have been reported.

Clinical Parameters, Work-up, and Treatment

Clinical signs for metastatic disease are usually a result of disruption of liver function. The clinical work-up should be the same as that described for primary liver cancer. However, treatment will differ between tumor types and is usually directed at palliation rather than curative intent.

Nonhematopoietic Primary Liver Tumors in Cats

Background

In cats, biliary carcinoma is the most common primary liver tumor, followed by hepatocellular carcinoma, hemangiosarcoma, and other sarcomas. An evaluation of 107 cats with nonvascular, nonhematopoietic liver tumors found 57 intra-hepatic bile duct tumors, of which 34 (60%) were benign. Hepatocellular carcinoma is less common in cats than in dogs and accounted for 25% of primary feline liver tumors. Tumors of the extrahepatic bile duct (9 of 107) or gallbladder (4 of 107) are usually malignant. Most cats affected with bile duct tumors are middle-age, ranging upward in age from 6 years. In a series of 21 cats with liver tumors, affected animals were older than 10 years of age. Sex predilection for bile duct tumors has not been resolved, because one study found male cats to be overrepresented, whereas another found the opposite to be true. In both studies, bile duct tumors were more common in domestic short hairs than in Siamese. The median age of cats affected with hepatocellular carcinoma is 11 years, and males are more commonly affected (11 of 17 [65%]). As is the case with biliary tumors, hepatocellular carcinomas also affect domestic short hairs more frequently. FeLV does not seem to play a role in nonhematopoietic liver tumors. Hepatic myelolipoma, an uncommon tumor consisting of adipose tissue and bone marrow elements, has been associated with diaphragmatic hernias in cats and may be associated with chronic hypoxia or trauma to the liver.

Clinical Parameters

Clinical signs of liver tumors include anorexia, lethargy, and weakness. Less commonly a patient may have presenting symptoms of vomiting, diarrhea, polydipsia, and ascites. In most cats a mass in the cranial abdomen or hepatomegaly can be detected on palpation.

Clinical Work-up

Hematologic abnormalities are less commonly detected in cats than in dogs with liver tumors. Liver enzyme elevations are less likely (possibly due to the short serum half-life of ALP in the cat) and are thought to be nonspecific for liver cancer. In cats with cystadenomas the most common abnormality is azotemia, without bilirubinemia and elevated liver enzyme levels, which is more indicative of another disease process.

Chest radiographs and abdominal ultrasonography are extremely valuable in assessing cats with a liver mass. Benign liver masses are most often cystic with several different compartments, whereas malignant tumors tend to be multilobular. One study found that benign bile duct adenomas involved multiple liver lobes in 50% (8 of 16) of

the cases, whereas the majority (7 of 9 [78%]) of bile duct carcinomas were widespread throughout the liver. Metastasis to the peritoneal surfaces, hepatic lymph nodes, and lungs is commonly encountered with malignant bile duct tumors in cats; less common sites include thoracic lymph nodes, diaphragm, spleen, urinary bladder, GI tract, and bone. Malignant transformation from benign to malignant lesions has also been reported. Of 18 cats with hepatocellular carcinoma, however, only 5 (28%) had evidence of metastasis to the hepatic lymph nodes, lung, or spleen.

Aspiration or biopsy (and prebiopsy evaluation) should be performed as outlined in the section on primary liver tumors in dogs. As is the case in dogs, cytologic evaluation from fine-needle aspiration has only a 44% correlation with histopathologic findings and should be interpreted with caution. In the case of cystadenomas, aspiration of cystic fluid characteristically produces a yellow to colorless transudate with a specific gravity of 1.001 to 1.008 and protein concentration less than 2 gm/dl, with the most common cell type being a macrophage. Although this finding is not diagnostic for hepatobiliary cystadenomas, it will permit one to rule out abscesses, hematomas, and parasitic cysts.

Treatment

In those cases where the liver mass is confined to a resectable portion of the liver and there is no evidence of metastasis, surgical resection is indicated.

Benign hepatobiliary cystadenomas prevail as the tumor type in older cats, and for this reason surgical resection with long-term control of disease is often possible (Figure 11-13). Surgical resection of a hepatobiliary cystadenoma involving both the left medial and lateral lobes of the liver resulted in long-term survival (over 18 months), with the patient still alive at time of publication. Long-term survivals, ranging from 12 to 44 months, with no postoperative complications were reported in five cats with surgical resections of hepatobiliary cystadenomas. This study also found that although complete surgical excision is preferable, even partial resection merits a good prognosis. In another report a 16-year-old cat lived 27 months after surgical excision of a myelolipoma and had no tumor recurrence.

To date there are no reports of adjuvant chemotherapy in cats with malignant tumors of the liver. Few data exist on the efficacy of chemotherapeutic

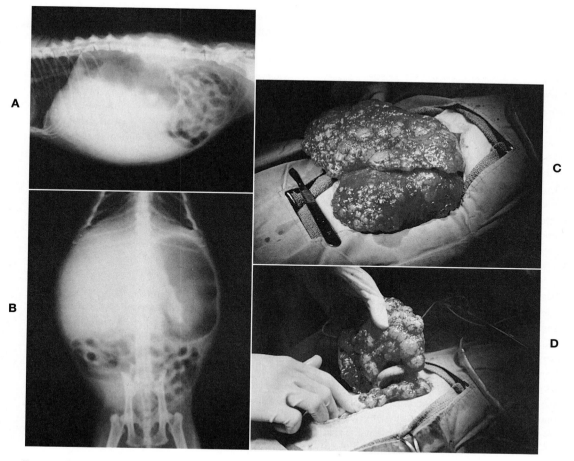

FIGURE 11-13 Biliary cystic hyperplasia in a 15-year-old cat. The cat was asymptomatic, and results of a complete blood count and biochemical profile were normal. **A,** Lateral and, **B,** ventrodorsal survey abdominal radiographs showing marked hepatomegaly and displacement of the stomach dorsally and to the left. **C** and **D,** Appearance of the liver at laparotomy. Multiple (polycystic) hepatic cysts were present throughout the liver. Treatment involved removal of two liver lobes to decrease the size of the liver. The polycystic disorder appears to be inheritable and runs a benign course in affected patients. (Courtesy Dr. Todd R. Tams.)

treatment of dogs with primary hepatic tumors. Doxorubicin and 5-FU have been recommended by some; however, efficacy is unknown.

Hematopoietic Liver Tumors in Cats
Background
Lymphoma is the most common hematopoietic tumor with liver involvement in the cat, followed by a variety of myeloproliferative neoplasias and mast cell tumors.

Clinical Parameters, Work-up, and Treatment
Clinical signs result from the infiltration and disruption of liver function. Diagnosis and treatment

for these tumors are similar to that which is described in the section on tumors of the GI tract.

Metastatic Liver Tumors in Cats
Background
Metastatic liver disease is less common in the cat. Although no specific tumor type is overrepresented, the most common metastatic tumor types include pancreatic carcinoma, intestinal carcinoma, and renal carcinoma.

Clinical Parameters, Work-up, and Treatment
Clinical signs for metastatic disease are usually a result of disruption of liver function. The clinical work-up should be the same as that described for

primary liver cancer. However, treatment will differ between tumor types and is usually directed at palliation rather than curative intent.

Exocrine Pancreas Tumors in Dogs
Background
Exocrine pancreatic tumors are uncommon. These tumors do not show a sex predilection and occur in older dogs. Cocker spaniels may be overrepresented, because this breed was seen in 3 of 14 cases reported in one study. Another series found that only spaniel breeds were affected in the cases reported. The most common histologic type is carcinoma arising from the ductal epithelium, with adenocarcinoma—which arises from the acinar cell—being the second most common.

Clinical Parameters
Nonspecific clinical signs such as weight loss, depression, and anorexia are often seen with pancreatic tumors. Although these tumors are thought to cause vomiting, this is a relatively uncommon finding; if vomiting does occur, it is usually at the terminal stages of disease when extrahepatic bile duct obstruction secondary to liver metastasis has occurred. Abdominal palpation may reveal a mass in the cranial abdomen, and abdominal fluid may also be present. In a report of three dogs with pancreatic carcinoma found on necropsy, panniculitis with subsequent subcutaneous swelling and shifting leg lameness over a period of months were the only clinical signs reported.

Clinical Work-up
A complete blood count, biochemical profile, urinalysis, chest and abdominal radiographs and abdominal ultrasound should be performed to evaluate the general health status of the patient, stage for metastasis, and assess the primary mass. In dogs with pancreatic carcinomas, half are solitary masses and the rest consist of multiple nodules throughout the pancreatic parenchyma. Metastases are common, occurring in over 92% of cases. The liver is most commonly affected (12 of 13) with the omentum (6 of 13) and regional lymph nodes (4 of 13) less frequently affected. Less commonly other visceral sites are sites for metastasis. For instance, in one case of pancreatic carcinoma associated with diabetes insipidus, metastasis to the pituitary gland was detected. Although it is unusual, no evidence of metastasis was seen in one series of three cases of pancreatic

carcinoma where panniculitis, subcutaneous swelling, and shifting leg lameness were clinically apparent for months. Blood work revealed marked elevations in levels of serum lipase and amylase in one of these cases, although no evidence of pancreatitis was seen. Hematologic abnormalities associated with pancreatic carcinoma may include elevated serum amylase and lipase levels; lipase levels of 25 times greater than normal are most likely to be diagnostic for exocrine pancreatic carcinoma.

Ultrasonography can be useful in detecting a pancreatic mass if the pancreas can be visualized despite shadowing from gas–filled GI structures. This will also permit evaluation of the liver for metastases, although definitive diagnosis requires biopsy.

Treatment
If a pancreatic mass is detected in a stable patient and there is no evidence of metastasis, exploratory laparotomy with intent to surgically resect the mass may be considered. However, due to the high rate of metastasis, the prognosis should be considered poor for control of disease.

Chemotherapy is not considered effective in the treatment of pancreatic carcinoma because there is a high incidence of de novo resistance to cytotoxic drugs.

Endocrine Pancreas Tumors in Dogs
Insulinoma (Beta Cell Tumor, Islet Cell Tumor)
Background
Insulinomas are functional secreting tumors that arise from the islet cells in the endocrine pancreas. In addition to the secretion of insulin and its precursors, insulinomas are now known to secrete pancreatic polypeptide, somatostatin, glucagon, serotonin, gastrin, and corticotropin. These tumors are most commonly carcinomas and most often present late in the course of disease with signs attributable to the resultant hypoglycemia. Insulinomas occur in older dogs, with no sex predilection reported.

Metastasis is common with insulinomas. At the time of diagnosis, evidence of metastasis is present in approximately 36% of the cases, with the most common sites being the lymph nodes and liver. Spread to the duodenum, mesentery, omentum, spleen, spinal cord, and kidney have also been reported.

The WHO staging scheme is as follows:

Stage I ($T_1 N_0 M_0$)   Tumor confined to pancreas only

Stage II ($T_1 N_1 M_0$)   Tumor in pancreas and regional lymph nodes

Stage III ($T_1 N_{0-1} M_1$)   Tumor in pancreas, lymph nodes, and distant metastatic sites (most commonly the liver)

Clinical Parameters

Clinical signs of insulinomas include seizures, collapse, generalized or caudal weakness, lethargy, ataxia, muscle fasciculations, bizarre behavior, polyphagia, exercise intolerance, shaking/trembling, polyuria/polydipsia, and weight gain. These clinical signs can be explained by hyperinsulinemia with resultant hypoglycemia and release of counter-regulatory hormones (catecholamines and glucagon in the early phase and cortisol and growth hormones in the later phase of disease). Because of the patient's ability to adjust to a chronic state of hypoglycemia, signs of hypoglycemia are often not seen, even with extremely low blood glucose levels. The rate of decrease in blood glucose, as well as the duration of hypoglycemia, is considered important in the development of clinical signs.

There are two types of presenting clinical signs: *neuroglycopenic* (seizures, weakness, ataxia, and lethargy) and *sympathetic* (behavioral changes, shaking/trembling, and muscle fasciculations). Neurologic signs are due to the reliance of the central nervous system on diffusion for glucose uptake (which is predictably low in periods of hypoglycemia) and its inability to utilize other forms of energy, such as fatty acids and ketone bodies. The sympathetic signs are related to an increased discharge of counter-regulatory hormones. There is no correlation between the severity of clinical signs and the stage of disease, however.

Clinical Work-up

Basic blood work and urinalysis, chest and abdominal radiographs, and abdominal ultrasound should be performed to diagnose and stage dogs with suspected insulinomas, to rule out other causes of hypoglycemia, and to evaluate for the presence of any concurrent disease. Blood work, urinalysis, and radiographs are usually unremarkable in the patient with insulinoma, with the exception of hypoglycemia and, rarely, elevated liver enzymes.

Abdominal ultrasound infrequently detects a mass on the pancreas, but other organ metastases and/or mesenteric lymphadenopathy may be evident. The diagnosis of insulinoma is based on demonstration of hyperinsulinemia in the face of hypoglycemia. There are several means by which one can achieve this, including the insulin-glucose, glucose-insulin, and amended insulin-glucose ratios. For the most part these ratios are not considered diagnostic because they are associated with a high number of false-positive results. For this reason, performing a paired insulin and glucose test is considered to be the most reliable method of diagnosing an insulinoma. This test is further described below.

One study describes the use of chromogranin A (CgA) and neuron-specific enolase (NSE) as a marker for canine and feline pancreatic islet cell tumors. The study found these assays to be sensitive in detecting tumors of neuroendocrine origin. Another report describes the use of fructosamine measurement, which may be helpful in conjunction with insulin measurement in diagnosing an insulinoma. Provocative testing has been described in the literature. Such tests include glucagon tolerance, glucose tolerance, tolbutamide tolerance, L-leucine, oral glucose tolerance, epinephrine tolerance, and the calcium infusion test. These tests use the administration of potentially dangerous substances and are expensive, time consuming, and most importantly not as accurate as the paired insulin-glucose tests.

Preferred Test Protocol. Most dogs will become hypoglycemic within 8 to 10 hours of fasting. Dogs should be fed at 5:00 PM, 8:30 PM, and midnight, then fasted thereafter. Blood glucose should be monitored starting at 8:00 AM the next morning. When serum glucose is 60 mg/dl, serum should be saved for insulin levels. This test will detect hyperinsulinemia in approximately 77% of patients. The remaining 23% will show insulin levels in the normal range, which is highly suggestive for but not diagnostic of insulinoma, and the test should be repeated.

Treatment

Surgical resection is the treatment of choice for insulinoma. Both lobes of the pancreas are affected with equal frequency, with the body of the pancreas affected less commonly. In a study of 39 dogs with insulinoma comparing surgical to medical treatment, 26 underwent exploratory celiotomy and partial pancreatectomy and the median survival was 381 days (range, 20 to 1758 days). Thirteen were treated medically and had a median survival of 74 days (range, 8 to 508 days). Twelve of the 13 dogs (92%) died or were euthanized because of clinical signs resulting from hypoglycemia.

Medical Management. Medical management should be approached in a stepwise fashion. Initially a reduction in exercise and concomitant dietary changes (frequent small feedings containing high protein and complex carbohydrates) is employed. Prednisolone can be introduced as signs of hypoglycemia worsen. Prednisolone has antiinsulin and hyperglycemic effects starting at a dose of 0.11 mg/lb (orally twice daily); the dose can be increased as needed up to 0.5 mg/lb (orally twice daily) when iatrogenic Cushing's disease becomes a risk.

Diazoxide has several beneficial effects in the treatment of insulinomas. It inhibits cell uptake of glucose, blocks calcium entry into beta cells, catalyzes the breakdown of glycogen to glucose, and enhances glucose synthesis. The initial dose is 2.3 mg/lb (orally twice daily), which may be increased to 13.6 mg/lb (orally twice daily) if required to control signs of hypoglycemia. Potential side effects include GI toxicity (vomiting, diarrhea, inappetence), hyperglycemia, diabetes, myelosuppression, and hypernatremia. Hydrochlorothiazide (0.9 to 1.8 mg/lb, orally once daily) can be added to potentiate the effects of diazoxide.

Octreotide acetate (somatostatin) can be given at 10 to 20 μg subcutaneously two to three times daily. Its efficacy is variable in the small subset of patients treated to date. Calcium channel blockers may be useful. Alloxan (29.5 mg/lb intravenously with concurrent fluid therapy) has been described in a small number of dogs. Streptozotocin, a nitrosurea compound, has also been reported in two dogs but is extremely nephrotoxic, can be hepatotoxic, and should be considered as a rescue agent only. Similarly, doxorubicin and streptozotocin, carboplatin, cyclophosphamide, tubercidin and mithramycin have all been used in humans, but with variable effects, and there is no data on canine patients to date. Radiation therapy has not been reported in dogs. The prognosis for long-term control of insulinoma in the dog is grave in those with metastatic disease, although the short-term control is good. Young dogs and those with very high serum insulin concentrations have shorter survival times. In one study the overall survival for dogs undergoing surgery for insulinoma was 10 to 14 months. Dogs in stages I and II tend to have similar survival times, although dogs in stage II

have recurrence of clinical signs earlier. More than 80% of dogs in stage III have recurrence of disease at 1 year. There is little doubt that surgery should be recommended for patients with suspect insulinomas and that many patients require concurrent medical management.

Glucagonoma
Background

A rare tumor of the pancreatic alpha-islet cells, glucagon-secreting tumors have been described in the dog in a number of case reports. A review of the characteristic syndrome, referred to as glucagonoma syndrome, cites no sex predilection.

Clinical Parameters and Work-up

Clinical signs described in the literature include skin lesions, referred to as superficial necrolytic dermatitis (SND) or metabolic epidermal necrosis (MEN). These lesions are characterized by mild to marked hyperkeratosis and fissuring of the footpads, erythema, and crusting plaques on the oral cavity, muzzle, limbs, abdomen, and genital areas. Staging for glucagonoma should include basic blood work, urinalysis, and thoracic and abdominal imaging. Biochemical abnormalities are variable and may include hyperglycemia, elevated liver enzyme levels, and nonregenerative anemia. A case report on one dog found hyperglucagonemia, hyperinsulinemia, and hypoaminoacidemia. Ultrasound findings are usually unremarkable, although a pancreatic mass was suggested in one of seven dogs reported.

Treatment

Surgical excision is the treatment of choice. Metastasis is common to the liver (three of four dogs [75%]) and/or mesenteric lymph node (one of four dogs [25%]). However, survival and resolution of disease is reported in one case. The major postoperative surgical complication in reported cases was bile duct obstruction and pancreatitis.

Medical management includes symptomatic therapy with intravenous amino acid administration. A 10% solution of crystalline amino acid solution, approximately 11.4 ml/lb of body weight, is administered over 6 to 8 hours and repeated every 7 to 10 days. Oral nutritional support with a high-quality protein diet should also be instituted. Supplementation with egg yolks (three to six daily), zinc, essential fatty acids, and prednisone have also been described. Somatostatin analogues have been used in humans and have resulted in remissions, although these drugs have not been evaluated in dogs.

Gastrinoma

Background

A rare tumor of the pancreatic islets, gastrinomas secrete gastrin and result in hypertrophic gastritis and subsequent peptic ulcers. This syndrome is referred to as Zollinger-Ellison syndrome. These tumors are usually small, discrete masses within the pancreas. Most are malignant and metastasize to the regional lymph nodes and liver.

Clinical Parameters and Work-up

Clinical signs of gastrinomas include chronic vomiting and weight loss. These signs are related to the hypersecretion of gastrin and consequent ulceration. A complete staging scheme should include a complete blood count, biochemical profile, urinalysis, and thoracic and abdominal imaging. Diagnosis involves the measurement of serum gastrin, demonstration of gastric hypertrophy and ulceration (via endoscopy), and increased secretion of gastric acid. Provocative testing with secretin or calcium is usually only indicated when gastrin levels are minimally elevated. A novel method of diagnosis described is the use of somatostatin-receptor scintigraphy.

Treatment

Although the course of gastrinomas tends to be chronic, early surgical resection can be attempted. Medical management is symptomatic and includes an H_2-receptor antagonist or omeprazole, and octreotide acetate. Ulcer therapy is described in detail in Chapter 5. Survival data is sparse; however, one dog treated with octreotide (10 to 20 µg subcutaneously three times daily) lived for 10 months, and two dogs treated with a combination of antacids and octreotide lived for 4.5 months.

Pancreatic Polypeptidoma (Vasoactive Intestinal Peptidoma, Somatostatinoma)

Background

Pancreatic polypeptidoma is a rare endocrine tumor of the pancreatic islet cell; pancreatic polypeptide hormone is elevated in 77% of dogs with endocrine polypeptideomas.

Clinical Parameters and Work-up

Clinical signs of vomiting, hypertrophic gastritis, and duodenal ulceration characterize this tumor. Basic blood work and urinalysis, chest and abdominal radiographs, and abdominal ultrasound should be performed to assess general health status, possibly diagnose a pancreatic mass, and stage the disease. These tests are usually unremarkable.

Because the signs are similar to those seen with gastrinoma, this is one case that would merit provocative testing with secretin and calcium. The result should be a normal gastrin level in response to these challenges. Further, failure to respond to H_2-receptor antagonist therapy should raise the index of suspicion that a polypeptidoma, rather than a gastrinoma, is responsible for clinical signs. Lastly, immunohistochemical staining of pancreatic biopsy specimen for pancreatic polypeptide will confirm the diagnosis.

Treatment

Surgical resection in a healthy patient with no evidence of metastasis should be attempted. Few data exist on survival times because of the rarity of this tumor. Individual cases where complete excision has been performed have resulted in long-term control and resolution of all clinical signs.

Exocrine Pancreatic Tumors in Cats

Background

Exocrine pancreatic carcinomas are similarly rare in the cat. No breed or sex predilection is reported, and affected cats are generally older.

Clinical Parameters

The clinical signs associated with exocrine pancreatic carcinomas in the cat are nonspecific, as in the dog; signs include anorexia, vomiting, and weight loss. Other clinical signs reported are lethargy, icterus, constipation, diarrhea, steatorrhea, pyrexia, dehydration, and a distended abdomen. In contrast to dogs, cats usually have larger and more easily palpated abdominal masses. A unique paraneoplastic alopecia has been reported in cats with pancreatic acinar carcinoma. This effect has not been recognized in dogs or humans to date and has no known etiology.

Clinical Work-up

A minimum database, chest and abdominal radiographs, and ultrasound of the abdomen should be performed to evaluate the general health status of the patient, stage for metastasis, and assess the primary mass. The results of routine blood work are usually unremarkable, although neutrophilia, anemia, hypokalemia, bilirubinemia, azotemia, hyperglycemia, and elevated liver enzyme levels have been reported. Serum lipase and amylase levels are rarely elevated.

Ultrasonography can sometimes detect a soft tissue density in the cranial abdomen, but determining whether the mass arises from the pancreas can be difficult. There may be effusion in the abdomen that can be aspirated, but this rarely provides a diagnosis because pancreatic carcinomas do not readily exfoliate into the peritoneum. This tumor can metastasize anywhere, but liver and intraabdominal nodes are commonly involved.

Treatment

Because diagnosis is usually made by exploratory laparotomy, if the patient is in good general health and there is no evidence of metastasis, an attempt at surgical resection can be considered. However, due to the highly malignant nature of this tumor (81% metastasis at the time of diagnosis), complete surgical excision is rarely achieved. Chemotherapy and radiation therapy have not been reported to be efficacious in pancreatic neoplasia.

Endocrine Pancreas Tumors in Cats
Insulinoma (Beta Cell Tumor, Islet Cell Tumor)
Background

Insulinoma is rare in the cat. It is a functional secreting tumor that arises from the islet cells in the endocrine pancreas. In addition to the secretion of insulin and its precursors, insulinomas are now known to secrete pancreatic polypeptide, somatostatin, glucagon, serotonin, gastrin, and corticotropin. Insulinomas are considered slow growing, are most commonly carcinomas, and often present late in the course of disease with signs attributable to the resultant hypoglycemia. Insulinomas occur in older cats.

Clinical Parameters

Clinical signs most commonly seen in cats are seizures, cutaneous twitching that progresses to muscle tremors, generalized ataxia, and focal tremors of the facial and appendicular musculature. These clinical signs can be explained by hyperinsulinemia with resultant hypoglycemia and release of counter-regulatory hormones (catecholamines and glucagon in the early phase and cortisol and growth hormones in the later phase of disease). Because of the patient's ability to adjust to a chronic state of hypoglycemia, signs of hypoglycemia are often not seen, even with extremely low blood glucose levels. The rate of decrease in blood glucose, as well as the duration of hypoglycemia, is considered important in the development of clinical signs.

There are two types of presenting clinical signs: *neuroglycopenic* (seizures, weakness, ataxia, and lethargy) and *sympathetic* (behavioral changes, shaking/trembling, and muscle fasciculations). The neurologic signs are due to the reliance of the central nervous system on diffusion for glucose uptake (which is predictably low in periods of hypoglycemia) and its inability to utilize other forms of energy such as fatty acids and ketone bodies. The sympathetic signs are related to an increased discharge of counter-regulatory hormones.

Clinical Work-up

Basic blood work and urinalysis, chest and abdominal radiographs, and abdominal ultrasound should be performed to diagnose and stage cats with suspected insulinomas and to rule out other causes of hypoglycemia. Blood work, urinalysis, and radiographs are usually unremarkable. Abdominal ultrasound infrequently detects a mass on the pancreas, but other organ metastases and/or mesenteric lymphadenopathy may be evident. The diagnosis of insulinoma is based on demonstration of hyperinsulinemia in the face of hypoglycemia. There are several means by which one can achieve this, including the insulin-glucose, glucose-insulin, and amended insulin-glucose ratios. For the most part these ratios are not considered diagnostic because they are associated with a high number of false-positive results. For this reason, performing a paired insulin and glucose test is considered to be the most reliable method of diagnosing an insulinoma. This test is further described in the earler section on endocrine pancreas tumors in the dog. However, it should be noted that the radioimmunoassay for insulin has not been validated in cats and so should be interpreted with caution.

One study describes the use of CgA and NSE as a marker for canine and feline pancreatic islet cell tumors and found these assays to be sensitive in detecting tumors of neuroendocrine origin. One report in the dog states that the use of fructosamine measurement may be helpful, in conjunction with insulin measurement, in diagnosing an insulinoma. Provocative testing has been described in the literature. Such tests include glucagon tolerance, glucose tolerance, tolbutamide tolerance, L-leucine, oral glucose tolerance, epinephrine tolerance, and the calcium infusion test.

These tests use the administration of potentially dangerous substances and are expensive, time consuming, and most importantly not as accurate as the paired insulin-glucose tests.

The metastatic behavior of insulinoma in the cat is unknown. Of three cases, only one had histologic confirmation. This mass was solitary and well encapsulated. No metastases were detected grossly. However, this patient developed hypoglycemia 7 months later, suggestive of incomplete surgical excision and recurrence or a metastatic lesion.

Treatment

Minimal information is available for treatment of insulinoma in the cat. However, in a stable patient with no evidence of metastasis, surgical resection can be attempted.

Medical management has not been described for the management of insulinoma in the cat. For a discussion of appropriate drugs for use in the dog, see the section on endocrine pancreas tumors in the dog.

Glucagonoma
Background

Rare tumors of the pancreatic alpha cells, glucagon-secreting tumors have been described in two cats. The typical lesions that are concomitant with a glucagonoma are SND or MEN and are characteristic of glucagonoma syndrome.

Clinical Parameters and Work-up

Clinical signs described in the literature include skin lesions and blood work abnormalities. In the cat, skin lesions are characterized by erythema and crusting plaques on the limbs, abdomen, and genital areas. A complete staging scheme should include basic blood work, urinalysis, and abdominal and thoracic imaging. In one tumor evaluated with immunohistochemical stains, glucagon was not evident in the cells of the carcinoma. Biochemical parameters included normal liver enzyme levels and hyperglycemia. Diagnosis is usually made by skin biopsy, exploratory celiotomy, and histopathologic evaluation of a pancreatic mass.

Treatment

Surgical resection of a glucagon-secreting tumor should be attempted in an otherwise healthy cat with no evidence of metastatic disease; however, because there are very few reports of this tumor to date, no specific recommendations can be made.

Medical management for glucagonoma syndrome has been described in the dog. For specifics, see the section on endocrine pancreas tumors in the dog.

Gastrinoma
Background

A rare tumor of the pancreatic islets, gastrinomas secrete gastrin and result in hypertrophic gastritis and subsequent peptic ulcers. This syndrome is referred to as Zollinger-Ellison syndrome.

Clinical Parameters and Work-up

Clinical signs of gastrinomas include chronic vomiting and weight loss, which is related to the hypersecretion of gastrin and consequent ulceration. The clinical work-up should include basic blood work, urinalysis, and abdominal and thoracic imaging. Diagnosis involves the measurement of serum gastrin, demonstration of gastric hypertrophy and ulceration, and increased secretion of gastric acid. Provocative testing with secretin or calcium is usually only indicated when gastrin levels are minimally elevated. A novel method of diagnosis described is the use of somatostatin-receptor scintigraphy.

Treatment

Although the course of gastrinomas tends to be chronic, early surgical resection can be attempted. Medical management is symptomatic and includes an H_2-receptor antagonist or omeprazole, and octreotide acetate. Ulcer therapy is described in detail in Chapter 5.

Pancreatic Polypeptidoma (Vasoactive Intestinal Peptidoma, Somatostatinoma)

This tumor is not reported in the cat.

REFERENCES

Oral and Salivary Gland Tumors

Bateman KE et al.: 0-7-21 radiation therapy for the treatment of canine oral melanoma, *J Vet Intern Med* 8:267, 1994.

Beck ER et al.: Canine tongue tumors: a retrospective review of 57 cases, *J Am Anim Hosp Assoc* 22:525, 1986.

Blackwood L, Dobson JM: Radiotherapy of oral malignant melanoma in dogs, *J Am Vet Med Assoc,* 209:98, 1996.

Bostock DE: Prognosis after surgical excision of canine melanomas, *Vet Pathol* 16:32, 1979.

Bostock DE, White RA: Classification and behavior after surgery of canine epulides, *J Comp Pathol* 97:197, 1987.

Bradley RL, MacEwen EG, Loar AS: Mandibular resection for removal of oral tumors in 30 dogs and 6 cats, *J Am Vet Med Assoc* 184:460, 1984.

Bradley RL, Sponenberg DP, Martin RA: Oral neoplasia in 15 dogs and 4 cats, *Semin Vet Med Surg (Small Anim)* 1:33, 1986.

Brooks MB et al.: Chemotherapy versus chemotherapy plus radiotherapy in the treatment of tonsillar squamous cell carcinoma in the dog, *J Vet Intern Med* 2:206, 1988.

Brewer WG Jr, Turrel JM: Radiotherapy and hyperthermia in the treatment of fibrosarcomas in the dog, *J Am Vet Med Assoc* 181:146, 1982.

Buhles WC, Theilen GH: Preliminary evaluation of bleomycin in feline and canine squamous cell carcinoma, *Am J Vet Res* 34:289, 1973.

Carberry CA, et al.: Salivary gland tumors in dogs and cats: a literature and case review, *J Am Anim Hosp Assoc* 24:561, 1988.

Carpenter JL, Andrews LK, Holzworth J: Tumors and tumor-like lesions. In Holzworth J, ed: *Diseases of the cat: medicine and surgery,* Philadelphia, 1987, WB Saunders.

Carpenter LG et al.: Squamous cell carcinoma of the tongue in 10 dogs, *J Am Anim Hosp Assoc* 29:17, 1993.

Ciekot PA et al.: Histologically low grade yet biologically high grade fibrosarcomas of the mandible and maxilla of 25 dogs (1982 to 1991), *J Am Vet Med Assoc* 204:610, 1994.

Cotter SM: Oral pharyngeal neoplasms in the cat, *J Am Anim Hosp Assoc* 17:917, 1981.

Delverdier M et al.: Les tumeurs de la cavite buccale du chien: etude anatomoclinique a partir de 117 cas, *Revue Med Vet* 142:811, 1991.

Dhaliwal RS, Kitchell BE, Marretta SM: Oral tumors in dogs and cats. I. Diagnosis and clinical signs, *Comp Cont Educ* 20:1011, 1998.

Dhaliwal RS, Kitchell BE, Marretta SM: Oral tumors in dogs and cats. II. Prognosis and treatment, *Comp Cont Educ* 20:1109, 1998.

Dubielzig RR, Goldschmidt MJ, Brodey RS: The nomenclature of periodontal epulides in dogs, *Vet Pathol* 16:209, 1979.

Elmslie RE, Potter TA, Dow SW: Direct DNA injection for the treatment of malignant melanoma. Proceedings of the Veterinary Cancer Society Fifteenth annual conference, 1995.

Elmslie RE, Sow SW, Potter TA: Genetic immunotherapy of canine oral melanoma. Proceedings of the Veterinary Cancer Society Fourteenth annual conference, 1994.

Evans SM et al.: Technique, pharmacokinetics, toxicity, and efficacy of intratumoral etanidaxole and radiotherapy for treatment of spontaneous feline oral squamous cell carcinoma, *Int J Radiat Oncol* 20:703, 1991.

Evans SM, Shofer F: Canine oral nontonsillar squamous cell carcinoma: prognostic factors for recurrence and survival following orthovoltage radiation therapy, *Vet Radiol* 29:133, 1988.

Evans SM, Thrall DE: Postoperative orthovoltage radiation therapy of parotid salivary gland adenocarcinoma in three dogs, *J Am Vet Med Assoc,* 182:993, 1983.

Fox LE et al.: Owner satisfaction with partial mandibulectomy or maxillectomy for treatment of oral tumors in 27 dogs, *J Am Anim Hosp Assoc* 33:25, 1997.

Gillette SM, Gillette EL: Radiation therapy for head and neck cancers, *Semin Vet Med Surg Small Anim* 10:168, 1995.

Goetz TE, Boulton CH, Ogilvie GK: Clinical management of progressive multifocal benign and malignant melanomas of horses with oral cimetidine, Proceedings of the American Association of Equine Practitioners 35th annual conference, 1989.

Goldschmidt MH: Benign and malignant melanocytic neoplasms of domestic animals, *Am J Dermatopathol* 7:203, 1985.

Gorman NT et al.: Chemotherapy of a recurrent acanthomatous epulis in a dog, *J Am Vet Med Assoc* 184:1158, 1984.

Guptill L et al.: Retrospective study of cisplatin treatment for canine malignant melanoma, Proceedings of the Veterinary Cancer Society thirteenth annual conference, 1993.

Hahn KA: Vincristine sulfate as single-agent chemotherapy in a dog and a cat with malignant neoplasms, *J Am Vet Med Assoc* 197:796, 1990.

Hahn KA et al.: Canine oral malignant melanoma: prognostic utility of an alternative staging system, *J Small Anim Pract* 35:251, 1994.

Hahn KA, Nolan ML: Surgical prognosis for canine salivary gland neoplasms. Proceedings of the Veterinary Cancer Society seventeenth annual conference, 1997.

Hammer A et al.: Salivary gland neoplasia in the dog and cat: survival times and prognostic factors. Proceedings of the Veterinary Cancer Society seventeenth annual conference, 1997.

Harvey HJ et al.: Prognostic criteria for dogs with oral melanoma, *J Am Vet Med Assoc* 178:580, 1981.

Heymann SJ et al.: Canine axial skeletal osteosarcoma: a retrospective study of 116 cases (1986 to 1989), *Vet Surg* 21:304, 1992.

Himsel CA, Richardson RC, Craig JA: Cisplatin chemotherapy for metastatic squamous cell carcinoma in two dogs, *J Am Vet Med Assoc* 189:1575, 1986.

Hogge GS et al.: Preclinical evaluation of a GM-CSF transfected melanoma vaccine in canines. Proceedings of the Veterinary Cancer Society sixteenth annual conference, 1996.

Hutson CA et al.: Treatment of mandibular squamous cell carcinoma in cats by use of mandibulectomy and radiotherapy: seven cases (1987–1989), *J Am Vet Med Assoc* 201:777, 1992.

Kapatkin AS et al.: Mandibular swelling in cats: prospective study of 24 cats, *J Am Anim Hosp Assoc* 27:575, 1991.

King GK, Bergman PJ, Haris D: Radiation oncology of head and neck tumors, *Vet Clin North Am Small Anim Pract* 27:101, 1997.

Knapp DW et al.: Cisplatin therapy in 41 dogs with malignant tumors, *J Vet Intern Med* 2:41, 1988.

Kraegel SA, Page RL: Advances in platinum compound chemotherapy. In Kirk RW, Bonagura JD, eds: *Current veterinary therapy* XII, Philadelphia, 1992, WB Saunders.

LaDue-Miller T et al.: Radiotherapy of canine non-tonsillar squamous cell carcinoma, *Vet Radiol Ultrasound* 37:74, 1996.

LaRue SM et al.: Shrinking-field radiation therapy in combination with mitoxantrone chemotherapy for the treatment of oral squamous cell carcinoma in the cat. Proceedings of the Veterinary Cancer Society eleventh annual conference, 1991.

Liu SK, Dorfman HD, Patnaik AK: Primary and secondary bone tumors in the cat, *J Small Anim Pract* 15: 141, 1974.

MacEwen EG: Update on macrophage activation to prevent metastasis. Proceedings of the twelfth annual conference of the American College of Veterinary Internal Medicine, 1994.

MacEwen EG et al.: Canine oral melanoma: comparison of surgery versus surgery plus *Corynebacterium parvum*, *Cancer Invest* 4:397, 1986.

MacEwen EG et al.: Combined L-MTP-PE and surgery for canine oral melanoma. Proceedings of the Veterinary Cancer Society fourteenth annual conference, 1994.

MacMillan R, Withrow SJ, Gillette EL: Surgery and regional irradiation for treatment of canine tonsillar squamous cell carcinoma: retrospective review of eight cases, *J Am Anim Hosp Assoc* 18:311, 1982.

McChesney SL et al.: Influence of WR 2721 on radiation response of canine soft tissue sarcomas, *Int J Radiat Oncol* 12:1957, 1986.

McChesney SL et al.: Radiotherapy of soft tissue sarcomas in dogs, *J Am Vet Med Assoc* 194:60, 1989.

Modiano JF, Ritt MG, Wojcieszyn J: The molecular basis of canine melanoma: pathogenesis and trends in diagnosis and therapy, *J Vet Intern Med* 13:163, 1999.

Moore AS et al.: Preclinical study of sequential tumor necrosis factor and interleukin-2 in the treatment of spontaneous canine neoplasms, *Cancer Res* 51:233, 1991.

Oakes MG et al.: Canine oral neoplasia, *Compend Cont Educ* 15:15, 1993.

Ogilvie GK et al.: Papillary squamous cell carcinoma in three young dogs, *J Am Vet Med Assoc* 192:933, 1988.

Ogilvie GK et al.: Efficacy of mitoxantrone against various neoplasms in dogs, *J Am Vet Med Assoc* 198:1618, 1991.

Ogilvie GK et al.: Toxicoses and efficacy associated with the administration of mitoxantrone to cats with malignant tumors, *J Am Vet Med Assoc* 202:1839, 1993.

Patnaik AK, Mooney S: Feline melanoma: a comparative study of ocular, oral and dermal neoplasms, *Vet Pathol* 25:105, 1988.

Postorino Reeves NC, Turrel JM, Withrow SJ: Oral squamous cell carcinoma in the cat, *J Am Anim Hosp Assoc* 29:438, 1993.

Poulet FM, Valentine BA, Summers BA: A survey of epithelial odontogenic tumors and cysts in dogs and cats, *Vet Pathol* 29:369, 1992.

Quigley PJ, Leedale AH: Tumors involving bone in the domestic cat: a review of fifty-eight cases, *Vet Pathol* 20:670, 1983.

Rassnick KM et al.: Use of carboplatin for treatment of dogs with malignant melanoma: 27 cases (1989-2000), *J Am Vet Med Assoc* 218(9):1444, 2001.

Ruslander DM et al.: Intravenous melphalan: phase II evaluation in dogs with malignant melanoma. Proceedings of the Veterinary Cancer Society thirteenth annual conference, 1993.

Salisbury SK, Lantz GC: Long-term results of partial mandibulectomy for treatment of oral tumors in 30 dogs, *J Am Anim Hosp Assoc* 24:285, 1988.

Salisbury SK, Richardson DC, Lantz GC: Partial maxillectomy and premaxillectomy in the treatment of oral neoplasia in the dog and cat, *Vet Surg* 15:16, 1986.

Schmidt BR et al.: Piroxicam therapy in canine oral squamous cell carcinoma. Proceedings of the American College of Veterinary Radiology/Veterinary Cancer Society, 1997.

Schwarz PD et al.: Mandibular resection as a treatment for oral cancer in 81 dogs, *J Am Anim Hosp Assoc* 27:601, 1991.

Shapiro W et al.: Cisplatin for treatment of transitional cell and squamous cell carcinomas in dogs, *J Am Vet Med Assoc* 193:1530, 1988.

Smith MM: Surgical approach for lymph node staging of oral and maxillofacial neoplasms in dogs, *J Am Anim Hosp Assoc* 31:514, 1995.

Spangler WL, Culbertson MR: Salivary gland disease in dogs and cats: 245 cases (1985–1988), *J Am Vet Med Assoc* 198:465, 1991.

Stebbins KE, Morse CE, Goldschmidt MH: Feline oral neoplasia: a ten year survey, *Vet Pathol* 26:121, 1989.

Straw RC et al.: Canine mandibular osteosarcoma: 51 cases (1980–1992), *J Am Anim Hosp Assoc* 32:257, 1996.

Theon AP, Rodriguez C, Madewell BR: Analysis of prognostic factors and patterns of failure in dogs with malignant oral tumors treated with megavoltage irradiation, *J Am Vet Med Assoc* 210:778, 1997.

Theon AP et al.: Analysis of prognostic factors and patterns of failure in dogs with periodontal tumors treated with megavoltage irradiation, *J Am Vet Med Assoc* 210:785, 1997.

Thrall DE: Orthovoltage radiotherapy of oral fibrosarcomas in dogs, *J Am Vet Med Assoc* 179:159, 1981.

Thrall DE: Orthovoltage radiotherapy of acanthomatous epulides in 39 dogs, *J Am Vet Med Assoc* 184:826, 1984.

Todoroff RJ, Brodey RS: Oral and pharyngeal neoplasia in the dog: a retrospective study of 361 cases, *J Am Vet Med Assoc* 175:567, 1979.

Vos JH, Van der Gaag I: Canine and feline oral pharyngeal neoplasms, *J Vet Med* 34:420, 1987.

Wallace J, Matthiesen DT, Patnaik AK: Hemimaxillectomy for the treatment of oral tumors in 69 dogs, *Vet Surg* 21:337, 1992.

Werner RE Jr: Canine oral neoplasia: a review of 19 cases, *J Am Anim Hosp Assoc* 17:67, 1981.

White RA: Mandibulectomy and maxillectomy in the dog: long term survival in 100 cases, *J Small Anim Pract* 32:69, 1991.

Withrow SJ et al.: Premaxillectomy in the dog, *J Am Anim Hosp Assoc* 21:45, 1985.

Wood CA et al.: Phase I evaluation of carboplatin in tumor bearing cats. Proceedings of the Veterinary Cancer Society Sixteenth annual conference, 1996.

Yoshida K et al.: The effect of intralesional bleomycin on canine acanthomatous epulis, *J Am Anim Hosp Assoc* 34:457, 1998.

Esophageal, Gastric, Intestinal, and Anal Sac Apocrine Gland Tumors

Bagley RS, Levy JK, Malarkey DE: Hypoglycemia associated with intra-abdominal leiomyoma and leiomyosarcoma in six dogs, *J Am Vet Med Assoc* 208:69, 1996.

Bellah JR, Genn PE: Gastric leiomyosarcoma associated with hypoglycemia in a dog, *J Am Anim Hosp Assoc* 32:283, 1996.

Berrocal A et al.: Canine perineal tumors, *J Am Vet Med Assoc* 36:739, 1989.

Birchard SJ, Couto CG, Johnson S: Nonlymphoid intestinal neoplasia in 32 dogs and 14 cats, *J Am Anim Hosp Assoc* 22:533, 1986.

Brick J, Rownigk W, Wilson G: Chemotherapy of malignant lymphoma in dogs and cats, *J Am Vet Med Assoc* 153:47, 1968.

Bruecker KA, Withrow SJ: Intestinal leiomyosarcomas in six dogs, *J Am Anim Hosp Assoc* 24:281, 1988.

Carb AV, Goodman DG: Oesophageal carcinoma in the dog, *J Small Anim Pract* 14:91, 1973.

Carpenter J, Holzworth J: Treatment of leukemia in the cat, *J Am Vet Med Assoc* 158:1130, 1971.

Carpenter JL, Andrews LK, Holzworth J: Tumors and tumor-like lesions. In Holzworth J, ed: *Diseases of the cat: medicine and surgery*, Philadelphia, 1987, WB Saunders.

Chen HH, Parris LS, Parris RG: Duodenal leiomyosarcoma with multiple hepatic metastases in a dog, *J Am Vet Med Assoc* 184:1506, 1984.

Church EM, Mehlhaff CJ, Patnaik AK: Colorectal adenocarcinoma in dogs: 78 cases (1973–1984), *J Am Vet Med Assoc* 191:727, 1987.

Comer KM: Anemia as a feature of primary gastrointestinal neoplasia, *Compend Contin Educ Pract Vet* 12:13, 1990.

Cotter S: Treatment of lymphoma and leukemia with cyclophosphamide, vincristine and prednisolone. II. Treatment of cats, *J Am Anim Hosp Assoc* 19:166, 1983.

Coughlin A: Carcinoid in canine large intestine, *Vet Rec* 130:499, 1992.

Couto CG et al.: Gastrointestinal lymphoma in 20 dogs: a retrospective study, *J Vet Intern Med* 3:73, 1989.

Cribb AE: Feline gastrointestinal adenocarcinoma: a review and retrospective study, *Can Vet J* 29:709, 1988.

Crystal MA et al.: Use of ultrasound-guided fine-needle aspiration biopsy and automated core biopsy for the diagnosis of gastrointestinal diseases in small animals, *Vet Radiol Ultrasound* 34:438, 1993.

Dorn AS et al.: Gastric carcinoma in a dog, *J Small Anim Pract* 17:109, 1976.

Elliott GS et al.: Surgical, medical and nutritional management of gastric adenocarcinoma in a dog, *J Am Vet Med Assoc* 185:98, 1984.

Esplin DG, Wilson SR: Gastrointestinal adenocarcinomas metastatic to the testes and associated structures in three dogs, *J Am Anim Hosp Assoc* 34:287, 1998.

Fonda D, Gualtieri M, Scanziani E: Gastric carcinoma in the dog: a clinicopathological study of 11 cases, *J Small Anim Pract* 30:353, 1989.

Fondacaro JV et al.: Feline gastrointestinal lymphoma: 67 cases (1988–1996), *Eur J Compar Gastroenterol* 4:23, 1999.

Gibbons GC, Murtaugh RJ: Cecal smooth muscle neoplasia in the dog: report of 11 cases and literature review, *J Am Anim Hosp Assoc* 25:191, 1989.

Gibbs C, Pearson H: Localized tumors of the canine small intestine: a report of twenty cases, *J Small Anim Pract* 27:507, 1986.

Goldschmidt MH, Zoltowski C: Anal sac gland adenocarcinoma in the dog: 14 cases, *J Small Anim Pract* 22:119, 1981.

Grooters AM, Johnson SE: Canine gastric leiomyoma, *Comp Cont Ed* 17:1485, 1995.

Hardy WD Jr et al.: A feline leukaemia virus and sarcoma virus-induced tumour-specific antigen, *Nature* 270:249, 1977.

Henroteaux M: L'adenocarcinoma du colon chez le chien, *Med Vet Quebec* 20:79, 1990.

Holmberg CA, Manning JS, Osburn BI: Feline malignant lymphomas: comparison of morphologic and immunologic characteristics, *Am J Vet Res* 37:1455, 1976.

Jeglum K, Whereat A, Young K: Chemotherapy of lymphoma in 75 cats, *J Am Vet Med Assoc* 190:174, 1987.

Jones BD, Jergens AE, Giolford WG: Diseases of the esophagus. In Ettinger SJ, ed: *Textbook of veterinary internal medicine*, ed 3, Philadelphia, 1989, WB Saunders.

Kapatkin AS et al.: Leiomyosarcoma in dogs: 44 cases (1983-1988), *J Am Vet Med Assoc* 201:1077, 1992.

Kerpsack SJ, Birchard SJ: Removal of leiomyomas and other noninvasive masses from the cardiac region of the canine stomach, *J Am Anim Hosp Assoc* 30:500, 1994.

Kleine LJ: Radiologic examination of the esophagus in dogs and cats, *Vet Clin North Am* 4:663, 1974.

Kosovsky JE, Matthiesen DT, Patnaik AK: Small intestinal adenocarcinoma in cats: 32 cases (1978-1985), *J Am Vet Med Assoc* 192:233, 1988.

Lawson DD, Pirie HM: Conditions of the canine oesophague-II vascular rings, achalasia, tumors, and perioesophageal lesions, *J Small Anim Pract* 7:117, 1966.

Leib MS, Fallin EA, Johnston SA: Endoscopy case of the month: abnormally shaped feces in a dog, *Vet Med*:762, 1992.

Lingeman CH, Garner FM: Comparative study of intestinal adenocarcinomas of animals and man, *J Natl Cancer Inst* 48:325, 1972.

MacDonald JM, Mullen HS, Moroff SD: Adenomatous polyps of the duodenum in cats: 18 cases (1985-1990), *J Am Vet Med Assoc* 202:647, 1993.

MacEwen EG: Feline lymphoma and leukemias. In Withrow SJ, MacEwen EG, eds: *Small animal clinical oncology,* ed 2, Philadelphia, 1996, WB Saunders.

Mahony OM et al.: Alimentary lymphoma in cats: 28 cases (1988-1993), *J Am Vet Med Assoc* 202:1593, 1995.

Matros L et al.: Megaesophagus and hypomotility associated with esophageal leiomyoma in a dog, *J Am Anim Hosp Assoc* 30:15, 1994.

McCaw D, Pratt M, Walshaw R: Squamous cell carcinoma of the esophagus in a dog, *J Am Anim Hosp Assoc* 16:561, 1980.

McClelland R: Chemotherapy in reticulum-cell sarcoma in five dogs and a cat and in mast cell leukemia in a cat, *Cornell Vet* 61:477, 1971.

McPherron MA et al.: Colorectal leiomyomas in seven dogs, *J Am Anim Hosp Assoc* 28:43, 1992.

Meuten DJ et al.: Hypercalcemia associated with an adenocarcinoma derived from the apocrine glands of the anal sac, *Vet Pathol* 18:454, 1981.

Mooney S et al.: Treatment and prognostic factors in lymphoma in cats: 103 cases (1977-1981), *J Am Vet Med Assoc* 194:696, 1989.

Mooney S et al.: Renal lymphoma in cats: 28 cases (1977-1984), *J Am Vet Med Assoc* 200:373, 1992.

Moore AS et al.: A comparison of doxorubicin and COP for maintenance of remission in cats with lymphoma, *J Vet Intern Med* 10:372, 1996.

Moore A et al.: Toxicity and efficacy of oral idarubicin administration to cats with neoplasia, *J Am Vet Med Assoc* 206:1550, 1995.

Murray M et al.: Primary gastric neoplasia in the dog: a clinico-pathological study, *Vet Rec* 120:79, 1987.

Ogilvie GK, Moore AS: Clinical briefing: lymphoma. In Ogilvie GK, Moore AS, eds: *Managing the veterinary cancer patient,* Trenton, NJ, 1995, Veterinary Learning Systems.

Ogilvie GK, Moore AS: Clinical briefing: mast cell tumors. In Ogilvie GK, Moore AS, eds: *Managing the Veterinary Cancer Patient,* Trenton, NJ, 1995, Veterinary Learning Systems.

Ogilvie G et al.: Toxicoses and efficacy associated with the administration of mitoxantrone to cats with malignant tumors, *J Am Vet Med Assoc* 202:1839, 1993.

Patnaik AK, Hurvitz AI, Johnson GF: Canine gastrointestinal neoplasms, *Vet Pathol* 14:547, 1977.

Patnaik AK, Hurvitz AI, Johnson GF: Canine gastric adenocarcinoma, *Vet Pathol* 15:600, 1978.

Patnaik AK, Hurvitz AI, Johnson GF: Canine intestinal adenocarcinoma and carcinoid, *Vet Pathol* 17:149, 1980.

Patnaik AK, Liu SK, Johnson GF: Feline intestinal adenocarcinoma: a clinicopathologic study of 22 cases, *Vet Pathol* 13:1, 1976.

Patnaik AK et al.: Surgical resection of intestinal adenocarcinoma in a cat, with survival of 28 months, *J Am Vet Med Assoc* 178:479, 1981.

Pennick D et al.: Ultrasonography of alimentary lymphosarcoma in the cat, *Vet Radiol Ultrasound* 35:299, 1994.

Pennick DG et al.: Ultrasonographic evaluation of gastrointestinal diseases in small animals, *Vet Radiol* 31:134, 1990.

Pennick DG et al.: The technique of percutaneous ultrasound-guided fine-needle aspiration biopsy and automated microcore biopsy in small animal gastrointestinal diseases, *Vet Radiol Ultrasound* 34:433, 1993.

Ridgway RL, Suter PF: Clinical and radiographic signs in primary and metastatic esophageal neoplasms of the dog, *J Am Vet Med Assoc* 174:700, 1979.

Rijnberk A et al.: Pseudohyperparathyroidism associated with perirectal adenocarcinomas in elderly female dogs, *Tijdschr Diergeneeskd* 103:1069, 1978.

Rivers BJ et al.: Canine gastric neoplasia: utility of ultrasonography in diagnosis, *J Am Anim Hosp Assoc* 33:144, 1997.

Rosol TJ et al.: Identification of parathyroid hormone-related protein in canine apocrine adenocarcinoma of the anal sac, *Vet Pathol* 27:89, 1990.

Ross JT et al.: Adenocarcinoma of the apocrine glands of the anal sac in dogs: a review of 32 cases, *J Am Anim Hosp Assoc* 27:349, 1991.

Roth L, King JM: Mesenteric and omental sclerosis associated with metastases from gastrointestinal neoplasia in the dog, *J Small Anim Pract* 31:28, 1990.

Saulter JH, Hanlon GF: Gastric neoplasms in the dog: a report of 20 cases, *J Am Vet Med Assoc* 166:691, 1975.

Scanziani E et al.: Gastric carcinoma in the Belgian shepherd dog, *J Small Anim Pract* 32:465, 1991.

Sellon RK, Bissonnette, Bunch SE: Long-term survival after total gastrectomy for gastric adenocarcinoma in a dog, *J Vet Intern Med* 10:333, 1996.

Sinclair CJ, Jones BR, Verkerk G: Gastric carcinoma in a bitch, *N Z Vet J* 27:16, 1979.

Slawienski MJ et al.: Malignant colonic neoplasia in cats: 46 cases (1990-1996), *J Am Vet Med Assoc* 211:878, 1997.

Squire R, Bush M: The therapy of canine and feline lymphosarcoma, *Bibl Haematol* 39:189, 1973.

Straw RC: Tumors of the intestinal tract. In Withrow SJ, MacEwen EG, eds: *Small animal clinical oncology,* ed 2, Philadelphia, 1996, WB Saunders.

Sullivan M et al.: A study of 31 cases of gastric carcinoma in dogs, *Vet Rec* 120:79, 1987.

Takiguchi M et al.: Esophageal/gastric adenocarcinoma in a dog, *J Am Anim Hosp Assoc* 33:42, 1997.

Theilen GH, Madewell BR: Tumors of the digestive tract. In Theilen GH, Madewell BR, eds: *Veterinary cancer medicine,* Philadelphia, 1979, Lea & Febiger.

Thompson JP et al.: Paraneoplastic leukocytosis associated with a rectal adenomatous polyp in a dog, *J Am Vet Med Assoc* 201:737, 1992.

Turk MA, Gallina AM, Russell TS: Nonhematopoietic gastrointestinal neoplasia in cats: a retrospective study of 44 cases, *Vet Pathol* 18:614, 1981.

Turrel JM, Theon AP: Single high-dose irradiation for selected canine rectal carcinomas, *Vet Radiol* 27:141, 1986.

Vail DM et al.: Feline lymphoma (145 cases): proliferation indices, cluster differentiation 3 immunoreactivity, and their association with prognosis in 90 cats, *J Vet Intern Med* 12:349, 1998.

Valerius KD et al.: Adenomatous polyps and carcinoma in situ of the canine colon and rectum: 34 cases (1982-1994), *J Am Anim Hosp Assoc* 33:156, 1997.

Watson DE, Mahaffey MB, Neuwirth LA: Ultrasonographic detection of duodenojejunal intussusception in a dog, *J Am Anim Hosp Assoc* 27:367, 1991.

White RA, Gorman NT: The clinical diagnosis and management of rectal and pararectal tumors in the dog, *J Small Anim Pract* 28:87, 1987.

Williams LE et al.: Response to chemotherapy in dogs with adenocarcinomas of the perineum: retrospective study 1985-1995. Proceedings of the Veterinary Cancer Society seventeenth annual conference, 1997.

Withrow SJ: Esophageal cancer. In Withrow SJ, MacEwen EG, eds: *Small animal clinical oncology,* ed 2, Philadelphia, 1996, WB Saunders.

Zwahlen CH et al.: Results of chemotherapy for cats with alimentary malignant lymphoma: 21 cases (1993-1997), *J Am Vet Med Assoc* 213:1144, 1998.

Hepatic and Pancreatic Tumors

Altschul M et al.: Evaluation of somatostatin analogues for the detection and treatment of gastrinoma in a dog, *J Small Animal Pract* 38:286, 1997.

Anderson NV, Johnson KH: Pancreatic carcinoma in the dog, *J Am Vet Med Assoc* 150:286, 1967.

Bjorling DE: Liver and biliary system. In Bojrab MJ, ed: *Current techniques in small animal surgery,* Baltimore, 1998, Williams and Wilkins.

Brooks DG et al.: Pancreatic paraneoplastic alopecia in three cats, *J Am Anim Hosp Assoc* 30:557, 1994.

Brown PJ et al.: Multifocal necrotizing steatitis associated with pancreatic carcinoma in three dogs, *J Small Anim Pract* 35:129, 1994.

Byrne KP: Metabolic epidermal necrosis-hepatocutaneous syndrome, *Vet Clin North Am Small Anim Pract* 29:1337, 1999.

Carpenter JL, Andrews LK, Holzworth J: Tumors and tumor-like lesions. In Holzworth J, ed: *Diseases of the cat: medicine and surgery,* Philadelphia, 1987, WB Saunders.

Caywood DD et al.: Pancreatic insulin-secreting neoplasms: clinical, diagnostic, and prognostic features in 73 dogs, *J Am Anim Hosp Assoc* 24:577, 1988.

Center SA et al.: Bile acid concentrations in the diagnosis of hepatobiliary disease in the dog, *J Am Vet Med Assoc* 187:935, 1985.

Davenport DJ, Chew DJ, Johnson GC: Diabetes insipidus associated with metastatic pancreatic carcinoma in a dog, *J Am Vet Med Assoc* 189:204, 1986.

Dial SM: Clinicopathologic evaluation of the liver, *Vet Clin North Am Small Anim Pract* 25:257, 1995.

Elie MS, Zerbe CA: Insulinoma in dogs, cats, and ferrets, *Comp Cont Ed* 17:51, 1992.

Eng J et al.: Cat gastrinoma and the sequence of cat gastrins, *Regul Pept* 37:9, 1992.

Evans SM: The radiographic appearance of primary liver neoplasia in dogs, *Vet Radiol* 28:192, 1987.

Feeney DA, Johnston GR, Hardy RM: Two-dimensional, gray-scale ultrasonography for assessment of hepatic and splenic neoplasia in the dog and cat, *J Am Vet Med Assoc* 184:68, 1984.

Feldman BF, Strafuss AC, Gabbert N: Bile duct carcinoma in the cat: three case reports, *Feline Pract* 6:33, 1976.

Fineman L et al.: Serum lipase concentrations in dogs with pancreatic carcinoma. Proceedings of the Veterinary Cancer Society fourteenth annual conference, 1994.

Fondacaro JV et al.: Diagnostic correlation of liver aspiration cytology with histopathology in dogs and cats with liver disease. Proceedings of the Seventeenth annual conference of the American College of Verterinary Internal Medicine, 1999.

Fry PD, Rest JR: Partial hepatectomy in two dogs, *J Small Anim Pract* 34:192, 1993.

Hammer AS, Sikkema DA: Hepatic neoplasis in the dog and cat, *Vet Clin North Am Small Anim Pract* 25:419, 1995.

Happe RP et al.: Zollinger-Ellison syndrome in three dogs, *Vet Pathol* 17:177, 1980.

Jones BR, Nicholls MR, Badman R: Peptic ulceration in a dog associated with an islet cell carcinoma of the pancreas and an elevated plasma gastrin level, *J Small Animal Pract* 17:593, 1976.

Kerwin SC: Hepatic aspiration and biopsy techniques, *Vet Clin North Am Small Anim Pract* 25:275, 1995.

Kosovsky JE et al.: Results of partial hepatectomy in 18 dogs with hepatocellular carcinoma, *J Am Anim Hosp Assoc* 25:203, 1989.

Kruth SA, Carter RF: Laboratory abnormalities in patients with cancer, *Vet Clin North Am Small Anim Pract* 20:897, 1990.

Kruth SA, Feldman EC, Kennedy PC: Insulin-secreting islet cell tumors: establishing a diagnosis and the clinical course for 25 dogs, *J Am Vet Med Assoc* 181:54, 1982.

Leifer CE, Peterson ME, Matus RE: Insulin-secreting tumor: diagnosis and medical and surgical management in 55 dogs, *J Am Vet Med Assoc* 188:60, 1986.

Love NE, Jones C: What's your diagnosis? *J Am Vet Med Assoc* 195:1285, 1989.

Lowseth LA et al.: Detection of serum α-fetoprotein in dogs with hepatic tumors, *J Am Vet Med Assoc* 199:735, 1991.

Magne ML: Primary epithelial tumors in the dog, *Comp Cont Ed* 6:506, 1984.

Magne ML, Withrow SJ: Hepatic neoplasia, *Vet Clin North Am Small Anim Pract* 15:243, 1985.

McCaw DL, da Silva Curiel JM, Shaw DP: Hepatic myelolipomas in a cat, *J Am Vet Med Assoc* 197:243, 1990.

McConnell MF, Lumsden JH: Biochemical evaluation of metastatic liver disease in the dog, *J Am Anim Hosp Assoc* 19:173, 1983.

McDonald RK, Helman RG: Hepatic malignant mesenchymoma in a dog, *J Am Vet Med Assoc* 188:1052, 1986.

Middleton DJ et al.: Duodenal ulceration associated with gastrin-secreting pancreatic tumor in a cat, *J Am Vet Med Assoc* 183:461, 1983.

Morrison W: Primary cancers and cancer-like lesions of the liver, biliary epithelium and exocrine pancreas. In Morrison W, ed: *Cancer in dogs and cats,* Philadelphia, 1998, Lippincott, Williams and Wilkins.

Myers NC, Andrews GA, Chard-Bergstrom C: Chromogranin A plasma concentration and expression in pancreatic islet cell tumors of dogs and cats, *Am J Vet Res* 58:615, 1997.

Ogilvie GK: Insulinoma in dogs. In Ogilvie GK, Moore AS, eds: *Managing the veterinary cancer patient,* Trenton, 1995, Veterinary Learning Systems.

Partington BP, Biller DS: Hepatic imaging with radiology and ultrasound, *Vet Clin North Am Small Anim Pract* 25:305, 1995.

Patel A, Whitbread JJ, McNeil PE: A case of metabolic epidermal necrosis in a cat, *Vet Dermatol* 7:221, 1996.

Patnaik AK: A morphologic and immunocytochemical study of hepatic neoplasms in cats, *Vet Pathol* 29:405, 1992.

Patnaik AK et al.: Canine hepatocellular carcinoma, *Vet Pathol* 18:427, 1981.

Peterson SL: Intrahepatic biliary cystadenoma in a cat, *Feline Pract* 14:29, 1984.

Post G, Patnaik AK: Nonhematopoietic hepatic neoplasms in cats: 21 cases (1983-1988), *J Am Vet Med Assoc* 201:1080, 1992.

Roth L, Meyer DJ: Interpretation of liver biopsies, *Vet Clin North Am Small Anim Pract* 25:293, 1995.

Schuh JC: Hepatic nodular myelolipomatosis (myelolipomas) associated with a peritoneopericardial diaphragmatic hernia in a cat, *J Comp Pathol* 97:231, 1987.

Steiner JM, Williams DA: Feline exocrine pancreatic disorders: insufficiency, neoplasia and uncommon conditions, *Comp Cont Ed* 19:836, 1997.

Straus E, Johnson GF, Yalow RS: Canine Zollinger-Ellison syndrome, *Gastroenterology* 72:380, 1977.

Strombeck DR: Clinicopathologic features of primary and metastatic disease of the liver in dogs, *J Am Vet Med Assoc* 173:267, 1978.

Tasker S et al.: Resolution of paraneoplastic alopecia following surgical removal of a pancreatic carcinoma in a cat, *J Small Animal Pract* 40:16, 1999.

Thoresen SI et al.: Pancreatic insulin-secreting carcinoma in a dog: fructosamine for determining persistent hypoglycemia, *J Small Animal Pract* 36:282, 1995.

Tobin RL et al.: Outcome of surgical versus medical treatment of dogs with beta cell neoplasia: 39 cases (1990-1997), *J Am Vet Med Assoc* 215:226, 1999.

Torres SM et al.: Resolution of superficial necrolytic dermatitis following excision of a glucagon-secreting pancreatic neoplasm in a dog, *J Am Anim Hosp Assoc* 33:313, 1997.

Trout NJ: Surgical treatment of hepatobiliary cystadenomas in cats, *Semin Vet Med Surg* 12:51, 1997.

van der Gaag I, et al.: Zollinger-Ellison syndrome in a cat, *Vet Q* 10:151, 1988.

Voros K et al.: Correlation of ultrasonographic and pathomorphological findings in canine hepatic diseases, *J Small Anim Pract* 32:627, 1991.

Wheeler SL: Endocrine tumors. In Withrow SJ, MacEwen EG, eds: *Clinical veterinary oncology,* Philadelphia, 1989, JB Lippincott.

Xu FN: Ultrastructural examinations as an aid to the diagnosis of canine pancreatic neoplasms, *Aust Vet J* 62:197, 1985.

Zerbe CA et al.: Pancreatic polypeptide and insulin secreting tumor in a dog with duodenal ulcers and hypertrophic gastritis, *J Vet Intern Med* 3:178, 1989.

12

ENTERAL AND PARENTERAL NUTRITION

Howard B. Seim III
Joseph W. Bartges

NUTRITIONAL SUPPORT

In order to provide complete patient care the clinician should include nutritional support as part of the therapeutic plan. Providing nutrition may accomplish several goals (Box 12-1).

We recommend the 2-step approach: step 1—the clinician assesses the PATIENT (What is the physiological state of the patient?), FEED (What nutrients am I concerned with and what diets are available to meet those concerns?), and MANAGEMENT (How will I administer nutrition?); step 2—the clinician formulates and initiates a feeding plan, including assessment and alteration of the plan as needed.

Importance of Providing Nutritional Support

A few days of food deprivation is not detrimental to healthy animals; however, it may be detrimental to a sick animal (Table 12-1). Animals are cyclic eaters. Short periods of food deprivation are not a problem because the body is able to use endogenous energy substrates such as glycogen. During prolonged food deprivation the body shifts to a hypometabolic state to conserve structural and functional proteins as much as possible. Thus glucose and fatty acids become the major energy sources. During periods of food deprivation associated with stress and illness, however, the body cannot utilize fatty acids or glucose efficiently. Therefore, amino acids are mobilized and used for gluconeogenesis, for DNA and RNA synthesis, and for acute phase protein production, and malnutrition can occur rapidly (Figure 12-1).

Indications for Nutritional Support

Whether nutritional support is indicated or not can usually be determined by taking a good history and performing a thorough physical examination (Box 12-2). In patients with acute weight loss the decrease in body weight likely reflects fluid

BOX 12-1   Goals of Nutritional Support

1. Minimize metabolic derangements
   a. Maintain hydration
   b. Attenuate acid–base disorders
   c. Attenuate electrolyte disturbances
   d. Provide disease-specific nutrients
2. Provide nutrients to facilitate recovery
   a. Suppress hypermetabolic response
   b. Reverse protein catabolism and negative nitrogen balance
   c. Maintain gastrointestinal tract integrity and function
   d. Optimize immune function
3. Maintain lean body mass and body weight
4. Avoid complications associated with refeeding

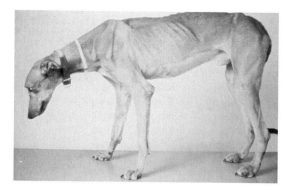

FIGURE 12-1 An adult male Greyhound with severe protein-calorie malnutrition.

loss (dehydration). If a critically ill patient has not eaten for 3 or more days, if there is evidence of increased nutrient demands (e.g., surgery, infection, fever), or if there is evidence for nutrient losses (e.g., vomiting, diarrhea, wounds), then nutritional support is indicated. Physical examination may reveal that nutritional support is indicated if the patient is underweight or cachectic, has decreased muscle mass, is generally debilitated, and has evidence for diseases associated with increased nutrient demands or excessive nutrient losses. Use of a body condition score can aid the clinician in determining the overall nutritional status of the patient (Table 12-2). The clinician should be careful not to overinterpret edema, ascites, or excessive body fat as representing adequate body mass. There are no good laboratory tests for aiding in assessment of nutritional status. Hypoalbuminemia is associated with increased morbidity and mortality; however, a normal serum albumin concentration does not rule out malnutrition.

Decisions on How to Provide Nutrition

There are 2 main "Golden Rules" of nutrition: (1) if the gut works, use it, and (2) keep it simple. As much of the gastrointestinal (GI) tract should be used as possible. Parenteral nutrition is limited to comatose or paralyzed patients or those with severe GI dysfunction such as intractable vomiting, malassimilation syndromes, severe pancreatitis, or peritonitis. Parenteral nutrition should be considered in patients in which provision of nutrients is not feasible using the enteral route. The clinician should use common sense in providing nutrition. Nutritional support should be an integral part of the therapeutic plan.

ENTERAL NUTRITIONAL SUPPORT

Enteral nutritional support is a practical, safe, easy, economic, physiologic, and well-tolerated technique with minimal morbidity; however, it requires

TABLE 12-1   Comparison of Simple Starvation and Stressed Starvation in Humans

Characteristic	Starvation	Stress
Cardiac output	−	++
Systemic vascular resistance	NC	− − −
Oxygen consumption	−	++
Resting energy expenditure	−	+++
Mediator activation	NC	++
Regulatory responsiveness	++++	+
Primary fuels	fat	mixed
Proteolysis	+	+++
Protein oxidation	+	+++
Branched-chain amino acid oxidation	+	+++
Hepatic protein synthesis	+	+++
Ureagenesis	+	+++
Glycogenolysis	+	+++
Gluconeogenesis	+	+++
Lipolysis	++	+++
Ketone body formation	++++	+
Rate of development of malnutrition	+	++++

From Cerra FB: How nutrition changes what getting sick means, *J Parenter Enteral Nutr* 14:164S, 1990.
NC, No change; −, decrease; +, increase.

BOX 12-2   Possible Indications for Nutritional Support

PATIENTS KNOWN TO BE PROTEIN-ENERGY MALNOURISHED

Any patient in critical care unit

Recent weight loss of ≥5% to 10% of body weight

Decreased food intake or anorexia for ≥3 to 5 days

Generalized loss of muscle mass or body fat

Generalized weakness and lethargy for ≥5 days

Hypoalbuminemia

Lymphopenia unassociated with severe stress or drug therapy

Presence of a nonhealing wound, delayed wound healing, or a decubital ulcer

Presence of a chronic, unrelenting fever or other signs of infection or sepsis

Poor body condition characterized by easily epilated hair and cracked nails

PATIENTS WITH CONDITIONS KNOWN TO CAUSE PROTEIN-CALORIE MALNUTRITION

Recent severe trauma or major surgery

Resection of ≥70% of the small intestine

Chronic vomiting or diarrhea

Protein-losing nephropathies

Increased nutrient needs with neoplasia

Peritonitis, pleuritis, or chylous effusion with effective, progressive drainage

Large wounds or burns, with persistent exudative losses

Use of drugs that promote catabolism

Chronic or massive hemorrhage

Cachexia

PATIENTS WITH CONDITIONS ASSOCIATED WITH POOR FOOD INTAKE

Fractures of the mandible or maxilla

Congenital hard- or soft-palate clefts

Recovery from major oral or nasal surgery

Severe generalized stomatitis, glossitis, pharyngitis, and esophagitis

Severe periodontal disease

Neurologic conditions associated with coma or seizures requiring sedation

Tetraplegia that prevents patient from eating

Bilateral cranial nerve V or XII palsies

Severe oropharyngeal or cricopharyngeal dysphagia

Megaesophagus

Esophageal stricture or foreign body

Following esophageal resection

Following extensive stomach disease, surgery, or resection

Following extensive intestinal surgery or resection

Anorexia with refusal to eat because of various metabolic diseases (e.g., renal failure, pancreatitis, hepatic failure)

Severe persistent vomiting

Withholding food for ≥3 to 5 days because of therapeutic or diagnostic procedures

TABLE 12-2   Body Condition Scoring System Based on a 5–Point or 9–Point Scale

Descriptor	Description	5 Point	9 Point
Cachectic	Ribs are easily palpated with no fat cover; bony structures are prominent and easy to identify; muscle tone and mass often decreased; little to no subcutaneous fat; hair coat often poor; pronounced abdominal tuck	1	1
Underweight	Ribs are easily palpated with little fat cover; abdominal tuck present; bony structures are palpable but not prominent; hair coat may be poor; muscle tone and mass may be good or slightly decreased	2	3
Ideal	Ribs are easily palpated, but fat cover is present; hourglass shape present and abdominal tuck is present, but not pronounced; bony prominences are palpable but not visible; some subcutaneous fat, but no large accumulations; muscle tone and mass good; hair coat quality is good	3	5
Overweight	Ribs are difficult to palpate due to overlying fat accumulation; hourglass shape is not prominent, and abdominal tuck is absent; subcutaneous fat obvious with some areas of accumulation; muscle tone and mass good; hair coat quality may be decreased; cannot identify bony prominences	4	7
Obese	Ribs are impossible to palpate due to overlying fat; hourglass shape is absent, and animal may have a round appearance; subcutaneous fat is obvious, and accumulations are present in the neck, tail-base, and abdominal regions; muscle tone and mass may be decreased; hair coat quality may be decreased	5	9

a functional GI tract. It is the preferred method to efficiently achieve nitrogen balance and accelerate wound healing. Simply put, "If the gut works, use it."

Indications

Enteral nutritional support is indicated in any patient with overt or impending protein-calorie malnutrition in which the GI tract is functional. Examples include patients in a hypermetabolic state (e.g., severe burn, sepsis, postsurgical stress, trauma, cancer); patients with chronic anorexia/malnutrition, as evidenced by greater than 10% loss of normal body weight and hypoalbuminemia; postoperative patients in whom 5 to 7 days of anorexia has occurred or is anticipated (e.g., oral, pharyngeal, esophagogastric, duodenal, pancreatic, or biliary tract surgery); postoperative cancer patients, particularly if chemotherapy is instituted; and patients with a mental status that prevents adequate self-feeding (e.g., head trauma, brain surgery). In virtually any situation in which the clinician has diagnosed protein-calorie malnutrition or can predict its occurrence, enteral nutritional support should be considered.

Contraindications

Enteral nutritional support may be contraindicated in several situations. Patients with adynamic ileus, small bowel obstruction, severe intrinsic small bowel disease (e.g., inflammatory bowel disease, diffuse intestinal lymphosarcoma), persistent vomiting or diarrhea, or severe malabsorption should have nutrients delivered by routes other than the GI tract. In addition, patients at risk for aspiration pneumonia (e.g., stupor or coma) should not be fed via the GI tract.

▌ROUTES OF ADMINISTRATION

As a general rule, the closer one comes to the oral route of food intake and digestion, the more efficient is the assimilation and digestion of nutrients and the greater the flexibility in formula composition. Conversely, the further aboral one gets, the less efficient is the assimilation and digestion of nutrients and the greater the care that must be taken when choosing formula composition. Route of administration also dictates feeding tube

---

BOX 12-3   Route of Administration Determines Tube Diameter

TUBE DIAMETER: 3.5 TO 5 FR
- Nasoesophageal
- Gastroduodenostomy
- Enterostomy

TUBE DIAMETER: ≥8 FR
- Orogastric
- Nasoesophageal (dogs >22 lb)
- Esophagostomy
- Pharyngostomy
- Gastrostomy

---

diameter; tube diameter in turn dictates usable feeding formulas because of varying formula viscosity and particulate matter size (Box 12-3).

The most common routes of administration for enteral alimentation include oral, nasoesophageal, pharyngostomy, esophagostomy, gastrostomy, gastroduodenostomy, and enterostomy. Each route has its indications, contraindications, advantages, disadvantages, and complications.

Oral

As a general rule, oral feeding is the method of choice if adequate amounts of nutrients can be consumed to meet the patient's protein and calorie needs. Several techniques have been used to successfully coax a patient to eat. Sending the patient home if the disease state permits and if owners are capable of managing the patient may prove successful. Petting and vocal reassurance is also helpful in stimulating patients to eat; however, it is time consuming (Figure 12-2). Highly palatable foods or food coverings (e.g., gravy) may stimulate appetite; adding water to food increases palatability for dogs (Figure 12-3). Warming foods to near but not above body temperature (e.g., with a microwave oven) will increase aroma and palatability. Nutrition may also be provided by syringe feeding, but the diet must be semiliquid in consistency and there is a risk of aspiration pneumonia (Figure 12-4). Drugs may be used successfully to stimulate appetite sometimes; however, if they do not work immediately, then more aggressive forms of nutritional support should be considered. A list of drugs and their recommended dosages are given in Table 12-3.

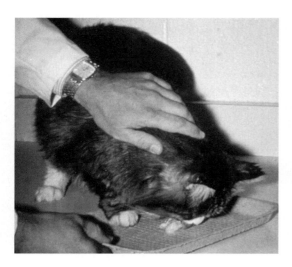

FIGURE 12-2 Petting and vocal reassurance may help stimulate oral intake of food.

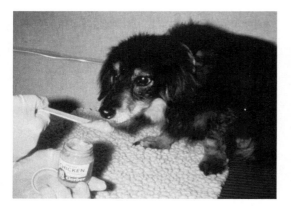

FIGURE 12-3 Using a variety of diets or highly palatable foods may stimulate appetite.

Appetite stimulant drugs are generally not adequate in promoting replacement of a patient's caloric needs; however, they may provide the stimulus necessary for the patient to resume eating. Appetite stimulants are contraindicated in patients suffering from severe malnutrition or in those patients that cannot tolerate the medication. Diazepam should be used cautiously in patients with preexisting liver disease because its use has been associated with inducing hepatocellular necrosis. Glucocorticoids stimulate appetite; however, they are catabolic and induce diuresis and hepatic lipid accumulation. Megestrol acetate may induce diabetes mellitus, adrenal suppression, and mammary neoplasia in cats. None of these drugs work consistently, and none have been evaluated in a controlled manner.

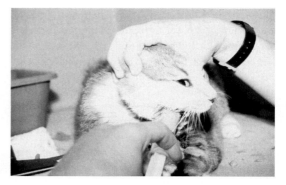

FIGURE 12-4 Syringe feeding a semiliquid diet to an adult cat.

In addition to appetite stimulants, patients may be force-fed by hand feeding or syringe feeding. Boluses of food in the oropharynx will stimulate swallowing. Using "meatballs" of canned food or using a syringe may accomplish this. Canned food gruels or convalescent canned veterinary products may be administered via syringe. Force-feeding is easy to perform; however, it may add additional stress to a sick patient. Furthermore, it is difficult to do for more than a couple of days, and it is difficult to meet nutritional needs of large dogs using this technique.

Orogastric Tube

Passing a feeding tube through the mouth into the distal esophagus or stomach is technically easy to do; however, it is usually stressful to adult dogs and cats (Figure 12-5). It is often used to provide nutrition to orphaned puppies and kittens. A 5 Fr infant feeding tube can be used for orphans weighing less than 300 g, an 8 to 10 Fr infant feeding tube can be used for orphans weighing over 300 g, or an appropriate-size, soft, male urethral catheter may be used. An appropriate size syringe should be used to avoid disconnecting the syringe from the feeding tube to refill it while feeding and to prevent administering formula too rapidly. Once weekly the feeding tube should be clearly marked to indicate the depth of insertion to ensure gastric delivery; that is, the distance from the last rib to the tip of the nose can be measured and marked off on the feeding tube as a guide. To insert an orogastric feeding tube in a neonatal puppy or kitten, the clinician passes the feeding tube through the mouth into the stomach. The feeding tube must be in the GI tract and not the respiratory tract

TABLE 12-3	Appetite Stimulants That Can Be Used in Cats (C) and Dogs (D)			
Agent	**Dose**	**Route**	**Frequency**	**Species**
Diazepam	0.5–1 mg/lb	PO	As needed	C
	0.05–0.1 mg/lb	PO	As needed	D
	0.025–0.05 mg/lb	IV	As needed	C, D
	0.5–2.0 mg	IV	As needed	C
Oxazepam	0.15–0.2 mg/lb	PO	As needed	C, D
	2–2.5 mg	PO	As needed	C
Flurazepam	0.05–0.1 mg/lb	PO	As needed	C
	0.05–0.25 mg/lb	PO	As needed	D
Chlordiazepoxide	2 mg	PO	As needed	C
Cyproheptadine	2 mg	PO	q8–12h	C
Prednisone	0.125–0.25 mg/lb	PO	q48h	C, D
Boldenone undecylenate	5 mg	IM/SQ	q7d	C
Nandrolone decanoate	10 mg	IM	q7d	C
	2.5 mg/lb (maximum 200 mg)	IM	q7d	D
Stanozolol	1–2 mg	PO	q12h	C, D
	25–50 mg	IM	q7d	C, D
Megestrol acetate	0.5 mg/lb	PO	q24h	D
B vitamins	1 ml/L fluids	IV	CRI	C, D
Cobalamin	0.25 mg/lb	SQ	q24h	C
	0.5 mg/lb	SQ	q24h	D
Elemental zinc	0.5 mg/lb	PO	q24h	C, D
Potassium	0.25–0.5 mEq KCl/lb	PO	q12h	C, D
	3 mEq K gluconate	PO	q6–8h	C, D
Interferon alfa-2b	3–30 IU	PO	q12h	C

PO, Orally; *IV,* intravenously; *IM,* intramuscularly; *SQ,* subcutaneously; *CRI,* constant rate infusion.

before feeding; it can often be palpated in the cervical esophagus. If an obstruction is felt while passing the tube before reaching the mark, the tube is in the trachea. After inserting the feeding tube to the premeasured mark, the clinician places the flared end of the tube in a glass of water and observes for bubbles while the neonate breathes. If the feeding tube has been inadvertently inserted into the respiratory tract, bubbles will appear in the water as the neonate breathes. If the tube is properly placed, then the neonate may be fed. When feeding, the clinician fills a syringe with warm formula and fits it to the feeding tube, being careful to expel any air in the tube or syringe, then aspirates back on the tube to make sure there is no residual formula remaining from the previous feeding. When certain that the tube is in the stomach, the clinician slowly administers the formula over a couple of minutes to allow sufficient time for slow filling of the stomach. Regurgitation of formula rarely occurs, but if it does, the feeding tube is withdrawn and feeding is interrupted until the next scheduled meal.

Nasoesophageal/Nasogastric Tube

Nasoesophageal tube placement is an easy, effective, and efficient means of providing enteral nutritional support (Figure 12-6). The availability of small-bore, soft polyvinyl and Silastic feeding

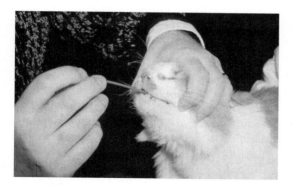

FIGURE 12-5 Orogastric feeding tube placement in an adult cat.

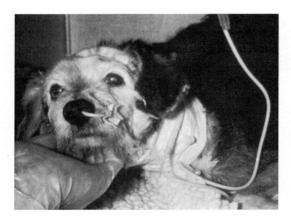

FIGURE 12-6 Use of a nasoesophageal feeding tube in an adult dog.

tubes (i.e., 3.5 to 5 Fr) and low-viscosity, nutritionally complete liquid diet formulations and patient tolerance of tube placement have made nasoesophageal tube placement a popular avenue for feeding malnourished patients. Nasoesophageal tube placement is indicated in any conscious patient with protein-calorie malnutrition that will not undergo oral, pharyngeal, esophageal, gastric, or biliary tract surgery.

Technique. Local nasal anesthesia, sedation, or light general anesthesia may be necessary for placement of a nasoesophageal tube in dogs and cats. In the majority of cases, topical anesthetic is all that is necessary for proper tube placement. In cats the clinician places 0.5 to 1 ml of 0.5% proparacaine hydrochloride (topical local anesthetic) or in dogs the clinician places 1 to 2 ml of 0.5% proparacaine or 2% lidocaine into the nasal cavity and tilts the head up to encourage the local anesthetic to coat the nasal mucosa (Figure 12-7, A). Application of local anesthetic is repeated to ensure adequate anesthesia of the nasal mucous membrane. If the patient will not tolerate nasal intubation (i.e., if excess stress is required to place the nasoesophageal tube, particularly with debilitated cats), light sedation or a light plane of anesthesia is induced.

Tube. An appropriate-size polyvinyl chloride feeding tube is selected. For cats a 5 Fr, 91-cm tube works best. For dogs between 4.5 and 22 lb, a 5 Fr, 91-cm tube is best, and an 8 Fr, 91-cm tube is best for dogs greater than 22 lb. The clinician estimates the length of tube to be placed in the esophagus or stomach by placing the tube from

the nasal planum along the side of the patient's body to the last rib (Figure 12-7, B). The distal end of the feeding tube may terminate in the thoracic esophagus or the stomach. Because of the small diameter of the tube, gastroesophageal reflux rarely occurs. If the tube is to terminate in the distal esophagus, the clinician pulls the tube back 1 to 2 cm. A tape butterfly is placed on the tube as a marker once the appropriate measurement has been taken. The tip of the tube is lubricated with 5% lidocaine viscous before passage. The patient's head is held in a normal functional position (i.e., avoiding hyperflexion or hyperextension).

Tube Placement—Cat. The clinician places the tube in the ventromedial aspect of the external nares (Figure 12-7, C) and passes it in a caudoventral medial direction into the nasal cavity (Figure 12-7, D). The tube will generally "drop" into the oropharynx and stimulate a swallowing reflex. When the patient swallows, the clinician flexes the patient's head to facilitate passage of the tube into the esophagus and passes the tube to the predetermined mark.

Tube Placement—Dog. The clinician identifies the prominent alar fold and directs the tube from a ventrolateral location in the external nares to a caudoventral and medial direction as it enters the nasal cavity. When the tube is introduced 0.5 to 1 cm inside the nostril, the clinician feels it contact the median septum at the floor of the nasal cavity. At this moment the clinician pushes the external nares dorsally to facilitate opening the ventral meatus, elevates the proximal end of the tube, and continues to advance the tube (Figure 12-8). Once the tube is inserted an additional 3 to 5 cm, the clinician discontinues pushing the nares dorsally. The clinician flexes the patient's head while continuing to insert the tube to facilitate passage through the nasopharynx into the esophagus and inserts the tube to the predetermined measurement mark.

Confirming Esophageal Placement. The clinician confirms esophageal placement by injecting 3 to 5 ml of sterile saline through the tube. If a cough is elicited, the tube is removed and replaced. Alternately, the clinician places 6 to 12 ml of air in the tube and auscultates for borborygmus at the xiphoid to confirm tube placement. Esophageal placement can also be confirmed by taking a lateral thoracic radiograph. If the patient

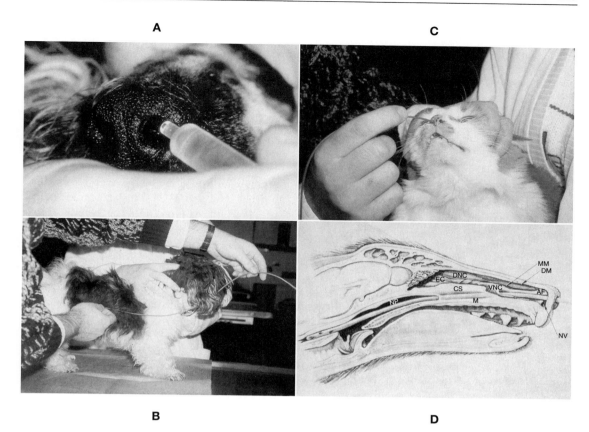

FIGURE 12-7 Nasoesophageal tube placement. **A,** Instillation of topical anesthetic into the nasal cavity. **B,** Estimation of length of tube to be inserted in the patient. **C,** The feeding tube is inserted into the ventromedial aspect of the nares. **D,** The feeding tube is inserted through the ventral meatus and nasopharynx into the esophagus. *NP,* Nasopharynx: *NV,* nasal vestibule; *CS,* cartilaginous septum; *M,* maxilla; *DM,* dorsal meatus; *MM,* middle meatus: *EC,* ethmoidal conchae; *VNC,* ventral nasal concha; *DNC,* dorsal nasal concha; *AF,* alar fold. (**D** from Crowe DT Jr: Clinical use of an indwelling nasogastric tube for enteral nutrition and fluid therapy in the dog and cat, *J Am Anim Hosp Assoc* 22:675, 1986.)

requires general anesthesia, tube placement can be determined visually.

Securing the Tube to the Patient. Once
the tube is properly inserted, the clinician should suture it to the nose and head to ensure that it will not be removed by the patient. The tube is secured to the lateral aspect of the nose with the preplaced butterfly tape and the zygomatic arch using 3-0 nylon suture (see Figure 12-6). An encircling suture and Chinese finger-trap friction suture (Figure 12-9, *A* and *B*) or cyanoacrylate glue may be used also. Although there may be concern about stimulating a feline's whiskers using this placement, clinical experience has not found this to be a problem. An Elizabethan collar should be used until it is determined if the patient will tolerate the presence of the tube. Many cats tolerate a nasoesophageal tube without an Elizabethan collar.

Tube Management. The clinician should
place a column of water in the tube and cap it with an infusion cap, three-way stopcock, or Christmas tree adapter when not in use; this prevents intake of air, reflux of esophageal contents, and occlusion of the tube by diet. Nasoesophageal tubes can be left in place for several weeks, are well tolerated, and are easily removed; the patient can drink and swallow around the tube; and repeated orogastric intubation is prevented.

Complications. Patients tolerate nasoesophageal
feeding tubes fairly well; however, several complications may occur. Premature removal is a common occurrence, particularly if the tube is irritating. Other complications include rhinitis, dacryocystitis, esophageal reflux, vomiting, aspiration pneumonia, and obstruction of the tube. In addition, patients may vomit or regurgitate the tube and inhale the

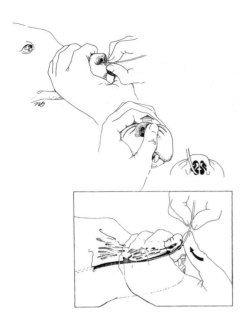

Figure 12-8 Nasoesophageal tube placement in dogs. The tip of the feeding tube is directed in a caudoventral-medial direction. The external nares are pushed dorsally to open the ventral meatus. (From Abood SK, Buffington A: Use of nasogastric tubes: indications, technique, and complications. In Kirk RW, Bonagura JD, eds: *Current veterinary therapy XI,* Philadelphia, 1992, WB Saunders.)

distal end, resulting in aspiration pneumonia if they are fed.

Pharyngostomy tube

Whenever it is necessary to provide nutritional supplementation to an anorexic patient (e.g., suffering protein–calorie malnutrition) or to patients

that are unable or reluctant to ingest food orally (e.g., cleft palate, mandibular or maxillary fractures, oral neoplasia), a pharyngostomy tube can be considered (Figure 12-10). Pharyngostomy tubes should not be used for nutritional management of patients with esophageal disorders (e.g., esophagitis, esophageal stricture, recent esophageal surgery, following esophageal foreign body removal, esophageal neoplasia). The major advantage of a pharyngostomy tube over a nasoesophageal/nasogastric tube is tube diameter; pharyngostomy tubes are generally 12 to 24 Fr, thus accommodating a wider variety of diets. Pharyngostomy tubes should terminate in the distal esophagus; they should never be placed through the lower esophageal sphincter. Generally, esophagostomy tubes are preferred over pharyngostomy because placement and use result in fewer complications.

Technique. Patients should be placed under general anesthesia and the trachea intubated. The patient is positioned in lateral recumbency with the side receiving the pharyngostomy incision uppermost. The clinician aseptically prepares a 4-cm-square area just caudal to the angle of the mandible. The mouth is held open with an oral speculum. The clinician premeasures and marks a 12 to 24 Fr polyvinyl chloride feeding tube from the exit point of the tube in the pharynx to the level of the seventh or eighth intercostal space, ensuring esophageal placement. The clinician places an index finger into the pharynx, near the base of the tongue, and palpates the epiglottis, arytenoid cartilages, and hyoid apparatus (Figure 12-11, *A*). The index finger is flexed toward the lateral aspect of the neck, and the junction of

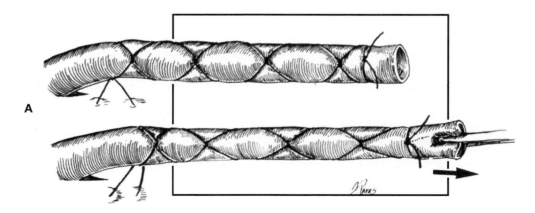

A

Figure 12-9 **A,** Schematic demonstrating placement of a Chinese finger-trap friction suture.

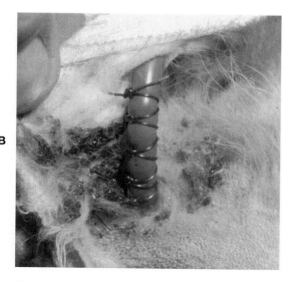

FIGURE 12-9, cont'd B, Chinese finger-trap friction suture used to secure a pharyngostomy feeding tube.

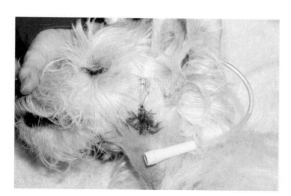

FIGURE 12-10 A pharyngostomy feeding tube in an adult male West Highland white terrier.

the intrapharyngeal ostium and laryngopharynx is identified; this is the proper location for the pharyngostomy tube exit (Figure 12-11, *B*). Enough pressure is gently applied to the lateral pharyngeal wall to create an externally visible bulge. An Eld device or large curved forceps (e.g., Carmalt or Doyen) should be used to maintain the bulge. A 1- to 2-cm skin incision is made over the bulge, and curved forceps are used to bluntly dissect subcutaneous tissue, pharyngeal muscle, and pharyngeal mucosa until the forceps become visible. If an Eld device is used, see esophagostomy tube placement for technique. The clinician uses forceps to grasp the tip of the pharyngostomy tube and pull it through the incision, into the oral cavity, and out of the mouth. The tip of the tube is rein-

serted into the mouth and passed into the mid-esophagus (i.e., premarked location on the feeding tube) (Figure 12-11, *C*). A stylet is generally not necessary for placement in the esophagus. The tube is secured to the patient's neck at its exit point with a Chinese finger-trap friction suture technique (see Figure 12-9, *A* and *B*). The clinician places a column of water in the tube and caps it with a 3-ml syringe when not in use; this prevents intake of air, reflux of esophageal contents, and occlusion of the tube by diet. When the tube is no longer required, the clinician cuts the Chinese finger-trap friction suture, pulls the tube, and allows the pharyngeal wound to heal by contraction and epithelialization.

Complications. If the pharyngostomy tube is placed ventral and medial to the intrapharyngeal ostium and laryngopharynx, partial airway obstruction, coughing, and gagging may result. If the tube is improperly placed (i.e., through the lower esophageal sphincter), reflux esophagitis and stricture may occur. Vomiting the tube has also been reported. Because of the lower incidence of complications, esophagostomy tubes are preferred.

Esophagostomy Tube

Esophagostomy tube feeding is indicated in anorexic patients with disorders of the oral cavity or pharynx or anorexic patients with a functional GI tract distal to the esophagus (Figure 12-12). Esophagostomy tube placement is contraindicated in patients with a primary or secondary esophageal disorder (e.g., esophageal stricture, following esophageal foreign body removal or esophageal surgery, esophagitis, megaesophagus).

Tube Placement. Patients should be placed under general anesthesia and the trachea intubated. The patient is placed in right lateral recumbency with left side uppermost. The tube can be placed on either the right or left side of the midcervical region; however, the esophagus lies slightly left of midline, making left-sided placement more desirable. The clinician aseptically prepares a 4-cm-square area along the left lateral midcervical area. The neck is slightly extended and the mouth held open with a mouth speculum. The clinician premeasures and marks a 14 to 24 Fr polyvinyl chloride or Silastic feeding tube (i.e., 20 to 24 Fr for dogs and 14 to 18 Fr for cats) from the level of the midcervical region (i.e., exit point of

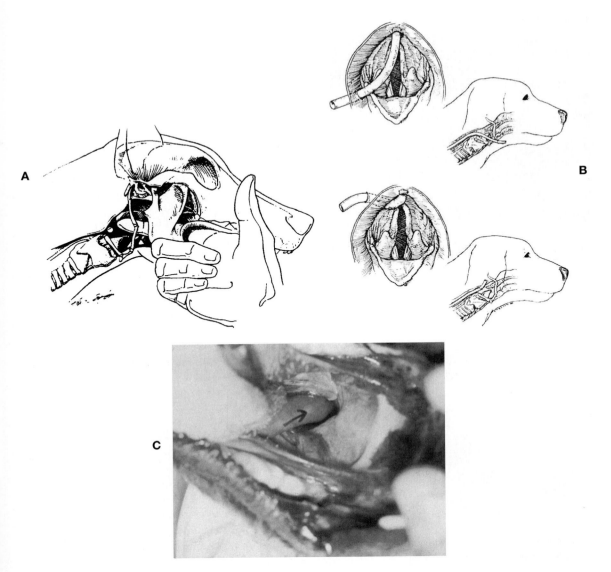

FIGURE 12-11 Pharyngostomy tube placement. **A,** Anatomic location for tube placement in the lateral pharyngeal wall. The white circle indicates the appropriate site for tube placement. (From Crowe DT Jr, Downs MO: Pharyngostomy complications in dogs and cats and recommended technical modifications: experimental and clinical investigations, *JAAHA* 22:493, 1986.) **B,** *Top:* Improper placement of the tube exiting cranial to the epihyoid cartilage results in interference with function of the epiglottis and hyoid apparatus. *Bottom:* Proper placement of the tube exiting caudal to the hyoid apparatus. (From Crowe DT Jr: Nutrition in critical patients: administering the support therapies, *Vet Med* 84:162, February 1989.) **C,** The tip of the feeding tube exiting the oral cavity is grasped with forceps and directed into the esophagus.

feeding tube) to the level of the seventh or eighth intercostal space, ensuring thoracic esophageal placement. The clinician enlarges the two lateral openings of the feeding tube or cuts off the distal rounded end of the feeding tube to encourage smoother flow of blended diets. There are two techniques that can be used to place esophagostomy tubes: one method involves using an Eld per-

cutaneous gastrostomy feeding tube placement device (Eld device), and the second involves using long curved forceps similar to pharyngostomy tube placement except caudal to the larynx.

Eld Gastrostomy Feeding Tube Placement Device Technique.

An Eld device can be used to place an esophagostomy feeding tube.

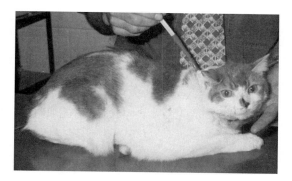

FIGURE 12-12 An esophagostomy feeding tube in an adult domestic shorthair cat.

The clinician places the oblique tip of the instrument shaft through the oral cavity and into the esophagus to the level of the midcervical region (i.e., equal distance between the angle of the mandible and thoracic inlet) and palpates the tip as it bulges the cervical skin. A small skin incision is made over the device tip (Figure 12-13, *A1, A2,* and *A3*). The clinician activates the spring-loaded instrument blade until it penetrates the esophageal wall, cervical musculature, and subcutaneous tissue and is visible through the skin incision. The clinician carefully enlarges the incision in the subcutaneous tissue, cervical musculature, and esophageal wall with the tip of a No. 15 scalpel blade to allow penetration of the instrument shaft (Figure 12-13, *B1* and *B2*). A 2-0 nylon suture is placed through

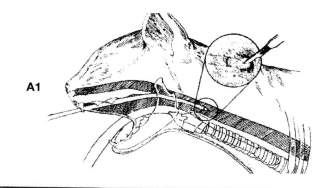

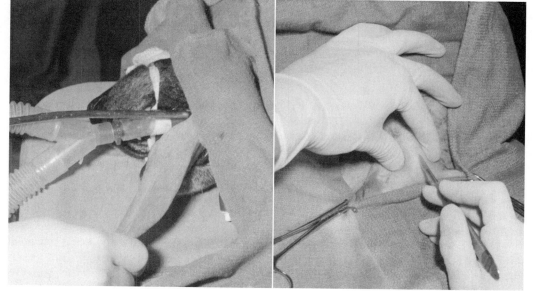

FIGURE 12-13 A, Esophagostomy tube placement: Eld PGFT applicator. 1, The applicator is passed through the oral cavity into the mid to proximal esophagus. A small skin incision is made in the lateral cervical region over the tip of the applicator. 2 and 3, Photographs illustrating these steps.

Continued

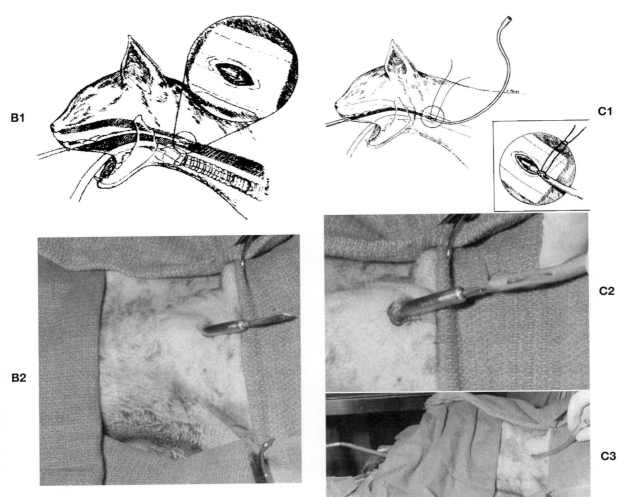

FIGURE 12-13, cont'd B, 1, The skin incision is enlarged in order to allow exteriorization of the applicator. 2, Photograph illustrating this step.

FIGURE 12-13, cont'd C, 1, The feeding tube is attached to the applicator blade and retracted into the esophagus. The applicator with the feeding tube attached is then removed, pulling the feeding tube through the oral cavity. 2 and 3, Photographs illustrating these steps.

the side holes of the feeding tube and through the hole in the instrument blade. The suture is tightened until the tip of the instrument blade and feeding tube tip are in close apposition (Figure 12-13, C1, C2, and C3). The instrument blade is retracted into the instrument shaft so the feeding tube tip just enters the instrument shaft (i.e., deactivating the instrument blade). Sterile water–soluble lubricant is placed on the tube and instrument shaft. The clinician retracts the instrument and pulls the feeding tube into the oral cavity to its predetermined measurement. The 2-0 nylon suture is removed to free the feeding tube from the instrument.

Curved Forceps Technique. Placement of an esophagostomy tube using curved forceps is

done in a manner similar to placement using the Eld device (Figure 12-14, A, B, and C). The patient is positioned in right lateral recumbency, and the curved end of the forceps is passed through the oral cavity into the midcervical esophagus. The ends of the forceps are palpated, and a skin incision is made over the end. The incision is continued through the subcutaneous tissue and esophagus, and the tips of the forceps are exteriorized. The distal end of the feeding tube is

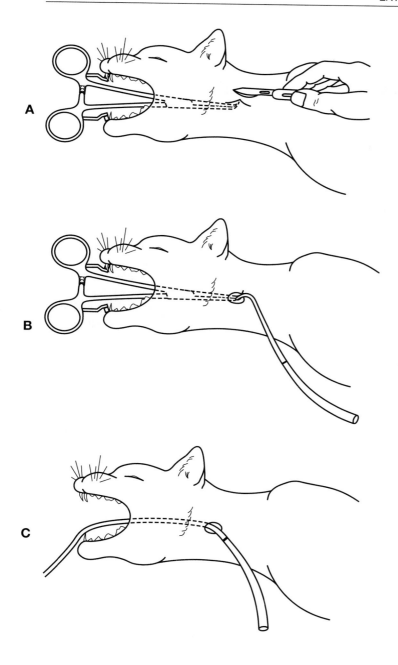

FIGURE 12-14 Esophagostomy tube placement: curved forceps. **A,** A long curved forceps is inserted through the oral cavity into the mid to proximal esophagus. The tip of the forceps is palpated, and a small skin incision is made over the tip. **B,** The incision is extended through the underlying subcutaneous tissue and musculature into the lumen of the esophagus, and the curved forceps are exteriorized through the incision. The feeding tube is grasped by the curved forceps. **C,** The forceps and feeding tube are retracted into the esophagus and out of the oral cavity. (From Levine PB et al.: Esophagostomy tubes as a method of nutritional management in cats: a retrospective study, *J Am Anim Hosp Assoc* 33:405, 1997.)

grasped with the forceps, and the forceps are retracted into the oral cavity.

Redirection of Tube. With either method, using the Eld device or using curved forceps, the distal end of the tube exits the oral cavity and the flared end of the feeding tube exits the midcervical esophagus. The next step is to redirect the distal end of the feeding tube so that it terminates in the thoracic esophagus. There are two methods that the clinician can use to accomplish this: one

involves using a stylet or hemostat to advance the distal tip of the catheter into the esophagus, and the second involves inserting a stylet down the shaft of the feeding tube. In the dog the clinician places a stylet through one of the side holes of the feeding tube and against its tip. The feeding tube is lubricated and advanced into the esophagus until the entire oral portion of the tube disappears. The clinician gently retracts the stylet from the oral cavity, being careful to ensure its release from the feeding tube (Figure 12-15, *A* and *B*). In the cat the

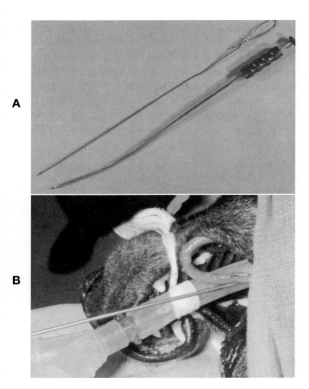

A

B

FIGURE 12-15 Esophagostomy tube placement: redirection of tube. **A,** Photograph of Eld PGFT applicator and stylet used to facilitate redirection of esophagostomy tube. **B,** The stylet is inserted through one of the side holes of the distal end of the esophagostomy tube and is used to redirect the feeding tube caudally in the esophagus.

clinician should NOT use a stylet. The feeding tube is simply advanced into the esophagus with fingers or a mosquito hemostat until the entire portion of the tube disappears. The clinician must be sure that the tube is placed to the level of its pre-measured mark. In the second technique an endo-tracheal tube stylet is passed into the proximal end of the feeding tube and is used to facilitate directing the distal end of the feeding tube in an aboral direction (Figure 12-16, *A* and *B1*). The end of the stylet should not protrude beyond the end of the feeding tube. The clinician gently retracts the feeding tube with the stylet inserted from the mid-cervical hole while placing gentle upward pressure on the tube (Figure 12-16, *B2*). As the feeding tube is slowly retracted, the distal end of the tube will be redirected toward the distal esophagus by sliding the distal end of the tube along the opposite esophageal wall. Once the

distal end of the feeding tube is directed toward the stomach, the tube can be inserted to the pre-measured mark (Figure 12-16, *B3*). The distal end of the feeding tube should terminate in the distal esophagus.

Securing the Tube. The clinician secures the tube to the cervical skin with a Chinese finger-trap friction suture of Novofil (see Figure 12-9, *A* and *B*). The exit point of the tube can be left exposed or loosely bandaged. A column of water is placed in the tube, and the exposed end capped with a 20-gauge hypodermic needle cap; this prevents intake of air, reflux of esophageal contents, and occlusion of the tube by diet. Most patients tolerate the tube without the need of an Elizabethan collar. Esophagostomy tubes can be removed immediately after placement or left in place for several weeks to months. The tube exit site should be periodically cleaned with an antiseptic solution. Tube removal is performed by cutting the Chinese finger-trap friction suture and gently pulling the tube. No further exit wound care is necessary; the hole seals in 1 to 2 days and heals in 3 to 5 days.

Advantages and Disadvantages.
Advantages of esophagostomy tube feeding include the following: the tube is easily placed;

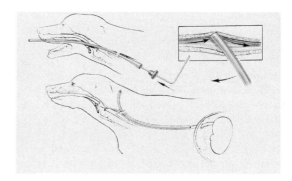

FIGURE 12-16 A, Esophagostomy tube placement: alternate technique for redirection of tube. A stylet is inserted into the lumen of the feeding tube so that the tip of the stylet is near but not through the end of the tube. The tube and stylet are slowly retracted while upward pressure is applied. The end of the feeding tube is redirected in the esophagus so that it can be inserted into the distal esophagus. (From Rawlings CR: Percutaneous placement of a midcervical esophagostomy tube: new technique and representative cases, *J Am Anim Hosp Assoc* 29:526, 1993.)

Continued

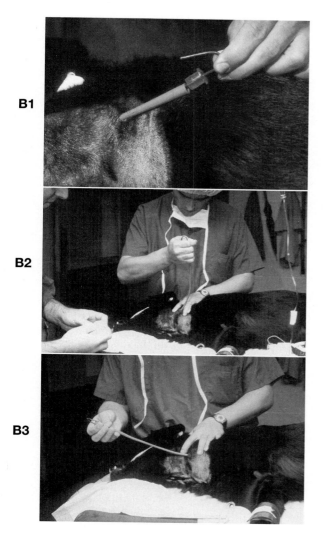

B1

B2

B3

FIGURE 12-16, cont'd B, Photographs illustrating redirection of the esophagostomy feeding tube. 1, The stylet is inserted into the lumen of the feeding tube so that the stylet tip is near but not through the end of the tube. 2, The feeding tube and stylet are slowly withdrawn so that the tip of the feeding tube can be redirected toward the thoracic esophagus. 3, The feeding tube and stylet are inserted caudally in the esophagus so that the end of the feeding tube terminates in the thoracic esophagus.

tubes are well tolerated by the patient; large-bore feeding tubes (greater than 12 Fr) can be used, allowing use of blended diets; tube care and feeding is easily performed by the owner; patients can eat and drink around the tube; and tube removal can be performed anytime after placement. Esophageal tube placement eliminates coughing, laryngospasm, or aspiration occasionally associated

with pharyngostomy tubes. The major disadvantage of an esophagostomy tube is the need for general anesthesia during placement.

Complications. Complications associated with esophagostomy tube placement include early removal by the patient or vomiting the tube. Two cases of esophageal perforation in cats have been reported. This was thought to be due to placement of the tube with a stylet. Esophageal perforation has not occurred since eliminating the stylet from placement protocol. Esophageal perforation has not been reported in the dog. No significant long-term complications have been reported (e.g., esophagitis, esophageal stricture, esophageal diverticulum, or subcutaneous cervical cellulitis). Reflux esophagitis can occur from improper tube placement (i.e., through the lower esophageal sphincter) or esophageal irritation from the tube itself (Figure 12-17). Midesophageal placement of silicone rubber tubes greatly reduces the incidence of esophageal injury and eliminates reflux esophagitis.

Gastrostomy Tube

Tube gastrostomy is indicated in anorexic patients with a functional GI tract distal to the esophagus or patients undergoing operations of the oral cavity, larynx, pharynx, or esophagus (Figure 12-18). Gastrostomy tube placement is contraindicated in patients with primary gastric disease (e.g., gastritis, gastric ulceration, gastric neoplasia) or disorders

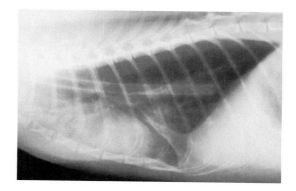

FIGURE 12-17 Lateral cervical radiograph of an esophagostomy feeding tube in an adult dog. The end of the feeding tube terminates in the thoracic esophagus and does not traverse the lower esophageal sphincter. (From Rawlings CR: Percutaneous placement of a midcervical esophagostomy tube: new technique and representative cases. *J Am Anim Hosp Assoc* 29:526, 1993.)

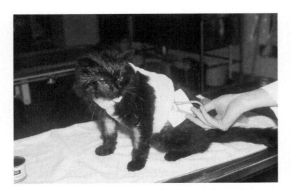

FIGURE 12-18 Percutaneous endoscopically placed gastrostomy feeding tube in an adult cat with idiopathic hepatic lipidosis.

causing uncontrolled vomiting and in comatose patients. Advantages of gastrostomy tube feeding include ease of tube placement, patient tolerance, use of large-bore feeding tubes, ease of tube care and feeding by the owner, and the fact that oral feeding can commence while the tube is in place. Disadvantages of gastrostomy tube feeding include the following: use of specialized equipment may be necessary (e.g., endoscope, special tube placement instruments), general anesthesia is required, feeding cannot be initiated the first 12 hours after tube placement, and, depending upon placement technique, tubes must remain in place for a minimum of 7 to 14 days before removal (in order to encourage adhesion formation between stomach and abdominal wall).

Tube Placement. Gastrostomy feeding tubes may be placed without visualization (using the stomach tube technique, Eld feeding tube placement device, or Cook feeding tube placement device) or with visualization (using endoscopy or surgery). Gastrostomy tubes placed surgically may be done with or without gastropexy. Gastrostomy tubes are usually placed under general anesthesia with the patient positioned in right lateral recumbency. For all techniques except placement through a midline laparotomy, the left paralumbar fossa is clipped and prepared aseptically. Drapes are not necessary unless a surgical approach is used. Gastrostomy feeding tubes should exit the left lateral abdominal wall approximately 1 to 2 cm caudal to the costochondral arch and approximately one third of the way dorsal from the ventral abdominal wall. This results in the tube being located along the gastric fundus cranial to the spleen and caudal to the liver.

Technique
Percutaneous Without Visualization
Placement of gastrostomy tubes with visualization is advised when possible because direct visualization is associated with potentially fewer complications; however, gastrostomy feeding tubes can be placed safely without visualization.

Stomach Tube Technique
A gastrostomy tube placement device can be prepared by purchasing a length of vinyl or stainless steel tubing from a hardware store (Figure 12-19, *A*). The length of the tubing is determined by measuring the distance from the nasal planum to the iliac crest and adding 15 cm. The outer diameter of the tube ranges from 1.2 cm (patients weighing less than 25 lb) to 2.5 cm for dogs weighing more than 55 lb. The distal tip of a stainless steel tube can be flared and deflected 45 degrees to the long axis of the tube to help displace the body wall laterally. The patient is anesthetized and positioned in right lateral recumbency. The lubricated tube is passed through the mouth and into the stomach. The tube is advanced until the end of the tube displaces the stomach laterally. Positioning the patient with its head over the edge of the table and lowering the proximal end of the tube will facilitate identifying the tube tip through the body wall (Figure 12-19, *B*). A stab skin incision is made over the distal end of the tube, and a 14-gauge hypodermic needle or an over-the-needle intravenous catheter is introduced percutaneously into the lumen of the tube while holding the distal tip of the tube between two fingers. Proper positioning of the catheter is confirmed by moving the hub from side to side and feeling the catheter tip strike the inside of the tube. A guide wire prepared from a monofilament banjo string or cerclage wire is threaded through the needle or catheter, into the tube, and out of the mouth of the patient (Figure 12-19, *C* and *D*). The tube and catheter are removed, and the wire is attached to a gastrostomy tube, which is secured (Figure 12-19, *E*). Securing the gastrostomy feeding tube to the wire is accomplished by cutting off the flared end of the mushroom-tipped catheter (Figure 12-19, *F*). An intravenous catheter or 5-ml pipette tip is fed over the wire at the oral cavity. Two V-shaped notches are then cut opposite each other at the proximal end of the gastrostomy tube. The feeding tube is tied to the wire, and the notched end of the feeding tube is planted firmly in the flared end of the intravenous catheter or pipette tip. The feeding tube and catheter/pipette tip are lubricated. A long

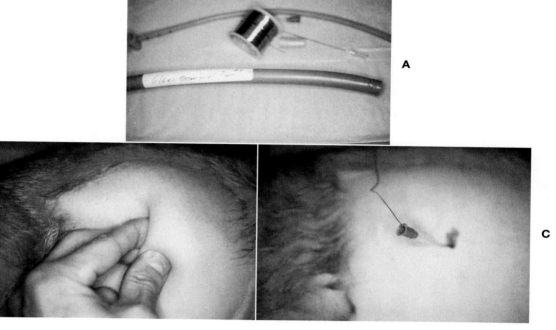

FIGURE 12-19 Gastrostomy tube placement without visualization: stomach tube. **A,** Equipment required to insert a gastrostomy feeding tube without visualization using a stomach tube. The stomach tube may be hard plastic or metal. A length of wire is also necessary for placement. **B,** The stomach tube is inserted through the oral cavity and esophagus into the stomach. The end of the tip in the stomach is palpated through the abdominal wall. **C,** An intravenous catheter has been inserted through a small skin incision into the lumen of the stomach tube, and a wire has been inserted into the catheter and lumen of the stomach tube. (**A-C** courtesy Dr. T. Glaus, Switzerland.)

Continued

piece of fishing line or Vetafil is placed through the side holes of the mushroom end of the feeding tube; this suture should not be tied. This provides a means to recover the feeding tube should problems arise. The tube is then pulled through the esophagus, into the stomach, and through the abdominal wall by placing tension on the wire at the abdominal wall exit site (Figure 12-19, *G* and *H*). The skin incision may need to be enlarged to facilitate passage of the feeding tube through the body wall and skin (Figure 12-19, *I*). The mushroom tip should be palpable through the body wall. The mushroom tip should not be pulled through the body wall. Once the feeding tube is secured, the suture placed through the side holes of the mushroom tip is removed by pulling on one end of the suture.

Eld Feeding Tube Device

Gastrostomy feeding tubes may be placed nonvisually using a device that facilitates placement. One device is the Eld percutaneous gastrostomy feeding tube applicator (Eld device) (Figure 12-20, *A*).

Placement of a gastrostomy feeding tube using the Eld device is performed in a manner similar to using the device to place an esophagostomy tube. The patient is anesthetized and placed in right lateral recumbency; the tube will exit the left lateral abdominal wall in the paralumbar fossa. The Eld device is passed through the oral cavity, down the esophagus, and into the stomach. Gentle downward pressure is applied to the handle to facilitate identification of the distal end of the Eld device in the stomach (Figure 12-20, *B*). When the distal end of the Eld device is positioned properly in the left paralumbar fossa, a small stab skin incision is made over the distal end. Then the spring-loaded plunger is pushed (Figure 12-20, *C*), resulting in the sharp point being thrust through the gastric and abdominal wall. A piece of suture (such as Vetafil) or monofilament fishing line is inserted through the hole in the pointed tip of the distal end of the Eld device (Figure 12-20, *D*), and the distal end is retracted into the outer sheath. The entire device is removed, pulling the suture or

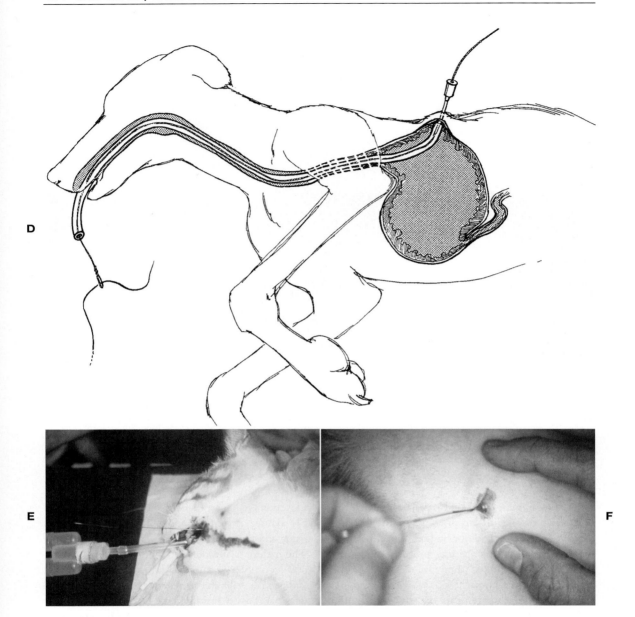

FIGURE 12-19, cont'd D, Schematic illustrating passage of the wire through the intravenous catheter and lumen of the stomach tube. **E,** The stomach tube is removed, but the wire is left in place. The wire now enters the lateral abdominal wall, passes through the stomach and esophagus, and exits the oral cavity. **F,** A tapered catheter is inserted on the end of the wire that exits the oral cavity, and the feeding tube is attached to the wire. (**E** and **F** courtesy Dr. T. Glaus, Switzerland.)

fishing line in an antegrade direction. This results in an end of the suture or fishing line exiting the oral cavity and the other end exiting the left abdominal wall. The gastrostomy tube is then secured to the suture exiting the oral cavity (Figure 12-20, *E*). Securing the gastrostomy feeding tube to the suture is accomplished by cutting off the flared end of the mushroom-tipped catheter. An intravenous catheter or 5-ml pipette

tip is fed over the wire at the oral cavity. Two V-shaped notches are then cut opposite each other at the proximal end of the gastrostomy tube. The feeding tube is tied to the suture, and the notched end of the feeding tube is planted firmly in the flared end of the intravenous catheter or pipette tip. The feeding tube and catheter/pipette tip are lubricated. A long piece of fishing line or Vetafil is placed through the side holes of the mushroom

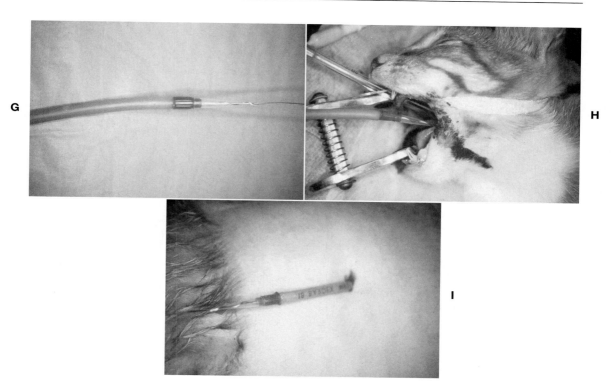

FIGURE 12-19, cont'd G, Tension is applied to the end of the wire that exits the lateral abdominal wall. **H,** The feeding tube is pulled into the oral cavity, esophagus, and stomach. **I,** The lateral abdominal wall skin incision is enlarged, and the feeding tube is exteriorized. (**G-I** courtesy Dr. T. Glaus, Switzerland.)

end of the feeding tube; this suture should not be tied. This provides a means to recover the feeding tube should problems arise. The tube is then pulled through the esophagus, into the stomach, and through the abdominal wall by placing tension on the suture at the abdominal wall exit site. The skin incision may need to be enlarged to facilitate passage of the feeding tube through the body wall and skin. The mushroom tip should be palpable through the body wall. The mushroom tip should not be pulled through the body wall. Once the feeding tube is secured, the suture placed through the side holes of the mushroom tip is removed by pulling on one end of the suture.

Cook Feeding Tube Placement Device

Use of a Cook feeding tube placement device (Cook device) is another technique for placing gastrostomy feeding tubes without visualization (Figure 12-21). The patient is anesthetized and placed in right lateral recumbency (Figure 12-22). The tube will exit in the left paralumbar fossa, and that area is aseptically prepared. The Cook device is passed through the oral cavity, down the esophagus, and into the stomach (Figure 12-23, *A*). The

distal end of the Cook device is angled and flared, and this end is palpated in the left paralumbar fossa. A stab skin incision is made over the flared end of the Cook device (Figure 12-23, *B*), and the application needle is passed through the stab incision and body wall into the lumen of the Cook device (Figure 12-23, *C*). Correct insertion of the needle

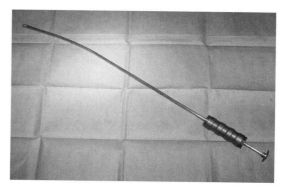

FIGURE 12-20 A, Gastrostomy tube placement without visualization: Eld percutaneous gastrostomy feeding tube (PGFT) applicator.

Continued

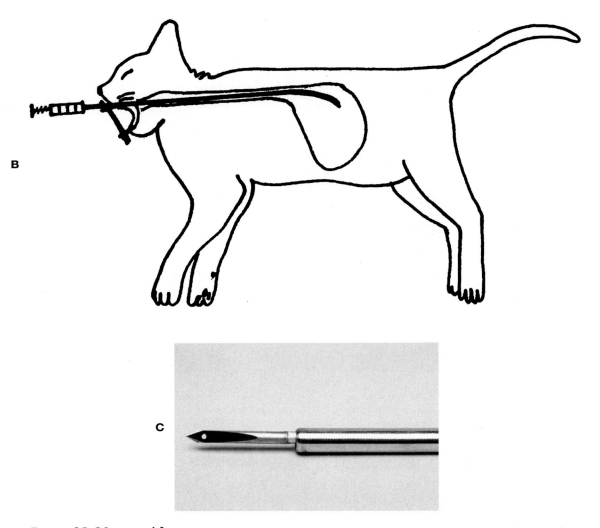

FIGURE 12-20, cont'd B, The applicator is inserted through the oral cavity and esophagus into the stomach. The tip of the tube is palpated through the lateral abdominal wall. **C,** When the spring-loaded plunger is depressed, a sharp, pointed end is exposed at the distal tip of the applicator. (**B** modified from *JorVet Eld gastrostomy tube applicator manual*, Jorgensen Laboratories, Loveland, Colo.)

is verified by tapping the needle against the inner wall of the lumen of the Cook device. If the flared end of the Cook device cannot be palpated in the gastric lumen or if the spleen appears to be overlying the end, a three-way stopcock can be attached to the proximal end of the Cook device and air can be injected to distend the stomach (Figure 12-23, *D*). A threaded wire supplied with the Cook device is inserted through the needle so that it exits the proximal end of the Cook device where it exits the oral cavity (Figure 12-23, *E*). The wire is fed so that the threaded end is inserted and exits at the mouth (Figure 12-23, *F*). The Cook device is then removed. The flared end of a mushroom-tipped feeding tube is cut off, and the remaining end of the feeding tube is inserted on the ribbed end of the tapered insertion device (Figure 12-23, *G*). The insertion device has a threaded end, which is attached to the threaded end of the wire exiting the mouth (Figure 12-23, *H*). A long piece of fishing line or Vetafil is placed through the side holes of the mushroom end of the feeding tube; this suture should not be tied. This provides a means to recover the feeding tube should problems arise. The insertion device and feeding tube are lubricated, and the tube is then pulled through the esophagus, into the stomach, and through the abdominal wall by placing tension on the wire at the abdominal wall exit site (Figure 12-23, *I*). The mushroom tip should not be pulled through the body wall (Figure

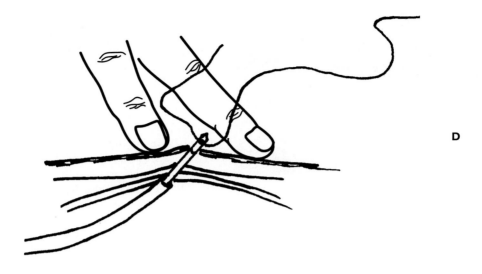

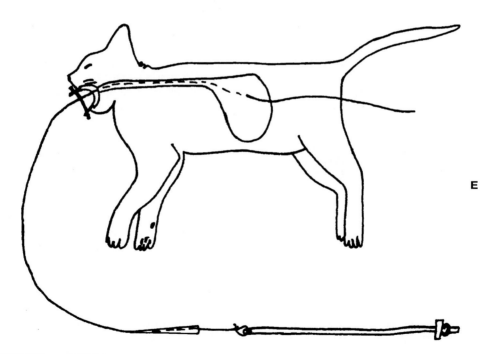

FIGURE 12-20, cont'd **D,** The sharp, pointed, distal tip of the applicator is thrust through the stomach and lateral abdominal wall. A piece of suture is threaded through the hole in the tip, and the tip is retracted into the body of the applicator. **E,** The applicator and attached suture are removed. The feeding tube is attached to the suture. (**D** modified from and **E** from *JorVet Eld gastrostomy tube applicator manual,* Jorgensen Laboratories, Loveland, Colo.)

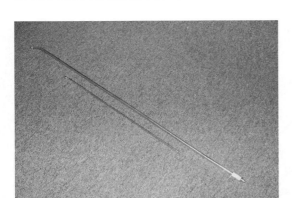

FIGURE 12-21 Gastrostomy tube placement without visualization: Cook feeding tube insertion device.

12-23, *J*). Once the feeding tube is secured, the suture placed through the side holes of the mushroom tip is removed by pulling on one end of the suture.

Advantages and Disadvantages. Advantages of gastrostomy feeding tube placement without visualization include ease of placement and low cost of placement. Disadvantages are the inability to perform surgical gastropexy to ensure an early and

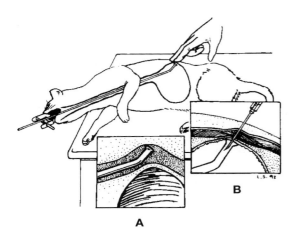

FIGURE 12-22 Gastrostomy tube placement without visualization: Cook feeding tube insertion device. The device is passed through the oral cavity and esophagus into the stomach with the patient in right lateral recumbency. **A,** The device is rotated 90 degrees counterclockwise so that it can pass freely over the base of the heart. **B,** The catheter needle is inserted through the skin into the flared end of the device at a 45-degree angle to parallel the distal end of the device. (From Mauterer JV Jr et al.: New technique and management guidelines for percutaneous nonendoscopic tube gastrostomy, *J Am Vet Med Assoc* 205[4]:574, 1994.)

permanent seal between the stomach wall and body wall and tube placement cannot be verified visually.

Percutaneous Endoscopic Placement
Percutaneous endoscopic tube placement is performed as described for percutaneous surgical placement without gastropexy with the exception that the suture is placed from the left flank out through the oral cavity with the aid of an endoscope. The clinician passes the endoscope into the stomach and insufflates the lumen with air (Figure 12-24, *A*). A 1-mm skin incision is made in the left flank 1 to 2 cm caudal to the last rib and approximately one third of the distance dorsally from the ventral abdominal wall. An 18-gauge hypodermic needle or an over-the-needle intravenous catheter is passed through the skin incision and into the stomach lumen (Figure 12-24, *B* and *C*). The clinician passes a strand of Vetafil through the needle into the stomach, retrieves it endoscopically (Figure 12-24, *D*), and brings it out through the mouth. Once the strand of suture is entering the left flank and exiting the oral cavity, the feeding tube is placed as described for percutaneous placement without visualization (Figure 12-24, *E-I*). A retrieval suture is also placed through the side ports of the mushroom-tipped catheter.

Advantages and Disadvantages. The advantage of endoscopic placement is direct visualization of tube placement during the procedure. The disadvantage is inability to perform surgical gastropexy to ensure an early and permanent seal between the stomach wall and body wall.

Percutaneous Surgical Placement With Gastropexy
General anesthesia and standard skin preparation of the left paralumbar fossa is performed. The clinician should instruct an assistant to pass a large-bore stiff plastic stomach tube (e.g., as for decompressing patients with gastric dilatation volvulus) into the stomach. The left flank area is palpated until the bulging end of the stomach tube can be palpated. The tube should be moved to a point 1 to 2 cm caudal to the last rib and 3 to 4 cm ventral to the transverse processes of lumbar vertebrae 2, 3, and 4 and grasped with thumb and finger (Figure 12-25, *A-C*). The clinician holds the stomach tube in this position and makes a 2-cm skin incision over the end of the tube. Subcutaneous tissues are bluntly dissected to expose the external abdominal oblique muscle. The external abdominal oblique muscle is bluntly dissected in the direction of its fibers to expose the internal abdominal

oblique muscle. This muscle is dissected in the direction of its fibers to expose the transversus abdominus muscle. The clinician dissects this muscle in the direction of its fibers and penetrates the peritoneum to expose the wall of the stomach over the tube, being careful not to enter the lumen of the stomach. One or two 3-0 Maxon stay sutures are placed in the exposed stomach wall to ensure that it will not fall back into the abdominal cavity. The orogastric tube can now be removed from the stomach. A purse-string suture is placed in the stomach wall around the proposed tube entry point using 3-0 Maxon. The clinician uses a No. 11 scalpel blade to enter the stomach, places a

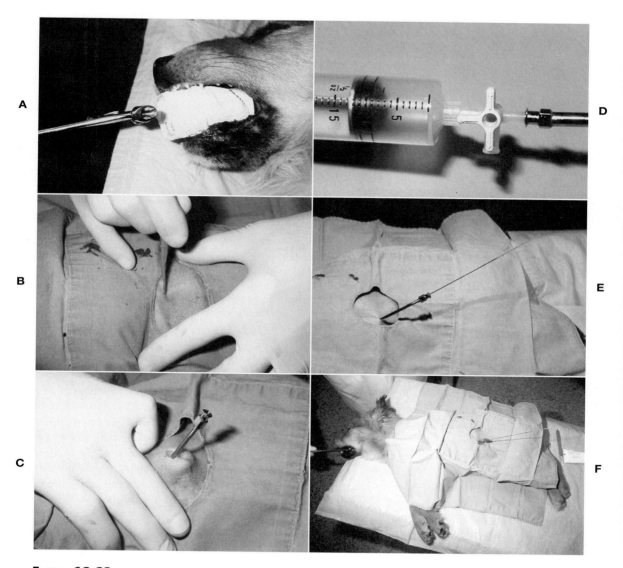

FIGURE 12-23 Gastrostomy tube placement without visualization: Cook feeding tube insertion device. **A,** The device is inserted through the oral cavity and esophagus into the stomach. **B,** A small skin incision is made over the left paralumbar fossa. **C,** The tip of the device located in the stomach is positioned under the skin incision, and the needle is inserted through the lateral abdominal wall and stomach wall into the lumen of the device. **D,** A three-way stopcock can be attached to the end of the device for stomach insufflation. **E,** The threaded wire is inserted through the needle into the lumen of the device until it is visualized at the end of the device inserted into the oral cavity. **F,** The wire extends from the left lateral abdominal wall through the stomach and esophagus, and exits the oral cavity. (**A-F** courtesy Dr. R. Bright, Colorado.)

Continued

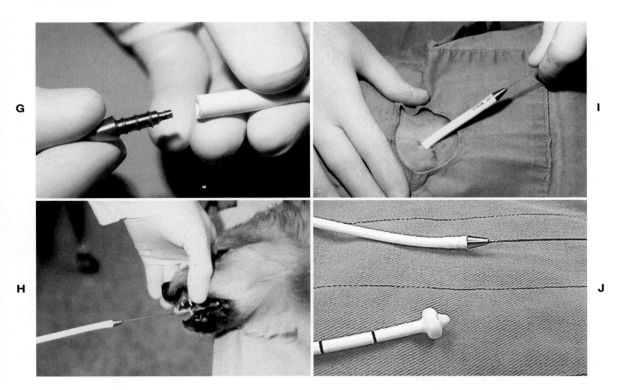

FIGURE 12-23, cont'd **G,** The flared end of the mushroom-tipped feeding tube is removed, and the remaining end of the feeding tube is attached to the ribbed end of the tapered insertion device. **H,** The tapered insertion device with the mushroom-tipped feeding tube is attached to the threaded end of the wire that exits the oral cavity. **I,** The wire is retracted through the abdominal wall, pulling the feeding tube through the oral cavity and esophagus into the stomach. **J,** The tapered insertion device aids in pulling the feeding tube through the stomach and lateral abdominal wall. (**G** courtesy Dr. R. Bright, Colorado.)

20 to 24 Fr Foley catheter 3 to 4 cm into its lumen, and inflates the bulb. The purse-string suture is secured around the Foley catheter to create an airtight and watertight seal. Gentle traction is placed on the Foley catheter to bring its bulb against the stomach wall and the stomach wall against the abdominal wall. Four or five simple interrupted sutures of 3-0 Maxon are placed from the stomach wall to the body wall to provide a firm gastropexy to the abdominal wall. The clinician closes subcutaneous tissues and skin around the exiting Foley catheter and secures the catheter to the skin with a Chinese finger-trap friction suture of No. 1 Novofil (Figure 12-26, *A-C*).

Advantages and Disadvantages. Advantages of the surgical technique include the following: the tube is easily placed, the stomach is easily found in an anoretic patient, tube placement is quick, no special equipment is needed to place the tube (i.e., endoscope or feeding tube placement device), surgical gastropexy ensures an immediate and long-

lasting seal between the stomach wall and body wall, and confirmation of proper tube placement is performed during placement. Feeding tubes can be safely removed at any time after placement. A disadvantage of this technique is the difficulty of palpating the orogastric feeding tube in the flank of obese patients. Also it requires a surgical and thus more invasive approach to placing a feeding tube.

Surgical Placement Through a Midline Laparotomy

The patient is aseptically prepared for a midline celiotomy. From a ventral midline laparotomy approach, the distal end of a 20 Fr Foley or Pezzer catheter is brought into the abdominal cavity through a stab incision in the left body wall. The ventral surface of the stomach is exteriorized, a purse-string suture is placed in the body of the stomach equidistant between the lesser and greater curvature, and a stab incision is made in the center of the purse-string suture with a No. 11 scalpel blade. The distal end of the feeding catheter is

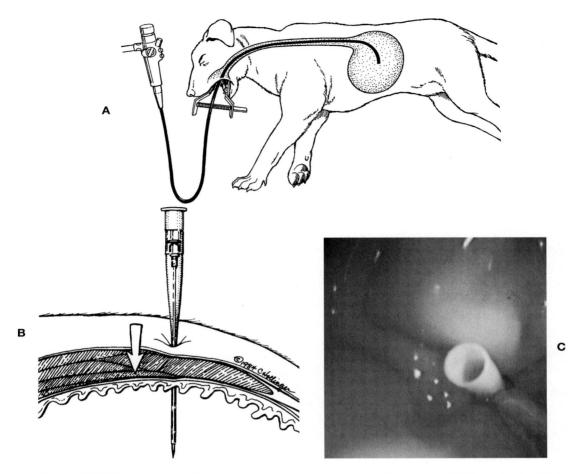

FIGURE 12-24 Gastrostomy tube placement: percutaneous endoscopic placement. **A,** With the dog in right lateral recumbency, the endoscope is inserted into the stomach and the stomach is distended with air. **B,** An over-the-needle catheter or hypodermic needle is placed transabdominally into the stomach lumen adjacent to the tip of the endoscope. **C,** Close-up of an endoscopic snare grasping a 2-inch catheter after the stylet has been removed. (**A** and **C** from Tams TR: *Small animal endoscopy*, ed 2, St. Louis, 1999, Mosby. **B** from Bright RM, Burrows CF: Percutaneous endoscopic tube gastronomy in dogs, *Am J Vet Res* 49[5]: 629, 1988.)   *Continued*

placed in the lumen of the stomach, and the purse-string suture is tightened around the catheter. The bulb (i.e., Foley) is inflated with saline, and gentle traction is placed on the catheter to bring the body of the stomach in close apposition to the left body wall. The stomach wall is sutured to the abdominal wall with four or five 3-0 Maxon sutures to provide an early permanent gastropexy. The feeding tube is secured to the skin with a Chinese finger-trap friction suture of No. 1 Novofil. The abdomen is closed routinely (Figure 12-27).

Advantages and Disadvantages. The advantage of gastrostomy tube placement via laparotomy is the ability to suture the stomach wall to the abdominal wall, creating an early permanent gastropexy. The major disadvantage is the need to perform a laparotomy to place the tube. This technique is generally performed when exploratory laparotomy is required for diagnosis or treatment of the patient's primary disorder.

Complications of Gastrostomy Feeding Tubes

Potential complications of gastrostomy feeding tubes relate to mechanical, GI, and metabolic complications. The most severe complication of gastrostomy tube placement is early removal with leakage of gastric contents into the abdominal cavity and subsequent generalized peritonitis.

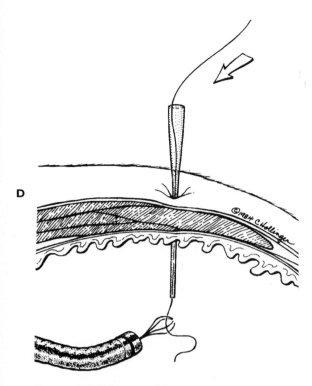

FIGURE 12-24, cont'd D, A strand of suture is inserted through the catheter into the stomach lumen and grasped with grasping forceps using endoscopic visualization. (From Bright RM, Burrows CF: Percutaneous endoscopic tube gastrostomy in dogs, *Am J Vet Res* 49[5]:629,1988.)

Ensuring firm placement of the feeding tube that results in an early and permanent gastropexy can prevent this complication. Peristomal infection can also occur if the tube is secured too tightly to the lateral abdominal wall or too loosely, resulting in rubbing of the tube in the gastrocutaneous fistula. GI complications include vomiting and diarrhea. Vomiting is often a result of preexisting disease or administration of food that is less than near body temperature or administering food too rapidly. Potential metabolic complications include intolerance to the diet, hyperglycemia due to stress-induced insulin resistance, and electrolyte imbalances. Protein intolerance may occur if too much protein is administered to a patient in renal or liver failure.

Low-Profile Gastrostomy Feeding Tubes. Low-profile gastrostomy feeding tubes (LPGFTs) can be used for long-term nutritional support (Figure 12-28, *A* and *B*). LPGFTs offer the advantage of exiting flush with the abdominal wall.

These feeding tubes are placed either surgically or percutaneously using a previously placed mushroom-tipped gastrostomy feeding tube. Surgical placement is through a midline celiotomy or through a left flank laparotomy. Placement can also be done using a previously placed gastrostomy feeding tube. A gastrostomy feeding tube is placed as described previously and left in place for 3 to 4 weeks to ensure adhesions between the stomach and body wall. The feeding tube is removed, and the depth of the fistula is measured (Figure 12-29, *A*). The appropriate LPGFT is chosen. The mushroom end of the LPGFT collapses with the aid of a stylet (Figure 12-29, *B*). The mushroom tip is collapsed and fed through the fistula into the gastric lumen. The stylet is removed, and the mushroom reexpands in the lumen. A cutaneous flange is inserted onto the LPGFT and used to secure the tube. LPGFTs have one or two internal valves to prevent reflux.

Advantages and Disadvantages. LPGFTs may be used for months to years in dogs and cats. Another advantage is that they lie flush with the skin; therefore bandage material is not required. Valves present in the LPGFTs prevent reflux of gastric contents. Disadvantages of LPGFTs include expense of the tubes, necessity for a previously placed gastrostomy tube or a surgical approach for placement, and the possibility of separating the adhesions while placing the LPGFT.

Percutaneous Gastroduodenostomy Tube

Percutaneous gastroduodenostomy is indicated in patients with severe gastroesophageal reflux, swallowing disorders, aspiration pneumonia, or persistent vomiting of gastric origin (Figure 12-30, *A*).

Technique. A percutaneous gastrostomy feeding tube is placed as described previously. A Pezzer catheter feeding tube is used, and the dome-shaped tip of the mushroom end is removed before placement. A strand of 2-0 silk suture is tied to the tip of an 8 to 10 Fr diameter, 60- to 110-cm, duodenal feeding tube with stylet. The duodenal tube is passed through the gastrostomy tube and into the stomach (Figure 12-30, *B*). The duodenal tube is visualized endoscopically, and the silk suture is grasped with biopsy forceps (Figure 12-30, *C*). The biopsy forceps are gently retracted into the endoscope port to pull the catheter tip against the endoscope. The clinician repositions the dog in left

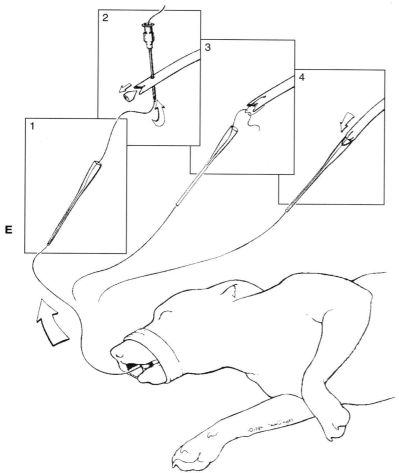

FIGURE 12-24, cont'd E, 1, The end of the suture that exits the oral cavity is passed retrograde through the lumen of an intravenous catheter or pipette tip. 2, The end of the feeding tube opposite the mushroom tip end is modified by removing a V-shaped piece. An 18-gauge hypodermic needle is passed transversely through the tube just under the trimmed portion. The suture and needle are removed as a unit. 3, The suture is tied in a square knot, with the knot pulled deep into the notched end of the feeding tube. 4, The end of the feeding tube is placed into the flared end of the catheter or pipette tip and kept under tension with traction on the suture exiting the lateral abdominal wall. **F,** The feeding tube is attached to the suture exiting the oral cavity. (**E** from Bright RM, Burrows CF: Percutaneous endoscopic tube gastrostomy in dogs, *Am J Vet Res* 49[5]:629,1988.)

Continued

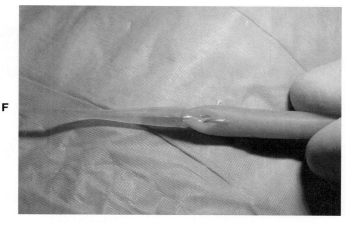

lateral recumbency, passes the endoscope through the pylorus and into the duodenum, advances the biopsy forceps to their full length, and releases the catheter (Figure 12-30, *D*). The biopsy forceps are replaced in the biopsy port, and the endoscope is slowly removed (Figure 12-30, *E*). The duodenal feeding tube is secured to the gastrostomy tube by seating the flanged end of the duodenal tube in the gastrostomy tube, and the duodenal tube stylet is slowly removed (Figure 12-30, *F*).

Advantages and Disadvantages. The advantage of this technique is placement of an enteral feeding tube without the need of laparotomy. Disadvantages include difficulty placing the tube in the duodenum, difficult placement in

Feeding tube

G1

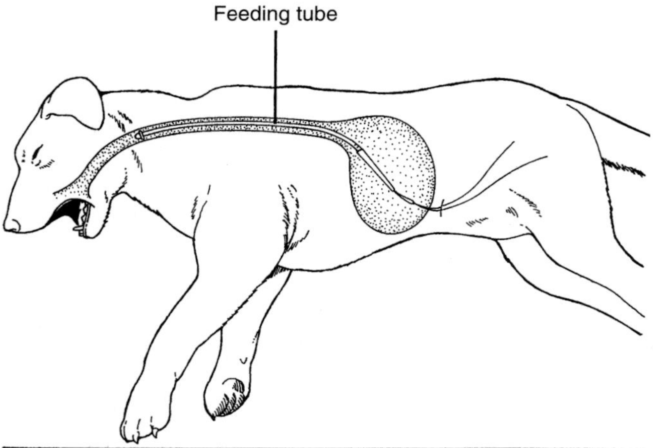

G2

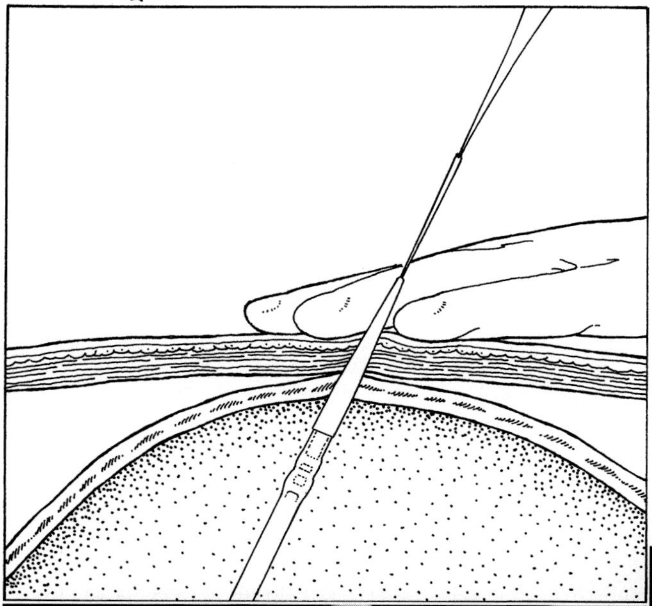

H

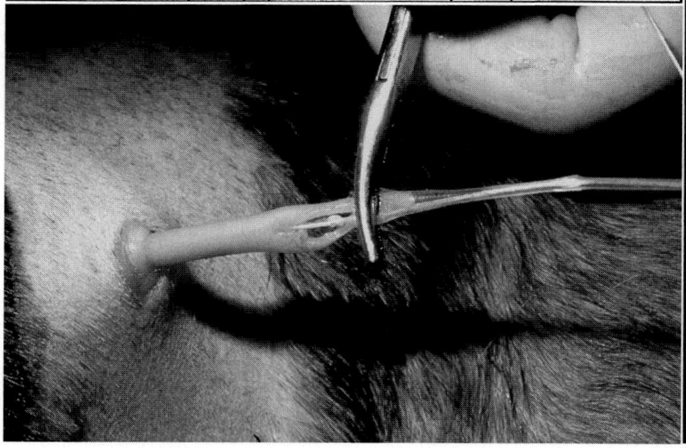

I

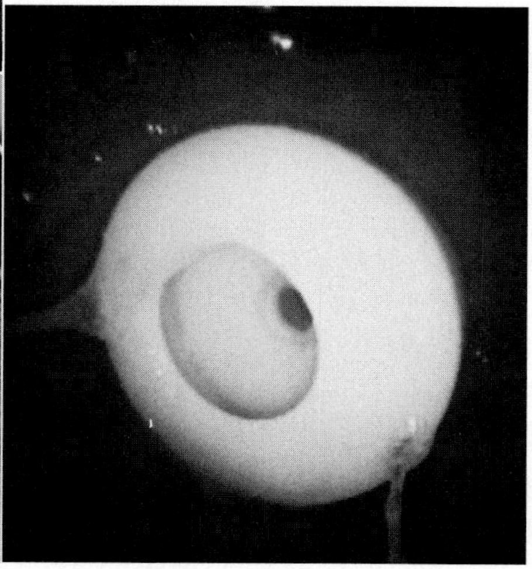

FIGURE 12-24, cont'd

G, 1, Traction is applied to the suture exiting the lateral abdominal wall, and the assembled feeding tube and catheter are pulled into the stomach, 2, and finally to the exterior. **H,** The feeding tube is exteriorized. **I,** Internal bumper of a PEG tube (Bard) after placement. (**G** and **I** from Tams TR: *Small animal endoscopy,* ed 2, St. Louis, 1999, Mosby.)

patients weighing less than 40 lb, migration of the tube from the duodenum, mechanical obstruction of the tube (e.g., kinking), specialized instrumentation necessary for placement, and the necessity of radiographic assessment for tube placement confirmation. This technique is technically demanding and is recommended only for veterinarians experienced in endoscopy.

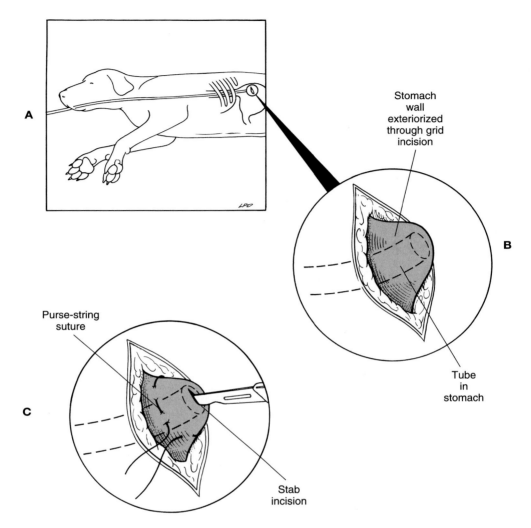

FIGURE 12-25 Percutaneous gastrostomy tube placement with gastropexy (cont'd in Figure 12-26). **A,** Pass a large-bore, stiff plastic stomach tube into the stomach. Palpate the end of the tube at the flank. **B,** Grasp the tube and move it to a point 2 to 3 cm caudal to the thirteenth rib and 2 to 3 cm distal to the transverse processes of the lumbar vertebrae. Secure the tube with thumb and finger, make an incision through the skin and subcutaneous tissue, and bluntly dissect the abdominal muscles to expose the gastric wall over the tube. **C,** Place a purse-string suture in the gastric wall around the tube and puncture the wall with a scalpel blade. (From Fossum et al.: *Small animal surgery*, ed 2, St. Louis, 2002, Mosby.)

Enterostomy (e.g., Duodenostomy or Jejunostomy) Feeding Tube

An enterostomy feeding tube is indicated in any patient undergoing oral, pharyngeal, esophageal, gastric, pancreatic, duodenal, or biliary tract surgery in which the intestinal tract distal to the surgical site is functional (Figure 12-31). Surgical patients with a neurologic status that may prevent postoperative feeding or patients with acute pancreatitis that are anticipated to be anorexic for more than 5 days may also be considered candidates for placement of an enterostomy feeding tube. Immediate feeding of a highly digestible, low-bulk diet in patients undergoing colonic surgery can be accomplished using an enterostomy tube. Patients with preexisting protein-calorie malnutrition that must undergo major abdominal surgery are considered candidates for early enteral hyperalimentation via enterostomy.

Technique. A celiotomy is required for placement of an enterostomy feeding tube. A 5 to 8 Fr diameter, 36-inch infant feeding tube in which

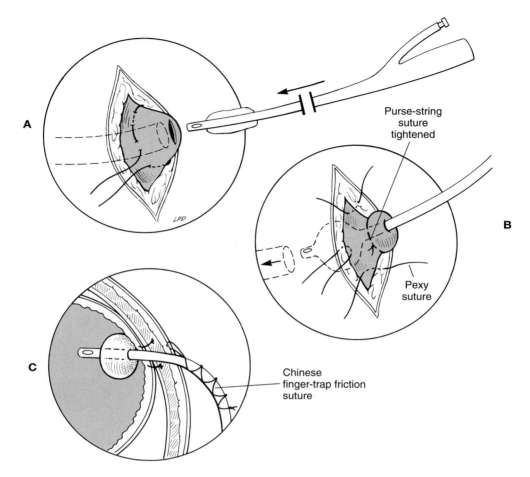

FIGURE 12-26 Percutaneous gastrostomy tube placement with gastropexy (cont'd from Figure 12-25). **A,** Place the Foley or Pezzer catheter into the lumen of the stomach and into the tube. **B,** Tighten the purse-string suture, remove the stomach tube, inflate the bulb of the Foley catheter, and suture the gastric wall to the abdominal wall. **C,** Note the proper tube placement of the inflated Foley catheter, the gastropexy, and the Chinese finger-trap friction suture to secure the tube in place. (From Fossum et al.: *Small animal surgery,* ed 2, St. Louis, 2002, Mosby.)

one end can be conveniently capped or a red rubber feeding tube is recommended. The distal tip of the feeding tube is brought into the abdominal cavity through a 2- to 3-mm stab incision on the right or left body wall using a No. 11 scalpel blade. The clinician selects a segment of small intestine, identifies the normal direction of flow of ingesta (i.e., oral to aboral), and ensures the selected segment can be easily mobilized to the feeding tube entrance location on the body wall. A 1- to 1.5-cm linear incision is made through the seromuscular layers of the antimesenteric border of the selected jejunal segment. A 10-gauge hypodermic needle or the point of a No. 11 scalpel blade is used, and the lumen of the jejunum is entered at the most aboral end of the incision. The distal end of the feeding tube is placed through the incision, and 10 to 12 inches of the tube is passed aborally in the lumen of the jejunum. The exiting portion of the tube is laid in the 1- to 1.5-cm seromuscular incision, and the tube is sutured in this "tunnel" by inverting the seromuscular layer over the tube with three or four interrupted Cushing sutures of 4-0 Maxon (Figure 12-32, *A-C*). The tube exit site of the jejunum is sutured to the exit site at the body wall with four to five simple interrupted sutures of 4-0 Maxon to provide a permanent enteropexy. The exiting feeding tube is secured to abdominal skin using a Chinese finger-trap friction suture of 2-0 Novofil. The clinician should be careful not to occlude the lumen of the tube when placing the finger-trap suture (Figure 12-33, *A-C*). The feeding tube exit site should be incorporated into a body bandage to prevent premature removal

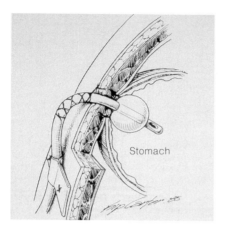

FIGURE 12-27 Gastrostomy tube placement: surgical placement through a midline laparotomy—cross section of the abdomen showing the gastropexy and position of the gastrostomy feeding tube. (From Crowe DT Jr: Enteral nutrition for critically ill or injured patients—part II, *Comp Cont Educ Pract Vet* 8:719, 1986.)

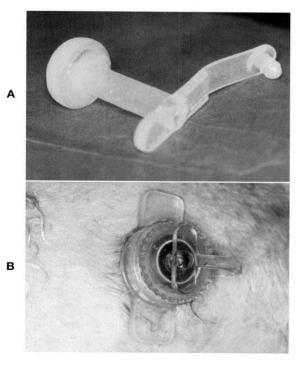

FIGURE 12-28 A, An example of a low-profile gastrostomy feeding tube. **B,** Low-profile gastrostomy feeding tube inserted in a male Collie with congenital megaesophagus.

by the patient, technical staff, or owner. Patients with an enterostomy feeding tube can be fed immediately postoperatively. A column of water should be kept in the tube between feedings to help prevent tube occlusion or reflux of intestinal contents into the tube.

Advantages and Disadvantages. Advantages of enterostomy feeding tubes include bypassing the upper GI tract while providing enteral nutritional support, decreased stimulation of pancreatic enzyme secretion, providing nutrition for enterocytes, and having fewer metabolic complications than parenteral nutrition has. Disadvantages of enterostomy feeding tube use include necessity of surgical placement, being limited to using liquid diets, necessity for more intensive monitoring because constant-rate infusion of diet is required, and potential for peritonitis with leakage or removal of the tube.

Complications. Complications include premature removal, tube-induced jejunal perforation, peritoneal leakage, and subcutaneous leakage. Tube-induced jejunal perforation is prevented by using soft rubber tubes designed for enterostomy feeding, not high-density polyethylene plastic tubes. Peritoneal leakage is prevented by paying close attention to include a 360-degree enteropexy. Passing 10 to 12 inches of tube into the jejunum and securely fixing the tube to skin with a Chinese finger-trap friction suture prevent subcutaneous leakage.

Gastrostomy-Enterostomy Tube Combination

Occasionally patients may require placement of gastrostomy and enterostomy feeding tubes (Figure 12-34). This combination of tubes is generally indicated for patients that present with vomiting as a major part of the history. These patients cannot initially be fed via a gastrostomy feeding tube immediately postoperatively. Therefore an enterostomy tube is placed and recommended for the initial feeding. A gastrostomy tube is also placed and used if the patient is still anorexic when the vomiting resolves.

Technique. Gastrostomy and enterostomy feeding tubes can be placed individually as described above. Alternatively, the enterostomy tube can be placed through the gastrostomy tube and into the jejunum. This technique is described below. The gastrostomy tube is placed as described above except for the following modifications. The distal end of the gastrostomy tube is cut off. A 5 Fr, 36-inch infant feeding tube (i.e., the tube used for

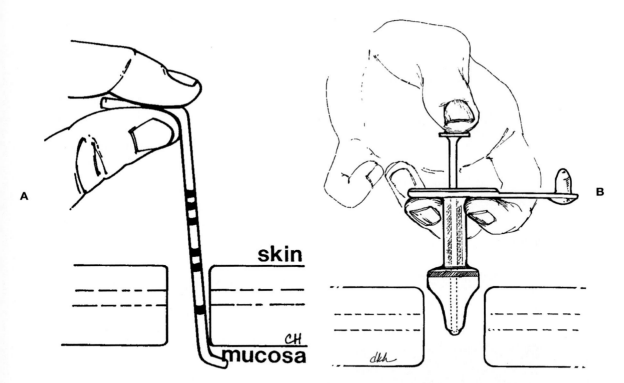

A **B**

skin

CH
mucosa

dkh

FIGURE 12-29 Low-profile gastrostomy tube placement. **A,** A stoma-measuring device placed into a gastrocutaneous fistula and withdrawn until the tip lies gently against the mucosa of the stomach. Circumferential lines indicate three depths (1.5, 2.6, and 4.3 cm) that correspond with the shaft length of the feeding tube. **B,** An obturator being advanced inward until the disk back apposes the base of the low-profile gastrostomy feeding tube. This elongates the mushroom tip, facilitating placement into the stomach. (Modified from Bright RM et al.: Use of a low-profile gastrostomy device for administering nutrients in two dogs, *J Am Vet Med Assoc* 207[9]:1184, 1995.)

enterostomy feeding) is passed through the gastrostomy tube so that it exits from its distal end. Before gastric placement of the gastrostomy tube, the exiting portion of the 5 Fr feeding tube is placed into the stomach lumen through the gastrotomy incision and manipulated into the duodenum and passed into the proximal jejunum. Once the enterostomy tube is placed 10 to 12 inches into the small intestine, the gastrostomy tube is placed into the gastrotomy incision and secured as described above in gastrostomy tube placement via laparotomy. The jejunostomy tube is secured to the gastrostomy tube to prevent tube migration.

Advantages and Disadvantages.
The primary advantage of combination tube placement is the ability to feed a vomiting patient immediately postoperatively via an enterostomy feeding tube and to continue feeding the patient into the stomach if the vomiting resolves but the patient remains anorexic. The primary disadvantage of combination gastrostomy-enterostomy tube placement is

the difficulty in passing the enterostomy tube in the small intestine. Care and patience is needed to encourage the small 5 Fr feeding tube to pass through the pylorus and into the small intestine.

Complications.
The major complication associated with combination gastrostomy-enterostomy tube placement is gastrostomy tube occlusion with diet fed in the enterostomy tube. Occasionally diet placed in the enterostomy tube will occlude the gastrostomy tube. It is important to encourage careful management of the enterostomy tube so that diet does not enter the gastrostomy tube.

CALCULATION OF NUTRITIONAL REQUIREMENTS

Once a decision is made that nutritional support is indicated and that the GI tract can be used, the number of calories (kilocalories), grams of protein,

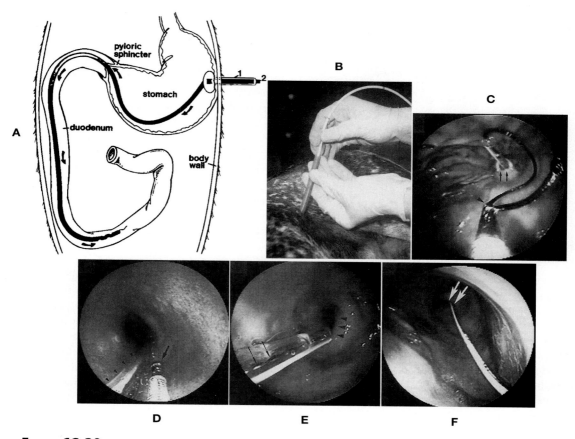

FIGURE 12-30 Percutaneous gastroduodenostomy tube placement. **A,** Ventrodorsal view of the abdomen of a dog, depicting the location of the percutaneous endoscopic gastrostomy (PEG) tube *(1)* and the percutaneous gastroduodenostomy (PEGD) tube *(2)*. The tip of the PEGD tube is at the caudal duodenal flexure. **B,** With the dog in right lateral recumbency, the enteral tube is pushed into the PEG tube after shortening the PEG tube and infusing it with 2.5 ml of water-soluble lubricant. **C,** Endoscopic view of the gastric fundus. The enteral tube is identified after pushing it through the cut end of the PEG tube *(arrows)*. The suture is grasped with a standard biopsy instrument *(large arrowhead)*. **D,** Endoscopic view of the duodenum. The dog is placed in left lateral recumbency to facilitate pyloric intubation. The endoscope is advanced aborally as far as possible. The biopsy forceps are advanced until moderate resistance is felt, then the suture is released. The biopsy forceps *(large arrow)* are retracted, leaving the enteral tube *(small arrowheads)* in the duodenum. **E,** Endoscopic view of the pylorus *(large arrowheads)*. The endoscope is gently retracted from the pylorus, while the enteral tube stylet *(thin arrows)* remains in place. **F,** Endoscopic view of the pyloric antrum. The endoscope is withdrawn from the stomach, while the remaining length of the enteral tube is pushed into the stomach and the stylet is removed, leaving the enteral tube in place. Arrows indicate where the enteral tube exits the pylorus. (From McCrackin MA et al.: Endoscopic placement of a percutaneous gastroduodenostomy feeding tube in dogs, *J Am Vet Med Assoc* 203[6]:792, 1993.)

and milliliters of water required by the animal is calculated.

Energy Requirements

There are several ways to estimate the amount of calories required by a patient. Illness energy requirements may be estimated by using a multiple of resting energy requirements or some fraction of maintenance energy requirements. In addition, energy requirements may be calculated using a linear or exponential formula. These formulas are presented in Table 12-4.

Although estimates overlap in patients weighing between approximately 2 and 20 kg (5 to 45 lb), in larger dogs the linear formula often overestimates

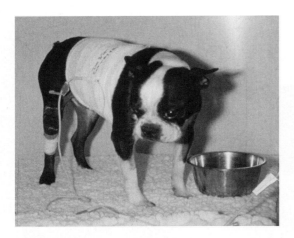

FIGURE 12-31 Use of a surgically placed enterostomy feeding tube in an adult Boston terrier.

energy requirements. As can be seen from the table, maintenance energy requirements are approximately two times resting energy requirements (RERs) for dogs and one and one-half times RERs for cats. In many patients that are ill, the stress of illness results in increased RERs; however, because of lack of physical activity, energy requirements during illness for most patients are less than maintenance. Numerous reports of critically ill humans indicate that metabolic rates are increased over RER: 25% to 35% postoperatively; 35% to 50% with trauma or cancer; 50% to 70% with sepsis; and 70% to 100% or more with major burns or head trauma. Energy requirements of critically ill humans rarely approach normal maintenance energy requirements. Based on data derived from humans, various factors have been suggested for estimating energy requirements of ill or injured animals. In most critically ill animals, the goal of nutritional support is to maintain body weight and body condition. Therefore a practical alternative to using a complex factoring system is to multiply the RER by a factor of 1.5 for dogs and cats. Alternatively, using the formula $100(BW_{kg}^{0.75})$ provides the same results as multiplying the RER by 1.5. The clinician should notice that this represents estimated maintenance energy requirements in cats. If cats are fed less than maintenance energy requirements, they are likely to lose weight.

Protein Requirements

After energy requirements are calculated, protein requirements should be estimated. Dietary protein is necessary to facilitate recovery from illness and injury. Protein requirements of ill or injured patients vary on a patient-by-patient basis. Variables include dietary energy content; dietary protein quantity and quality; and individual patient differences reflecting species, life stage, and type, degree, and stage of injury or illness. Protein requirements of critically ill dogs and cats have not been determined. Unless a patient has compromised renal or hepatic function, intake of dietary protein should meet maintenance protein requirements. Adequate protein intake is necessary to facilitate recovery to provide structural protein for repair of injured tissues, and to optimize immune function. For maintenance, diets should provide a minimum of 4 g of protein per 100 kcal of metabolizable energy (16% of energy as protein) for dogs and 6 g of protein per 100 kcal of metabolizable energy (25% of energy as protein) for cats. Taking into account availability, digestion, and absorption of enterally provided protein, requirements may be estimated at 4 g/BW_{kg} for dogs and 6 g/BW_{kg} for cats. In patients with liver or renal failure, less protein should be provided, and in patients with hypoalbuminemia or protein loss through the GI tract or through loss of protein-rich fluids (e.g., peritonitis), protein intake should be increased; protein intake should be decreased with protein-losing nephropathy. Protein of high biologic value should be used in critically ill patients. Special importance has been ascribed to metabolism of specific amino acids in nutritional support, and they have been added to commercially available convalescent diets. Arginine is an essential amino acid for dogs and cats and is important in wound healing, immune function, and promoting a positive nitrogen balance. Glutamine is a principal nutrient for enterocytes and is important in nitrogen metabolism. Branched-chain amino acids, valine, leucine, and isoleucine, decrease trauma- and sepsis–induced muscle catabolism and improve nitrogen retention. Taurine is an essential amino acid in cats and is important for cardiac function.

Fluid Requirements

It is important to maintain adequate hydration when providing nutritional support. Fluid is provided in prepared liquid diets or added to canned pet foods to make a gruel for enteral nutrition. Dogs and cats require 50 to 100 ml of water per kilogram of body weight for daily maintenance, depending on environmental temperature, type of food, and level of activity. Canned pet foods typically contain

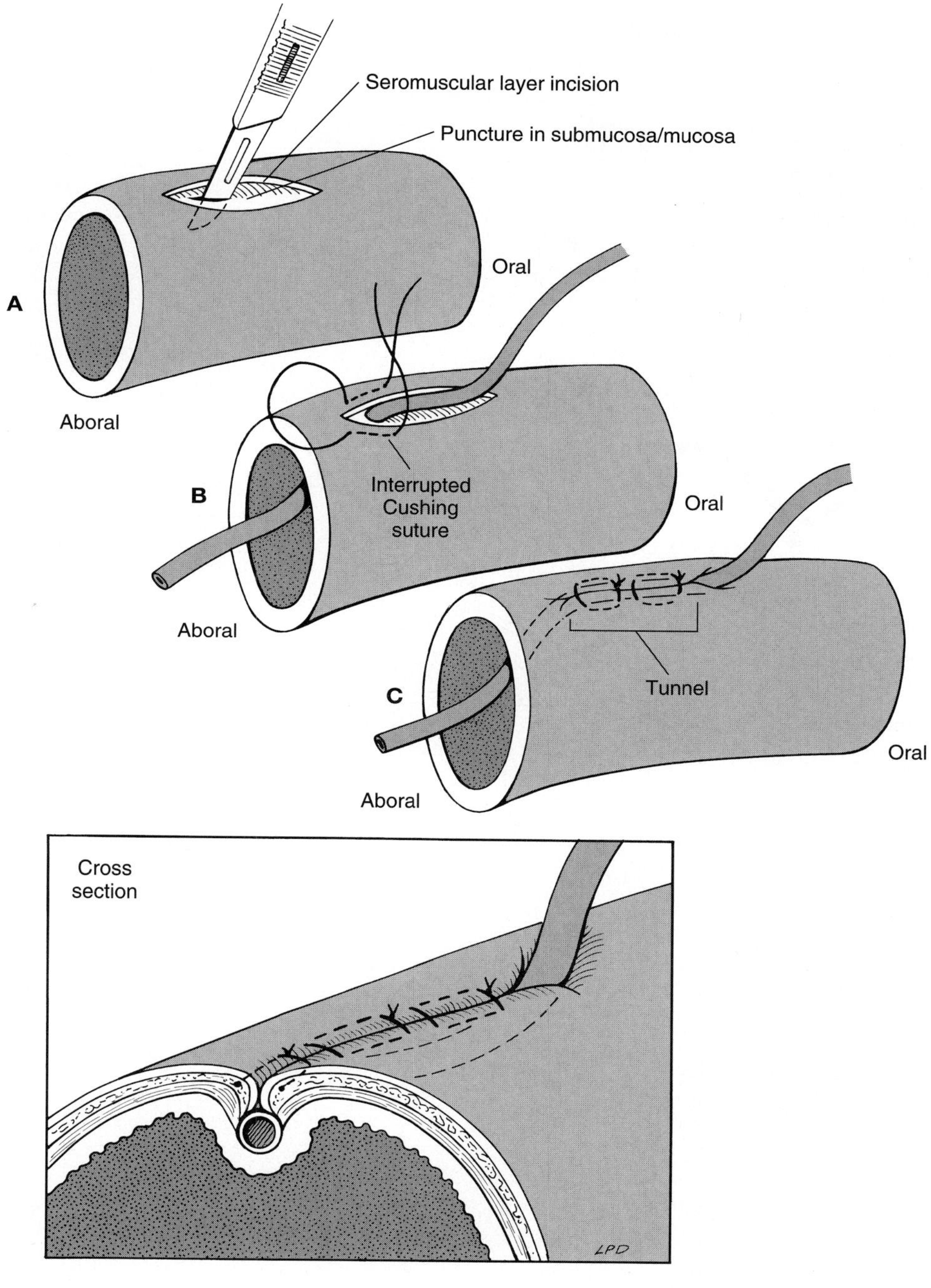

FIGURE 12-32 Placement of an enterostomy tube. **A,** Make a 1- to 1.5-cm linear incision in the seromuscular layers of the antimesenteric border of the selected jejunal segment; use the tip of a scalpel blade to puncture a hole in the aboral aspect of the seromuscular incision. **B** and **C,** Place the distal end of the feeding tube through the incision; lay the exiting portion of the tube in the 1- to 1.5-cm seromuscular incision and construct a "tunnel" by inverting the seromuscular layer over the tube with three or four Cushing sutures of 4-0 absorbable material. (From Fossum et al.: *Small animal surgery,* ed 2, St. Louis, 2002, Mosby.)

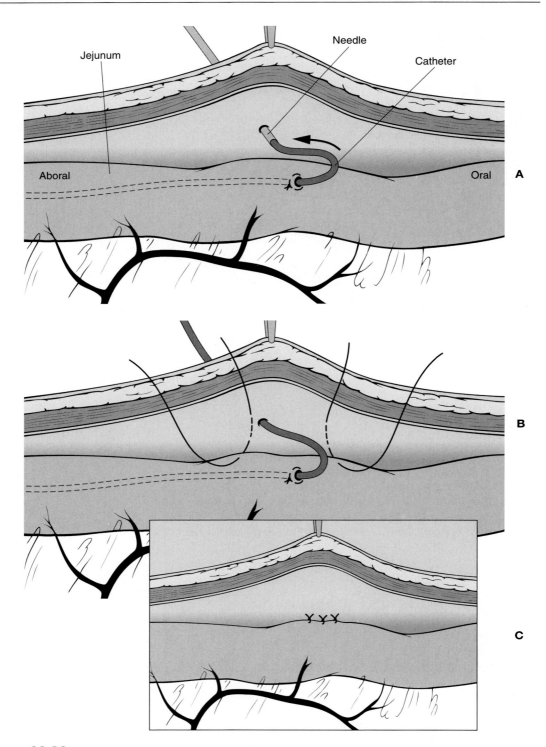

FIGURE 12-33 A, The catheter is exteriorized through a separate stab incision in the body wall. **B** and **C,** The jejunum is attached to the peritoneum with three to four simple interrupted sutures of 3-0 or 4-0 absorbable suture material. (From Fossum et al.: *Small animal surgery,* ed 2, St. Louis, 2002, Mosby.)

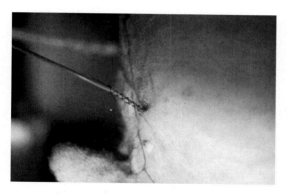

FIGURE 12-34 Combination of enterostomy feeding tube (red rubber feeding tube in foreground) and gastrostomy feeding tube (mushroom-tipped feeding tube in background) in an adult male West Highland white terrier with acute pancreatitis and hiatal hernia.

70% to 85% water. Normal daily fluid requirements are approximately equal to daily caloric requirements. Patients affected with diseases associated with excessive fluid losses (e.g., polyuria, diarrhea, vomiting, and third spacing of fluids) require more than calculated normal fluid amounts. Abrupt changes in body weight usually reflect hydration status; therefore fluid intake can be adjusted to maintain body weight. Fluid requirements should be met as part of nutritional support. A general recommendation is to mix water and canned diet in a 1:1 ratio to meet maintenance energy requirements for most patients.

Vitamins and Minerals

Little is known about vitamin and mineral status in critically ill patients, although deficiencies have been observed in veterinary medicine. One study in humans indicated that micronutrient deficiency was common (64% of 284 patients examined) in a wide variety of illnesses. Use of well-balanced diets should provide adequate amounts of micronutrients, especially when pet foods are used. Human enteral products may not provide adequate amounts. Oversupplementation should be avoided because excess vitamins and minerals may compromise the patient (e.g., iron supplementation may worsen bacterial infection and oxygen free radical production).

METHODS OF PROVIDING NUTRITION ENTERALLY

Feeding Into the Stomach

When feeding into the stomach (i.e., oral, nasogastric/nasoesophageal, esophagostomy, pharyngostomy, or gastrostomy), the quantity of diet fed is determined by the patient's stomach capacity. In normal dogs and cats, stomach capacity is approximately 80 ml of fluid per kilogram of body weight. However, anorexic patients can accommodate only 30 to 40 ml of fluid or liquid diet per kilogram of body weight when feeding begins. A gradual increase in volume over a 2- to 3-day period will generally allow the stomach to accommodate larger volumes of nutrients. A minimum of three feedings daily should be used; however, if vomiting and abdominal distention occur, the volume should be reduced and the number of feedings per day increased. When using 5 Fr or smaller feeding tubes (i.e., nasoesophageal or nasogastric tubes), only liquid diets may be administered. When using 8 Fr feeding tubes, convalescent diets with a homogeneous consistency may be used if diluted. When using larger-bore feeding tubes, blended canned diets may be used (Figure 12-35). The volume of food administered per feeding is determined by the caloric requirements and the consistency of the gruel. To calculate the amount of food to administer, the clinician divides the energy requirements of the patient by the caloric density of the food. Although the amount of water administered using canned products can be calculated by multiplying the volume of food to be administered by the moisture

TABLE 12-4	**Formulas Used to Estimate Energy Requirements**	
	Linear Formula	**Exponential Formula**
Resting energy requirements	$30(BW_{kg} + 70)$	$70(BW_{kg}^{0.75})$
Maintenance energy requirements	Dog: $2[30(BW + 70)]_{kg}$	Dog: $132(BW_{kg}^{0.75})$
	Cat: $1.5[30(BW_{kg} + 70)]$	Cat: $100(BW_{kg}^{0.75})$

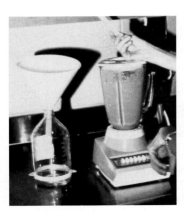

Figure 12-35 Blended canned diets can be administered through large-bore feeding tubes.

content of the diet, an alternative is to mix 1 part food with 1 part water. This usually exceeds the daily fluid requirements of the patient. Although starter regimens have been recommended (e.g., feeding one third of calories on day 1, two thirds of calories on day 2, and full caloric intake on day 3), we recommend feeding full caloric intake on day 1. It is necessary to feed the total amount of diet and water divided over 6 to 8 feedings on day 1, however. On day 2, the volume of administered diet per feeding can be increased and the frequency of feedings can be decreased to four to six times. On day 3, the number of feedings can usually be decreased to 3.

Feeding Into the Small Intestine

When feeding into the small intestine (i.e., gastroduodenostomy or enterostomy), the clinician must carefully regulate the rate and volume of diet to avoid overdistention. Each patient is unique in the amount of fluid the small intestine will accommodate; therefore a guideline for feeding via enterostomy tube is presented. Enterostomy tube feeding is usually done by constant-rate infusion rather than bolus feeding. Because of this, the day is divided into two 12-hour cycles and the liquid diet is administered via constant-rate infusion over 8 to 10 hours, providing 2 to 4 hours to rest the GI tract. During the first 12-hour cycle, one quarter of the calculated diet is administered over 8 to 10 hours and then discontinued for 2 to 4 hours. If the patient tolerates the rate, one half of the daily calculated amount of diet is administered over the next 8 to 10 hours, again discontinuing for 2 to 4 hours. After that, one half of daily calculated diet requirements is administered per each 12-hour cycle, providing 2 to 4 hours of GI rest.

It is difficult to decrease the infusion time of diet to less than 8 hours or to bolus feeding, although both have been reported in enterostomy-fed patients.

Monitoring Tube-Fed Patients

Body weight and physical examination should be monitored daily while the patient is hospitalized. The tube site should be cleaned every day or every other day. Blood work should be performed as deemed necessary for optimum care of the patient (Box 12-4).

Transition From Tube Feeding to Oral Feeding

When the patient begins to eat voluntarily or is able to eat voluntarily, the clinician should consider making a transition from tube feeding to oral feeding. This should be done over several days. If the tube is not interfering with oral consumption of food, the clinician should leave it in for a few extra days to use if the patient is not consuming enough diet or if the patient stops eating again.

General Complications of Tube Feeding

Three types of complications can occur during the course of enteral nutritional support: mechanical, GI, and metabolic.

Mechanical Complications. Mechanical complications include inadvertent tube placement or displacement in the trachea (nasogastric/nasoesophageal, esophagostomy, pharyngostomy) or peritoneal cavity (gastrostomy, gastroduodenostomy, jejunostomy), gut perforation by the feeding tube

BOX 12-4	Protocol for Monitoring Tube-Fed Patients

1. Verify position of feeding tubes:
   Continuous feeding: at least once a day
   Bolus feeding: before each meal
2. Monitor vital signs at least once a day initially, then as necessary
3. Weigh patient daily
4. Check urine glucose or blood glucose concentrations every 6 to 12 hours initially, then once a day
5. Monitor fecal frequency and consistency daily
6. Perform other laboratory tests as necessary

(gastroduodenostomy, jejunostomy), regurgitating or vomiting the tube (nasogastric, esophagostomy, pharyngostomy), esophageal irritation (nasogastric/nasoesophageal, esophagostomy, pharyngostomy), infection at the tube exit site, occlusion with diet, or tube removal by the patient.

Inadvertent placement of feeding tubes in the trachea or peritoneal cavity can be prevented by careful attention during tube placement. A small amount of sterile aqueous contrast material should be injected through the feeding tube and an x-ray film taken if there is any question of tube location (Figure 12-36, *A-C*).

The possibility of gut perforation can be virtually eliminated by the use of small-bore Silastic or soft rubber gastroduodenostomy and jejunostomy feeding tubes.

Premature tube removal by the patient can be prevented by use of an adequate mechanical restraint device (e.g., bandaging and Elizabethan collar) and secure attachment of the tube to its exit site (i.e., Chinese finger-trap friction suture technique). Patient tolerance has been enhanced by the use of appropriate-size soft rubber feeding tubes. Cats do not tolerate large amounts of bandaging material. Alternatives to using bandage material include use of Ace bandages, use of a "sweater" made from stockinette, or use of "onesies" (sleeveless T-shirts with snaps used with neonatal humans). Most cats and many dogs do not require Elizabethan collars or excessive amounts of mechanical restraint devices.

Esophagitis secondary to nasogastric/nasoesophageal, esophagostomy, and pharyngostomy tube placement has been reported; however, use of Silastic, soft rubber, or soft polyvinyl feeding tubes prevents esophageal irritation. Also, midesophageal placement effectively eliminates reflux esophagitis.

Proper tube management can prevent infection at the tube exit. The area should be kept clean and covered with a bandage. Care should be taken when feeding the patient to keep diet formula from contaminating the exit site. Rhinitis secondary to nasogastric/nasoesophageal tube placement can be prevented by use of small-bore soft rubber feeding tubes.

Small- and large-diameter feeding tubes may become occluded with diet. Using a commercial liquid diet rather than a blenderized diet best prevents this problem in small-bore feeding tubes (i.e., 3.5 to 5 Fr). Taking care to flush diet out of the tube when feeding is complete and capping the tube to maintain a column of water will help prevent GI reflux and tube occlusion. If a tube becomes occluded, the use of a carbonated liquid (e.g., sparkling water, cola) can be infused into the tube. It is felt that the effervescence of the liquid will help encourage removal of clogged material. If this is unsuccessful, tube replacement may be necessary.

Gastrointestinal Complications. GI complications include vomiting, cramping, abdominal distention, and diarrhea. The most common causes are feeding too rapidly, feeding too large a volume, and feeding diets with high osmolality. Treatment is directed at decreasing the rate and volume fed or diluting the diet to a more acceptable osmolality. In addition, diet should be warmed to near body temperature before infusion because administration of cold diets may cause cramping and GI upset.

Metabolic Complications. Hyperglycemia secondary to rapid absorption of glucose is the most common metabolic complication; however, it occurs rarely in veterinary patients. Insulin may be used to control hyperglycemia. Regular insulin may be administered IV or as SQ boluses (0.12 U/lb q4-6h). Alternatively, NPH insulin may be administered as follows:

Dog: 0.25 to 0.45 IU/lb NPH insulin SQ q12h
Cat: 0.12 IU/lb NPH insulin SQ q12h

In most instances, complications can be prevented by proper tube placement technique, use of appropriate-diameter soft rubber feeding tubes, use of proper diets, carefully calculated feeding schedules, and proper tube management during and between feedings.

PARENTERAL NUTRITIONAL SUPPORT

Nutrition can be provided intravenously to meet part or all of a patient's nutritional needs (Figure 12-37, *A* and *B*). Either all of the nutritional needs may be met (so-called total parenteral nutrition [TPN]), or some of the nutritional needs may be met (so-called partial parenteral nutrition [PPN]). Actually, even with TPN, nutritional requirements are not completely met; however, most of the major nutrient requirements may be met. Components used in formulating parenteral nutrition include a protein source in the form of amino

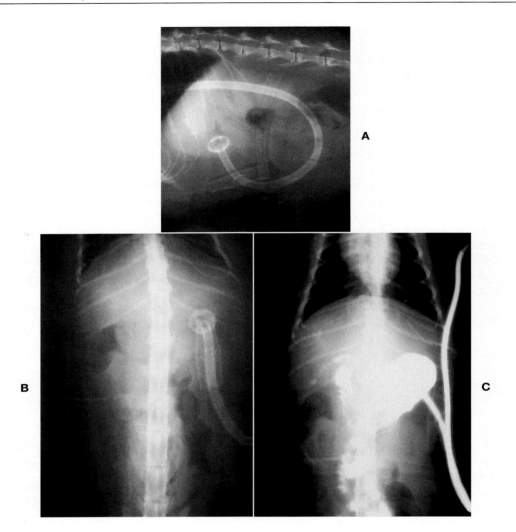

FIGURE 12-36 A, Survey lateral abdominal radiograph of an adult cat with a mushroom-tipped percutaneous endoscopic gastrostomy feeding tube. **B,** Survey ventrodorsal abdominal radiograph of the adult cat in **A.** **C,** Ventrodorsal abdominal radiograph of an adult cat with a mushroom-tipped percutaneous endoscopic gastrostomy feeding tube. Diluted iodinated contrast medium has been injected into the tube, which is positioned on the left abdominal wall. Contrast fills the stomach and has entered the small intestine.

acids, a carbohydrate source in the form of dextrose, a lipid source in the form of long-chain fatty acids, electrolytes, minerals, trace elements, and vitamins (Figure 12-38). Amino acids are commonly supplied as an 8.5% solution with or without electrolytes (4.25% to 10% solutions are available), dextrose is commonly supplied as a 50% solution, and lipids are commonly supplied as a 20% emulsion (10% solutions are also available). If electrolytes are not contained in the amino acid solution, an electrolyte solution designed for use with parenteral nutrition can be used (TPN electrolytes providing 16.1 mg sodium chloride per milliliter, 16.5 mg calcium chloride per milliliter, 74.6 mg potassium chloride per milliliter, 25.4 mg magnesium chloride hexahydrate per milliliter, and 121 mg sodium acetate per milliliter) and potassium phosphate (224 mg of monobasic potassium phosphate per milliliter and 236 mg dibasic potassium phosphate per milliliter) may be added as a source of phosphate. Vitamins and trace elements are also available for use. We routinely use a B-vitamin complex in the parenteral solution (1 ml/L of TPN). Vitamin K cannot be given intravenously and is administered subcutaneously at 0.25 mg/lb once a week.

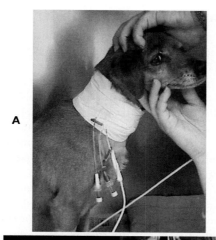

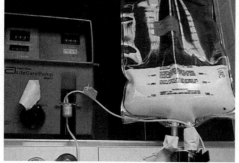

FIGURE 12-37 A, Total parenteral nutrition (TPN) being administered to an adult male Dachshund with an insulinoma. A triple lumen jugular catheter has been inserted, and the TPN is the white solution flowing through the bottom infusion line. **B,** TPN admixture bag for the dog described in **A.** TPN is administered using an infusion pump.

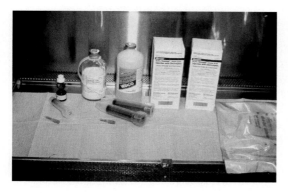

FIGURE 12-38 TPN components (clockwise from left): TPN multivitamin (brown bottle), lipid (white solution in glass bottle), 50% dextrose (plastic bottle), amino acids (two boxes), all-in-one admixture bag, and syringes and needles.

Total Parenteral Nutrition

Nutritional requirements are calculated in the same way as described for enteral nutrition. We calculate energy requirements, protein requirements, and then water requirements. The lipid and dextrose (nonprotein calories) provide energy. Usually the lipid component provides 40% to 60% of the nonprotein calories, and the dextrose component provides the remainder of the calculated caloric requirements. A 20% lipid emulsion provides 2 kcal/ml, and a 50% dextrose solution provides 1.7 kcal/ml. Protein requirements are then calculated as described previously. For maintenance, 4 g/100 kcal of energy intake for dogs and 6 g/100 kcal of energy intake for cats is required; more or less can be provided depending on protein status and disease state. An 8.5% amino acid solution provides 0.085 g of protein per milliliter. We add 20 ml of TPN electrolyte solution per liter of TPN solution and 5 ml of potassium phosphate per liter of TPN solution. The amino acid solution is also available as a balanced electrolyte solution; however, it is more expensive than amino acid solutions without added electrolytes. B vitamins may be added at 1 ml per liter of solution. If additional electrolytes are required, for example, KCl, they may be added. If additional fluids are required, for example, lactated Ringer's solution (LRS), they may either be added to the TPN solution or they may be administered through a separate intravenous catheter. Magnesium may be added to parenteral solutions; however, magnesium chloride is the salt of choice to add and not magnesium sulfate because the sulfate form is not compatible with parenteral solutions.

The resultant osmolality of TPN is usually 800 to 1200 mOsm/kg; therefore TPN solution must be administered through a centrally placed catheter to avoid thrombophlebitis. The 8.5% amino acid solution is approximately 800 mOsm/kg; therefore 4.25% amino acid solution is close to isotonicity. The 50% dextrose solution is approximately 2000 mOsm/kg (Table 12-5); therefore 5% dextrose is approximately isotonic. The lipid emulsion does not exert tonicity; therefore it is not included in the calculation of osmolality.

Partial Parenteral Nutrition

With partial parenteral nutrition, all of the calculated nutritional requirements are not met. This may occur if less than the calculated amount of formula is administered, if components of the parenteral nutrition are not administered, or if components are diluted to allow administration through a peripheral vein. If the clinician is administering parenteral nutrition through a peripheral vein (such as a cephalic or saphenous vein), the solution must be isotonic. It is difficult to meet protein needs with 4.25% amino acid solution, and difficult to meet caloric needs using 5% or 10% dextrose. Often PPN is administered to dogs infected with parvovirus to provide some calories or protein. In most instances we use TPN.

TABLE 12-5	Parenteral Glucose Solutions	
Glucose Concentration (%)	Caloric Content (kcal/L)	Osmolarity (mOsm/L)
5	170	253
7.7	262	388
10	340	505
20	680	1010
30	1020	1515
40	1360	2020
50	1700	2525
60	2040	3030
70	2380	3535
100	3400	5050

Formulation and Administration

When compounding parenteral nutrition solution, it is critical that aseptic technique be adhered to (Box 12-5). The dextrose and lipid are excellent media for bacteria, and there are no bacteriostatic or bactericidal properties to parenteral solutions. If pharmacists prepare parenteral nutrition solutions, they will use a laminar flow hood to minimize the risk of bacterial contamination. We compound parenteral nutrition solutions in an operating room suite after gowning and gloving in (Figure 12-39). Tops to bottles are prepared aseptically as if it were a surgical site. Although infrequent, sepsis and bacteremia can occur with TPN administration (in humans on long-term TPN administration, the incidence is 3% to 5%).

We place single-, double-, or triple-lumen catheters in the jugular vein for administration of TPN. If a single-lumen catheter is inserted, it should only be used for TPN administration. If a double- or triple-lumen catheter is used, one port is dedicated for TPN solution administration and the other port(s) may be used for administering other fluids, administering medication, or collecting blood samples. The jugular catheter must be placed as aseptically as possible. It is possible to administer TPN through a single-lumen jugular catheter that is inserted into a cephalic vein, which terminates in the subclavian vein or cranial vena

---

BOX 12-5	Prevention, Diagnosis, and Therapy Protocols for Sepsis Associated With Parenteral Nutrition

PREVENTION PROTOCOL

Prepare and handle parenteral solutions aseptically.

Use aseptic technique to place intravenous catheters.

Ensure strict aseptic management of dressing and infusion apparatus.

Change bandage covering intravenous catheter at least every other day.

Maintain a closed system.

Do not inject medications or blood products, measure central venous pressure, or draw blood through the catheter.

Use a specialized team or individual to manage therapy.

Appropriately treat concurrent infections.

DIAGNOSIS AND TREATMENT PROTOCOLS

Suspect sepsis if the patient develops a fever.

Monitor closely for any indication of source and/or progression toward septic shock/endotoxemia.

Monitor blood parameters for predictive changes of sepsis.

If no source of fever can be found within 24 hours after detection, culture the blood, parenteral nutrition solution, and catheter. Pending culture results, use Gram stain to examine the solution and catheter, if it is removed.

Catheter may be removed and replaced over a guide wire pending culture results if continued feeding or vascular access is desired.

If the bacteriologic culture of the catheter is positive, remove the replacement catheter.

Begin empiric antibiotic therapy until culture results return.

Allow 24 to 48 hours for bacteremia to resolve before a new catheter is placed.

Specific antibiotic therapy is initiated according to culture and sensitivity results.

Continue specific, symptomatic, and supportive treatment appropriate for the patient's clinical status.

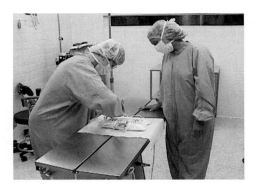

FIGURE 12-39 Veterinary nurses aseptically preparing TPN solution.

cava, or a catheter inserted into the femoral vein, which terminates in the caudal vena cava. Aseptic catheter management is imperative. As few people should handle the catheter or the TPN solution as possible. Tubing connections should be scrubbed before connecting, and the connections should be taped together to prevent them from accidentally separating. If the lines become disconnected, then all tubing should be discarded. Some recommend discarding the TPN solution as well in this instance.

Once the TPN is formulated and compounded, the daily amount is calculated and is administered as a constant-rate infusion. The volume of TPN solution that must be administered over the 24-hour period determines the rate. Usually the administered volume meets or slightly exceeds the daily fluid requirement; therefore additional fluids are not needed. However, if a patient is losing more fluid than maintenance (e.g., ascites, polyuric diseases, or peritonitis), then additional fluids must be administered. To begin TPN, one half of the calculated rate (milliliters per hour) is administered for the first 8 to 12 hours; supplemental fluids will need to be administered to meet daily fluid requirements. At the end of this period

the clinician should measure levels of blood glucose, blood urea nitrogen (BUN), packed cell volume (PCV), and total solids and examine the plasma or serum for lipemia or hemolysis. If the findings are normal, the rate of TPN is increased to full and the supplemental fluids are decreased or discontinued. After an additional 8 to 12 hours (which is usually in the morning), a complete blood count, serum biochemical analysis, and urinalysis should be performed (Box 12-6). The TPN solution can be adjusted as needed based on these results. Laboratory evaluation should be performed as needed depending on the underlying disease; however, renal function, electrolyte concentrations, and acid-base status should be evaluated every 3 to 4 days. Blood work should be repeated anytime an unexpected turn for the worse occurs. A bottle of TPN solution may be used for 3 days and occasionally 4 days. If used for more than 3 or 4 days, the risk of bacterial contamination increases and the lipid emulsion begins to break down. Breaking down of the emulsion results in a "brown scum" that adheres to the glass bottle; this process is called caramelization.

Once the patient begins eating or is well enough to begin eating, TPN may be discontinued. This is accomplished by decreasing the rate to one half of the calculated maintenance rate for 8 to 12 hours. TPN can be discontinued after this point is reached. If TPN is discontinued too quickly, hypoglycemia may occur.

Complications of Parenteral Nutrition

Complications associated with parenteral nutrition may be classified as mechanical or metabolic (Table 12-6). Mechanical complications include accidental removal of the venous catheter, accidental disconnection of lines, kinking of the

BOX 12-6	Protocol for Monitoring Patients Receiving Parenteral Nutrition

1. Vital signs, including temperature, pulse, and respiration (TPR), mucous membrane color, and capillary refill time every 6 to 12 hours
2. Body weight every 24 hours
3. Blood glucose level every 6 to 12 hours initially, then at least every 24 to 72 hours
4. Serum electrolyte concentrations every 24 hours for the first 2 to 3 days, then at least one to two times a week

5. Serum urea nitrogen concentration 12 hours after beginning parenteral nutrition, then at least one to two times a week
6. Packed cell volume, total solids, platelet count, and plasma color and turbidity every 24 hours for 2 to 3 days, then at least once a week
7. Complete blood cell count and serum biochemical profile at least one to two times a week, more often if indicated

catheter or lines, occlusion of the lines or catheter, or using a bottle of parenteral solution for too long. There are several metabolic complications that can occur and have been described; however, the most common ones are hypoglycemia, hyperglycemia, hyperlipidemia, metabolic acidosis, and potassium imbalances. Fortunately, these are not usually severe. As mentioned before, trace element and/or mineral deficiency may occur. In one study of dogs and cats receiving TPN for 1 to 14 days,

clinical signs of mineral or trace element deficiencies were not apparent. In that study 46% of cases experienced mechanical problems (e.g., break in infusion line or catheter dysfunction), 16% developed clinical sepsis, and metabolic complications (e.g., glucose, lipid, protein, electrolyte, or acid-base imbalances) occurred in approximately 50% of the cases but did not result in clinical problems. Mechanical and septic complications can be minimized by practicing aseptic technique when

TABLE 12-6	Complications, Predisposing Factors, Prevention, and Therapy Related to Parenteral Nutrition		
Complication	**Predisposing Factors**	**Prevention**	**Therapy**
Hyperglycemia	Diabetes mellitus, stress, glucocorticoids, rapid glucose infusion	Consider enteral nutrition, insulin therapy with diabetes mellitus; monitor blood and urine glucose	Decrease infusion rate; change to a lower dextrose/higher lipid infusion, insulin
Hypoglycemia	Abruptly stopping dextrose solution	Taper feedings; monitor blood glucose levels	Intravenous or oral carbohydrate
Hypokalemia	Insulin therapy, diuretic therapy, vomiting, diarrhea, rapid dextrose infusion, chronic renal disease in cats, metabolic alkalosis	Monitor serum K^+	Supplement K^+; correct or control underlying cause
Hyperkalemia	Metabolic acidosis, renal failure	Monitor serum K^+	Sodium bicarbonate if acidotic; decrease K^+ content of solution; increase dextrose infusion; glucose and insulin administration; administer diuretics that promote K^+ excretion
Hypophosphatemia	Diabetes mellitus, insulin therapy	Monitor serum phosphorus	Supplemental phosphorus; stop insulin if possible; stop feedings
Hypomagnesemia	Diuretic therapy, malabsorption	Monitor serum Mg^{2+}	Supplemental Mg^{2+}
Hypocalcemia	Hypoalbuminemia, hypomagnesemia, hyperphosphatemia	Monitor serum Ca^{2+}	Supplemental Mg^{2+} if low; monitor ionized Ca^{2+}; supplemental Ca^{2+}; increase serum protein
Edema	Low Na^+/low carbohydrate diet, cardiac disease, hypoalbuminemia	Avoid high carbohydrate/high Na^+ diets	Correct Na^+ intake; increase serum protein; treat underlying cardiac disease
Abnormal liver function test results	Stress, infection, excessive intake of carbohydrate, anorexia (cats)	Monitor liver enzymes	Decrease intake of dextrose/increase lipid; decrease feedings
Metabolic acidosis	Diarrhea, renal failure, excessive amino acid intake	Monitor serum total CO_2 or blood gas values; avoid excessive amino acid infusion	Increase acetate and decrease Cl^- in solution; decrease amino acid intake; sodium bicarbonate therapy

TABLE 12-6	Complications, Predisposing Factors, Prevention, and Therapy Related to Parenteral Nutrition—cont'd		
Complication	**Predisposing Factors**	**Prevention**	**Therapy**
Metabolic alkalosis	Vomiting	Monitor CO_2 or blood gas values; control vomiting	Increase Cl^- and decrease acetate in solution
Hypovolemia	Gastrointestinal or renal losses, fluid loss in body cavities	Monitor hydration status; quantitate fluid loss	Increase intake of fluid
Hyponatremia	Gastrointestinal loss, fluid overload, diuretics	Monitor serum Na^+; discontinue diuretics; monitor hydration	Supplemental Na^+
Hyperlipidemia	Diabetes mellitus, glucocorticoids, rapid or excessive lipid infusion	Monitor plasma turbidity	Decrease rate or amount of lipid infused, treat underlying metabolic cause(s) of lipid intolerance

placing the intravenous access line and by careful handling of the infusion system. Monitoring serum biochemical parameters and adjusting the TPN rate or formulation as needed may minimize metabolic complications.

REFERENCES

Abood SK, Buffington CA: Improved nasogastric intubation technique for nutritional support in dogs, *J Am Vet Med Assoc* 199:577, 1991.

Abood SK, Buffington CA: Use of nasogastric tubes: indications, technique, and complications. In Kirk RW, Bonagura JD, eds: *Current veterinary therapy XI,* Philadelphia, 1992, WB Saunders.

Abood SK et al.: Nutritional support of hospitalized patients. In Slatter D, ed: *Textbook of small animal surgery,* ed 2, Philadelphia, 1993, WB Saunders.

Armstrong PJ: Enteral feeding of critically ill pets: the choices and techniques, *Vet Med* 87:900, 1992.

Armstrong PJ, Lippert AC: Selected aspects of enteral and parenteral nutritional support, *Semin Vet Med Surg (Small Anim)* 3:216, 1988.

Bartges JW: Nutritional support. In Lipowitz AJ et al., eds: *Complications in small animal surgery,* Baltimore, 1996, Williams & Wilkins.

Brady LJ et al.: Influence of prolonged fasting in the dog on glucose turnover and blood metabolites, *J Nutr* 107:1053, 1977.

Bright RM: Percutaneous tube gastrostomy with and without endoscopy. Proceedings of the fourth annual forum of the American College of Veterinary Internal Medicine, 1986.

Bright RM, Burrows CF: Percutaneous endoscopic tube gastrostomy in dogs, *Am J Vet Res* 49:629, 1988.

Carnevale JM et al.: Nutritional assessment: guidelines to selecting patients for nutritional support, *Comp Cont Educ Pract Vet* 13:255, 1991.

Cerra FB: How nutrition intervention changes what getting sick means, *J Parenter Enteral Nutr* 14:164S, 1990.

Crowe DT: Nutritional support for the seriously ill or injured patient: an overview, *J Vet Emerg Crit Care* 1:1, 1985.

Crowe DT: Clinical use of an indwelling nasogastric tube for enteral nutrition and fluid therapy in the dog and cat, *J Am Anim Hosp Assoc* 22:675, 1986.

Crowe DT, Downs MO: Pharyngostomy complications in dogs and cats and recommended technical modifications: experimental and clinical investigations, *J Am Anim Hosp Assoc* 22:493, 1986.

Fulton RBJ, Dennis JS: Blind percutaneous placement of a gastrostomy tube for nutritional support in dogs and cats, *J Am Vet Med Assoc* 201:697, 1992.

Haskins SC: A simple fluid therapy planning guide, *Semin Vet Med Surg (Small Anim)* 3:227, 1988.

Howe PE et al.: Fasting studies. VI. Distribution of nitrogen during a fast of 117 days, *J Biol Chem* 11:103, 1912.

Lippert AC: Parenteral nutrition. In: DiBartola SP, ed: *Fluid therapy in small animal practice,* Philadelphia, 1992, WB Saunders.

Lippert AC, Fulton RBJ, Parr AM: A retrospective study of the use of total parenteral nutrition in dogs and cats, *J Vet Intern Med* 7:52, 1993.

Lippert AC et al.: Total parenteral nutrition in clinically normal cats, *J Am Vet Med Assoc* 194:669, 1989.

McCrackin MA et al.: Endoscopic placement of a percutaneous gastroduodenostomy feeding tube in dogs, *J Am Vet Med Assoc* 203:792, 1993.

Rawlings CA: Percutaneous placement of a midcervical esophagostomy tube: new technique and representative cases, *J Am Anim Hosp Assoc* 29:526, 1993.

Remillard RL, Martin RA: Nutritional support in the surgical patient, *Semin Vet Med Surg (Small Anim)* 5:197, 1990.

Remillard RL, Thatcher CD: Parenteral nutritional support in the small animal patient, *Vet Clinic North Am Small Anim Pract* 19:1287, 1989.

Sanderson SS, Bartges JW, Osborne CA: Management of anorexia. In Kirk RW, Bonagura JD, eds: *Current veterinary therapy XIII*, Philadelphia, 1999, WB Saunders.

Tennant B, Willoughby K: The use of enteral nutrition in small animal medicine, *Comp Cont Educ Pract Vet* 15:1054, 1993.

Thatcher CD, Hand MS, Remillard RL: Small animal clinical nutrition: an iterative process. In Hand MS et al., eds: *Small animal clinical nutrition,* ed 4, Topeka, Kan, 2000, Mark Morris Institute.

INDEX

Page numbers followed by f indicate figures; t, tables; b, boxes.